Handbook of FAQs on
Basic Genetics and
Common Genetic
Disorders
for Students

Handbook of FAQs on
Basic Genetics and Common Genetic Disorders
for Students

Chief Editor

Komal Uppal

DCH, DNB (Paediatrics), FSIAMG, PGCCMGC

Medical Scientist

Division of Genetics, AIIMS, New Delhi

Co-Editor

Seema Kapoor

MD (Paediatrics)

Director Professor (Division of Genetics)

Department of Paediatrics

Maulana Azad Medical College, New Delhi

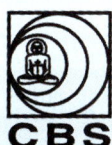

CBS

CBS Publishers & Distributors Pvt Ltd

New Delhi • Bengaluru • Chennai • Kochi • Kolkata • Mumbai

Hyderabad • Jharkhand • Nagpur • Patna • Pune • Uttarakhand

Handbook of FAQs on
Basic Genetics and Common Genetic Disorders
for Students

ISBN: 978-93-90709-89-2

Copyright © Editors and Publisher

First Edition: 2022

Published by Satish Kumar Jain and produced by Varun Jain for

CBS Publishers & Distributors Pvt Ltd
4819/XI Prahlad Street, 24 Ansari Road, Daryaganj, New Delhi 110 002, India
Ph: 011-23289259, 23266861, 23266867   Website: www.cbspd.com
Fax: 011-23243014   e-mail: delhi@cbspd.com; cbspubs@airtelmail.in

Corporate Office: 204 FIE, Industrial Area, Patparganj, Delhi 110 092, India
Ph: 011-4934 4934   Fax: 011-4934 4935   e-mail: publishing@cbspd.com; publicity@cbspd.com

Branches

- Bengaluru: Seema House 2975, 17th Cross, K.R. Road, Banasankari 2nd Stage, Bengaluru 560 070, Karnataka, India
  Ph: +91-80-26771678/79   Fax: +91-80-26771680   e-mail: bangalore@cbspd.com
- Chennai: 7, Subbaraya Street, Shenoy Nagar, Chennai 600 030, Tamil Nadu, India
  Ph: +91-44-26680620, 26681266   Fax: +91-44-42032115   e-mail: chennai@cbspd.com
- Kochi: 42/1325, 1326, Power House Road, Opposite KSEB, Power House, Ernakulum-682018, Kochi, Kerala, India
  Ph: +91-484-4059061-67   Fax: +91-484-4059065   e-mail: kochi@cbspd.com
- Kolkata: 147, Hind Ceramics Compound, 1st Floor, Nilgunj Road, Belghoria, Kolkata 700056, West Bengal, India
  Ph: +91-9096713055/7798394118, 9836841399   e-mail: kolkata@cbspd.com
- Mumbai: PWD Shed, Gala No. 25/26, Ramchandra Bhatt Marg, Next to JJ Hospital Gate No. 2
  Opp. Uninon Bank of India, Noorbaug, Mumbai-400009, Maharashtra, India
  Ph: +91-22-66661880/89   e-mail: mumbai@cbspd.com

Representatives

• **Hyderabad**	0-9885175004	• **Jharkhand**	0-9811541605	• **Nagpur**	0-9421945513
• **Patna**	0-9334159340	• **Pune**	0-9623451994	• **Uttarakhand**	0-9716462459

Printed at: Nutech Print Services India, Faridabad, India.

Contributors

Chief Editor
Komal Uppal
DCH, DNB (Paediatrics), FSIAMG, PGCCMGC
Medical Scientist
Division of Genetics, AIIMS, New Delhi
email: uppalkomal3@gmail.com

Co-Editor
Seema Kapoor
MD (Paediatrics)
Director Professor (Division of Genetics)
Department of Paediatrics
Maulana Azad Medical College, New Delhi
email: drseemakapoor@gmail.com

Prajnya Ranganath
MD (Paediatrics), DM (Medical Genetics)
Associate Professor and Head
Department of Medical Genetics
Nizam's Institute of Medical Sciences
Hyderabad, Telangana
Adjunct Scientist
Diagnostics Division, Centre for DNA
Fingerprinting and Diagnostics, Hyderabad
email: prajnyaranganath@gmail.com

Inusha Panigrahi
MD (Paediatrics), Dip NB DM (Medical Genetics)
Professor
Genetic Metabolic Unit
Department of Paediatrics
APC, PGIMER, Chandigarh
email: panigrahi.inusha@pgimer.edu.in; inupan@yahoo.com

Neerja Gupta
MD, DM (Medical Genetics)
Associate Professor
Division of Genetics
Department of Paediatrics
AIIMS, Ansari Nagar, New Delhi
email: neerja17@gmail.com; neerja17aiims@gmail.com

Kausik Mandal
MD (Paediatrics), DM (Medical Genetics)
Additional Professor
Medical Genetics
SGPGIMS, Lucknow
email: mandal.kausik@gmail.com

Deepti Saxena
MS (Obstetrics & Gynaecology), DM (Medical Genetics)
Assistant Professor
Department of Medical Genetics
Sanjay Gandhi Postgraduate
Institute of Medical Sciences
Raibareli Road, Lucknow
email: saxenadrdeepti@gmail.com

Chaitanya A Datar
MBBS, MD (Medical Genetics)
Clinical and Metabolic Geneticist
Bharati Hospital, Pune
and KEM Hospital, Pune
Surya Hospital and
Aditya Birla Memorial Hospital, Pune
email: dr.cdatar@gmail.com

Qurratulain Hasan
PhD, FNASc
Senior Consultant and Head
Department of Genetics and
Molecular Medicine
Kamineni Hospitals, LB Nagar
Hyderabad, Telangana
email: qhasan 2013@gmail.com

Kuldeep Singh
MD (Paediatrics), DM (Medical Genetics)
Dean Academics
Head, School of Public Health and
Head, Department of Paediatrics
All India Institute of Medical Sciences, Jodhpur
email: kulpra@hotmail.com; kulpra@gmail.com

Usha R Dutta
PhD [Human Molecular Genetics], DAAD Fellow
Cytogeneticist
Diagnostics Division Centre for DNA
Fingerprinting and Diagnostics
(Ministry of Science & Technology, GoI)
Inner Ring Road, Uppal
Hyderabad, Telangana
email: usha@cdfd.org.inushadutta@hotmail.com

Seema Thakur
MS (Ob-Gyn), DM (Medical Genetics)
Senior Consultant
Genetic and Fetal Medicine
Fortis Hospital, Delhi-NCR
Rainbow Children Hospital, Delhi
email: Seematranjan@gmail.com

Meenakshi Lallar
MS (Ob-Gyn), DM (Medical Genetics)
Clinical Geneticist
Prime Imaging and Prenatal Diagnostics
Sector 24 D, Chandigarh
Consultant
Geneticist Medgenome, Bangalore
email: meenakshilallar@gmail.com

Divya Agarwal
MBBS, MD (Paediatrics), DM (Medical Genetics)
Consultant
Medical Genetics, Max Hospital
Gurgaon, Haryana
email: dr.divya2512@gmail.com

T Karthik Bharadwaj
MD (Paediatrics), DNB (Medical Genetics)
Principal
Clinical Geneticist
CSIR—Center for Cellular and Molecular Biology
Hyderabad, Telangana
email: karthikt@ccmb.res.in

Gayatri N
DGO, DNB (OBG), DNB (Medical Genetics)
Consultant
Medical Geneticist
Fernandez Hospital
Hyderabad, Telangana
email: drgayatri@gmail.com

Surya Balakrishnan
DNB (Internal Medicine), DNB (Medical Genetics)
Senior Clinical Geneticist
CCMB, Hyderabad
email: gierra@gmail.com

Mounika Endrakanti
MBBS, MD (Paediatrics), DM (Medical Genetics)
Senior Resident
All India Institute of Medical Sciences
New Delhi
email: mounika1404@gmail.com

Suresh Thomas MD (Paediatrics)
Professor and Head
Department of Paediatrics
Kamineni Institute of Medical Sciences
Narketpally, Nalgonda, Telangana
email: drsureshthomas@gmail.com

Shruti Bajaj MD (Paediatrics)
Fellowship Clinical Genetics (MUHS)
Consultant
Clinical Geneticist
Sir HN Reliance Foundation Hospital
Mumbai, Maharashtra
email: info@geneticsinindia.comdrshru.a@gmail.com

Sarah Bailur
MBBS, DNB (Paediatrics), FICG, FSIAMG
Paediatrician and Clinical Geneticist
Kamineni Hospitals, LB Nagar
Hyderabad, Telangana
email: medicosarah@gmail.com

Manisha Goyal
MBBS, DGO, Fellowship Medical Genetics and Fetal Medicine.
Postgraduate Diploma in Ultrasonography
Medical Geneticist
Centre of Rare Disease
JK Lone Hospital
SMS Medical College
Jaipur, Rajasthan
email: manidr2000@gmail.com

Snehal Patil MBBS, DCH
Fellowship Clinical Genetics (MUHS)
Senior Resident
SMBT Institute of Medical Sciences
and Research Center
Dhamangaon Igatpuri, Nasik, Maharashtra
email: sneh.doc@gmail.com

Ami Shah
DNB (Paediatrics), Fellowship Clinical Genetics (MUHS)
Consultant
Nanavati Super Specialty Hospital
Mumbai, Maharashtra
email: drami.rajesh.shah@gmail.com

Suvarna Ghanashammagar
DNB (Paediatrics)
MGM Medical College
N-6, CIDCO, Aurangabad, Maharashtra
email: drsuvarnamagar@gmail.com

Risha Nahar Lulla
MSc (Med Gen), PhD (Gen Genomics)
Consultant, IBM Watson Health
Hyderabad, Telangana
email: rishanahar@gmail.com

Syeda Zubeda
PhD (Genetics)
Scientific Officer
Department of Genetics
Kamineni Hospitals, LB Nagar
Hyderabad, Telangana
email: zubeda.syeda@yahoo.co.in

Priyanka Srivastava PhD
Assistant Professor
Genetic Metabolic Unit
Department of Paediatrics
Postgraduate Institute of Medical Education
and Research (PGIMER)
Sector-12, Chandigarh
email: srivastavapriy@gmail.com

Aruna Priya Kamireddy
MSc, Human Genetics [PhD]
Research Scholar
Kamineni Hospitals
LB Nagar, Hyderabad
email: aru.priya10@gmail.com

Gayatri R Iyer
PhD
Human Genetics and Senior Research Fellow
DST INSPIRE Fellow
Kamineni Hospitals
Hyderabad, Telangana
email: gaya3riyer@gmail.com

Varuna Vyas
MBBS, MD (Paediatric Endocrinology)
Assistant Professor
AIIMS, Jodhpur, Rajasthan
email: drvaruna.vyas@gmail.com

Soma Santosh Kumar DCH, DNB (Paediatrics)
Assistant Professor
Department of Paediatrics
Kamineni Institute of Medical Sciences
Narketpally, Nalgonda, Telangana
email: santoshsoma880@gmail.com

Meenakshi Bothra Gupta
MD (Paediatrics)
Assistant Professor
Department of Paediatrics
Maulana Azad Medical College
email: meenakshibothra@gmail.com

Siyaram Didel MD (Paediatrics)
Assistant Professor
AIIMS, Jodhpur, Rajasthan
email: drdsram2001@gmail.com, didelsr@aiimsjodhpur.edu.in

Shreya Tanneru
MBBS, MD (Paediatrics)
Assistant Professor
Department of Paediatrics
Kamineni Institute of Medical Sciences (KIMS)
Nalgonda, Telangana
email: drshreyatanneru@gmail.com

Irene Mathews
MD (Dermatology, Venereology and Leprology), DNB, SCE
Post-Doctoral Fellowship in Paediatric Dermatology
JIPMER, Puducherry
email: irenemathews7@gmail.com

Jerene Mathews
MD, Fellowship (Paediatric Dermatology)
Assistant Professor
Department of Dermatology
Believers Church Medical College
Thiruvalla, Kerala
email: jerenemathews7@gmail.com

Yashodhara Bhattacharya MSc (Biomedical Genetics),
Post Graduate Diploma in Medical and Genetic Counseling
Genetic Counselor
Redcliffe Lifesciences
Kolkata, West Bengal
email: y.bhattacharya12@gmail.com

Divya Kumari
Senior Research Fellow (SRF)
Genetic Metabolic Unit
Department of Paediatrics
APC, PGIMER, Chandigarh
email: kumari.divya093@gmail.com

Foreword

It gives me great pleasure to provide this introduction to the first editon of the *Handbook of FAQs on Basic Genetics and Common Genetic Disorders for Students*. This book is a unique compilation of important concepts related to medical genetics in a question and answer format. Though the primary intent behind the effort is to provide a ready reference to undergraduate and postgraduate medical students to help them attempt questions related to medical genetics in examinations, it also serves the much bigger purpose of elucidating the principles and practice of medical genetics to medical students at an early stage in their career.

Introducing the concepts of medical genetics and highlighting the relevance of this subject to medical practice to students, right from their undergraduate training period is imperative in this field of genetic diagnostics and molecular therapy in recent years. Apart from the so-called 'pure genetic disorders' which are known to be caused by chromosomal abnormalities and genetic mutations, a growing number of multifactorial disorders including diabetes, hypertension, malignancies, autoimmune diseases, psychiatric disorders and many others, are being identified to have genetic contributory factors in their causation. These chromosomal disorders and monogenic diseases, as well as multifactorial disorders can affect all body organs and organ systems. Therefore, all medical practitioners, irrespective of their field of specialization, need to understand the basic conceps of genetics as well as be aware about these recent advances.

Unfortunately, at present, very little emphasis being given to genetics in undergraduate medical teaching and postgraduate medical training. Though genetics is a part of the medical curriculum, it is often mistakenly considered to be a non-clinical research area, not relevant to clinical practice. Students also get put-off by the so-called 'complex terminology' and 'hard-to-grasp' concepts of medical genetics.

This book is an attempt to simplify the concepts of genetics, highlight the importance and relevance of the subject in medical practice, and inculcate an interest in the subject in medicos early in their career. I congratulate the editorial team for this wonderful and timely effort. I am sure this book would prove to be of great help to medical students not just in their estimations but also in their practice.

Dr Prajnya Ranganath
MD (Paediatrics), DM (Medical Genetics)
Associate Professor and Head
Department of Medical Genetics
Nizam's Institute of Medical Sciences
Hyderabad

Preface

Genetics is an essential subject in the field of human science. In the last two decades due to various advancements in diagnostics and therapeutic genomic techniques, the whole world has got transformed. But the medical students are still lagging behind in understanding the fundamental concepts of genetics and common genetic disorders. Even though the chapters on the basic information related to genetics are introduced at the middle school level but still the foundational knowledge of the medical students about genetics is not satisfactory.

Because of this reason, students are not very comfortable in writing the answers related to genetics in the examinations.

In view of the above, via this book, an attempt is made to bridge the gap between the low level and the expected level of knowledge of students about the subject and to facilitate them to develop the required knowledge base, and skills to write correct answers in the examination. This book will be having a wide variety of questions and their answers based on basic cellular and molecular genetics, common genetic disorders, conventional and advanced diagnostic techniques, treatment and prevention of genetic disorders and recent advances in the genetics. To prepare these questions and answers various expert contributors, some of whom being eminent teaching faculty in medical colleges, with their vast knowledge about the subject and understanding the needs of the students, have spent a lot of time and energy.

With the objective of providing comprehensive and basic information on genetics—almost all the FAQs related to genetics which are frequently asked in the examinations have been covered in a simple and easy language in this book. Hopefully, the book will be friendly and a single window solution for students to revise the subject before the examinations.

Any suggestion to improve the book will be greatly acknowledged.

Komal Uppal

Acknowledgments

I would like to thank:

- Dr Suresh Thomas who motivated me to compile and publish the book with the stated objective.
- Dr Prajnya Ranganath who inspired me a lot to move further in the field of genetics.
- Dr Anne Hasan who always motivated me to take initiative to increase understanding of the basic genetics concepts of medical students.
- Co-editor, Dr Seema Kapoor, without her contributions this book would not have come to being.
- Dr Madhulika Kabra for continuous guidance and support.
- Various authors and colleagues, who have contributed to this book and also thankful to all my past and present pediatric teachers, clinical geneticists and to all my patients.
- My family members, especially my kids Bhrigu and Diza Uppal, for giving me free time so that I can focus on this book.
- Mr Vicky and Miss Shruti for editing, formatting and designing the content.

I acknowledge the contribution of CBS Publishers & Distributors, Mr Satish Kumar Jain Chairman and Managing Director and Mr Sunil Dutt Promotion and Development Manager for their efforts to publish this book on time.

I have made all the attempts to acknowledge all the sources of information and relevant illustrations. If something has left out unintentionally, I apologize for that.

Komal Uppal

Contents

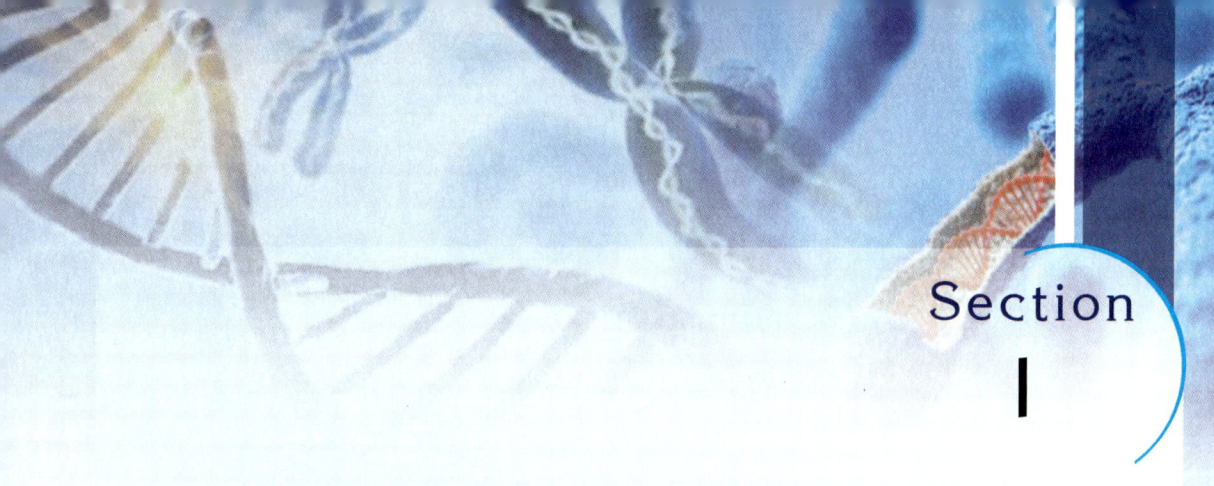

Basic Genetics

- Basic Introduction to Cellular and Molecular Biology and the Human Genome

- Mutation and Polymorphism

- Chromosomal Abnormalities and their Mechanism

- Pattern of Inheritance: Mendelian Inheritance

- Non-Mendelian Inheritance

Basic Introduction to Cellular and Molecular Biology and the Human Genome

Komal Uppal, Shreya Tanneru, Suresh Thomas, Priyanka Srivastava, T Karthik Bharadwaj

Q 1. Define medical genetics, hereditary and congenital terms.

Ans. **Medical genetics** is a branch of science related to the study of human genetic disorders and includes various genetics applications like pedigree analysis, genetic diagnosis, treatment and genetic counseling in clinical practice. Due to various advances in the genetic field, now it has moved from the Human Genome Project to the study of the whole genome, functional genetic studies, gene therapy and to reveal the association of various polymorphism with multifactorial diseases.

➲ **Hereditary:** The transmission of any trait from one generation to next generation.

➲ **Congenital:** Any abnormality presents in an individual from birth due to either prenatal or perinatal insult.

Q 2. What is the impact of genetic disorders in the medicine?

Ans. The impact of genetic disorders in medicine.

➲ The genetic disorders now are not limited only to one subject rather it has become a part of all the subjects in medicine like pediatrics, obstetric and gynecology, surgery, general medicine, neurology, oncology, etc. So all the physicians and medical students from all specialities should be aware of basic concepts of genetics.

➲ Due to changing paradigm like increasing burden of genetic disorders from newborn to old age group including multifactorial

diseases, increased diagnostic, therapeutic, preventive (prenatal testing) and genetic counseling facilities, along with healthcare providers, public should also be aware of the basic nature, genetic etiology, available diagnostic, therapeutic and preventive measures of the genetic diseases to reduce the burden of these diseases in the family and the society.

➲ The limitations of genome sequencing, prenatal diagnosis, gene therapy, preimplantation genetic testing, cell-free DNA analysis in maternal blood and various ethical issues in medical genetics have raised many challenging questions which require expert geneticists and genetic counselors to clear doubts of the public in future.

Q 3. Write about the role of pediatrician in genetic disorders.

Ans. The role of a pediatrician in genetic disorders is multifold:

1. **Suspecting and identifying a genetic disorder in a child:** Most of the genetic disorders manifest during infancy/childhood. The pediatrician can identify phenotypical features of a particular genetic condition as accurately as possible. The clinical acumen of a pediatrician is especially helpful in identifying single gene disorders that show variable expressivity.

2. **Confirmation of a genetic condition** becomes difficult in a resource limited setting and due to financial constraints of

the parents. Based on the type of genetic condition suspected, the appropriate genetic testing like chromosomal analysis, FISH (fluorescent *in situ* hybridization), single gene sequencing, whole exome sequencing, etc. has to be ordered for the confirmation of diagnosis.

Prenatal diagnosis of a disease helps a family decide about the continuation/termination of pregnancy. **Predictive testing** is done in presymptomatic patients with a significant family history of a genetic condition (this is helpful in genetic disorders that have age dependent penetrance).

3. **Genetic counseling:** Pediatrician plays a vital part in the counseling of the parents to understand the natural history of the disease, prognosis, the risk of recurrence of the condition in future pregnancies and the options available for prenatal testing.

4. Once diagnosed, the pediatrician plays a major role in the management and follow-up of the patient. Therapeutic options include dietary manipulation, enzyme replacement therapies, organ transplantation. In conditions with no cure, the parents have to be taught how to best manage the condition at home, the complications to look for and advised to follow-up regularly.

Q 4. Write a note on the changing pattern of genetics in pediatric medicine.

Ans. Changing pattern of genetics in pediatric medicine: The role of genetics in diagnosing and management of a disorder occurring during childhood has improved immensely over the past few decades. Earlier, many disorders went undiagnosed due to lack of awareness and availability of adequate testing methods. The research in this field has helped us better understand the etiology of the conditions, has made counseling, specific treatment, recurrence risk analysis and planning for future pregnancies much easier.

Few developments in the field of genetics:

1. A normal newborn screening program for genetic, metabolic disorders is the norm in many urban areas today.

2. Although prenatal screening was previously available, noninvasive prenatal testing by using cell-free fetal DNA or fetal cells in maternal blood is becoming increasingly available.

3. Preimplantation genetic diagnosis can be done to select unaffected embryos in couples opting for *in vitro* fertilization.

4. Inborn errors of metabolism are now being easily diagnosed using tandem mass spectrometry.

5. Apart from testing a child with signs and symptoms, predictive genetic testing (performing a test in a person who is at risk of developing a disorder) for age-dependent disorders has also come into play.

6. Some of the metabolic disorders can be treated after definitive diagnosis.

7. After testing the variants, target therapy can be given.

8. Stem cell therapy and gene therapy under trial will be the future of therapeutic medicine for untreatable disorders.

CELLULAR BIOLOGY
Komal Uppal

Q 5. Show the diagrammatic representation of cell structure.

Ans. Human body consists of approximately 100 trillion cells where genetic material resides in nucleus and in the cytoplasm protein synthesis occurs. When cell is seen under electron microscope various small structures seen in the cell as shown in Figure 1.1.

Q 6. Write about the cell cycle.

Ans. Cell cycle: Human body develops from zygote by hundreds of mitotic divisions including both nuclear and cytoplasm division. Before mitotic division the cell contents become double in interphase period (G1, S, G2). The mitosis and interphase period progress alternatively in the form of a cycle called cell cycle. The various phases of a cell cycle are shown in Figure 1.2.

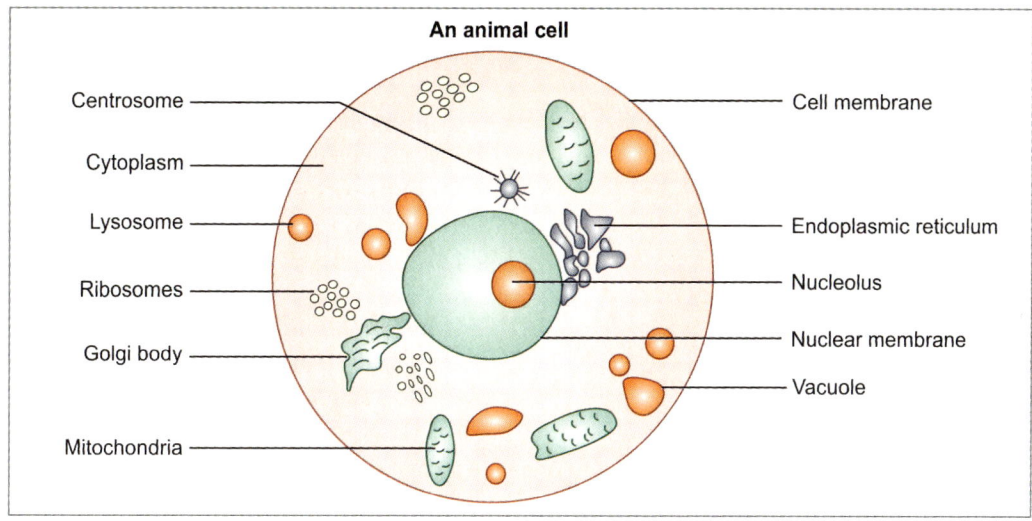

Figure 1.1: Cell structure

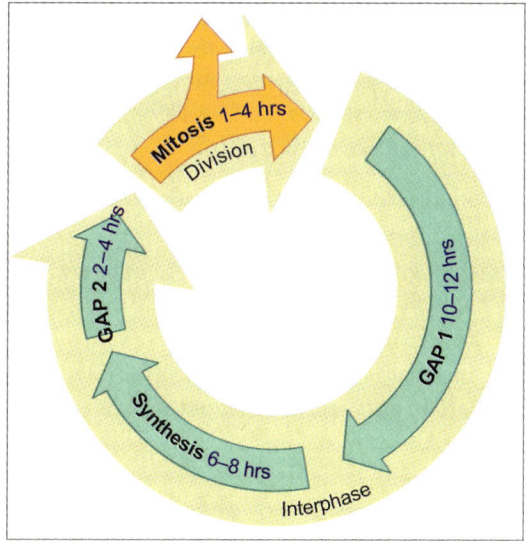

Figure 1.2: Phases of the cell cycle

1. **G1:** RNA and protein formation occur, and the cell can rest here for hours, days or years. In this phase, cell has one diploid copy of genetic material.
2. **G0:** Neurons and red blood cells do not divide and rest in G0 phase. Hepatocytes rests here for some time and then enter in G1 and continue on the cell cycle.
3. **S phase:** DNA synthesis and replication happen which prepare the chromosome for

attachment to the mitotic spindle. In this phase, cell contains two copies of diploid genetic material.

4. **G2 phase:**
    ⮕ DNA repair and cell apoptosis happen here by various checkpoints to check if there was any damage occurred to DNA during the cycle.
    ⮕ Cell becomes ready to enter into mitosis.
    ⮕ Chromosome becomes dense thread-like structures.
    ⮕ Sister chromatid exchange happens here.

The length and the rate of the cell cycle depends upon cell type and various cell cycle regulators like cyclins. In rapidly dividing cells it lasts for hours like skin or gut mucosal cells and in other cells it lasts for months to years.

Q 7. Write about mitosis cell division with the help of diagram.

Ans. Mitosis: The type of division in which two diploid daughter cells are formed from one diploid cell involving division of the nucleus and cytoplasm. It occurs in zygote and other somatic cells like marrow cells and skin tissues. It is a part of cell cycle and takes 1–2 hours to complete. It has following stages (Figure 1.3):

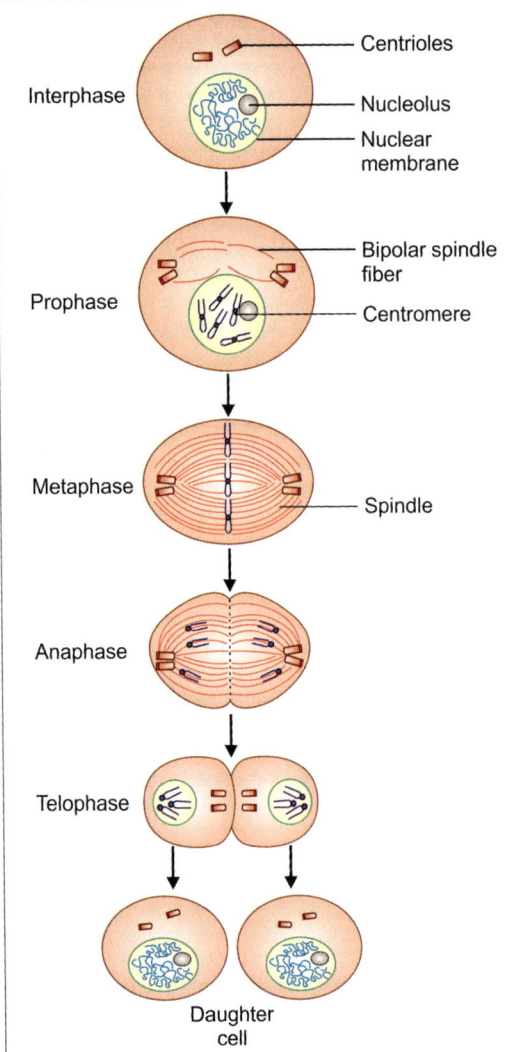

Figure 1.3: Phases of mitotic division

1. **Prophase:**
   - Chromosomes look dense and coiled in light microscope.
   - Sister chromatids remain attached to centromere.
   - Nuclear membrane disappears.
   - Spindle fiber formation from centriole situated in opposite direction of the cell.
   - Pulling of the two sister chromatids by spindle fibers opposite to each other.
2. **Metaphase:**
   - Chromosomes are maximally condensed and easily detectable.
   - Chromosomes arranged along the equatorial plane of the cell in the center of the spindle.
3. **Anaphase:** Two sister chromatids separate and move to opposite sides of the cell in equal number by longitudinal division of the chromosome.
4. **Telophase:**
   - Nuclear membrane appears around both the 23 pairs of chromosomes.
   - Spindle fibers disappear.
   - Chromosomes decondense.
   - Cytoplasm divides into two parts leading to formation of two diploid daughter cells similar to parent cell.

Q 8. Write about meiosis cell division with the help of diagram.

Ans. Meiosis leads to formation of haploid gametes (secondary oocyte and spermatocyte) from diploid cell (oogonia or spermatogonia) in two parts of division—meiosis I and II. However, DNA replication occurs only once.

Meiosis I (reduction division) Figure 1.4:

1. **Prophase I:**
   - Chromosomes become clear after condensation and sister chromatids joined at centromere.
   - Homologous chromosomes come opposite to each other (synapsis process) called bivalent.
   - Crossing over happens between homologous chromosomes and exchange of chromatid occurs leading to recombinant homologous chromosome formation (except between X and Y chromosomes in males).
   - The recombinant chromosomes separate to opposite side of cell except at the point of crossing over. This is called chiasmata.
   - Spindle formation starts and nuclear membrane disappears.
2. **Metaphase I:**
   - Chromosomes arranged along the equatorial plane of the cell in the center of the spindle.

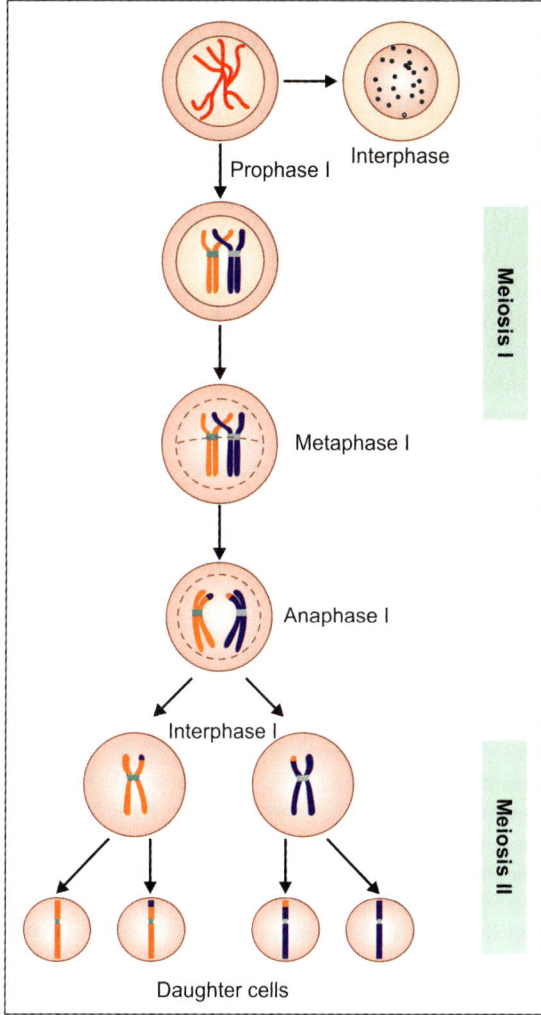

Prophase I   Interphase

Meiosis I

Metaphase I

Anaphase I

Interphase I

Meiosis II

Daughter cells

Figure 1.4: Phases of meiotic division

3. **Anaphase I:**
   - Homologous chromosomes move to opposite sides of the cell after disappearance of chiasmata.
   - Centromere does not divide.
   - Half of the parent cell chromosomes (22 autosomes and one sex chromosome) move towards each side.
4. **Telophase I:**
   - Two daughter cells are formed with half the number of chromosomes at opposite side (one secondary oocyte and one polar body or two secondary spermatocytes).

Meiosis II: Like in mitosis, in meiosis II, two daughter cells form from each secondary gamete. As a result, a total of four cells (sperms) are formed in males and one ova and 3 polar bodies are formed in females.

Q 9. Write the clinical relevance of both mitosis and meiosis in medicine.

Ans.   Clinical relevance of mitosis:
Mitosis normally maintains the number of chromosomes and prevents the loss or gain of genome in a cell. But due to faulty division it can lead to various genetic disorders such as:
1. **Nondisjunction after fertilization or in placenta:** It leads to mosaicism as in Down syndrome.
2. **Malignancy:** Abnormal separation of chromosomes can lead to cytogenic abnormal malignancies as in colon cancer.

Clinical relevance of meiosis:
Meiosis normally maintains the number of chromosomes in a species by reducing the chromosome number to half. The clinical significance of meiosis is:
- **Genetic diversity** due to crossing over between chromatids and gene shuffling.
- **Individual with specific features** due to recombinant chromosomes.
- **Nondisjunction** leads to fetal abnormality and spontaneous abortions and various aneuploidies (Down syndrome) and polyploidy abnormalities.
- **Unequal recombinations** lead to variations in response to medicines, thalassemia or sexual disorders.
- **Malignancy:** Abnormal crossing over in somatic tissue leads to malignancy.

MOLECULAR BIOLOGY AND HUMAN GENOME
KOMAL UPPAL, SHREYA TANNERU, SURESH THOMAS, PRIYANKA SRIVASTAVA, T KARTHIK BHARADWAJ

Q 10. What is chromosome?
Ans. Chromosomes are thread-like structures composed of compact DNA (deoxyribose nucleic acid) present in the nucleus of a cell.

These can be seen clearly in metaphase stage of mitosis. There are 46 chromosomes in human species. These contain all the genes which have the entire genetic information for the expression of genes for formation of proteins needed for cell functioning and cell survival. Any alteration in the chromosomes or genes leads to clinical impact on the health of an individual.

Q 11. Diagrammatically represent the chromosome structure.

Ans. Chromosome structure:

⮑ Chromosome structure is much more complex than DNA structure. DNA gets coiled and folded further to form chromosome. The length of each chromosome varies from each other but roughly it is less than half a millimetre.

⮑ After primary coiling of DNA, secondary coiling around histone leads to formation of nucleosome which forms a solenoid.

⮑ Tertiary coiling of solenoid around non-histone protein results in chromatin fiber formation which further extends and forms the loop chromatin fibers.

⮑ Chromatin fibers have 100 kbp of DNA.

⮑ These are seen as chromosome threads in metaphase stage under light microscope (Figure 1.5).

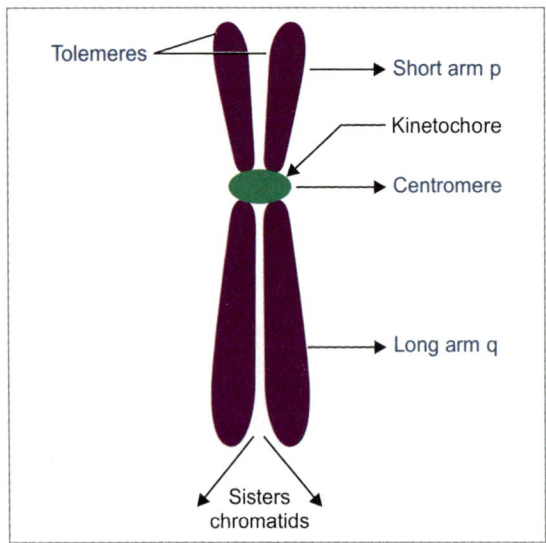

Figure 1.5: Chromosome threads (sister chromatids) in metaphase stage under light microscope

⮑ Chromosome has two similar strands called sister chromatids formed during S phase in DNA replication.

⮑ These two strands are joined at point called centromere.

⮑ Centromere divides the chromosome into p (short arm) and q (long arm).

⮑ Centromere helps in movement of chromosome during cell division.

⮑ Tip of the chromosome is called telomere which contains many tandem repeats of DNA sequence.

Based on the size and centromere location chromosomes are categorized into Figure 1.6:

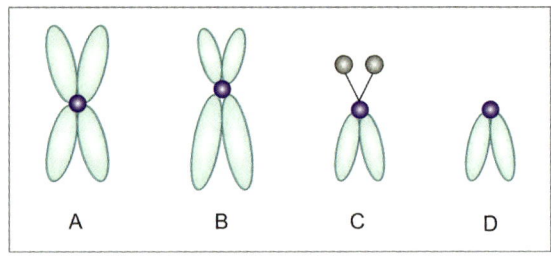

Figure 1.6: Chromosome categorization: (A) Metacentric (chromosome 1, 3, 16, 19, 20); **(B)** Submetacentric (chromosome 2, 4, 5, 6, 7, 8, 9, 10, 11, 12, 17, 18 and X); **(C)** Acrocentric (chromosome 13, 14, 15, 21, 22 and Y); **(D)** Telocentric

a. **Metacentric:** Centromere at center of the chromosome.

b. **Submetacentric:** Centromere at intermediate position of the chromosome.

c. **Acrocentric:** Centromere near the end of the chromosome. It contains stalk-like structure called satellite which leads to formation of nucleolus and rRNA.

d. **Telocentric:** Centromere at the end of the chromosome. In humans there is no telocentric chromosome.

Q 12. Write the classification of chromosome.

Ans. Based on the size, centromere location and presence or absence of satellites, chromosomes are classified into A-G groups (Figure 1.7).

⮑ 46 chromosomes are divided into 22 pairs of autosomes and one pair of sex chromosomes X and Y.

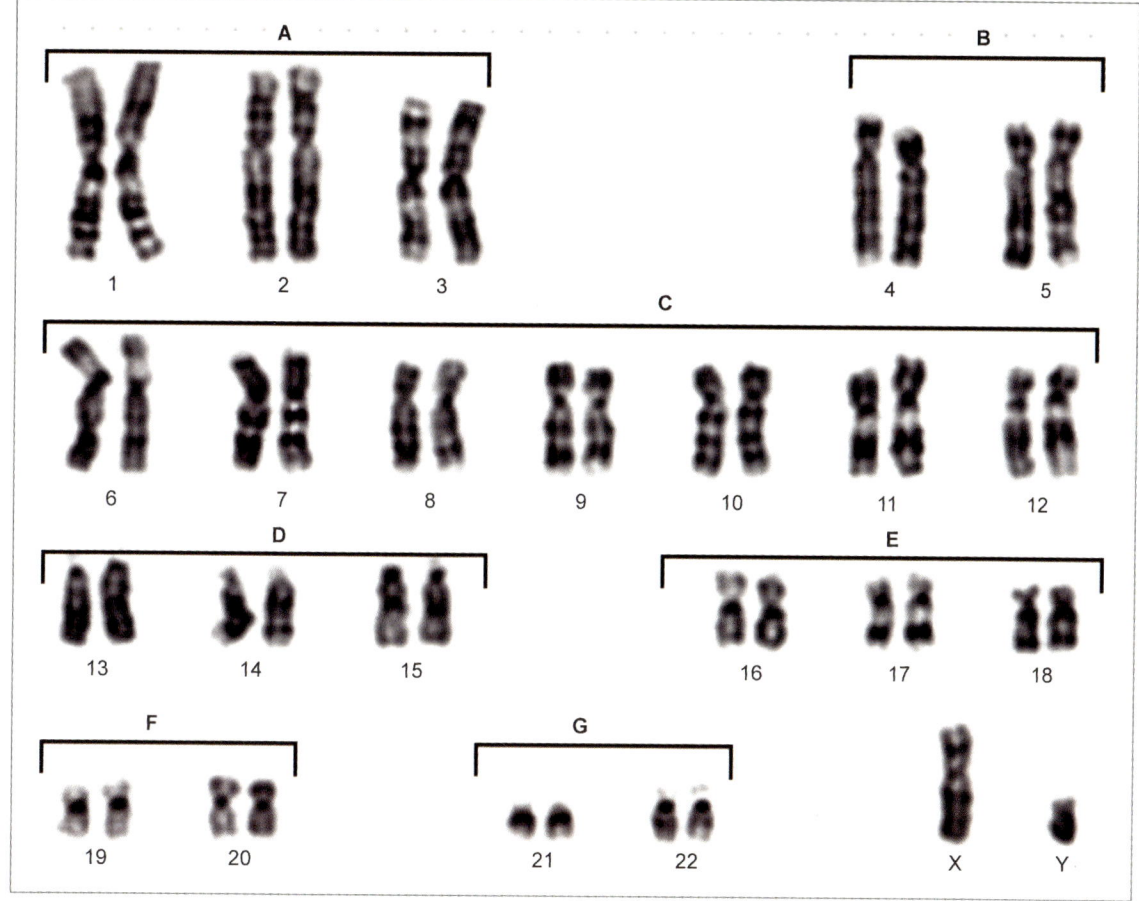

Figure 1.7: Chromosome classification A-G Group (A, 1–3; B, 4–5; C, 6–12 X; D, 13–15; E, 16–18; F, 19–20; G, 21–22 Y) (*Courtesy:* Dr Usha Dutta, CDFD, Hyderabad)

- Females have two X and males have one X and one Y chromosomes.
- Y chromosome is smaller than X chromosome. Genes on Y chromosome are very less in number as compared to autosomes and X chromosome and are responsible for sex determination (SRY) and spermatogenesis process.
- At the ends of X and Y chromosomes (Xp, Xq, Yp, Yq), there are regions called pseudoautosomal regions (PAR) (Figure 4.13, Chapter 4) which undergo meiotic pairing during meiosis I, like autosomal chromosomes and do not undergo inactivation like other X chromosome genes.
- Somatic cells are diploid, and gametes are haploid in number.

- One chromosome in each of the pair is inherited from one of the parents and these are called homologous chromosomes.
- In chromosomes, there can be euchromatin (lightly stained on banding and active) or heterochromatin (darkly stained and inactive) regions based on the chromatin fibers.

Q 13. What is X chromosome inactivation (lyonization)?

Ans. Lyonization: The process of random inactivation of one of the X chromosomes in a female is called lyonization or X chromosome inactivation. It is caused by epigenetic mechanism which leads to silencing of the genes on that inactivated X chromosome and results in equal dosage of genes in both males and females. This random inactivation starts in the embryonic period under the effect of XIST gene in the X inactivation center (XIC) located on inactivated proximal Xq chromosome. XIST gene expresses itself only in the inactive X chromosome but remains silent in active X chromosome. Any extra X chromosome either in male or female will get inactivated. Because of this process, females act as mosaic, as in some cells paternal X chromosome genes express and in others maternal X chromosome genes (Figure 1.8).

Lyonization generally leads to monoallelic expression from one X chromosome's genes. But 15% of the genes show biallelic expression, as in PAR region (Figure 4.13), genes on both X chromosomes do not undergo inactivation, so there is equal biallelic expression from both the X chromosomes. Secondly, in Turner syndrome there is biallelic expression for some of the genes, if all the genes on X chromosome gets inactivated, then all females will present as Turner phenotype.

Clinical consequences of X chromosome inactivation

- In X-linked recessive disorders, manifestation of the symptoms depends upon the proportion of cells with mutated genes on active X chromosome (skewed inactivation).
- X chromosome with structural abnormality always get inactivated. So, it has less effect on the phenotype of an individual as compared to abnormal autosome.
- In X-autosome translocation, there is always non-random inactivation in order to reduce the deleterious phenotypic effect of translocation abnormality.
- The genes which escape inactivation leads to variable clinical phenotype in normal and carrier females of X-linked recessive disorders.

Q 14. What is sex chromatin or Barr body? What is its clinical significance?

Ans. Barr body is an inactive, darkly stained, condensed one of the X chromosomes in a female which can be seen at one side of the nucleus of the somatic cells in interphase stage (Figure 1.8). The number of Barr bodies is always one less than total X chromosome. *Example:* In normal female, there will be one Barr body and in male there will no Barr body. So, it is used for sex determination by taking sample from buccal mucosa.

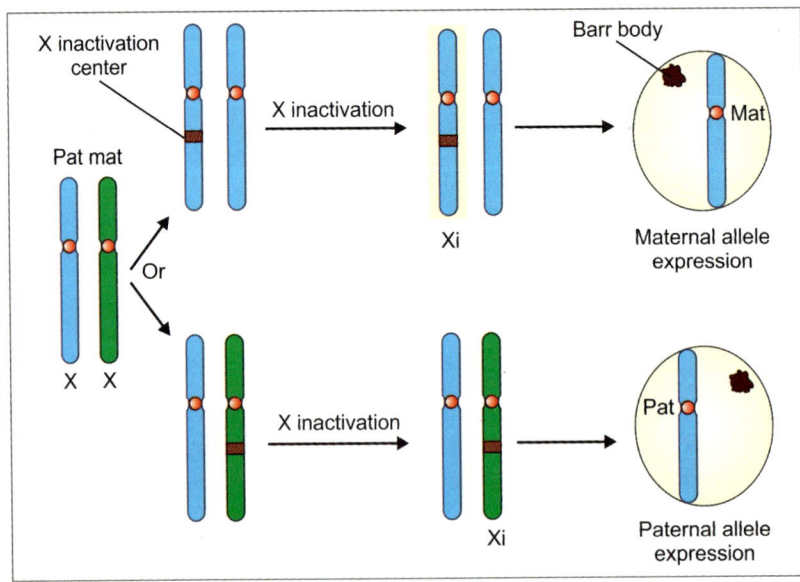

Figure 1.8: X chromosome inactivation shows in some cells paternal X chromosome genes express and in others maternal X chromosome genes

Q 15. What is DNA? Diagrammatically represent the structure of DNA.

Ans. DNA (deoxyribose nucleic acid) is a hereditary unit of humans and other organisms. It is found in the nucleus (nuclear DNA) and mitochondria (mitochondrial DNA) ineukaryotes. DNA is made up of nucleotides and each nucleotide is made up of three components (Figure 1.9):

   i A nitrogen-containing base (cytosine [C], guanine [G], adenine [A], thymine [T])

  ii. A five-carbon sugar: Deoxyribose

 iii. A phosphate group.

DNA structure was given by Watson and Crick

- Two polypeptide chains form a double helix by coiling around each other.
- One end is called 3′ and the other end is 5′.
- 5′ end of each strand is a phosphate group and a 3′ end is a hydroxyl group. Both are connected by phosphodiesterase bond.
- The two DNA strands are antiparallel to each other.
- The nucleotide bases are joint by hydrogen bonds (A = T, G ≡ C).

Q 16. Explain DNA replication.

Ans. DNA replication: DNA can replicate or make two identical copies/replicas of the original DNA molecule.

Basic rules of replication:

- Semiconservative
- Starts at the 'origin'
- Synthesis always occur in 5′ to 3′ direction
- Can be uni- or bi-directional.

Mechanism of replication (Figure 1.10): It occurs in S phase of cell cycle. It has three major steps—initiation, elongation and termination.

1. **Initiation:** DNA synthesis starts at particular sites known as origins.
   - The double helix of DNA unzip with the help of an enzyme called **helicase** which breaks the hydrogen bonds (A = T, G ≡ C) holding the complementary bases of DNA together.
   - Two single strands of DNA create a replication fork after separation.
   - The two separated strands will act as templates for synthesis of the new DNA strands.

2. **Elongation:** DNA polymerase binds to RNA primer made by primase enzyme and then keeps on adding new complementary nucleotide bases to the strand of DNA in the 5′ to 3′ direction called the leading strand.
   - The other strand called lagging strand is oriented away from the replication fork in the 5′ to 3′ direction as pieces called the

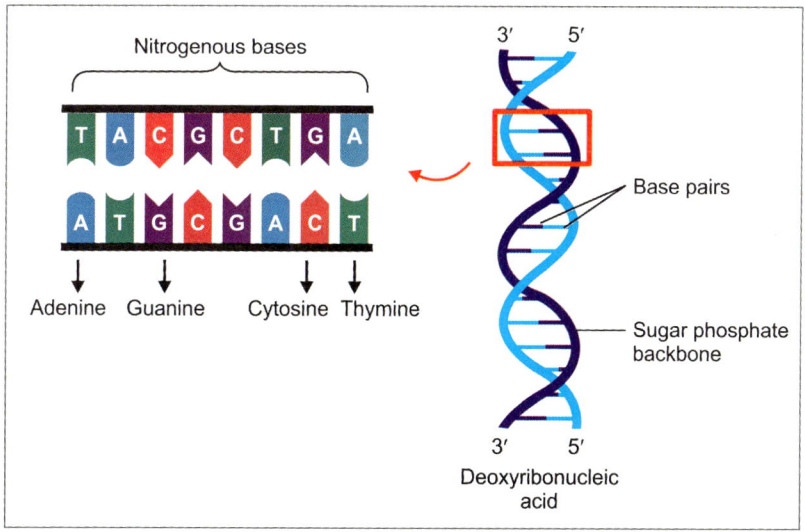

Figure 1.9: Structure of DNA

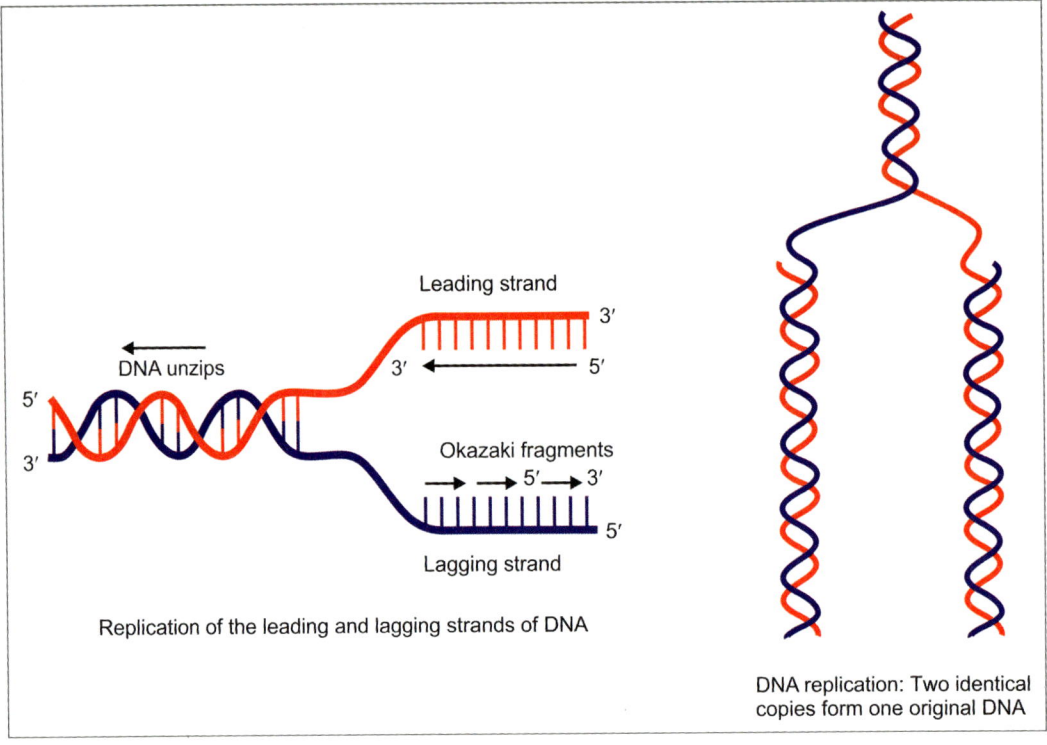

Leading strand

3′

DNA unzips

3′ ← 5′

5′

3′

Okazaki fragments

5′ → 3′

5′

Lagging strand

Replication of the leading and lagging strands of DNA

DNA replication: Two identical copies form one original DNA

Figure 1.10: DNA replication

Okazaki fragments which joined up later on by enzyme ligase.

3. **Termination:**
   - The resulting two DNA molecules consist of one new and one old chain of nucleotides. This is called semi-conservative replication.
   - After replication, the newly synthesized DNA automatically winds up into a double helix structure.

Q 17. Write about different types of DNA sequences and their clinical significance.

Ans. Three types of DNA sequences:

A. **Non-repetitive DNA:** They occur as a single copy in a haploid genome.

B. **Highly repetitive DNA:** These sequences occur in multiple copies in the genome. These are short tandem repeat sequences of 5–10 bps, which accounts for 10% of the total genome. It is further classified as:
   - *Satellite DNA:* These are 200 bp long and located in pericentromeric or telomeric heterochromatin region.
   - *Minisatellite:* These are represented by 5–50 tandem repeats of 15 base pairs. They are classified as VNTRs (variable number tandem repeats), basically used in DNA fingerprinting.
   - *Microsatellite:* These are formed of about 100 repeats of 2–5 bps (simple tandem repeats, STRs). They are used in crime detection and non-paternity identification.

C. **Moderately repetitive DNA:** These include short (150 to 300 bp) sequences or long ones (5 kbp) amounting to about 40% and 1–2% of the total genome, respectively. Their main function is gene regulation. It includes:

Interspersed repetitive DNA: They can jump from one place to another in the genome and are known as mobile elements or transposable elements. They are scattered throughout the genome and can cause pathogenic mutations due to unequal recombinations. They are of two types:

- *LINE (Long Interspersed Nuclear Elements)*: Up to 7,000 base pairs
- *SINE (Short Interspersed Nuclear Elements)*: 10–500 base pairs (the Alu-I family in primates).

Q 18. What is mitochondrial DNA? Write differences between mitochondrial and nuclear DNA.

Ans. Mitochondrial DNA is found in mitochondria. It is small, circular and consists of 16.5 kb (Table 1.1).

TABLE 1.1: Differences between mitochondrial and nuclear DNA

Mitochondrial DNA	Nuclear DNA
o Mitochondrial DNA is found inside mitochondria	o Nuclear DNA is found inside the nucleus

o It contains only
  • 37 genes
  • 2 rRNA
  • 22 tRNAW
  • 13 enzymes for oxidative phosphorylation
	o It contains ~25,000 genes.

o mtDNA is circular in shape	o It is linear in shape
o It is inherited from mother only	o It is inherited from both mother and father
o It contains only 1 chromosome	o It consists of 46 chromosomes
o mtDNA is responsible for metabolic activities	o Nuclear DNA is responsible for genetic make-up of a human being

Q 19. Define gene, housekeeping gene, pseudogene and novel gene.

Ans. Gene: A sequence of nucleotides in DNA/RNA constituting the physical and functional unit of heredity is called a gene. Human genome is estimated to have about 20000–25000 of such genes. Genes can be coding genes; get transcribed into RNA which gets translated into proteins. But in some instances, RNA (noncoding, i.e. tRNA, rRNA, miRNA, snoRNA, lncRNA) is the functional product of a gene.

Housekeeping genes: These genes are extremely essential for normal cellular function and maintenance and are thus, expressed continuously at constant rate in all the cells of an organism. For example, ATPases, RNA, polymerases, etc.

Pseudogenes: These are DNA sequences share close similarity with a functional gene but are otherwise inactive due to defective/incomplete duplication. Some might have regulatory functions. They can be:

- **Unprocessed pseudogenes** which retain their exon-intron structure.
- **Processed** ones arise out of integration of cDNA into the genome after reverse transcription and are thus, devoid of exon-intron structure.

Because of the sequence similarities, variations in these genes are falsely picked up as variations in the functional genes and are thus a common cause of false positives in diagnostics.

Novel gene: Novel gene in literal sense means new genes. However, it might be an entirely newly discovered protein-coding functional genetic sequence or might just produce a functional RNA or might be a known gene associated with a disease that has been newly discovered. They have important evolutionary role in diversification of organisms.

Q 20. Explain the structure of a gene with the help of diagram.

Ans. Gene is the functional unit of heredity constituting a complex structure (Figure 1.11)
Structure of gene:

- In eukaryotes, genes are frequently interrupted by non-coding sequences.
- The coding portions of the genes are exons, while the non-coding sequences are called introns.

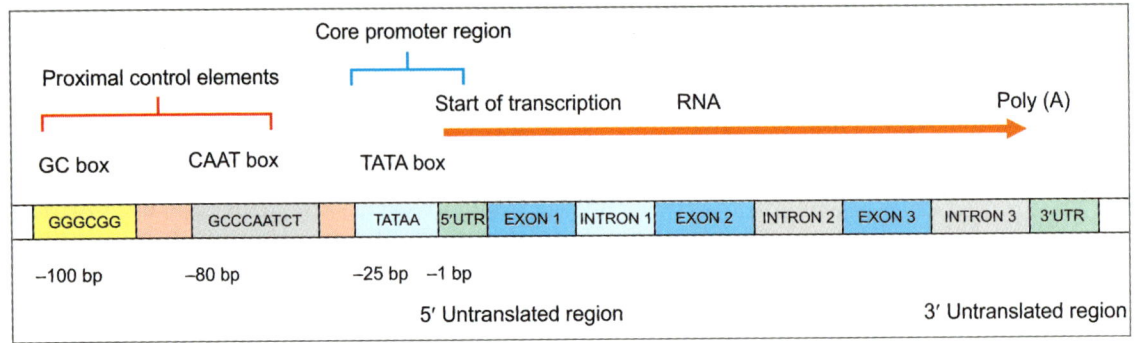

Figure 1.11: Schematic diagram showing the structure of a gene (*Courtesy:* Dr Usha Dutta, CDFD, Hyderabad)

- Genes are of varying lengths with different proportions of coding exons and introns.
- Exons are flanked by transcribed 5′ untranslated region—start site and 3′ untranslated stop site—having Poly A tail. These are important regulators of translation.
- DNA sequences for transcription towards 5′ are called upstream sequences and towards 3′ are called downstream sequences.
- Slightly upstream of the first exon, usually within 25–100 bases, sequences called promoter regions (the TATA and CAAT box). It is responsible for binding of various transcription initiation factors to the DNA strand.
- Other regulatory regions-enhancers, silencers and locus control regions are present upstream, downstream and sometimes within the gene itself.
- Initially, the entire genic sequence from the transcription start site is transcribed to pre-mRNA (pre-messenger RNA) which further undergoes downstream processing to form mature mRNA.

Q 21. What is the function of a gene?
Ans. Function of a gene: The function of genes is to get transcribed into RNA which in turn gets translated into various structural and functional proteins for the differential expression of a gene and functioning of different cells.

DNA → RNA → Protein

This is the principle of life. This whole process consists of various steps (Figure 1.12):

1. **Transcription** is the conversion of DNA to RNA. One strand of DNA is called template or antisense strand and the other strand is called sense strand. At the promoter region of the sense strand, enzyme RNA polymerase II and various other transcription initiation factors binds. Initially, the entire gene including the introns is transcribed to form pre-mRNA (pre-messenger RNA).

2. **Post-transcription modifications:** Pre-mRNA undergoes further downstream processing including 5′ capping, polyadenylation and splicing to form mature mRNA.
   i. **5′ capping** is done by addition of methylated guanine at the 5′ end which helps in transport of mRNA into the cytoplasm, ribosomal attachment and prevention from degradation.
   ii. **Poly A tail addition:** At the 3′ end, transcription stops after certain sequences in the 3′UTR are encountered by the RNA polymerases. A polyA tail is then added which serves a role in transport, translation and stabilization of the mRNA.
   iii. **Splicing** is the removal of intronic sequences from the transcript, prior to translation and the exons together form the mature RNA.

3. **Translation** is the conversion of mature RNA into protein in the cytoplasm.

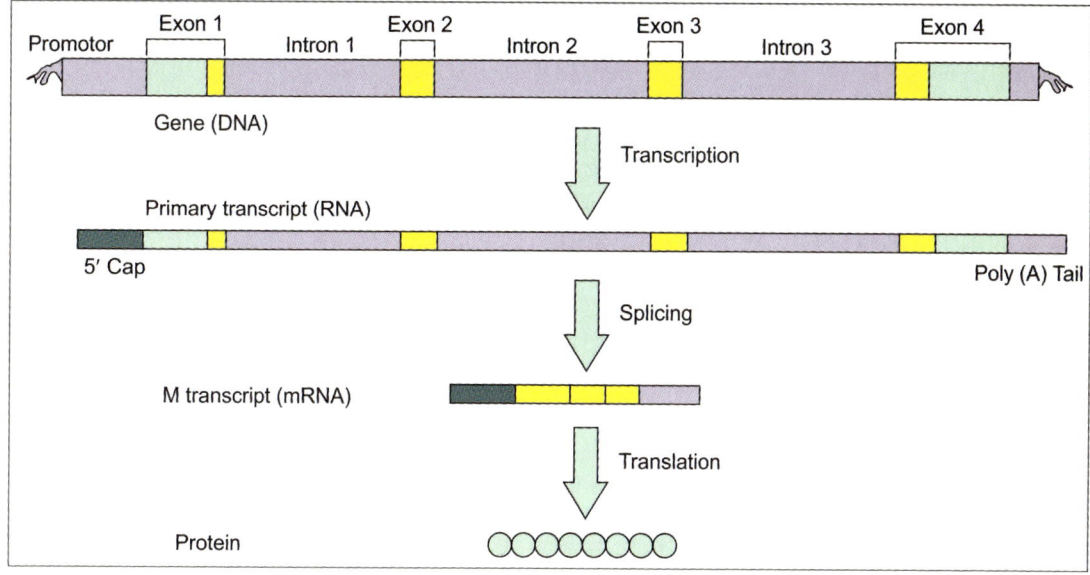

Figure 1.12: Process of protein synthesis from DNA

Polypeptide chains form at ribosomes with the help of rRNA, tRNA, aminoacyl tRNA synthetase enzyme and peptidyl transferase enzyme.

4. **Post-translation modification:** These polypeptide chains further undergo various modifications like hydroxylation, methylation, glycosylation or proteolysis to become structural and functional proteins.

Genes responsible for the formation of structural and functional proteins are constitutively expressed for survival and metabolism of a cell. Some genes can be switched on or off depending upon the presence of an inducer or repressor determined by the requirements of a cell. Expression of genes in various combinations results in differences in structure and physiology of an organism determining its response to environmental challenges and therefore its survival. Any change in DNA or protein synthesis process can result in disruption of gene function and thus disease/death or can lead to development of new traits, thus resulting in evolution.

BIBLIOGRAPHY

1. Emery & Rimoin's Principles & Practice of Medical Genetics, 7th edition.
2. Nelson's Textbook of Pediatrics, 21st edition.
3. Thompson & Thompson, Genetics in Medicine, 8th edition.

Mutation and Polymorphism

Syeda Zubeda

Q 1. Definitions

Ans.

1. **Genotype** is the genetic composition of an individual which describes the state of two copies (alleles) of a gene at a given locus on the chromosome.

   Example: If the eye color of an individual is green, then the two different alleles for the gene will be: G-Green color and g-Black color.

   The three genotypes will be:
   a. GG: Homozygote
   b. Gg: Heterozygote
   c. G or g: Hemizygote.

2. **Phenotype** is the external/observable expression of a trait. The phenotype of an individual depends upon the genotype and its environmental interaction.

   Examples: Eye color, skin color, height of an individual, etc.

3. **Locus** is the specific reference position where a gene is located on the chromosome. If it gives the information of many genes, it is called loci.

4. **Allele** is one of the two possible genetic sequences for a given gene at a particular locus on the chromosome.

   Example: For describing the height of a tree, the two alternate sequences/alleles can be represented as T and t for the trait.

   ○ *Wild type allele* is the allele of a particular gene which remained unchanged from our ancestors or through the evolutionary process and is seen in majority of healthy individuals.

   ○ *Variant or mutant allele* is the alternate sequence of the DNA instead of wild type, present in the gene due to change in the DNA nucleotide sequence.

5. **Mutations** are changes in the genetic material of an organism, which affects the normal organization (sequence, structure or function) of gene or the entire chromosome.

6. **Novel mutation** is the alternate sequence of the DNA different from the wild type which was not reported earlier and is identified in the genomic sequence during a research or a diagnostic test.

7. **Polymorphism** is the frequency of two or more variants in a given population greater than 1%, indicating that it is present due to normal evolution and has no major effect on phenotype.

Q 2. What is mutation? Explain how mutations arise in genetic material (or explain the basic pathogenesis of mutation).

Ans. **Mutation** is the inheritable change in the genetic material of an organism, which affects the normal organization (sequence, structure or function) of gene or the entire chromosome. Mutations that cause changes in one sequence or that is limited to a small locus in the gene can be termed small gene mutations and those that cause big alterations at chromosomal level are called large chromosomal mutations. These changes in the DNA subsequently affect the RNA and protein. The mutations that cause a positive effect are beneficial are likely cause of evolution and those which cause a disease are called pathogenic mutations.

Mutations can arise in genetic material due to:

1. **Natural factors:** Defect in DNA replication, DNA repair mechanism and chromosomal anomalies during cell division can lead to mutations which can be pathogenic or benign. The frequency of these mutations in a specific population depends upon the process of natural selection, genetic drift, gene flow and the rate of mutation. The rate of mutation depends upon the size and site of gene, parental gender and age.
   Example: Achondroplasia *de novo* mutation rate is more in advanced aged fathers.

2. **Environmental factors:**
   ⊃ *Mutagens* like chemicals, dyes, form aldehydes, benzene compounds, food adulterants, tobacco, etc. can cause both chromosomal and DNA mutations.
   ⊃ *Radiations:* Natural and artificial ionizing radiations like X-rays, gamma rays, alpha, beta and neutron particles from diagnostic and therapeutic radioactive interventions and occupational exposure can lead to somatic and germline mutations. It depends upon the dose and time of exposure to radiations. More the dose and exposure, more will be the rate of mutation but, small doses can also lead to variations in DNA. One chest X-ray exposure dose during diagnostic intervention is 0.1 mSv (unit of radiation average dose per year) and recommended dose exposure is 15 mSv per year. So, during diagnostic intervention or occupational exposure, risk and benefit of the procedure should be balanced to prevent occurrence of mutations.

Q 3. Write about different types of mutations.

Ans.

I. **Mutations based on tissue involved:**
   ⊃ *Somatic mutations* happen during mitotic division in somatic tissues after differentiation of the zygote in somatic and gonadal tissues. It does not transmit to future generation and can be diagnosed from somatic tissue by molecular test.
   Example: Segmental neurofibromatosis or cancer mutations.
   ⊃ *Germline mutations* get transmitted from the parental germ cells and present both in somatic and germ cells. It can be diagnosed in the peripheral blood by molecular tests and can be further transmitted to next generation.
   Example: Sickle cell anemia.

II. **Mutations based on the level and mechanism observed in a cell's DNA:**

1. GENE LEVEL

a. **Mutations in coding regions:** Point mutations or small-scale mutations caused due to base substitutions where one base sequence is substituted with another resulting in the change in one codon in the RNA sequence.

Mechanisms for point mutations: (Figure 2.1 A to C)
i. **Base substitutions:** At gene level:
   o **Transitions:** Adenine (A) is substituted by Guanine (G) (A-G), switch between two purines or a substitution of Cytosine (C) to Thymine (T) (C–T), switch between two pyrimidines.
   o **Transversion:** Either A/G are substituted by C/T, i.e. either a purine is replaced by pyrimidine or a pyrimidine is replaced by a purine.
   o **Mispairing:** Normally in DNA, A pairs with T and G pairs with C. During mispairing, non-Watson-Crick pairing occurs wherein A pairs with C and T pairs G.

ii. **Frameshift mutations:** The reading frame (three bases forming an amino acid) in the RNA shifts due to insertions or deletion of one or two bases leads to many different changes in the codons that code for the protein.
   Example: Hereditary motor and sensory neuropathy occurs due to insertion and Duchenne muscular dystrophy due to deletion of exon.

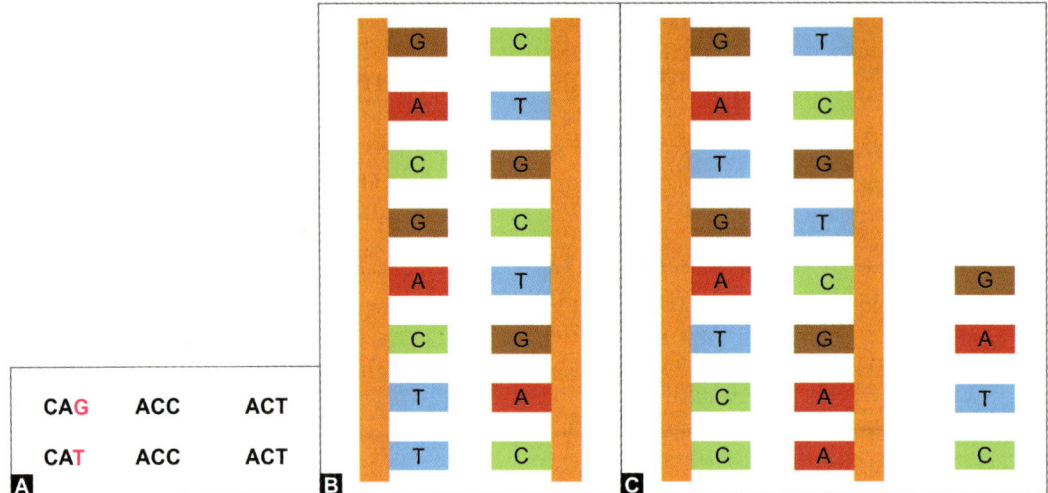

Figure 2.1: (A) Point mutation; (B) Normal nucleotide base pairing; (C) Mispairing of nucleotide base pairs (A–C, G–T)

b. **Mutations in non-coding regions** like promoter region, splice sites, miRNA, siRNA and various regulatory sites also lead to severe phenotypic manifestations.

2. TRIPLET REPEAT DISORDERS (See Chapter 16 for detail)

These occur due to expansion and instability of triplet repeat sequence (CAG CAGCAG). *Example*: Huntington disease.

3. CHROMOSOMAL LEVEL (LARGE SCALE) ABERRATIONS (See Chapter 3 for detail)

Various structural or numerical aberrations may affect more than one gene and can cause severe disease.

a. **Structural aberrations:**

i. **Deletions:** Deletions of large parts of chromosomes are usually caused due to heat or radiation, viruses, chemicals or even due to errors in recombination, etc. These cannot be reverted as the segment is lost permanently.

ii. **Duplications:** These result from doubling of chromosomal segments.

iii. **Insertions:** These can cause the increase in the genetic information.

iv. **Inversions:** The genetic information is not changed in amount, but it is inverted and rearranged and affects gene expression.

v. **Translocations:** They occur when a segment of one chromosome transfers to another chromosome and attaches there.

b. **Numerical aberrations: Aneuploidy and polyploidy** cause the change in the number of the chromosomes.

Q 4. What are structural effects of mutation on the protein products?

Ans. Structural effects of mutations on the proteins: There can be minimal to lethal consequences of mutations on the structure of the protein products by two ways (Figure 2.2):

➲ **Synonymous or silent mutations:** A single base pair substitution preferably at the third nucleotide in the triplet sequences wherein the final amino acid is not changed and there is no alteration in the protein features.

➲ **Nonsynonymous mutations:** When the substitution of a nucleotide(s) results in change in the amino acid or its sequence from the original triplet which it was supposed to code for, it leads to nonsynonymous mutation. It can result in abnormal protein function and can lead to disease.

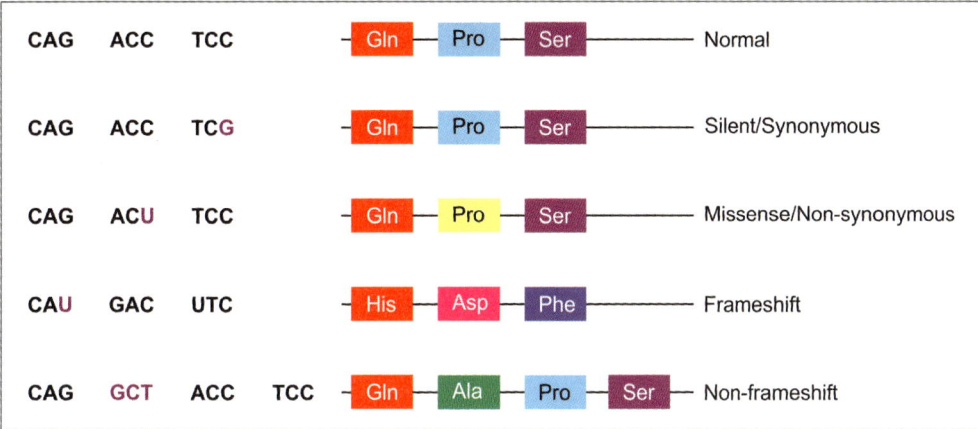

Figure 2.2: Structural effects of mutations on the protein products

- *Missense mutations:* Alteration of one single amino acid sequence that leads to abnormal structure of the protein.
  Example: Most of the structural hemoglobinopathies
- *Frameshift:* Complete downstream amino acid sequence of the polypeptide changes leading to frame out mutation.
  Example: Duchenne muscular dystrophy.
- *Nonsense mutation:* An introduction to stop codon may abruptly stop the polypeptide synthesis leading to incomplete protein product.

Q 5. What are functional effects of mutation on the protein products?

Ans. Functional effects of mutations on the proteins: There can be minimal to lethal consequences of mutations on the function of the protein products. Loss or gain of the function of the protein product is the ultimate functional effect due to mutations.

1. **Loss of function mutations** is the changes due to which the protein activity can get reduced or is completely lost. When there is decreased protein activity, it is called hypomorph (the change) and the complete loss of the protein activity is caused due to null allele or amorph. Loss of function mutations in metabolic disorders show autosomal recessive or X-linked recessive pattern of inheritance as there is one normal allele to compensate the protein activity.

2. **Haploinsufficiency** is the phenomenon leading to reduced enzyme production due to heterozygous genotype. It results in disease symptoms due to presence of only one normal copy of the gene.
   Example: Familial hypercholesterolemia. When there is homozygous mutation leading to the complete loss of function of protein, there is a much severe kind of phenotypic presentation.

3. **Gain of function mutations:** Either there will be an increase in the gene expression, or a completely new function is exhibited due to gain of function mutations. This can happen due to activation of a point mutation or increased gene dosage effect.
   Example: The increase in the number of triplet repeats causing Huntington's disease and HER-2 overexpression leading to HER-2 positive breast cancer.

4. **Dominant negative effect:** When a mutation present in heterozygous state produces a protein product which interferes with the protein product of normal allele and causes complete loss of protein activity, it is called dominant negative effect.
   Example: Osteogenesis imperfect.

Q 6. Describe polymorphisms, different types of polymorphism and its role in human genetics.

Ans. Polymorphism: The genomic sequences of different individuals when compared with each other, will be same at many loci. They are monomorphic. But some loci will differ in their nucleotide sequence, which are called polymorphic sections or polymorphisms. The factor which distinguishes these variants being referred to as mutants or polymorphism is their frequency in the population. If the frequency of the variant allele is less than 1% in the population, it is called mutant allele and if its frequency is higher than 1%, it is called a polymorphism.

The different types of DNA polymorphisms are:

1. **Single nucleotide polymorphisms (SNPs):** It is a sequence of DNA on which humans vary by one nucleotide. They can be synonymous or nonsynonymous.

2. **Tandem repeat polymorphisms:** It consists of a series of nucleotides that are repeated in tandem (i.e. one time after another).
   Example: Microsatellite, simple sequence repeat (SSR), or short tandem repeat (STR), minisatellite, variable number of tandem repeats (VNTR) and mobile repeats like Alu and long interspersed elements (LINE).

3. **Structural polymorphisms:** Structural variants involve deletions or insertions of a nucleotide sequence (also called a copy number variant), inversions, and translocations.

Polymorphic variants can be non-pathogenic and can be used for various purposes in human genetics:

➲ For gene mapping by linkage analysis
➲ Forensic medicine—for crime detection and paternity confirmation
➲ HLA matching of tissues.

Q 7. What do you mean by genotype-phenotype correlation? Explain with example.

Ans. In some **single gene disorders** like sickle cell disease, fragile X syndrome, muscular dystrophy, genetic change (genotype) responsible for a specific disease can be identified based on the clinical examination.

But for the complex diseases and due to genetic heterogeneity sometimes it becomes difficult to identify the etiological mutation on clinical basis. The variants found on whole genome sequence of an individual or whole exome sequencing gives a lot of genetic data and the exact sequence change to find out which one is actual causative or is associated with the disease is a challenging task. For identifying the actual association, different phenotypic details of the proband are taken and are correlated with the obtained genetic changes one by one based on their function, pathogenicity and mode of inheritance. This association between the genotype and responsible phenotype of an individual is called genotype–phenotype correlation.

Example: Larsen syndrome is a rare genetic disorder that has been associated with a wide variety of different symptoms caused by mutations of the FLNB gene.

Q 8. Explain genetic and clinical heterogeneity.

Ans. **A. Genetic heterogeneity** means different variations at genomic sequence/different genetic mechanism which will result in similar phenotypes. There are two types of genetic heterogeneity:

1. **Allelic heterogeneity:** Different variations at the same locus in the same gene resulting in similar phenotype is called allelic heterogeneity.
   Allelic diversity is also an important consideration in disorders, such as retinitis pigmentosa, cystic fibrosis, hemophilia, and β-thalassemia. Direct mutation analysis in these disorders for only a subset of specific mutations may fail to detect a different disease-causing mutation in a particular family, who may have critical genetic counseling implications for many individuals within that pedigree.

2. **Locus heterogeneity:** This can be defined as mutations at two or more genetic loci that produce similar phenotypes (either biochemical or clinical). This is relevant since genetic heterogeneity can present problems for heterozygote detection. Example: Hearing loss can occur with

different homozygous mutations in genes MYO6 and SCL26A5.

- ○ *Double heterozygotes:* Hearing loss due to autosomal recessive homozygous mutations in two different genes cause parents to be affected but their child who is heterozygous for each mutation does not manifest the disease.

B. Clinical heterogeneity: It is defined as very different biochemical or clinical phenotypes due to the presence of more than one mutation within the same gene. *Example:* Different mutations of RET proto-oncogene cause different human diseases like papillary thyroid carcinomas, multiple endocrine neoplasia type 2, Hirschsprung's disease and congenital disorder of enteric nervous system.

Q 9. What are different DNA repair pathways? Write about their mechanism and different disorders associated with it.

Ans. DNA repair mechanism occurs in every organism from bacteria to humans. If the DNA got damaged, it gets repaired by various mechanisms involving various enzymes like

- ○ DNA photolyase for thymine dimer formation
- ○ DNA repair endonucleases for cleavage
- ○ Endonuclease excise the nucleotides
- ○ Glycosylases to cleave glycosidic bonds
- ○ DNA polymerase for replication
- ○ DNA ligase for sealing the gaps.

Various DNA repair mechanisms are given in Table 2.1.

TABLE 2.1: Various DNA repair mechanisms

Type of DNA repair	Mechanism	Disorders
Light	Light dependent repair or photo reactivation cleaves thymine dimers, cytosine dimers and cytosine-thymine dimers in prokaryotes	—
Nucleotide	Excision repair thymine dimers, damaged base (S)	○ Xeroderma pigmentosum (XP) ○ Cockayne syndrome (CS) ○ Trichothiodystrophy (TTD)
Base excision repair	Replaces the abnormal base	○ Cancer predisposition ○ Colorectal cancer ○ Immunological defects
Mismatch repair	Excise and replace the mismatches in nucleotide after replication	Mismatches in hMLH1 and hMSH2 genes cause sporadic colorectal carcinomas
Post-replication repair	Rec A protein binds to the single strand at the gap in the template strand and mediate pairing with homologous and non-homologous segment of the sister double helix	○ Bloom syndrome due to BLM gene ○ Breast cancer (BRCA1, 2)

BIBLIOGRAPHY

1. Emery & Rimoin's Principles & Practice of Medical Genetics, 7th edition.
2. Nelson's Textbook of Pediatrics, 21st edition.
3. Thompson & Thompson, Genetics in Medicine, 8th edition.

Chromosomal Abnormalities and their Mechanism

Chapter 3

Priyanka Srivastava

Q 1. What is the incidence/prevalence of chromosomal abnormalities?

Ans. Incidence of chromosomal anomalies depends upon the mode of presentation. Some common examples are as follows:

Mode of presentation	Incidence of chromosomal anomalies
Spontaneous abortions	50%
Single malformation in fetus (detected by ultrasound)	5–10%
Multiple malformations	10–30%
Stillbirths or neonatal deaths	5–6%
Live borns	0.5–1%

Q 2. Write about the clinical consequences of different chromosomal abnormalities.

Ans. Clinical consequences:
The common clinical consequences of chromosomal anomalies are:

- **Stillbirth:** Aneuploidies and large segmental imbalances can cause embryonic death or stillbirth.
- **Mental retardation/intellectual disability:** Trisomies, microdeletions and microduplications which are tolerated by nature may cause birth of children with intellectual disability.
Example: Trisomy 21 (Down syndrome), trisomy 18 and 13.

- **Multiple malformations:** Various aneuploidies and structural chromosomal anomalies can cause congenital malformation.
Example: 22q11.2 microdeletion.
- **Hypogonadism and ambiguous genitalia:** Sex chromosome anomalies can lead to disorder of sexual development.
Example: 45, X (Turner syndrome); 47, XXX; 47, XXY (Klinefelter syndrome); 47, XYY.
- **Reproductive failure:** Infertility and recurrent abortions can happen if parents are carriers of balanced chromosomal rearrangements (3–6%).
- **Cancer:** Various somatic chromosomal imbalances are found in cancers like hematological malignancies.

Q 3. Enumerate different types of chromosomal abnormalities.

Ans. Chromosomal abnormalities are of two types (Flowchart 3.1):
- **Structural abnormalities:** Changes in the structure or morphology of chromosomes are called structural abnormalities.
- **Numerical abnormalities:** Changes in the number of chromosomes are known as numerical abnormalities. It can be aneuploidy or polyploidy.
- **Mixoploidy:** Mixoploidy refers to the presence of two or more populations of cells of different genotype developed from a single or different zygote.

Flowchart 3.1: Classification of chromosomal abnormalities

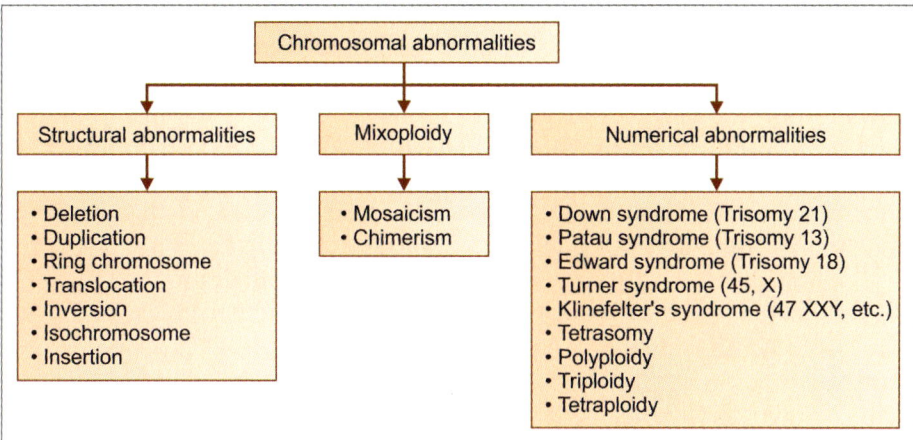

Q 4. **Describe the mechanism of various numerical chromosomal abnormalities and give one example of each abnormality.**

Ans. Numerical abnormalities:

Changes in the number of autosomal and sex chromosomes are known as numerical abnormalities, i.e. aneuploidy or polyploidy.

A. **Aneuploidy:** Extra or missing chromosome due to nondisjunction in mitosis or meiosis results in aneuploidy (Figure 3.1). When an organism is having an exact multiple of the haploid chromosome number (n), it is called a euploid.

Two common types of aneuploidy are:

⊃ *Monosomy* occurs when an organism has only one copy of a chromosome instead of two copies. *Example:* 45, X (Turner syndrome) (Figure 3.2).

⊃ *Trisomy* occurs when an organism has extra third copy of an autosomal or sex chromosome instead of two. These

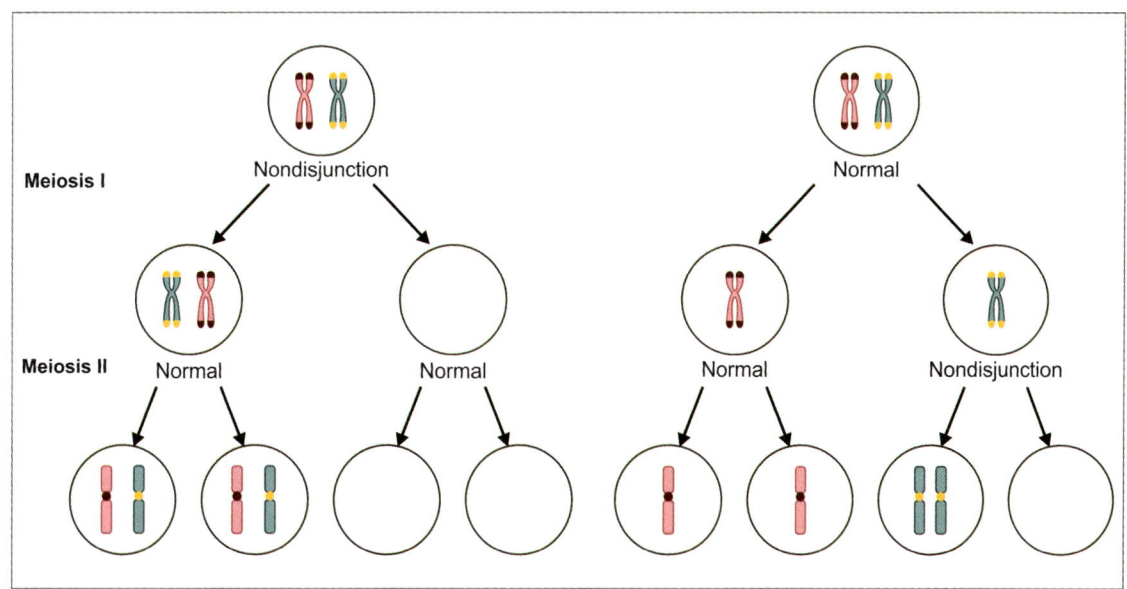

Figure 3.1: Meiosis I (left) and meiosis II (right) nondisjunction give rise to disomic and nullisomic gametes

represent about 0.3% of all live births. In early pregnancy, all the fetuses with trisomies of autosomal chromosome 8, 19 and 16 abort spontaneously. If they survive with trisomies of chromosomes like chromosome 21, 13 and 18, they will have multiple malformations, intellectual disability and short life. *Examples:* Down syndrome (Figure 3.2), 47, XXY (Klinefelter syndrome); 47, XYY; and 47, XXX.

B. **Polyploidy:** Organisms with more than two complete sets of chromosomes are said to be polyploid.

　⊃ *Triploidy and Tetraploidy:* Besides normal diploid (2n) number of chromosomes, two other euploid chromosome complements are occasionally present: Triploid 69, (3n) and tetraploid 92, (4n). Triploid and tetraploid fetuses generally do not survive.

Q 5. Explain the different structural chromosomal abnormalities and their mechanisms and give example of each abnormality.

Ans. Structural abnormalities:

Changes in the structure or morphology of chromosome are called structural abnormalities, resulting from single or multiple breaks on the chromosome causing different types of rearrangements. These can be either balanced or imbalanced. Balanced abnormalities do not cause any abnormal phenotype in the carrier individual, but these abnormalities can lead to gamete formation with imbalanced chromosomal abnormalities responsible for spontaneous pregnancy loss (30–50% which depends on the type of chromosomal structural abnormality, chromosome involved and the size of the chromosome segment involved in the imbalanced rearrangement) or abnormal phenotypic (5–10%) in their offspring.

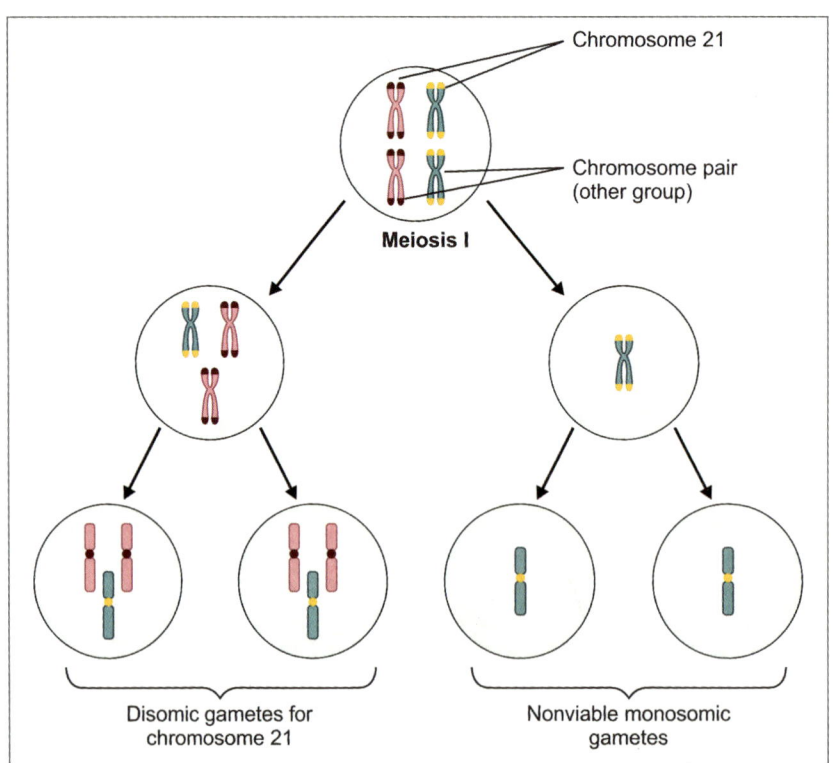

Figure 3.2: Down syndrome: The extra chromosome comes from the mother due to non-disjunction (failure of separation) of chromosomes during meiosis I

Structural abnormality can occur in several ways:

DELETIONS: A large or sub-microscopic portion of the chromosome can be missed or deleted (partial monosomy). Individuals with very large deletions do not survive and sub-microscopic deletions are responsible for intellectual disability (Figure 3.3).

o **Terminal deletion:** At the distal end of chromosome.

o **Interstitial deletion:** Intervening segment between two break points gets lost.

Example: Wolf-Hirschhorn syndrome (4p deletion) and Jacobsen syndrome (terminal 11q deletion).

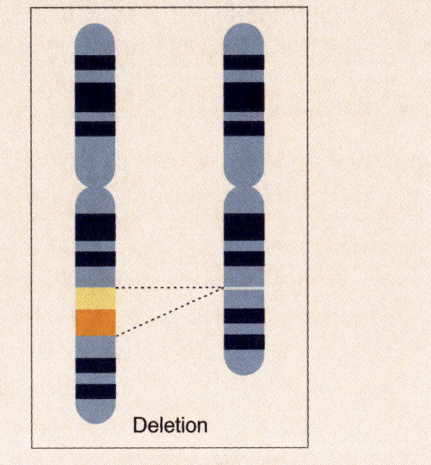

Deletion

Figure 3.3

DUPLICATIONS: A portion of the chromosome is duplicated (partial trisomy), resulting in extra genetic material (Figure 3.4).

Example: Duplication of the region containing gene PMP22 on chromosome 17 causing Charcot-Marie-Tooth disease type 1A.

o **Tandem duplication:** Duplication can occur either of the adjacent part of chromosome or in reverse manner. It can happen at the terminal end of chromosome also.

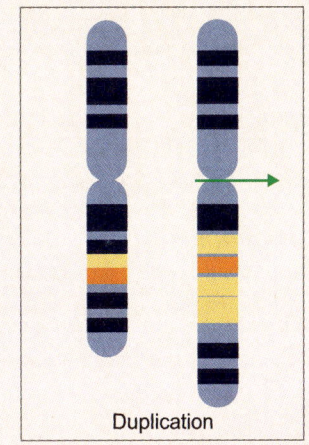

Duplication

Figure 3.4

TRANSLOCATIONS: A portion of one chromosome is transferred to another chromosome. It is mainly of two types.

o **Reciprocal translocation:** Exchange of segments from two different chromosomes (Figure 3.5a).

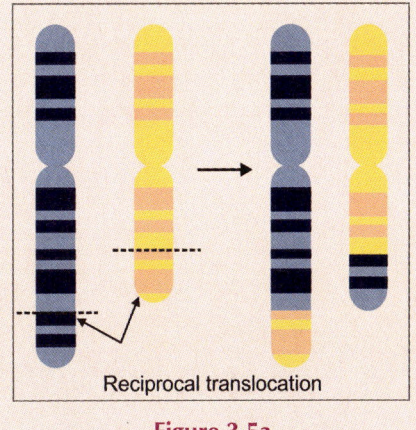

Reciprocal translocation

Figure 3.5a

○ **Robertsonian translocation:** It happens due to breakage of chromosome at or near the centromere of acrocentric chromosome and transfer of part of one acrocentric chromosome to another acrocentric chromosome (Figure 3.5b).

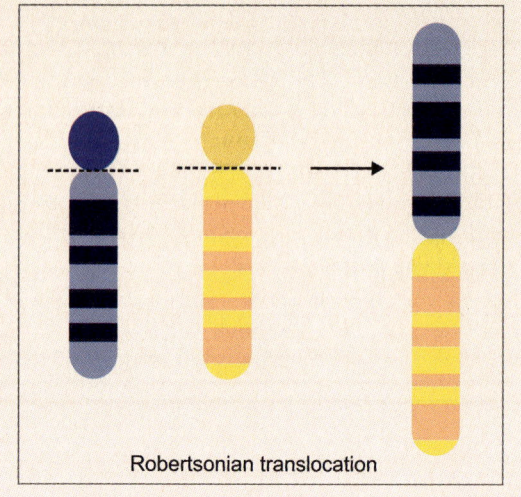

Robertsonian translocation

Figure 3.5b

SEGREGATION PATTERN OF TRANSLOCATIONS
Individuals carrying balanced translocations have a greater risk of producing gametes with unbalanced combinations of chromosomes. This depends on the segregation pattern during meiosis I. During meiosis I, homologous chromosomes synapse with each other. For the translocated chromosome to synapse properly, a translocation cross/quadrivalent must form. The segregation depends upon the length of segments involved in translocation. The three different types of segregation and outcome of each are:

  i. **Alternate Segregation (Figure 3.6a)**

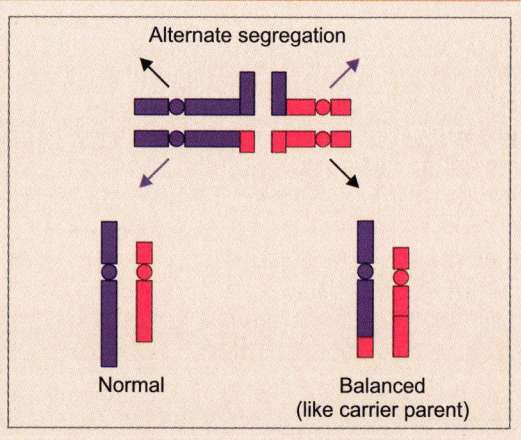

Alternate segregation

Normal   Balanced
                (like carrier parent)

Figure 3.6a

 ii. **Adjacent 2 Segregation (Figure 3.6b)**

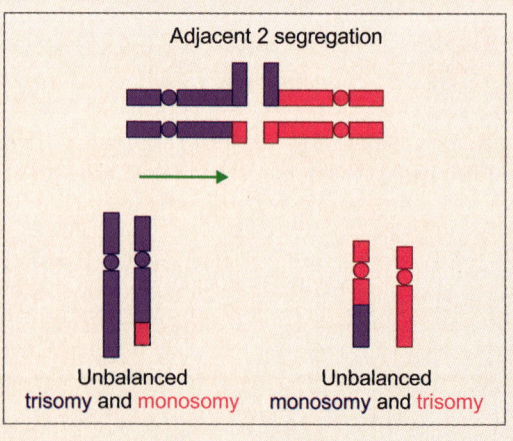

Adjacent 2 segregation

Unbalanced   Unbalanced
trisomy and monosomy   monosomy and trisomy

Figure 3.6b

iii. **Adjacent 1 Segregation (Fig. 3.6c)**

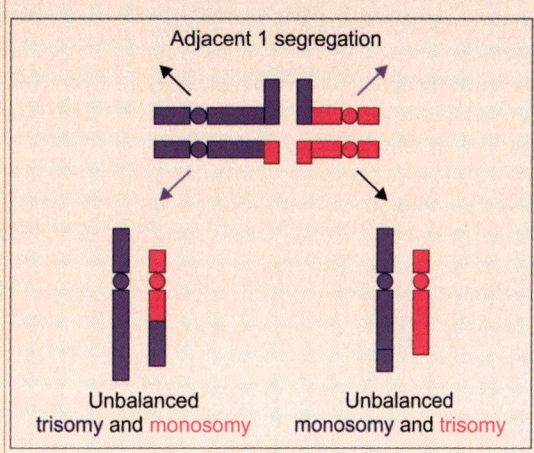

Figure 3.6c

INVERSIONS: A portion of the chromosome breaks off, reverses end to end and reattaches. Balanced carriers of inversion can lead to formation of gametes with unbalanced rearrangement during segregation in the meiosis and lead to severe consequences.

Inversions can be of two types:

○ **Pericentric** includes the centromere. Risk of birth defects increases with the size of inversion in offspring (Figure 3.7a).

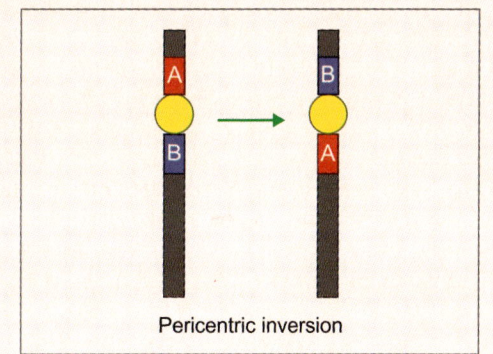

Pericentric inversion

Figure 3.7a

○ **Paracentric** excludes the centromere. It has very low risk of abnormal phenotype (Figure 3.7b).

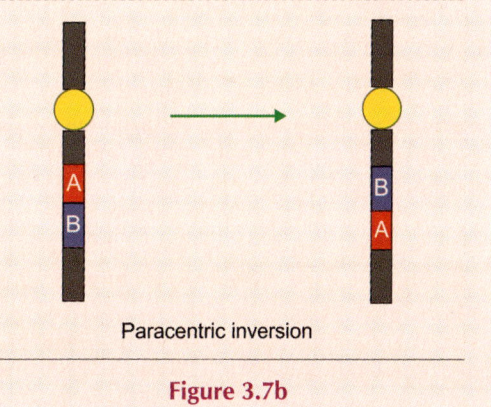

Paracentric inversion

Figure 3.7b

RING CHROMOSOMES: A portion of a chromosome breaks off and fuses together to form a circle or ring with or without loss of genetic material. It becomes unstable in mitosis, leads to mosaicism and monosomy in some cells (Figure 3.8a).

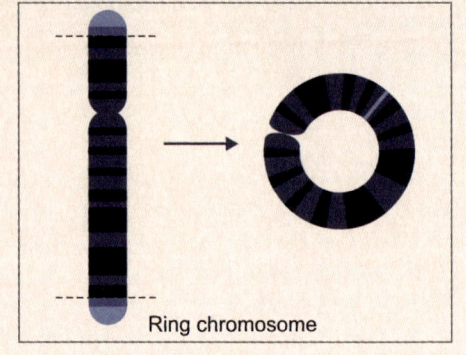

Ring chromosome

Figure 3.8a

ISOCHROMOSOMES: It is mirror image of one of the arms of the chromosome due to deletion of one arm leads to unbalanced abnormality.
Example: i(Xq) in some individuals with Turner syndrome (Figure 3.8b).

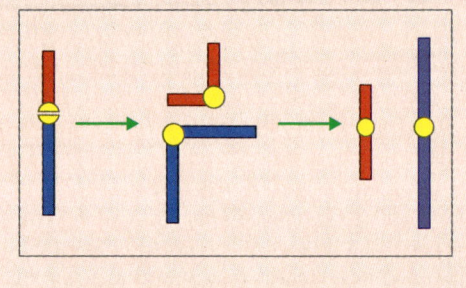

Figure 3.8b: Isochromosome

Q 6. Difference between balanced and unbalanced structural abnormality.

Ans. Structural abnormalities can be balanced or unbalanced (Table 3.1).

Q 7. Explain chimeras (mixoploidy) with example.

Ans. **Chimeras** are composed of two or more different population of genetically distinct cells from different zygotes (Figure 3.9). Human chimeras are of two types:

1. **Blood chimeras:** During bone marrow transplant, a person will have their own bone marrow destroyed and replaced with bone marrow from another person.

2. **Dispermic chimeras:** These are very rare and result from fusion of two zygotes into one individual.

Q 8. Write about different types of mosaicism and their clinical significance. What is the inheritance pattern of mosaicism?

Ans. **Mosaicism:** Mosaicism refers to the presence of two or more populations of cells of different genotypes developed from a

TABLE 3.1: Difference between balanced and unbalanced structural abnormality	
Balanced structural abnormalities	*Unbalanced structural abnormalities*
No overall gain or loss in the chromosomal dosage though rearranged.	Information is additional or missing.
The major consequence is the production of gametes with incomplete or partially duplicated sets of chromosomes.	It can affect many genes and, consequently, have severe effects on the individual. *Example:* Cri du chat, WAGR syndrome, etc.
It includes inversions and translocations.	It includes deletions, duplications or insertions of a chromosomal segment.

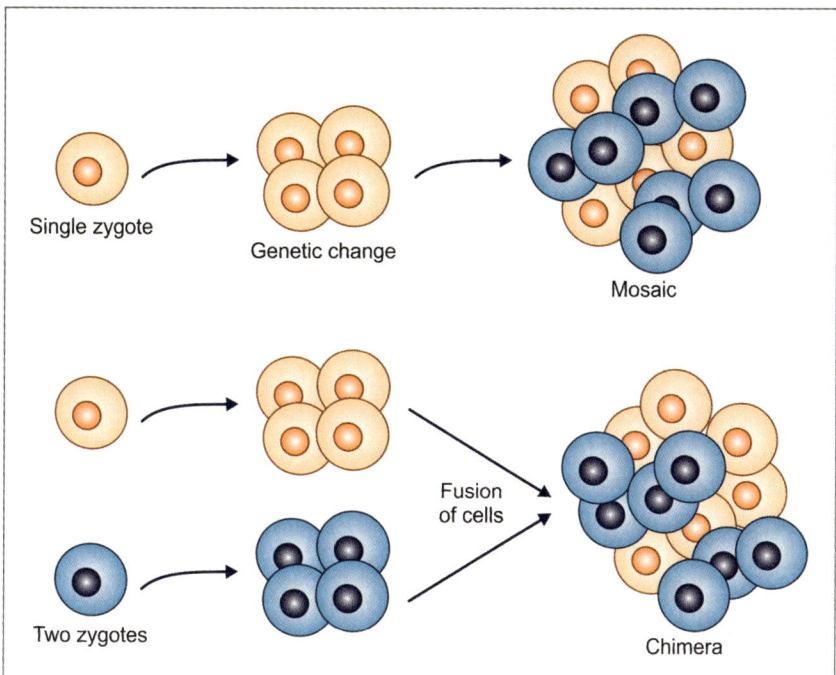

Figure 3.9: Pictorial presentation of mosaic and chimera

single zygote due to a mutation during early development. This can occur in any type of cell (Figure 3.10).

Types of mosaicism

Germline and somatic

A. **Germline mosaicism:** Mosaicism presents in germline cells where some gametes carry a mutation, but others are normal due to a sporadic mutation.

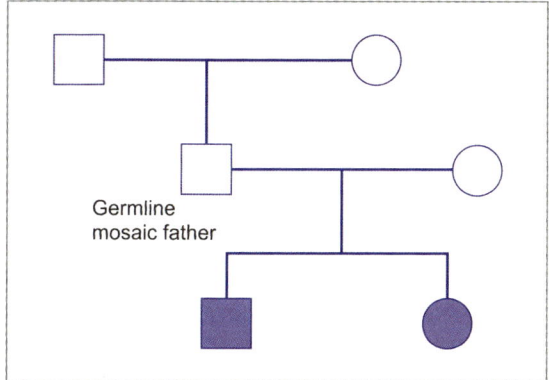

Figure 3.10: Pedigree of germline mosaicism for an autosomal dominant condition

Clinical significance: A germline mosaic mutation is commonly seen in autosomal dominant osteogenesis imperfecta and X-linked disorders like Duchenne muscular dystrophy. It is significant because it can pass to the offspring.

➲ Mostly people are not aware of germline mutations until they have affected children because the germline mosaicism will be present in all the cells of the child.

➲ Below in the pedigree (Figure 3.10), the father is unaffected with no mutation in his blood cells. It is very rare to have sporadic mutations in two children. The most likely cause of the children being affected is germline mosaicism in the father.

B. **Somatic mosaicism:** It refers to occurrence of two genetically different population of cells in the somatic cells of the body.

➲ It may or may not affect the individual or may affect only a portion of the body (segmental mosaicism).

➲ The expression of phenotypes depends on number and type of cells affected.

- These do not pass onto progeny.

Examples:

- Most of the cancers can arise from somatic mutations in genes.
- Down syndrome and neurofibromatosis (NF).

Mosaicism during Prenatal diagnosis:

- **True mosaicism:** Mosaicism present in the fetal tissue.

- **Pseudomosaicism:** It generally arises due to artefact in cells during cytogenic analysis of prenatal sample and is not present in the fetal sample.
- **Placental mosaicism:** When the placental tissue shows mosaicism for any abnormality (trisomy) in karyotype which is not apparent in fetus. It creates a discrepancy in chromosomal make-up of the placental cell and fetal cells.

BIBLIOGRAPHY

1. Emery & Rimoin's Principles & Practice of Medical Genetics, 7th edition.
2. https://en.wikibooks.org/wiki/Structural_ Biochemistry/Nucleic_Acid/DNA/DNA_ structure# Major_and_Mi nor_Grooves.
3. Thompson & Thompson, Genetics in Medicine, 8th edition.

Pattern of Inheritance: Mendelian Inheritance

Meenakshi Lallar, Komal Uppal, Surya Balakrishnan

AUTOSOMAL DOMINANT INHERITANCE
MEENAKSHI LALLAR

Q 1. Definitions

Ans. A. Dominant and recessive

Dominant and recessive are the terms used to describe a trait based on the presence of dominant allele (A) or recessive allele (a) of the gene on both autosomes and sex chromosomes (X-linked dominant and X-linked recessive, Y has very few genes).

a. **Dominant:** There are two copies of each gene, one inherited from each parent. Dominant trait is the one in which one copy of gene can express itself over the other (AA or Aa) and manifests most of the time in heterozygous state (one normal copy and one mutated copy) or rarely in homozygous state (both copies are mutated).
   Pure dominant are those phenotypes which manifest with similar features both in homozygous and heterozygous state.
   Incomplete dominant are those phenotypes which are less severe in heterozygous state and more severe in homozygous state.

b. **Recessive:** A recessive trait is expressed only when both copies of a gene are mutated and present in recessive form (aa). It is expressed in homozygous state.

c. **Semi-dominance** where a dominant allele under certain conditions behaves partially like recessive allele leading to variability in severity of phenotypes.

Example: Several X-linked diseases like OTC deficiency and Fabry disease, are classically classified as X-linked recessive but a significant number of carrier females exhibit the phenotype.

B. Zygosity

Zygosity of a particular gene tells us whether the two copies of the gene at a given locus are same or different.

Example: In thalassemia, the *HBB* gene has two alleles: The wild type (w) and the mutant (m).

a. **Homozygous:** Homozygosity means that at a particular locus the two copies of the gene (alleles) are same.
   Example: Homozygous for mutant allele-thalassemia patient—m/m, homozygous for wild allele—normal—w/w

b. **Heterozygous:** Heterozygous means that at a particular locus the two copies of the gene (alleles) are different.
   Example: Thalassemia carrier—m/w
   This person has both wild and mutant allele of *HBB* gene.
   Carrier: The individuals who are heterozygotes for alleles/genes that cause autosomal recessive diseases are known as carriers.

c. **Hemizygous:** Hemizygous means that at a particular locus there is only one copy of a gene. As males have a single X chromosome, all genes on X chromosome in males are referred to as hemizygous.

Example: For G6PD gene mutations, as males have one X chromosome, they will always be hemizygous (as only one X = one allele, XY), while the females can be heterozygous or homozygous (XX, two X chromosomes).

d. **Compound heterozygous:** Different types of mutations in a single gene causing the same disease is called compound heterozygous. It shows diversity in mutant alleles. In thalassemia, there are more than 200 mutations reported in HBB gene. If one mutant allele is m and another common mutated allele is m1.

Then, homozygote thalassemia patient would be having alleles—(m/m) or (m1/m1). But a compound heterozygote thalassemia patient would be—m/m1 allele.

Q 2. Enumerate classical/mendelian forms of genetic inheritance.

Ans. Mendelian inheritance

Mendelian inheritance is the pattern of inheritance that follows the mendelian laws. According to this, each gene has two alleles— dominant and recessive alleles. The alleles are randomly assorted and segregated in the progeny or germ cells. This is only applicable to diseases caused by single/both autosomal and sex-linked genes. The different forms of mendelian inheritance are:

Mode of mendelian inheritance	Common disease examples
Autosomal dominant (AD)	Neurofibromatosis, achondroplasia
Autosomal recessive (AR)	Thalassemia, cystic fibrosis
X-linked dominant	Incontinentia pigmenti
X-linked recessive	Duchenne muscular dystrophy, hemophilia

Q 3. Enumerate non-classical/non-mendelian forms of genetic inheritance.

Ans. Non-mendelian inheritance:

Non-mendelian forms of inheritance are the patterns of inheritance that do not follow the classic mendelian laws. These include:

- **Mitochondrial inheritance:** The transmission of genetic disease through inheritance of mitochondrial genes is called mitochondrial inheritance. It shows a unique feature of inheritance, i.e. maternal inheritance.

- **Uniparental disomy (UPD):** If we inherit both the chromosomes of a homologous pair from one parent and none from other it is called uniparental disomy.
  Example: Uniparental disomy for chromosome 15 causes Prader-Willi or Angelman syndrome depending upon uniparental disomy of maternal and paternal genes, respectively.

- **Genomic imprinting:** The parent of origin effect in differential gene expression is called genomic imprinting. *Example:* Angelman syndrome, Prader-Willi syndrome, Beckwith-Wiedemann syndrome and Silver-Russell syndrome.

- **Mosaicism:** Mosaicism refers to more than one genetic cell lines in an organism arising due to aberrant post-zygotic mitotic cell divisions. The commonest type of mosaicism is chromosomal mosaicism.
  Example: Turner females with karyotype— 45X[20]/46, XX[30]

- **Triplet repeat disorders:** The disorders caused by increase in number of triplet repeats in the gene are called triplet repeat disorders (dynamic mutations).
  Example: Fragile X syndrome and Huntington chorea.

- **Digenic/oligogenic inheritance:** Digenic or oligogenic inheritance are mechanisms that involve inheritance of a trait because of involvement of two or more genes to manifest the disease. Mutation in one gene does not cause the disease.
  Example: Retinitis pigmentosa.

Q 4. Describe the various symbols used in pedigree chart.

Ans. Figure 4.1.

Q 5. What is autosomal dominant inheritance? Write the unique features and draw the pedigree of autosomal dominant inheritance.

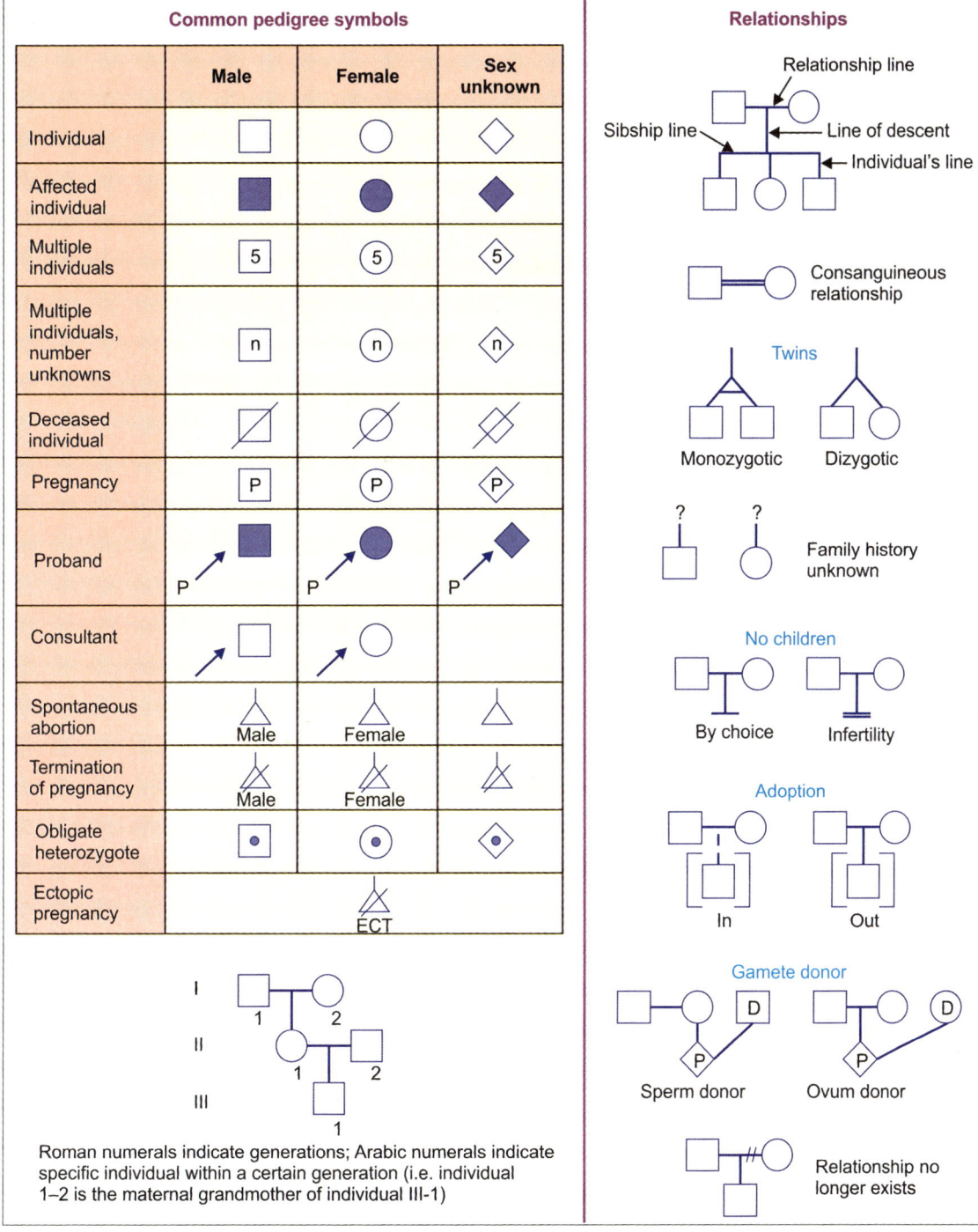

Figure 4.1: Diagram depicting the common symbols used in a pedigree chart.
[Symbols *adapted from* Bennett RL, French KS, Resta RG, Doyle DL. Standardized human pedigree nomenclature: update and assessment of the recommendations of the National Society of Genetic Counselors. J Genet Couns. 2008; 424–33]

Ans. Autosomal dominant (AD) inheritance refers to mode of inheritance which occurs due to mutations in the genes on autosomes and the mutated copy of gene dominates over the normal copy.

Here, the individual manifests in heterozygous state.

UNIQUE FEATURES OF AD MODE OF INHERITANCE (Figure 4.2)
1. Males and females are equally affected and both are at 50% risk to get the mutation.
2. Vertical transmission by both males and females is possible.
3. Every affected person (usually) has an affected parent (sometimes present with subtle manifestations).
4. Unaffected parents (usually) do not have affected children except in case of *de novo* and gonadal mosaicism.
5. Male to male transmission is possible.
6. *De novo* mutations can cause various sporadic disorders.

Q 6. What is the mechanism of dominance?
Ans. Mechanism of AD inheritance
The two alleles for each loci should additively contribute to the phenotype. Mostly, this is true and hence, for AR diseases, disease effects are seen only when both alleles are mutated, i.e. there is loss of function.

However, three main theories to explain disease mechanism in AD diseases are summarized below:

1. **Haplo insufficiency:** When one allele is null (due to termination/frameshift mutations), then the other allele produces only half of required product/protein. If this is not enough for function, it leads to disease. *Example:* For most microdeletion syndromes like 22q11.2, dosage haplo insufficiency of deleted genes leads to disease phenotype.

2. **Dominant negative:** In this disease mechanism, a mutant allele product adversely affects the normal, wild-type gene product. Example is osteogenesis imperfecta (OI). Here, collagen type I contains a triple helical segment in which glycine is in every third position. If glycine is replaced the helix disrupts and leads to disturbed helical folding resulting in overprocessing by the enzymes responsible for post-translational modification of (pro) collagen type I.

3. **Gain of function:** Increased or abnormally constitutive protein activity leading to overexpression of an allele depicts dominance due to gain-of-function mutation. *Example:* Achondroplasia. The mutation-induced FGFR3 activation suppresses proliferation and alters the

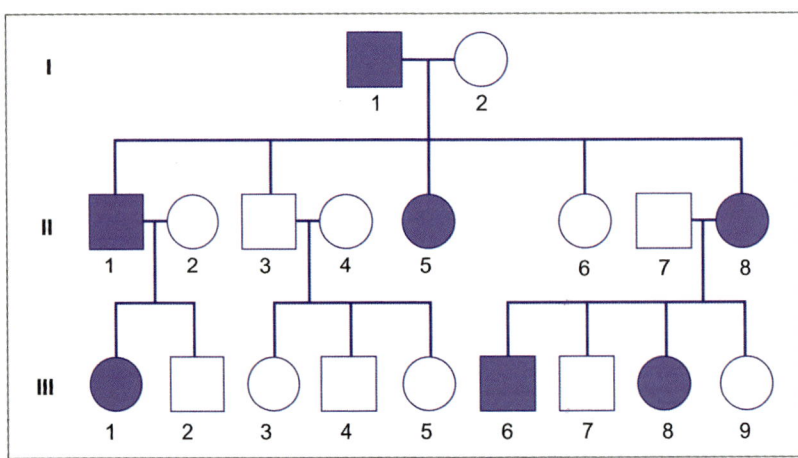

Figure 4.2: Autosomal dominant pedigree showing its unique features and 50% recurrence risk in progeny

hypertrophic differentiation of growth plate chondrocytes, leading to achondroplasia.

Q 7. Give examples of autosomal dominance inheritance disorders.

Ans. The common examples of AD mode of inheritance are:

Neuro-logical	Huntington disease, neurofibromatosis, tuberous sclerosis
Cardiac	*MYH7* related hypertrophic cardiomyopathy, long QTc syndrome.
Gastro-enterology	Familial adenomatous polyposis (FAP), hemochromatosis
Genito-urinary	ADPKD, Wilms tumor
Skeletal	Achondroplasia, osteogenesis imperfecta
Connective tissue	Marfan syndrome, Ehlers-Danlos syndrome
Metabolic	Porphyria, familial hyper-cholesterolemia
Hemato-poietic	Hereditary spherocytosis, von Willebrand's disease
Endocrinal	Maturity onset diabetes of the young (MODY)
Malignancies	Hereditary breast and ovarian carcinoma, (HBOC-BRCA1, BRCA2 related), multiple endocrinal neoplasia (MEN1, 2)

Q 8. What is recurrence risk in autosomal dominant inheritance?

Ans:
- There is 50% risk to both sons and daughters of an autosomal dominant affected person as the affected parent has 50% chance of passing the disease—causing allele to the offspring in each pregnancy as shown in pedigree (Figure 4.2).
- But certain modifications/deviations of AD mode of inheritance should be always kept in mind during risk assessment like anticipation, triplet repeat disorders, penetrance, incomplete penetrance and variable expressivity.

Q 9. Definitions

Ans.

1. **Anticipation** is a phenomenon where the onset of disease occurs at an earlier age in the offspring than that in the parents or the disease occurs with increasing severity in subsequent generations. It is seen in autosomal dominant repeat expansion diseases as the repeats expand when they are passed down.

   Examples:
   a. *Congenital myotonic* dystrophy occurs due to triplet repeat CTG expansion in maternal meiosis and leads to severe neonatal form of myotonic dystrophy when the allele is transmitted from the asymptomatic mother.
   b. *Huntington disease* also shows anticipation due to expansion of the CAG trinucleotide repeat into the range associated with Huntington disease (36 repeats or more).

2. **Penetrance:** Penetrance means whether an individual with a mutation (i.e. heterozygote for mutant allele) will manifest signs and symptoms of the disease or not.

$$\text{Penetrance} = \frac{\text{Total number of individuals having signs and symptoms}}{\text{Total number of individuals having mutation}}$$

3. **Reduced/incomplete penetrance:** Reduced/incomplete penetrance means that few individuals in spite of carrying the mutant allele will not show the disease phenotype; but such individuals can pass on the disease allele to the next generation and have affected children. This is also termed skipped generation. The disease skips the generation due to reduced penetrance but appears in offspring as shown in Figure 4.3.

   III-1 and III-3 being affected due to incomplete penetrance, i.e. individual II-1 has the mutation but does not show the phenotype.

4. **Clinical variability or variable expressivity:** This is another important feature of diseases with AD mode of inheritance

where different individuals with same mutation, even of same family, have different signs/phenotype of the disease. It can be interfamilial or intrafamilial.

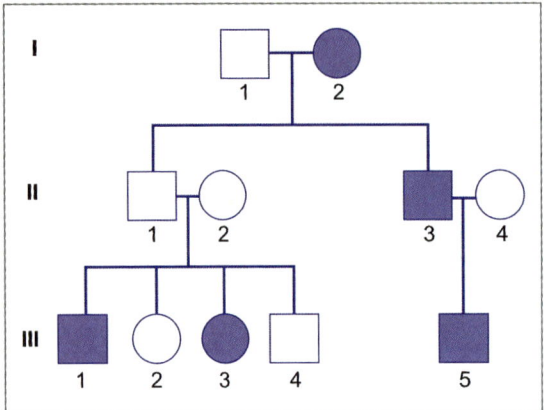

Figure 4.3: Pedigree shows LMNA gene associated with Emery-Dreifuss muscular dystrophy segregating in a family

Example: In tuberous sclerosis, among individuals from same family, some may have severe phenotype of intellectual disability, seizures while others might just have few hypomelanotic patches or adenoma sebaceum with completely normal intelligence and no seizures. This represents intrafamilial variable expressivity of mutated *TSC1* and *TSC2* genes (Figure 4.4).

5. **Pleiotropy:** Pleiotropy refers to different and unrelated systemic effects or multiorgan changes that occur due to mutation in a single gene.

Example: In tuberous sclerosis, the mutation in *TSC2* and *TSC1* gene cause effects ranging from skin changes to structural brain abnormalities and to structural renal abnormalities, etc. (Figure 4.4)

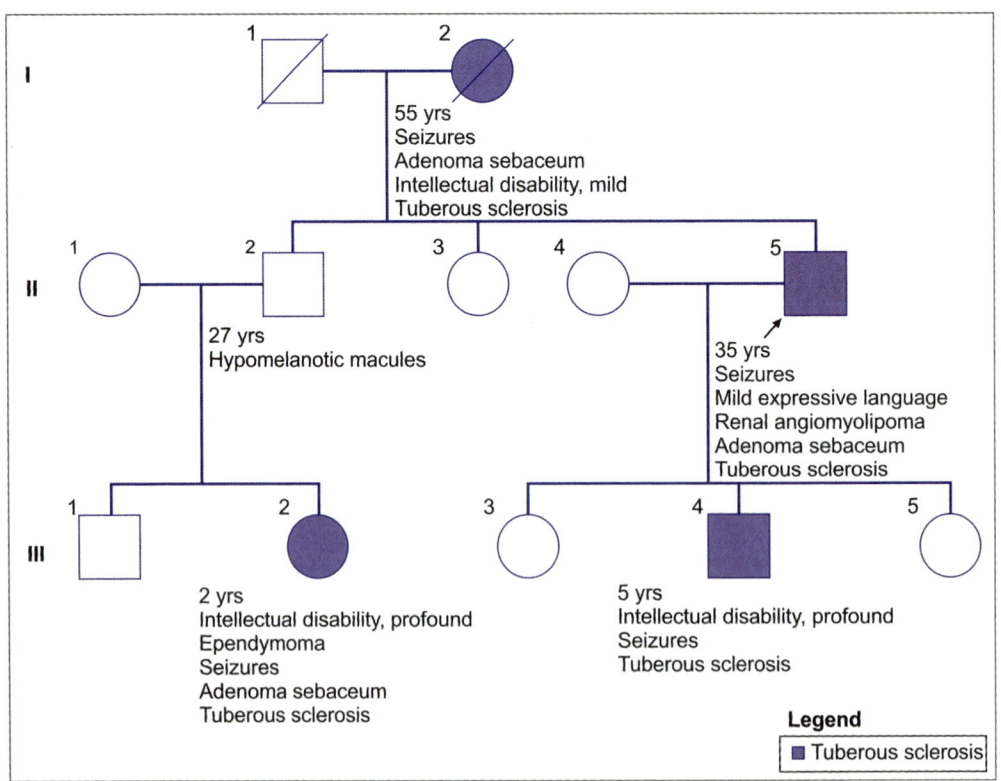

Figure 4.4: Three generations pedigree showing a family affected with tuberous sclerosis showing variable expressivity. II-5 has mild language delay while the offspring, III-4 has profound intellectual disability

Q 10. What do you mean by *de novo* mutations?

Ans. *De novo* mutation is a mutation that arises for the first time and is not inherited from either of the parents. The mutation may arise either during gametogenesis in ova or sperm or occurs postzygotically in very early stages. The exact timing of a *de novo* mutation cannot be deciphered. Generally many of the autosomal diseases begin as *de novo* and then segregate in the families.

Example: Achondroplasia, Marfan syndrome, neurofibromatosis and nonsyndromic autism like intellectual disability phenotypes arise due to *de novo* mutations in genes associated with brain signalling pathways, etc.

Example: In Figure 4.5, II-2, seeing the pedigree, the mode of inheritance can be *de novo* or autosomal recessive. The expressed phenotype gives clue to the mode of inheritance.

Here, only a single child is affected with non-specific phenotype of intellectual disability, autism. So by doing molecular diagnosis to ascertain the mutant gene in the proband and parents, we can establish the genetic etiology and mode of inheritance (*de novo*, inherited AD, AR).

Q 11. What do you mean by reproductive fitness?

Ans. Reproductive fitness means the ability of mutant individual to pass the disease genes to subsequent generations. If reproductive fitness of a genetic disease is high, then that disease will be able to run in families like Marfan disease. However, if reproductive fitness of a disease is low or zero, meaning the disease is very severe and affected individuals are unable to reproduce, then all new cases in the population will be accounted for by *de novo* mutations and the disease will not be able to run in families.

Example: Lobar holoprosencephaly, Type II achondrogenesis.

Q 12. Explain co-dominance with the help of an example.

Ans. **Co-dominance:** This means that instead of one allele being dominant over the other and being exclusively expressed, both the alleles are co-expressed.

The classic example is AB blood group antigens on RBC surface leading to AB blood group.

AUTOSOMAL RECESSIVE INHERITANCE
Komal Uppal

Q 13. What is autosomal recessive inheritance? Draw the pedigree of autosomal recessive inheritance.

Ans. Autosomal recessive means when both the alleles of a gene on autosome chromosomes are mutant and are recessive to normal allele.

Autosomal recessive inheritance is the transmission of two recessive mutant alleles; one from each of the asymptomatic

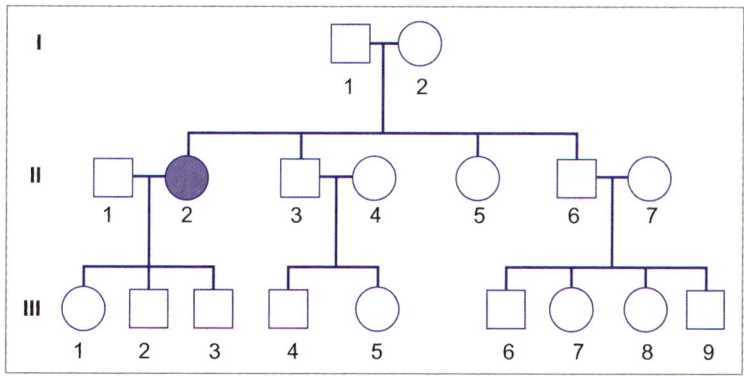

Figure 4.5: *De novo* mutation in II-2 individual having intellectual disability and autism

heterozygous parent (carriers of the mutant allele) to their offspring and manifestation of disease in the offspring who is in homozygous state for that mutant allele (Figure 4.6).

In homozygous state of autosomal recessive inheritance, due to mutant alleles in the gene, there is decreased or complete loss of function of the gene end product, so the disease manifestations occurs but in carrier state, the normal gene copy compensates for decreased function of the mutant allele so it does not become pathogenic.

Q 14. Write the unique features and give some examples of autosomal recessive disorders.

Ans. Unique features of autosomal recessive inheritance

1. There is equal chance for both male and female to be affected.
2. There is horizontal transmission of the disease, i.e. the disease is generally seen in siblings of the proband.
3. In each sibling of the proband, the risk for recurrence is 25%.
4. Parents of the proband will be asymptomatic carriers.
5. In some conditions, there can be history of consanguinity, but it is not must.

Examples of autosomal recessive disorders

1. **Hematological disorders:** Thalassemia, sickle cell disease
2. **Metabolic disorders:** Galactosemia, phenylketonuria, homocystinuria, glycogen and lysosomal storage diseases, alkapto-nuria, hemochromatosis, Wilson disease.
3. **Neurological disorders:** Spinal muscular atrophy and Friedreich's ataxia, neurogenic muscular atrophies
4. **Endocrine abnormalities:** Congenital adrenal hyperplasia
5. **Respiratory disorders:** Cystic fibrosis

Q 15. What is the recurrence risk of autosomal recessive disorder in the next child of a couple whose first child is affected with the disorder?

Ans. The recurrence risk of autosomal recessive disorder in the next child of a couple whose first child is affected with the condition depends upon the genotype of both the parents.

The following diagrams show the different genotypic status of parents and the recurrence risk in their next child.

1. When both the parents are carriers for mutant allele (Figure 4.7)

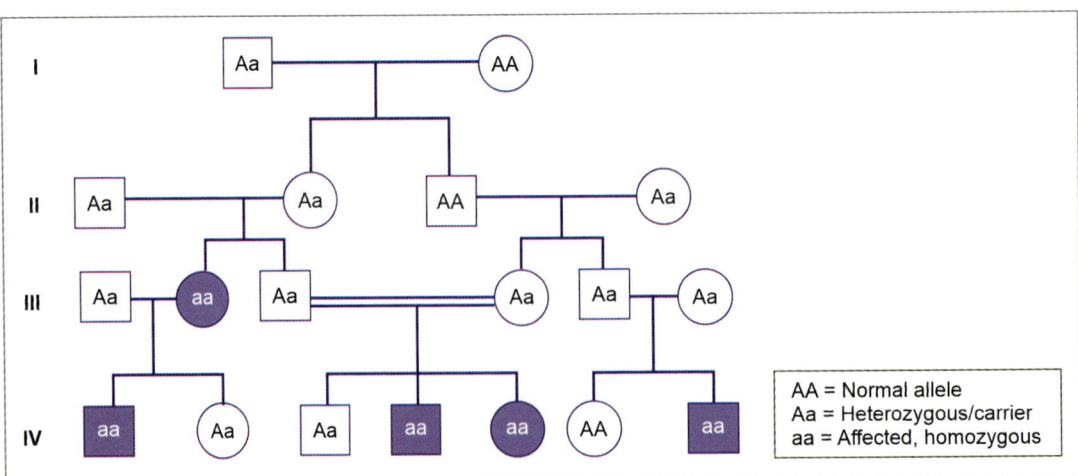

AA = Normal allele
Aa = Heterozygous/carrier
aa = Affected, homozygous

Figure 4.6: Pedigree of autosomal recessive inheritance

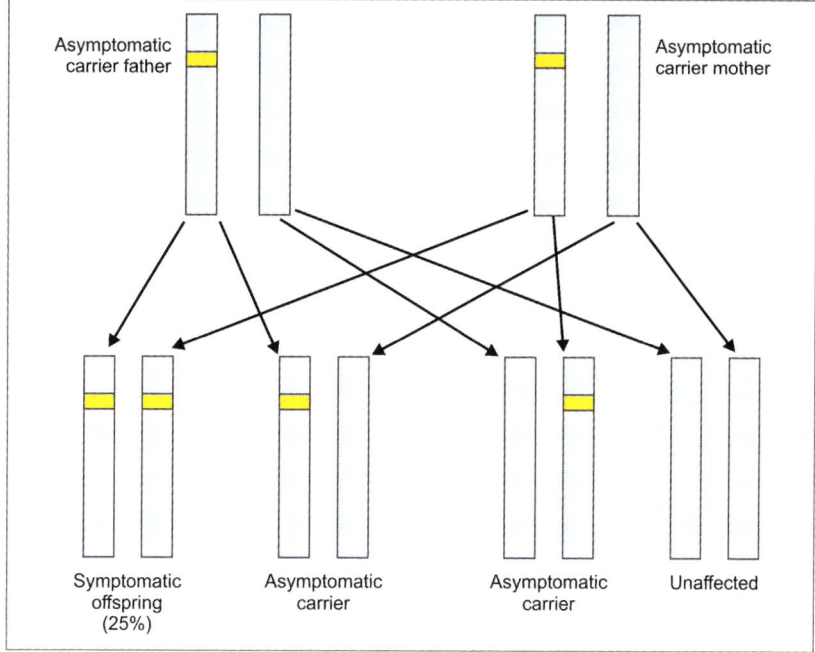

Figure 4.7: Recurrence risk in the next child when both parents are carriers

The recurrence risk in the next child in the above condition is 1 in 4, i.e. 25% with each pregnancy because each child gets 50% of mutant allele from each of the parent.

2. When one parent is affected with the autosomal recessive disorder and the other parent is carrier for the same mutant allele (Figure 4.8)

The recurrence risk in the next child in the above condition will be 50% with each pregnancy as it depends on whether the spouse transmits a mutant allele or normal allele.

3. When one parent is affected with the autosomal recessive disorder and the other parent is normal (Figure 4.9)

There is no chance of recurrence risk in the next child in the above condition as the spouse will never contribute the mutant allele.

Q 16. What can be the recurrence risk of autosomal recessive disorder in other family members of a couple whose first child is affected with autosomal recessive disorder?

Ans. The recurrence risk of autosomal recurrence disorder in the other family members of a couple whose first child is affected with an autosomal recessive disorder depends upon the following factors:

➲ The carrier status of the family members of the couple and their spouses (whether the spouse is a close relative or an unrelated person) (Figure 4.10).

➲ **Consanguinity:** The high-risk of recurrence in case of consanguineous marriages depends upon the degree of relationship among the partners.

➲ The carrier frequency for the same autosomal recessive disorder in the population (to which spouse belongs if the spouse is an unrelated person), which can be calculated by Hardy-Weinberg formula:

$$p^2 + 2pq + q^2 = 1$$

p^2 = homozygous frequency for dominant allele (AA)

q^2 = homozygous frequency for recessive allele (aa)

2pq = Carrier frequency (Aa)

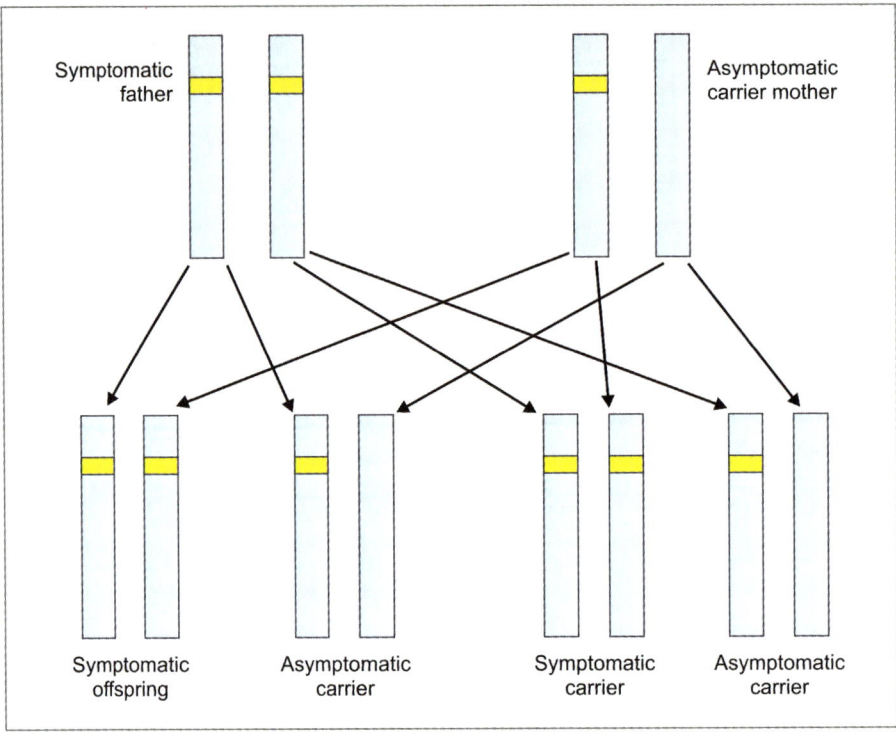

Figure 4.8: Recurrence risk in the next child when one parent is affected and the other parent is carrier

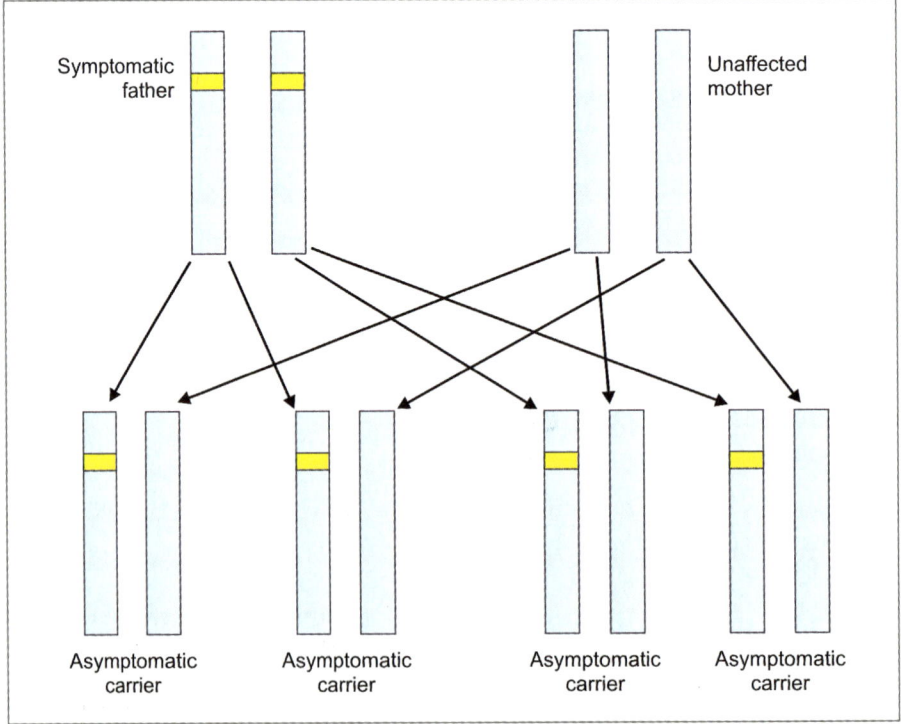

Figure 4.9: Recurrence risk in the next child when one parent is affected and the other one is normal

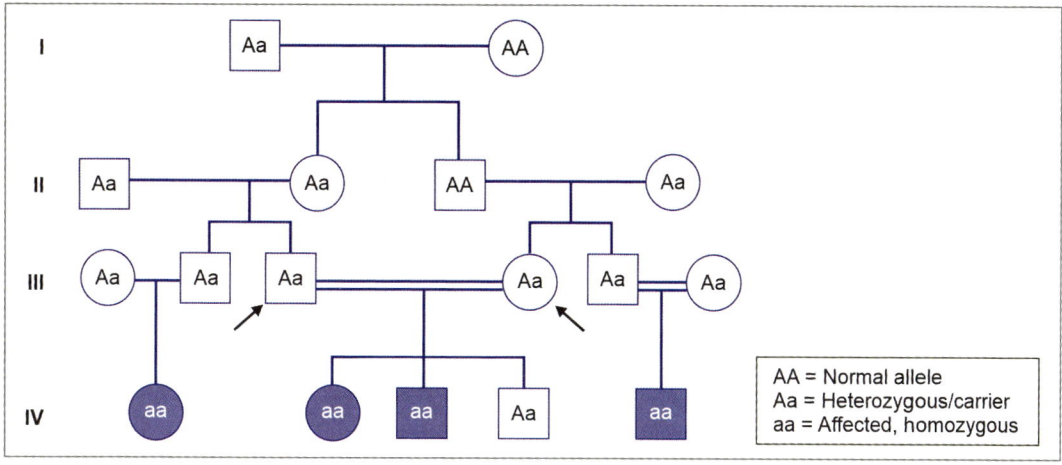

Figure 4.10: Recurrence risk of autosomal recessive disorder in the other family members of the proband

Q 17. What is the importance of detecting carrier status of parents or other relatives of a patient affected with autosomal recessive disorder?

Ans.

Importance of detecting carrier status of parents of an affected child	To know the carrier status of the parents (Figure 4.11: II-3 and II-4) of a patient affected with autosomal recessive disorder is important because the recurrence risk in their next child for the same disorder is 25% if the parents are asymptomatic carriers for the same mutation as of proband.
Importance of detecting carrier status of the relatives of an affected child	The detection of carrier status of other relatives (either paternal or maternal as in Figure 4.11: II-2 and II-5) of the proband is important because their risk of being carrier is 50% for the same mutation as of proband. If they are asymptomatic carriers and their partner to whom they get married is also heterozygous for that mutation (whether their spouse is a close relative or is an unrelated person from the population where the prevalence of that disorder is high, like thalassemia in Mediterranean and south east Asian regions), the risk of having the affected child for them becomes significant.

Q 18. Define pseudodominance inheritance. Give example and draw the pedigree chart.

Ans. Pseudodominance inheritance means when the transmission of a known autosomal recessive disorder appears to be inherited as autosomal dominant disorder. It happens when a homozygous individual for an autosomal recessive disorder gets married to an asymptomatic carrier for the same disorder. In this condition they have 50% chance of having either an affected offspring or an asymptomatic heterozygous child because each of the parent will contribute 50% of mutant allele to their offspring (Figure 4.12).

Example of this inheritance is sickle cell disease and nonsyndromic autosomal recessive hearing loss due to GJB2 gene mutation.

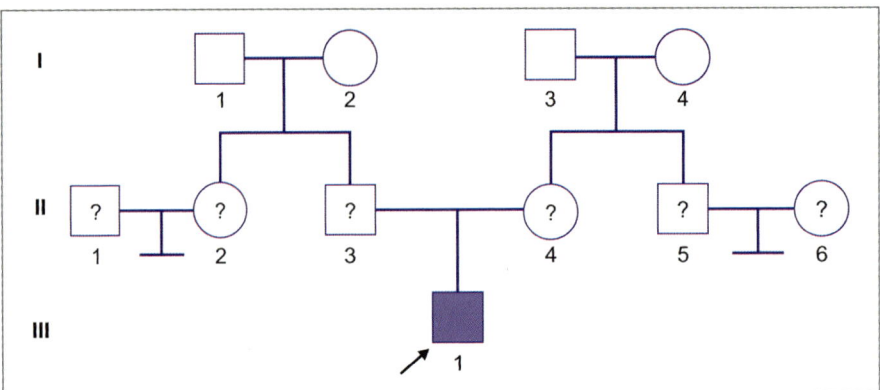

Figure 4.11: Unknown carrier status of parents and other relatives of proband. Hence, to know the carrier status, of parents, other relatives of the proband and their spouses if one partner is an asymptomatic carrier, the carrier detection testing is advised. If both the partners are heterozygous for the same mutation, they should be advised for prenatal testing to assess the risk in their future generations

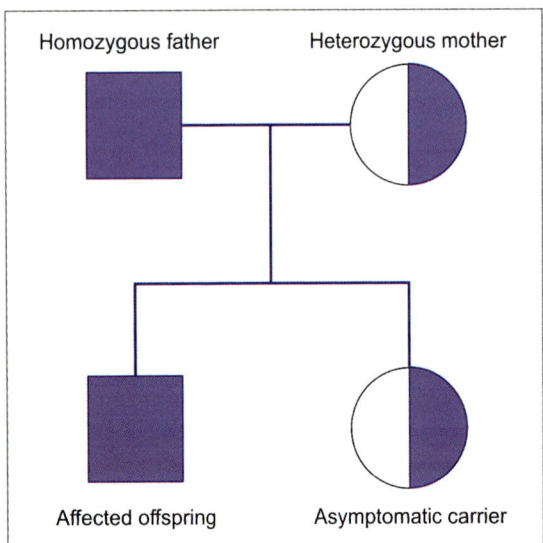

Figure 4.12: Pseudodominance inheritance of nonsyndromic autosomal recessive hearing loss due to GJB2 gene mutation

Q 19. Define pseudoautosomal inheritance. Give example and draw the pedigree chart.

Ans. Pseudoautosomal inheritance means the transmission of a disease which occurs due to presence of mutation at the pseuoautosomal region (PAR)Xp,Xq and Yp,Yq on tips of sex chromosomes X and Y respectively (Figure 4.13). This is similar to how autosomal dominant inheritance pattern happens and shows the unique feature of male to male transmission.

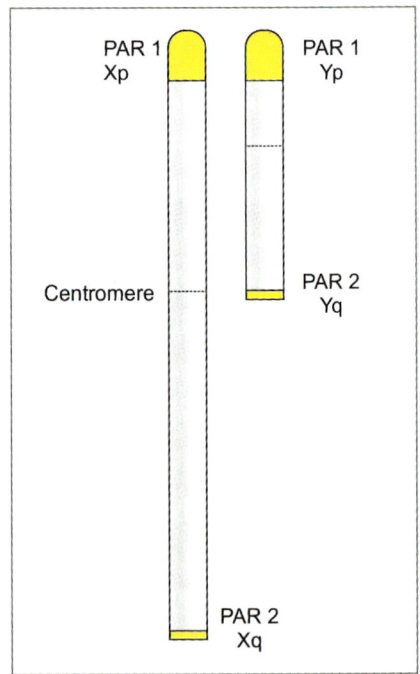

Figure 4.13: The pseudoautosomal regions, PAR1 and PAR2, at the tips of Xp-Yp and Xq-Yq respectively

The pseudoautosomal inheritance happens because of meiotic pairing between homologous genes at the PAR regions. (Normally, meiotic crossover happens between X-linked loci between the two homologous X chromosomes of the females.)

Due to meiotic paring there can be transfer of genes from Xp and Xq to Yp and Yq chromosomes respectively both in affected male and affected female. This transfer of genes from Xp to Yp in affected males makes the possibility of male to male transmission of a mutant gene like an autosomal dominant inheritance.

Example: Leri-Weil Dyschondrosteosis, a rare form of skeletal dysplasia, exhibits both autosomal dominant and X-linked recessive inheritance. Mutation in the SHOX gene which is located in the Xp and Yp pseudoautosomal regions is responsible for this disorder to be inherited as autosomal dominant (Figure 4.14).

Q 20. What do you mean by consanguinity?
Ans. Consanguinity: Marriage between two closely blood related individuals who are having at least one common ancestor. It is seen that the offspring of consanguineous married couples are at more risk for getting genetic disorders like congenital malformations and autosomal recessive disorders such as hearing disorder or learning disability because they share same disease gene from the common ancestor. Though the incidence of consanguineous marriages has been decreased than before but, in some communities in India, first cousin marriages are still relatively common.

Q 21. What is the relationship between consanguinity and autosomal recessive disorders? Explain with the help of example that consanguinity is more likely to be associated with rare autosomal recessive genetic disorders than common genetic disorders.
Ans. Generally, it is inferred that all autosomal recessive disorders are associated with consanguinity, but it is not always true. Consanguinity is more responsible for rare autosomal recessive disorders like xeroderma pigmentosa, alkaptonuria, galactosemia, etc. as compared to common disorders like thalassemia, sickle cell disease and cystic fibrosis.

For instance, a consanguineous couple in a family who is harboring a rare autosomal recessive disease gene like xeroderma pigmentosa, there is more chance of them being carriers for the same disease gene as they inherit it from the common ancestor. They can transmit this disease gene to their offspring. Thus, their offspring can be homozygous for

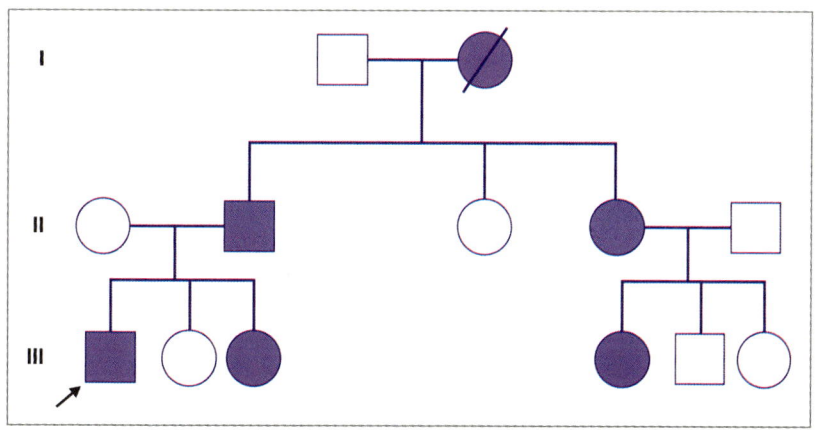

Figure 4.14: Mutation in the SHOX gene in Leri-Weil dyschondrosteosis. The male with the pointing arrow has got mutation on his Y chromosome from his father and his father has got mutation from X chromosome of his mother

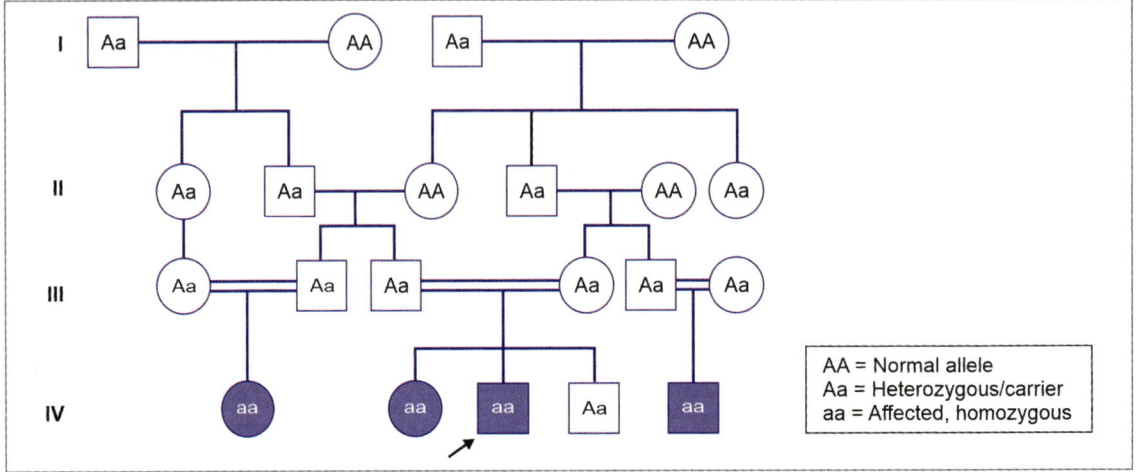

Figure 4.15: Pedigree showing consanguineous relationship responsible for rare autosomal recessive disorders like xeroderma pigmentosum

that disease gene and can manifest the disease (Figure 4.15).

While in the case of common genetic disorders like thalassemia, most of the cases are from non-consanguineous couples because the disease gene for it is so common in the general population that each partner of the non-consanguineous marriage can be a carrier for it by chance. Hence, the principle is made that in majority of the rare autosomal recessive disorders, couple would be consanguineous and for most of the common disorders, consanguinity is not essential.

Q 22. What is the risk of genetic abnormality in the offspring of a consanguineous couple?

Ans. The risk of having affected child in these couples depend upon the degree of blood relation and the proportion of genes shared. In relation to genetic disorders, consanguinity up to the fifth generation is significant. Closer the relationship, more the chance of having genetic disorders in the future generations as shown below. The risk of having affected offspring to a couple who are first cousins is 6–8%, almost double the risk in general population (3–4%).

RISK OF GENETIC DISORDERS IN RELATION TO DEGREE OF CONSANGUINITY

Level of consanguinity	Percentage sharing of genes	Percentage risk of genetic disorder in the next generation
First degree ○ Child-parent ○ Sister-brother	50%	50%
Second degree maternal or paternal ○ aunt-nephew ○ uncle-niece	25%	5–10%
Third degree First cousins	12.5%	6–8%

X-LINKED RECESSIVE, X-LINKED DOMINANT INHERITANCE AND Y-LINKED INHERITANCE

Surya Balakrishnan

Q 23. What is X-linked recessive inheritance and draw the pedigree?

Ans: X-linked recessive inheritance: X-linked recessive inheritance refers to the inheritance pattern followed by recessive genes present on the X chromosome (Figure 4.16).

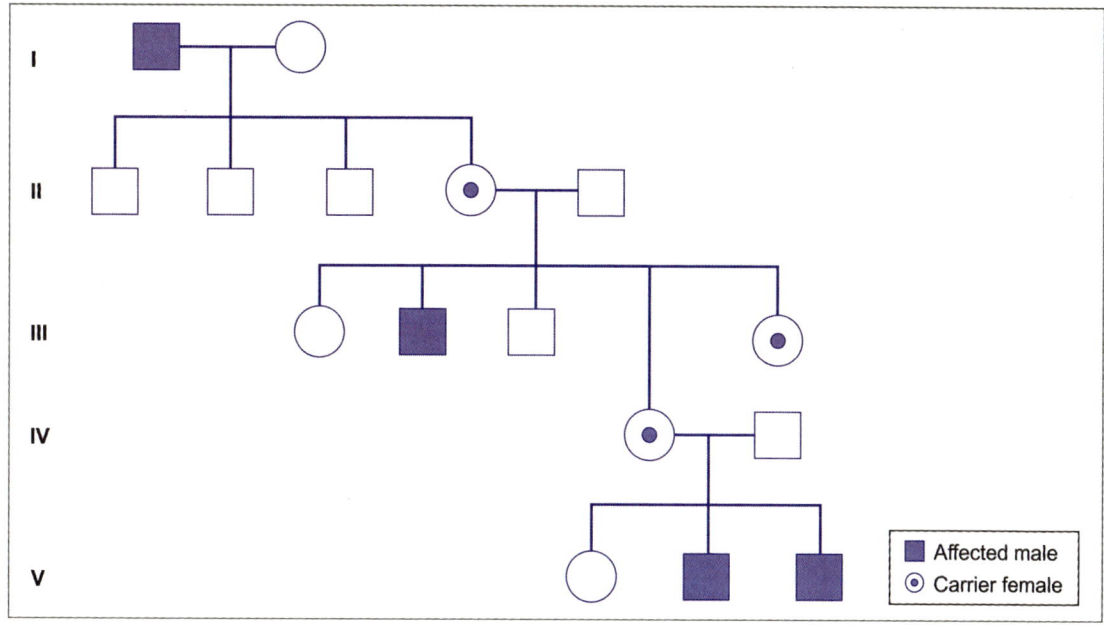

Figure 4.16: Pedigree showing X-linked inheritance where affected male is transmitting the diseased gene to his daughter who further transmits it to his grandson

Males have a single X chromosome, while females have two X chromosomes. The unequal distribution of X chromosomes between the two sexes is rendered functionally equal by a process called lyonization.

Lyonization refers to the random inactivation of extra X chromosome in all cells in females. All females have only one functionally active copy of X chromosome and are usually mosaics, with cells showing inactivation of either paternal X or maternal X in different proportions.

Q 24. Write the unique features and examples of X-linked recessive inheritance.

Ans. Unique features of X-linked recessive inheritance

➲ Shows **diagonal** or **Knight's move** pattern, since disease is transmitted to males via unaffected female carriers.

➲ Males are **hemizygous** for X chromosome associated genes. So, in majority of cases X-linked recessive disorders manifest in males.

➲ Females with a single mutated allele are termed obligate carriers and usually do not manifest any symptoms, except under special circumstances.

➲ For women being asymptomatic, reasons are:

- the function of the defective X chromosome may be compensated by the normal X
- defective X chromosome may be preferentially silenced by lyonization.

➲ Affected males can transmit the mutated allele to all daughters rendering them obligate carriers, while the disease cannot be transmitted to the sons. Note that the reproductive fitness (ability to reproduce and transfer genes to their children) of affected males may be low.

➲ Sons of a carrier female have 50% chance of being affected with disease, while daughters have 50% chance of being carriers.

➲ There is no male to male transmission of disease.

Examples of X-linked recessive disorders

- **Ophthalmological disorders:** Ocular albinism, red green color blindness
- **Muscular disorders:** Duchenne muscular dystrophy, Becker's muscular dystrophy
- **Bleeding disorders:** Hemophilia A and B, Wiskott-Aldrich syndrome.
- **Metabolic disorders:** Fabry's disease, Hunter's disease, Menkes disease, adreno-leucodystrophy
- **Neurological disorders:** Mental retardation, Fragile X syndrome.
- **Hemolytic anemia:** Glucose-6-phosphate dehydrogenase (G6PD) deficiency.

Q 25. What is the recurrence risk of X-linked recessive disorder in the next child and other family members of a couple whose first child is affected with X-linked recessive disorder?

Ans. The recurrence risk of X-linked recessive disorder in the next offspring and other family members of the couple whose first child is affected depends on whether mutation is present in the father, mother or other family members of the affected child or not.

- If father of the affected child or any male family member is affected (Figure 4.17).
- In case, the mother of the affected child or any female family member is a carrier (Figure 4.18).
- If a mother is carrier and father is affected, which is extremely rare (Figure 4.19).

Q 26. How will you do genetic counseling for parents of a child who is affected with X-linked recessive disorder?

Ans. *See* question 8: X-linked recessive disorders in Chapter 8.

Q 27. How will you do prenatal management for subsequent pregnancy for a couple whose first child is affected with X-linked recessive disorder?

Ans. Prenatal Diagnosis: Prenatal testing refers to testing of the fetus during early pregnancy to find out if the baby carries the same genetic defect identified in the family.

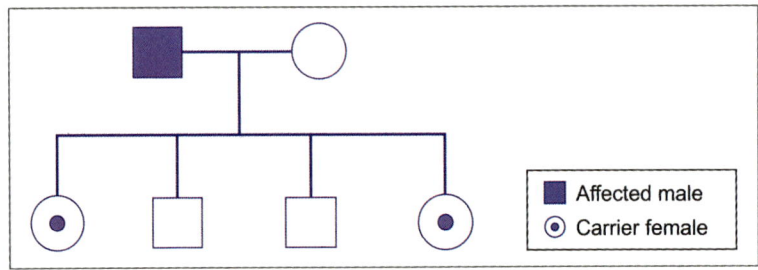

Figure 4.17: Affected father transmitting mutant gene to all the daughters rendering them obligate carriers and no son is affected

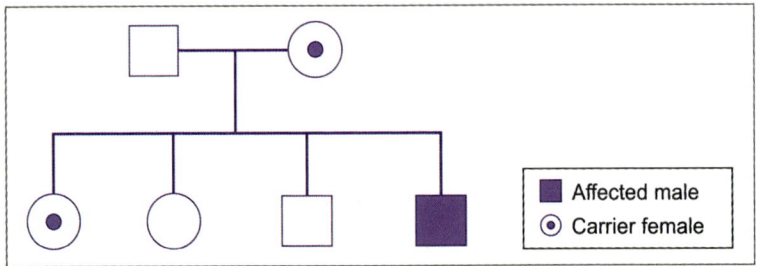

Figure 4.18: Recurrence risk when mother of the affected child is carrier. Sons have 50% chance of being affected with disease, while daughters have 50% chance of being carriers

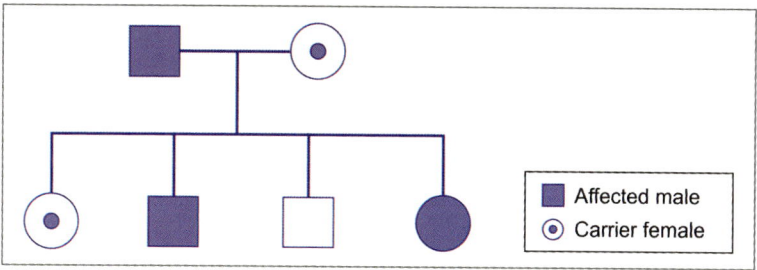

Figure 4.19: Recurrence risk when mother is a carrier and father is affected. Both daughters and sons have 50% chance of being affected

- Once a genetic defect is identified in the family, pregnant women, who are at-risk of passing the disease to their offspring must be identified.
- Prenatal testing may be performed in them till up to 20 weeks of pregnancy between 11–13 weeks and 16–18 weeks via chorionic villus sampling and amniocentesis after informed consent.
- If fetal sample shows the same mutation identified in the family, parents must be informed, counseled regarding the possible outcomes of pregnancy and options available including termination of pregnancy.

Q 28. Explain the conditions in which a carrier female can manifest X-linked recessive disorders.

Ans. A carrier female usually does not manifest disease symptoms except under the following circumstances:

a. **Skewed inactivation:** Normally X chromosome inactivation is random, but it can become selective in some cases where one of the X is mutated, so that the normal X can function. If this selective inactivation is impaired, the normal X may be silenced and the mutated X remains active. The proportion of cells with functional mutant X, decides the severity of symptoms. Nevertheless, the disease is mostly less severe than that seen in affected males (Figure 4.20).

b. **Turner syndrome or Xp or Xq deletion:** Women with Turner syndrome and females with Xp or Xq deletion also have partial copy of second X chromosome and may lead to manifestation of disease.

c. **Translocation of an X chromosome with an autosome:** In a translocation, the mutated X chromosome bearing portions of the autosome is preferentially maintained in the active state, since autosomal genes are usually critical for human viability (Figure 4.21). The translocation itself can delete or disrupt important genes and may cause additional clinical features.

d. **Phenotypic female:** Under virilization in males in genetic defects involving androgen biosynthesis and androgen action with normal 46,XY complement causes a female phenotype where apparent females manifest disease symptoms, as severe as that of affected males.

e. **Monozygotic twins:** Monozygotic female twins, both carriers for X-linked disease, where one twin manifests the disease and the other remains asymptomatic due to differences in the X inactivation.

Q 29. What is X-linked dominant inheritance?

Ans. X-linked dominant inheritance refers to the inheritance pattern followed by dominant genes on the X chromosome. Mutation in a single copy is sufficient to cause disease and the presence of a normal X chromosome cannot rescue the phenotype (Figure 4.22). However, severity of the phenotype is diminished in females due to the protective effect conferred by lyonization.

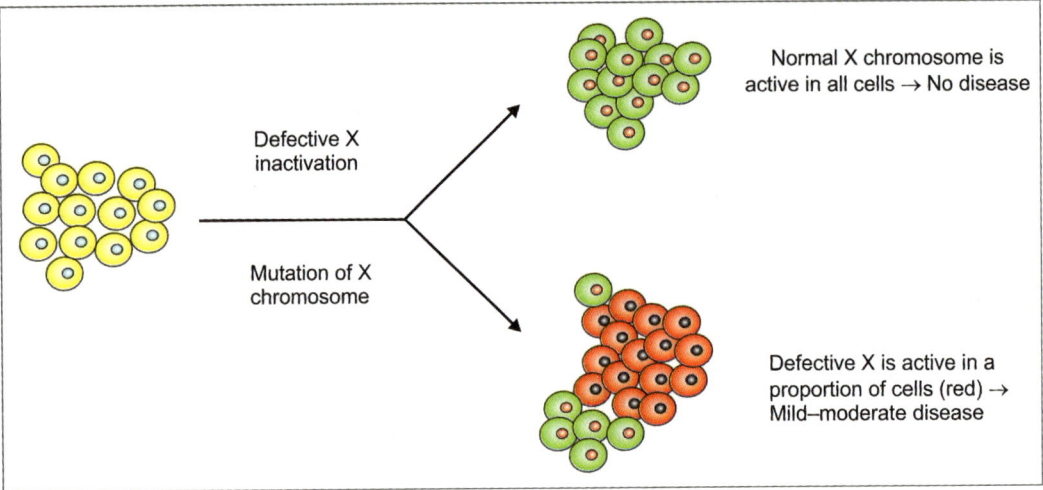

Figure 4.20: Skewed inactivation responsible for manifestation of disease in females with X-linked recessive disorders

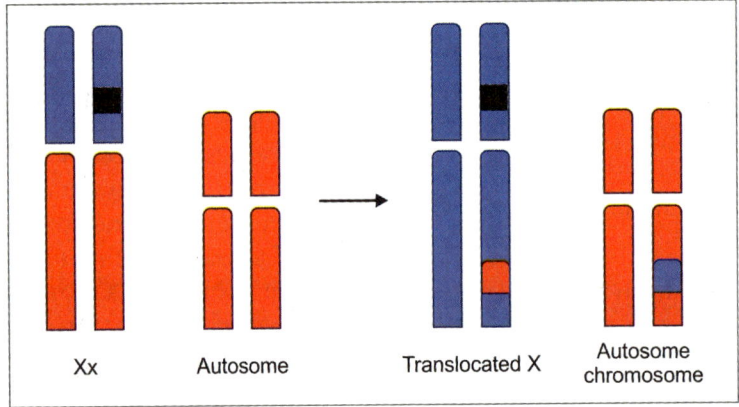

Figure 4.21: Translocation of an X chromosome with an autosome responsible for manifestation in female for X-linked recessive disorders

Q 30. Write the unique features and give examples of X-linked dominant disorders.

Ans. Unique features of X-linked dominant inheritance

- Females have a less severe phenotype due to the effects of lyonization. There are few exceptions to this rule.
- There is no male to male transmission of disease.
- Affected males can transmit the disease to all daughters, but not to their sons.

- Affected females can transmit the disease to both sons and daughters and the risk of disease in each is 50%.
- Family history may reveal an increased number of affected females, since male offspring with X-linked dominant mutation may develop severe disease and may not survive.
- Affected males with lethal mutations, if live born, tend to be mosaic for the genetic condition.

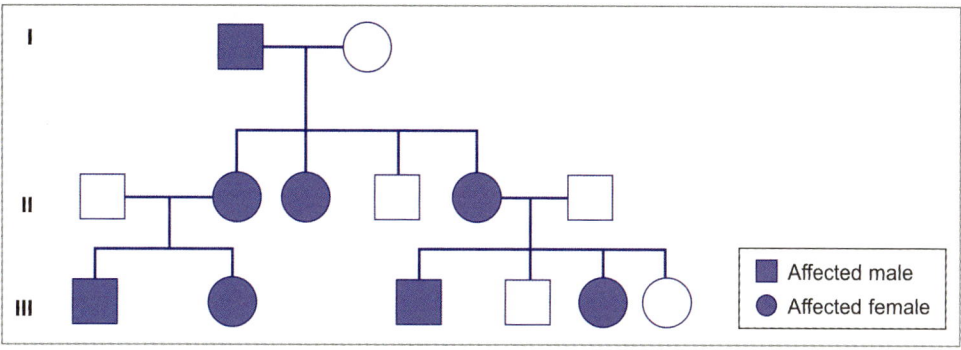

Figure 4.22: Pedigree showing X-linked dominant inheritance

🔎 **NOTE:** The recessive and dominant X-linked disorders are distinguished based on the clinical expression of symptoms in a woman with heterozygous mutations. Due to the effects of lyonization, the clinical picture is on a continuum, ranging from nil symptoms to disease of varying severity. Thus, all women with heterozygous mutations are neither completely recessive nor completely dominant. Therefore, disorders associated with X chromosome, are to be simply termed 'X-linked disorders'.

Examples of X-linked dominant disorders

⊃ **Metabolic disease:** Vitamin D resistant/ hypophosphatemic rickets, ornithine carbamoyl transferase deficiency
⊃ **Neurological disorder:** Rett syndrome, Aicardi syndrome, Coffin-Lowry syndrome
⊃ **Cutaneous disorders:** Incontinentiapig-menti, Goltz syndrome.

Q 31. What is recurrence risk of X-linked dominant disorder in the next child of a couple whose first child is affected with X-linked dominant disorder?

Ans. The recurrence risk of X-linked dominant disease in the next child of a couple whose first child is affected with X-linked dominant disorder is shown below which further depends on whether mutation is *de novo* or is present in the mother or the father of the affected child.

⊃ **In *de novo* X-linked dominant conditions,** the recurrence risk in next child is usually negligible.

⊃ **In a mother with heterozygous mutation,** there is 50% risk of disease in each child, irrespective of the gender (Figure 4.23).
⊃ **In an affected male with hemizygous mutation** (Figure 4.24).

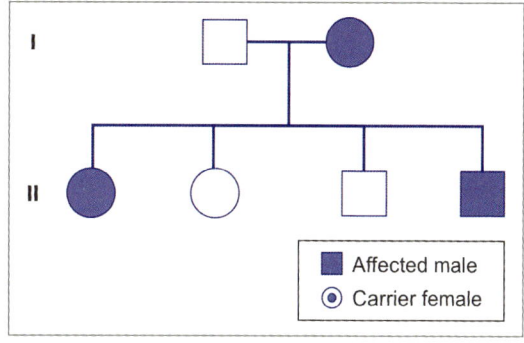

Figure 4.23: 50% risk in each offspring of heterozygous dominant mother

⊃ **X-linked conditions with lethal mutations** usually lead to spontaneous abortion of male conceptus. Live born male offspring tend to be mosaic for the condition.
⊃ In a mosaic state, the risk of disease is primarily dependent on the level of germline mosaicism and type of disorder.

Q 32. Why are X-linked dominant disorders lethal in males and only manifest in females? How do X-linked disorders transmit to the next generation?

Ans. The X chromosomes have highly active regions (euchromatin) and encompass more than 800 genes, many of which code for highly conserved proteins. Mutations in these genes

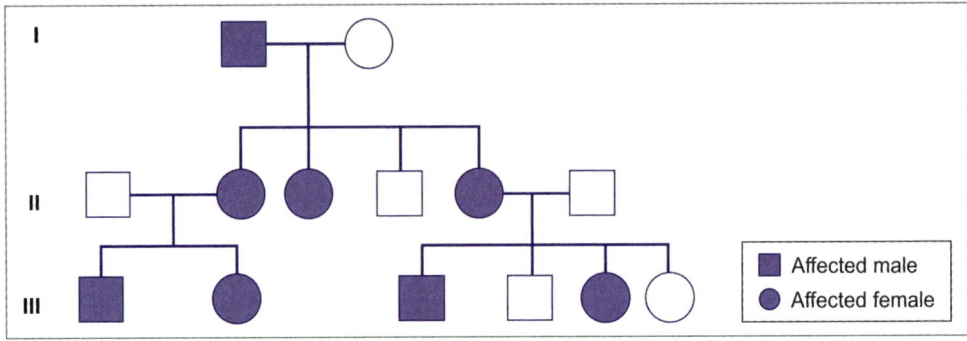

Figure 4.24: Pedigree shows the risk of transmission of X-linked dominant disease from an affected male with hemizygous mutation is 100% among daughters and 0% among sons

lead to abnormalities in these critical proteins which may lead to severe impairment of normal function.

◦ Male offsprings, being hemizygous for X chromosome, are unable to compensate for the lost function and thus, invariably manifest the disease. The reduced viability of such male conceptus prevents transmission of lethal mutations in nature and accounts for the relatively greater number of affected females within families.

◦ In a female, the defective X chromosome may be preferentially silenced by lyonization and the lost/abnormal function may also be compensated by the normal X chromosome. Therefore, the disease is less severe in women, even in mutations affecting critical genes. So, these conditions are transmitted to next generation by affected females.

Q 33. Write the difference between autosomal dominant and X-linked dominant inheritance.

Ans.

Autosomal dominant	X-linked dominant
Involves an autosomal chromosome	Involves an allosome or sex chromosome
Incidence is equal among males and females	Disease incidence shows a relative excess among females since male offspring with hemizygous lethal mutations are usually non-viable

Disease equally severe among both sexes	Disease less severe in females because of lyonization
50% recurrence risk of disease in each offspring, irrespective of gender	In heterozygous females, risk of disease is 50% among both sexes. Affected males can transmit the disorder to all daughters.
Male to male transmission seen	Male to male transmission not seen
May have reduced penetrance	X-linked diseases are usually fully penetrant

Q 34. Explain sex-influenced and sex-limited inheritance with examples.

Ans.

Sex-influenced inheritance	Sex-limited inheritance
The conditions which are autosomal disorders and can occur in both sexes, but preferentially affects one sex more than the other. This is mainly attributable to the hormone dependent differential gene expression or differences in genetic imprinting, based on the parent of origin.	The genetic conditions which manifest in a particular sex, where the target organs are present.

Example: Gout is more common among males, while systemic lupus erythematosus is more common among women.	Example: 5-alpha reductase gene mutations cause developmental sex disorders in males but do not cause any phenotype in females, since they lack the end organs, on which the enzyme acts.

Q 35. What is Y-linked inheritance? Draw the pedigree and give example of this inheritance.

Ans. It is the inheritance pattern followed by genes present on the Y chromosome and is also termed 'Holandric inheritance'. It is a type of sex-linked inheritance. It shows following features:

- ➲ Y chromosome is present only in males and disease related to Y chromosome manifests only in males (Figure 4.25).
- ➲ The disease is passed on from father to son only, provided the reproductive fitness of the affected father is preserved.
- ➲ Male infertility is a well-known Y-linked condition.

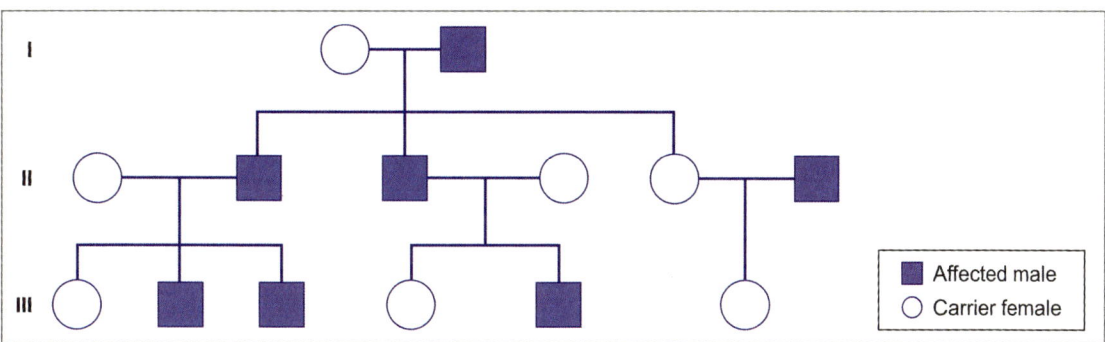

Figure 4.25: Y-linked inheritance where male to male transmission of a disease occurs

BIBLIOGRAPHY

1. Adam MP, Ardinger HH, Pagon RA, et al. editors. GeneReviews® [Internet]. Seattle (WA): University of Washington, Seattle; 1993–2020. Available from: https://www.ncbi.nlm.nih.gov/books/NBK1116/.

2. Emery & Rimoin's Principles & Practice of Medical Genetics, 7th edition.
3. Genetic Clinics, IAMG.
4. Nelson's Textbook of Pediatrics, 21st edition.
5. Thompson & Thompson. Genetics in Medicine, 8th Edition.

Non-Mendelian Inheritance

Gayatri R Iyer, Chaitanya A Datar

Q 1. Why non-mendelian inheritance is called so?

Ans. The inheritance pattern of phenotype/trait caused by genes that do not follow mendelian laws of inheritance is called non-mendelian inheritance, because they are not conventional and have unique pattern of inheritance, e.g. mitochondrial inheritance shows maternal inheritance and multifactorial inheritance observed in complex disorders wherein multiple genetic and environmental factors give rise to a trait.

Q 2. Write the unique features of mtDNA.

Ans. Mitochondrial DNA is circular with 16,569 base pairs. There are 2 to 10 circular DNA strands inside a mitochondria and number of mitochondria per cell could range from 10–10,000. mt DNA can undergo high frequency of mutations (5–10 times more common than nuclear DNA) and shows unique features.

Unique features of mt DNA (Figure 5.1)

➲ **Replicative segregation:** During each cell division, mt DNA amplification occurs in each mitochondria and it distributes randomly in the newly formed mitochondria. Further these new mitochondrias distribute themselves randomly in the daughter cells. This process is called replicative segregation. Because of this process, based on the presence of mutated or normal mt DNA, an individual can show clinical variability.

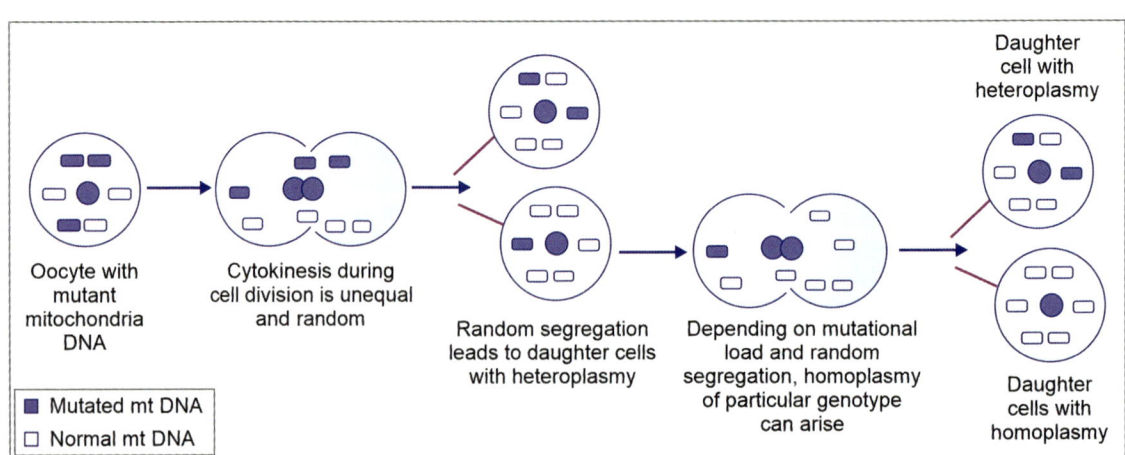

Figure 5.1: Cytokinesis giving rise to heteroplasmy, replication segregation and homoplasmy in mitochondrial inheritance

○ **Heteroplasmy:** The phenomenon of getting by chance a mixture of mitochondria with normal or mutated DNA in a cell during cell division is called heteroplasmy.

○ **Homoplasmy:** When identical copies of mtDNA, that is either all mutated or normal DNA is passed onto the daughter cell by chance, it is called homoplasmy.

○ **Mitochondrial genetic bottleneck:** The reduction in mtDNA in the oocyte and further development of normal or mutated mt DNA in oocyte is called mitochondrial genetic bottleneck.

Q 3. Write the unique features of mtDNA inheritance.

Ans. The mitochondrial inheritance does not show mendelian inheritance rather it follows maternal inheritance pattern (transmission of mitochondrial disorders is possible from mother not from father) because only the egg contains the mitochondria in the cytoplasm and the sperm shed their mitochondria before injecting their pronucleus into the ovum. Because of unique features of mtDNA, it shows distinct features which are as follows:

Unique Features of mt DNA Inheritance (Figure 5.2)

○ Mitochondrial inheritance shows maternal inheritance pattern.

○ All the offspring of a female having homoplasmic mutated mitochondria will be affected.

○ Father having homoplasmic mutation will not transmit the disease to any of the child.

○ The clinical symptoms of a mitochondrial disorder in an individual depend upon the relative proportion of mutated and normal mitochondria in a heteroplasmic mutation.

○ Due to special features of mtDNA like replicative segregation, bottleneck phenomenon and heteroplasmy genetic counseling related to clinical phenotype is a big challenge for mitochondrial disorders.

Q 4. How nuclear DNA interacts with mitochondrial DNA and modifies the phenotype of mitochondrial disorder?

Ans. The mitochondrial DNA consists of 37 genes coding for 13 polypeptides, 22 tRNA and 2 rRNA. These polypeptides are the enzymes involved in the respiratory chain

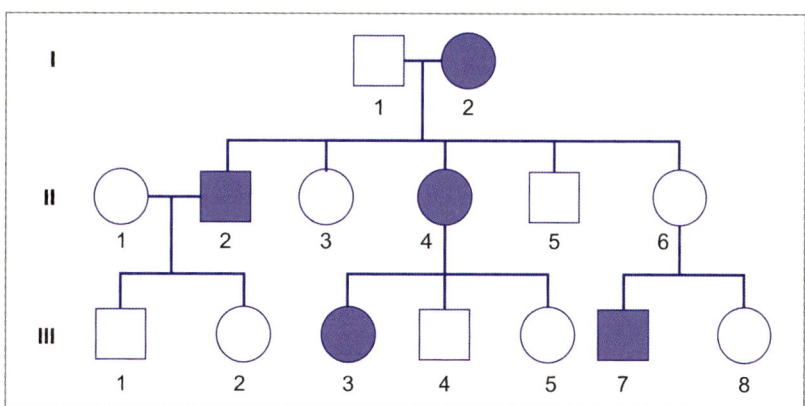

Figure 5.2: Pedigree showing mitochondrial inheritance: Individual I.2 carries mtDNA mutation and is affected, her offsprings II.2, II.4 also are affected. III.1 and 2 are not affected since affected male does not transmit the condition, III.3 is affected since her mother II.4 transmitted the disease. III.7 inherits the condition despite the mother being unaffected is because of heteroplasmy, the mutated mtDNA load is adequate to cause the disease. The mother II.6 though harbored the mutation; the load was less. Examples of mitochondrial diseases— LHON, MERRF, MELAS

complex for the production of energy for cells. The mitochondria is not self-sufficient by itself, it requires other proteins to make a functional respiratory chain complex, for mitochondrial replication, its integrity and transcription which are coded by the nuclear genome.

Mutated mtDNA are propagated differentially in different tissues depending on the nuclear coded protein machinery, indicating nuclear genes play a role in driving mutated mtDNA into heteroplasmy or homoplasmy depending on tissue type. Some of the disorders arising due to mitochondrial defects following autosomal inheritance also show interaction between nuclear DNA and mtDNA.

Example:
- Leigh's disease a mitochondrial disorder caused by nuclear gene *SURF1* follows autosomal recessive inheritance.
- Nuclear DNA can play a role in decreasing the severity of Lebers hereditary optic neuropathy (LHON) symptoms in a person who has inherited LHON mtDNA mutation.

Q 5. Enumerate some of the common mitochondrial disorders.

Ans. The common mitochondrial disorders are as follows:
- **Leber hereditary optic neuropathy (LHON):** Acute visual loss possibly due to optic nerve involvement.
- **Leigh disease:** Neuroregression of mile stones, developmental delay, seizures, respiratory problems.
- **Myoclonic epilepsy and ragged red fibers (MERRF):** Myoclonic epilepsy, ragged red fibers in skeletal muscle and other neurological symptoms.
- **Kaerns-Sayre syndrome:** Progressive external ophthalmoplegia, pigmentary retinopathy, heart block, ataxia, muscle weakness, deafness.
- **MELAS:** Myopathy, encephalomyopathy, lactic acidosis stroke-like episodes
- **NARP:** Neuropathy and retinopathy
- **DAD:** Diabetes and deafness

Q 6. What is digenic/oligogenic inheritance? Give some examples.

Ans. Digenic or oligogenic inheritance a non-mendelian inheritance is a mechanism that involves inheritance of a trait because of involvement of two or more gene to manifest the disease. Mutation in one gene does not cause the disease.

Digenic inheritance is of two types—
i. **True digenic:** Variants in two genes are necessary to cause the condition.
ii. **Composite digenic:** Variant in one gene can cause the condition, however, a variant in second gene significantly affects the phenotype.

Examples:
- *Bardet-Biedl syndrome:* Two genes involved are BBS1 + BBS2
- *Retinitis pigmentosa:* ROM1 + RDS
- *Acute necrotizing encephalopathy:* RANBP2 + CPT2

Q 7. Explain briefly about epigenetics (gene silencing) and its mechanism and its role in human genetic diseases.

Ans. There are two forms of information in the genome of the cell.
i. **Genetic information** that provides the building block for the synthesis of proteins needed for the cellular function.
ii. **Epigenetics** that provides instruction on how, when and where this genetic information should be used.

Epigenetics is a mechanism which does not lead to change in the DNA sequence yet alters the gene expression. All the genes cannot be active at the same time. It is due to mechanism of epigenetics which involves reversible changes in the genetic material which regulates the gene expression. Despite developing from a single zygote with two gametes, function of every cell in our body is defined like blood cells are not expressed in hair and hair cells are not expressed in eyes. This spaciotemporal expression of genes is regulated by epigenetics. X inactivation in human genome is a well-recognized event due to epigenetics.

Epigenetic regulation is facilitated by two mechanisms at two levels—acetylation and methylation at histone and DNA level.

1. Histone acetylation leads transcription and eventually translation
2. Histone methylation facilitates gene expression
3. DNA methylation is a mechanism by which the gene is always silenced. The methylation happens at the CpG islands which comprises long stretches of C and G nucleotides. Methyl is attached to the cytosine bases at the 5th position.

The clinical disorders due to alteration in gene expression as a result of epigenetics are as follows:

a. **Parental imprinting disorders:** Abnormal methylation of imprinted genes can lead to disorders such as Angelman and Prader-Willi syndromes.
b. **Malignancies:** Aberrant methylation like hypomethylation can cause leukemias and lymphomas or hypermethylation of tumor suppressor genes can silence it and give rise to carcinoma like colon cancer.
c. **Fragile X syndrome:** Methylation at the promoter region occurs when there is a large CGG expansion, leading inactivation of the gene and causing the clinical phenotype.

Q 8. Explain genomic imprinting (parent of origin imprinting) and its mechanism and write the names of some genomic imprinting disorders.

Ans. Genomic imprinting: Genomic imprinting is an epigenetic mechanism by which few genes are exclusively expressed from one allele depending on parent of origin. There are about 200 genes which are expressed from a single parent indicating only one copy is expressed and the other is silenced. These do not show pattern of classical mendelian inheritance in which genes inherited from both parent express equally.

Significance: This mechanism was evolved in mammals to discourage parthenogenesis (same gender fertilization) to conserve and promote heterosexual sexual reproduction as same gender conception gives rise to abnormal conceptional tissues. Imprinting confers a functional change in particular allele at the time of gametogenesis determined by the sex of the parent. This imprint lasts for one generation and is then removed, so that an appropriate imprint can be re-established in the germ cells of the next generation (Figure 5.3).

Mechanism: Most of the mechanisms of genomic imprinting were not well understood

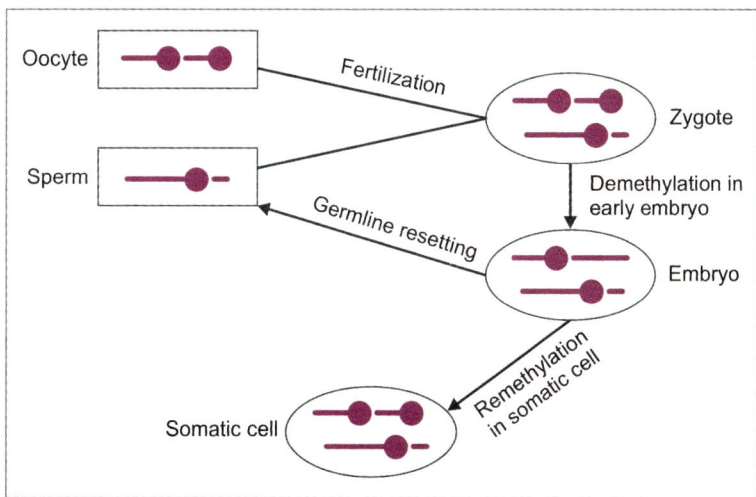

Figure 5.3: Genomic imprinting maintenance in germline and somatic cells

but the most understandable mechanism of it is the methylation of the cytosine of CpG islands (clusters of cytosine and guanine dinucleotides at promoter region) at the 5th position making it a 5′ methylcytosine. It can block the transcription and silence the gene expression under the control of imprinting control regions (ICR), usually located near these imprinted genes to enable their differential expression. Direct DNA methylation of ICR can also switch on or off a gene.

Examples of imprinting disorders: Since only single allele is active and the other is silenced, if the active allele undergoes aberrations like mutation, deletion, duplication, uniparental disomy, it would lead to various imprinting disorders. The examples of common imprinting disorders in genetics are as:

1. Prader-Willi syndrome
2. Angelman syndrome
3. Beckwith-Wiedemann syndrome
4. Silver-Russell syndrome

Q 9. What is uniparental disomy? Describe its mechanism.

Ans. Uniparental disomy (UPD) is a pheno-menon, which happens in diploid organisms when both the homologous chromosomes are transmitted from a single parent. Depending on its origin it is either called maternal uniparental disomy or paternal uniparental disomy. For example, if there is UPD of chromosome 7 of maternal origin, it is remarked as mat UPD7.

Mechanism: The possible mechanism of UPD is as follows (Figure 5.4):

1. **Trisomy or monosomy rescue in a zygote:** A trisomic or a monosomic conceptus is not viable for gestation and thus gives rise to a 46,XX or 46,XY embryo by chromosome loss or duplication respectively.

   a. *Trisomic rescue:* A gamete arises because of nondisjunction having both parental chromosomes in one gamete and if it gets fertilized with a normal gamete, it gives trisomic zygote but due to faulty selection in trisomy rescue, the normal gamete with single chromosome may be knocked out and the zygote will be containing both chromosomes from one parent and UPD may arise which is heterodisomy. It happens during Meiosis stage 1 (Figure 5.4).

   b. *Monosomic rescue:* Occasionally UPD may arise by fertilization of a monosomic gamete followed by duplication of the chromosome from the other gamete (monosomy rescue). This mechanism results in uniparental isodisomy, occurs duirng Meiosis stage 11.

2. **UPD in rare cases:** It could also arise by fertilization of a monosomic gamete with adisomic gamete, resulting in either isodisomy or heterodisomy.

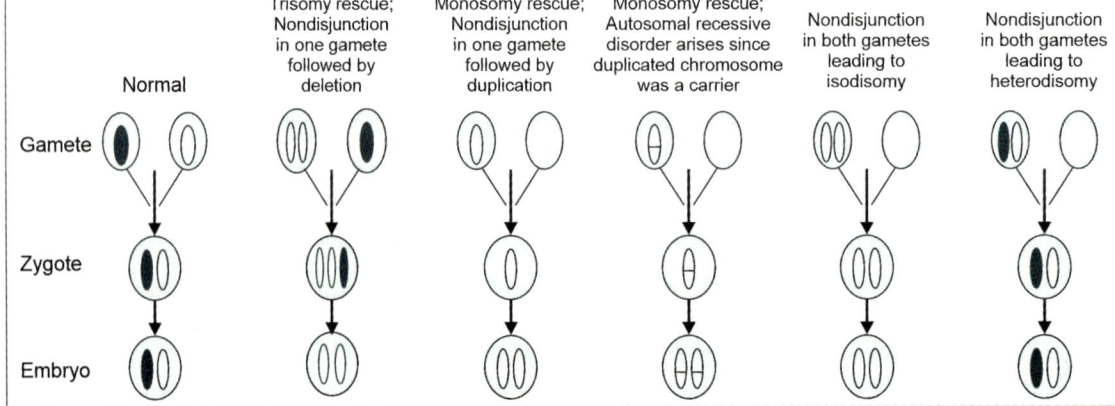

Figure 5.4: Mechanisms that give rise to uniparental disomy and types of uniparental disomy

Q 10. Enumerate some of the diseases which are caused by uniparental disomy?

Ans. UPD as such does not cause a disorder except in two situations, in either case, the recurrence in the subsequent pregnancy is less likely.

1. The parent who contributed the chromosome is carrier for an autosomal recessive disorder like cystic fibrosis and the offspring becomes homozygous for that mutation. It occurs only in case of isodisomy, not with heterodisomy (Figure 5.4).

2. The chromosome in disomy harbors imprinted genes which are essential for gestation, growth, development and intellect. Disomy would render absent active copy of an imprinted gene and give rise to conditions like Prader-Willi syndrome (mat UPD 15), Angelman syndrome (pat UPD 15) and Beckwith-Wiedemann syndrome, Russell-Silver syndrome.

Q 11. What do you mean by triplet repeat mutations (unstable/dynamic mutations)?

Ans. (*See* Chapter 16)

Q 12. What do you mean by multifactorial inheritance?

Ans. Some of the genetic disorders do not follow classical mendelian patterns of inheritance each time. Rather they are caused by various genes interacting with other genes as well as variety of environmental factors which act together to trigger or exacerbate the disease process.

Thus, the final phenotype of these conditions depends on these gene-gene or gene-environment interactions and such disorders follow multifactorial or complex inheritance patterns (Figure 5.5).

Examples of Gene–Environment Interactions:
- **Food intake:** Diabetes (sugar), hypercholesterolemia (oils and fats), congenital malformations (vitamin deficiencies)
- **Addictions:** Cancer (tobacco)

- **Radiations/chemical carcinogens:** Cancer **Gene–Gene interactions** are more complex and difficult to ascertain and to prevent or mitigation. Example: Schizophrenia, Alzheimer's disease, etc.

Recent evidence has suggested the role of epigenetic modifications in causing multifactorial diseases such as neural tube defects.

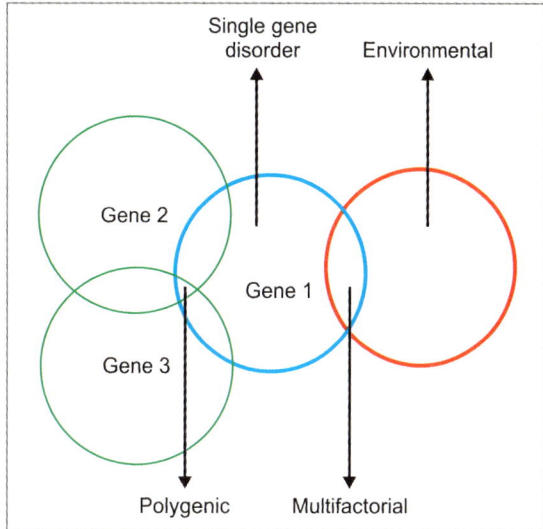

Figure 5.5: Gene–Gene and Gene–Environment interactions

Q 13. Name some common disorders that show multifactorial inheritance.

Ans. Common disorders showing multifactorial inheritance patterns:

Gene–Gene interactions:
- Autism spectrum disorder
- Alzheimer's disease
- Schizophrenia
- Multiple sclerosis
- Hirschsprung's disease.

Gene–Environment interactions:
- Congenital malformations: Neural tube defects, congenital heart disease
- Cleft lip-palate
- Congenital dislocation of hip
- Pyloric stenosis
- Asthma
- Epilepsy

- Cancer
- Diabetes mellitus
- Coronary artery disease
- Hypertension
- Bipolar disorder.

BIBLIOGRAPHY

1. Emery & Rimoin's Principles & Practice of Medical Genetics, 7th edition.

2. Thompson & Thompson, Genetics In Medicine, 8th edition.

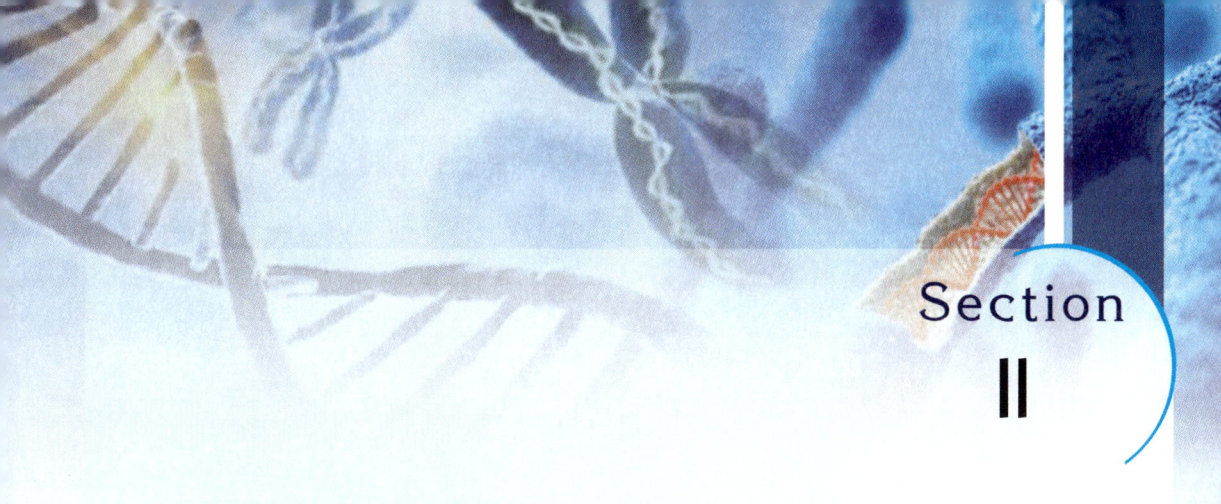

Laboratory Diagnostic Techniques

➲ Genetic Test: Cytogenetic Analysis and Molecular Genetic Analysis

Genetic Test: Cytogenetic Analysis and Molecular Genetic Analysis

Chapter 6

Usha R Dutta, Aruna Priya Kamireddy , T Karthik Bharadwaj, Deepti Saxena

GENETIC TEST
Usha R Dutta

Q 1. Define genetic testing.

Ans. Any medical test done to check for changes in the genetic material at the level of chromosomes, DNA, RNA and proteins leading to genetic abnormalities is genetic testing. These tests help in making the association between the genotype and phenotype in an individual or the possible occurrence of the disease in the family.

Q 2. How will you classify genetic tests? Write about diagnostic genetic test.

Ans. Based on the clinical indication and the level of abnormality in the genetic material genetic tests can be classified into three groups:

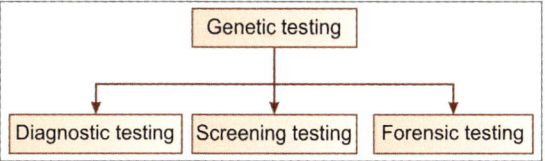

Diagnostic Testing

It is used to identify different types of mutations causing various human genetic diseases in the reproductive, prenatal, postnatal, newborn, childhood and adulthood periods. Different types of diagnostic tests are available based on the level of genetic abnormality.

Chromosomal testing

To detect chromosomal abnormalities various tests are:

- **Karyogram:** To detect abnormalities in the number of chromosomes (like Down syndrome) and structure of chromosomes (like translocations).
- **Fluorescence *in situ* hybridization (FISH):** A molecular cytogenetic technique to identify abnormalities involving few specific regions of chromosomes (like micro deletions and duplications).

Molecular genetic testing

The DNA is tested to identify variations in single genes or in known regions of a gene causing a genetic disorder. The variations can be small changes like a single base pair loss/gain or any other change in the DNA sequence.

Molecular tests based on the type of mutation

Index case testing

- **Multiplex ligation-dependent probe amplification (MLPA):** Duchenne muscular dystrophy, the gene deletion can be tested.
- **Sanger sequencing:** For Thalassemia, mutations can be detected by single gene molecular analysis.
- **Next generation sequencing based multi-gene panels, exome sequencing or the whole-genome analysis:** For a phenotype

like skeletal dysplasia or intellectual disability where the candidate gene for the disease is not known.

Prenatal testing

To check for targeted defective genes.

Pharmacogenetic test

It is done to know the relation between genetic constitution of an individual, and therapeutic and side effects of a drug.

Q 3. Write a note on screening and forensic genetic tests.

Ans. Screening Genetic Testing: Screening genetic test is done to know whether a person is at risk or not to have the genetic disorder before the appearance of symptoms of the disease. The common screening tests done are of the following types:

- **Predictive and presymptomatic testing:** It offered to asymptomatic people with a family history of genetic disorders to provide information about the risk of developing the disease. For example, Huntington disease.
- **Preimplantation testing:** This detects the genetic changes in an embryo *in vitro* before implantation.
- **Predispositional testing:** To reduce the risk of developing disease in a person by modifying the environmental factors, by screening surveillance or by taking treatment.
  Example: Breast cancer, hypertension, diabetes mellitus and coronary artery disease.
- **Carrier testing:** Offered to individuals who have a family history of a genetic disorder and carry a diseased gene.
- **Biochemical genetic testing:** The testing of proteins or enzymes causing metabolic disorders due to a defective protein or loss/gain of a protein. In some cases where the protein is not formed, the accumulated precursor protein in the pathway can be estimated.

Example: Newborn-screening to identify the metabolic disorders and for early intervention of some treatable disorders.

- **Prenatal screening testing:** Prenatal screening is done to identify the fetuses at high-risk to have a congenital abnormality or genetic disorder.

Forensic testing: Microsatellites, the highly repetitive DNA sequence, are unique to every individual and are used to establish the biological relation (maternity/paternity) and are also used in crime detection.

Q 4. What are the limitations of genetic testing?

Ans. Although genetic testing is a helpful tool in the identification of genetic disorders, there are several limitations which need to be taken into consideration while offering a test.

- No genetic test either cytogenetic or molecular is 100% accurate. *For example*, in cytogenetics, there could be 2–3% error either due to sample degradation or due to technical problems.
- Genetic tests cannot predict the severity of the disease and age of onset.
- There is no treatment for many genetic disorders which are diagnosed. *For example*, newborn-screening panels diagnose various metabolic disorders but many of them cannot be treated.
- Genetic testing can lead to complex emotional, social, health insurance and financial consequences. *Example:* Predictive testing of Huntington's disease creates anxiety and tension in the family.
- The test may not detect all the mutations that cause disease, as some tests lack sensitivity. For example, the panels for cystic fibrosis.
- Incidental finding in the tests is also a big concern.
- Genetic tests have limitation of diagnosing all the disease as all the genes that cause diseases have not been identified as of now.

Q 5. Write the special considerations which must be kept in mind while ordering a genetic test.

Ans. Genetic tests are very expensive and time consuming and hence, these tests should be ordered by an experienced geneticist.

The following considerations should be always kept in mind while ordering a genetic test.

1. A proper clinical evaluation with the detailed pedigree should be taken to decide which genetic test has to be sent; whether cytogenetic, biochemical or molecular.
2. The geneticist should explain in detail the possible outcome of the results, risks and limitations of the test.
3. A geneticist should be well aware of the applications and limitations of all the genetic tests.
4. Genetic tests should be offered to patients with some indications of a genetic disorder or familial inheritance.
5. While ordering a prenatal test, the patient should be made aware of the details of procedures, its limitations, the risk of miscarriages and time limit, and only then, an informed consent should be taken.
6. The confidentiality of genetic test results, proper quality assurance and standard guidelines should be maintained in the testing laboratories.

CYTOGENETIC ANALYSIS
Usha R Dutta

Q 6. Define cytogenetic analysis and enumerate the different types of tests for analysing chromosomes.

Ans. Cytogenetics is the study of all 23 pairs of homologous chromosomes structure arranged according to size, position of the centromere and the type of banding in a low resolution and the identification of numerical and structural chromosomal aberrations that cause the diseases.

The different cytogenetic tests include:

1. G-banding method and other cytogenetic banding techniques to identify chromosomes.

2. Molecular cytogenetic techniques with increased resolution such as
   a. Fluorescence *in situ* hybridization (FISH).
   b. Comparative genomic hybridization (CGH).

Q 7. What are different clinical indications for cytogenetic analysis?

Ans. The cytogenetic study can detect all numerical and large structural rearrangements on many tissues but most commonly used tissue is the peripheral blood. Certain clinical indications for which cytogenetic test should be performed are:

Reproductive Indications

⊃ **Recurrent miscarriages, stillbirth or infertility:** Evaluation of any couple with more than 2 miscarriages to rule out presence of balanced reciprocal translocations or marker chromosomes.

⊃ **Primary/secondary amenorrhea:** For Turner syndrome or Turner mosaic cases.

Pediatric Indications

⊃ **Dysmorphic features, developmental delay and/or multiple congenital anomalies:** To rule out any structural or numerical abnormalities like trisomy 21.

⊃ **Short stature or abnormal growth suggestive of sex chromosomal anomalies:** Turner syndrome or Klinefelter syndrome.

⊃ **Intellectual disability:** This can be due to imbalance in the genome. Karyotype can yield a diagnosis in 2.5–3% and microarray can give a diagnosis in 20% of unexplained intellectual disability patients.

⊃ **Disorders of sexual development (DSD):** The ambiguity of the sex would be revealed by chromosomal analysis.

⊃ **Possible balanced translocation carriers:** cytogenetic testing can detect balanced translocation, partial trisomy or partial monosomy.

⊃ **Hematological malignancies:** In acute lymphocytic leukemia to identify translocation between chromosome t (12 : 21) and other cytogenic abnormalities.

Prenatal Diagnostics Indications

- **Abnormal results of prenatal screening test:** Indicative of the possible risk of aneuploidies, especially trisomies.
- **Advanced maternal age:** Checks for increased risk of trisomies.
- **Fetal anomalies** detected through ultrasound.

- **Family history of chromosomal anomalies:** To check the reoccurrence of the same anomaly running in the family.

Q 8. What do you mean by karyogram, karyotype and ideogram?

Ans. **The term karyogram** refers to systematic arrangement of the 44 autosomes and 2 sex chromosomes either by digital imaging or photography (Figures 6.1 and 6. 2).

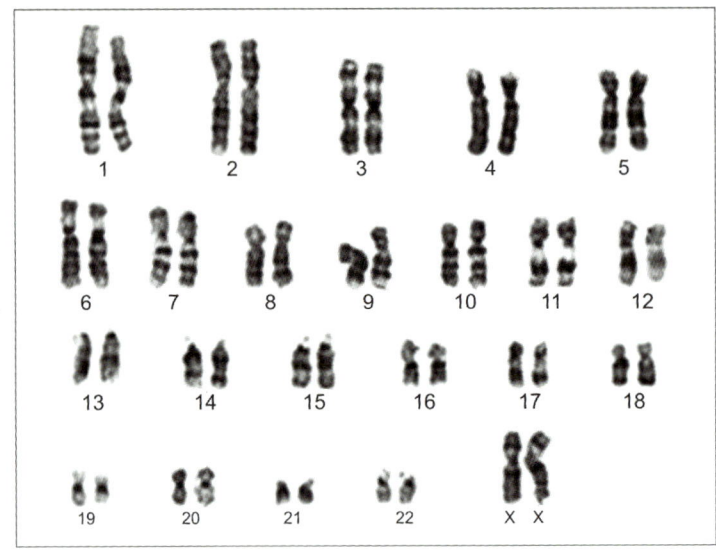

Figure 6.1: The karyogram showing normal female chromosome. The karyotype is 46,XX

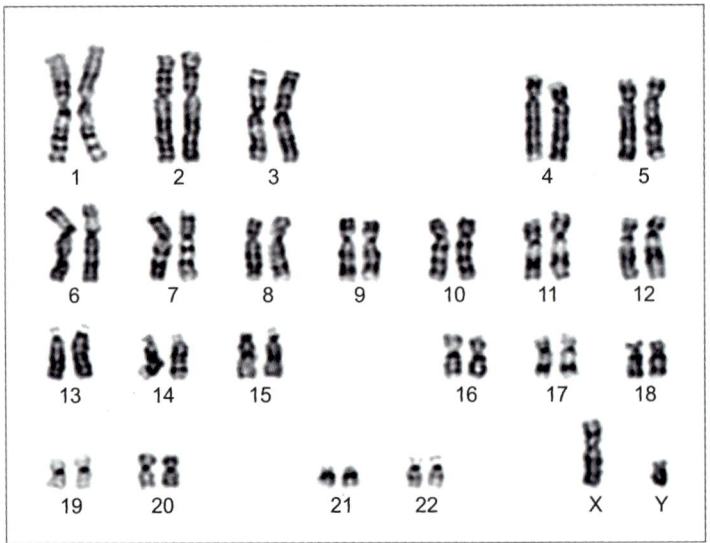

Figure 6.2: The karyogram showing normal male chromosome. The karyotype is 46,XY

In the karyogram, chromosomes are identified based on the size, banding pattern and centromeric position.

Karyotype is the written description of the normal or abnormal chromosomal complement of an individual in a standard arranged form as per the International System for Human Cytogenetic Nomenclature (ISCN) guidelines.

For example: 46,XX and 46,XY are the karyotypes.

Ideogram is a schematic diagrammatic representation of all the 23 chromosomes showing all the bands and sub-bands. Each chromosome can be individually identified based on the band level. The ISCN guidelines show 5 ideograms for each chromosome from 300 to 850 bands per haploid set (BPHS). The 550 BPHS ideogram is shown in Figure 6.3.

In simple terms, when a cytogenetic report of a normal female 46,XX along with the digital image is read, then the digital image is the karyogram and the result 46,XX is the karyotype.

Q 9. Write the procedure for chromosomal preparation.

Ans. The chromosomes are prepared from different types of live dividing tissues like T lymphocytes from peripheral blood, bone

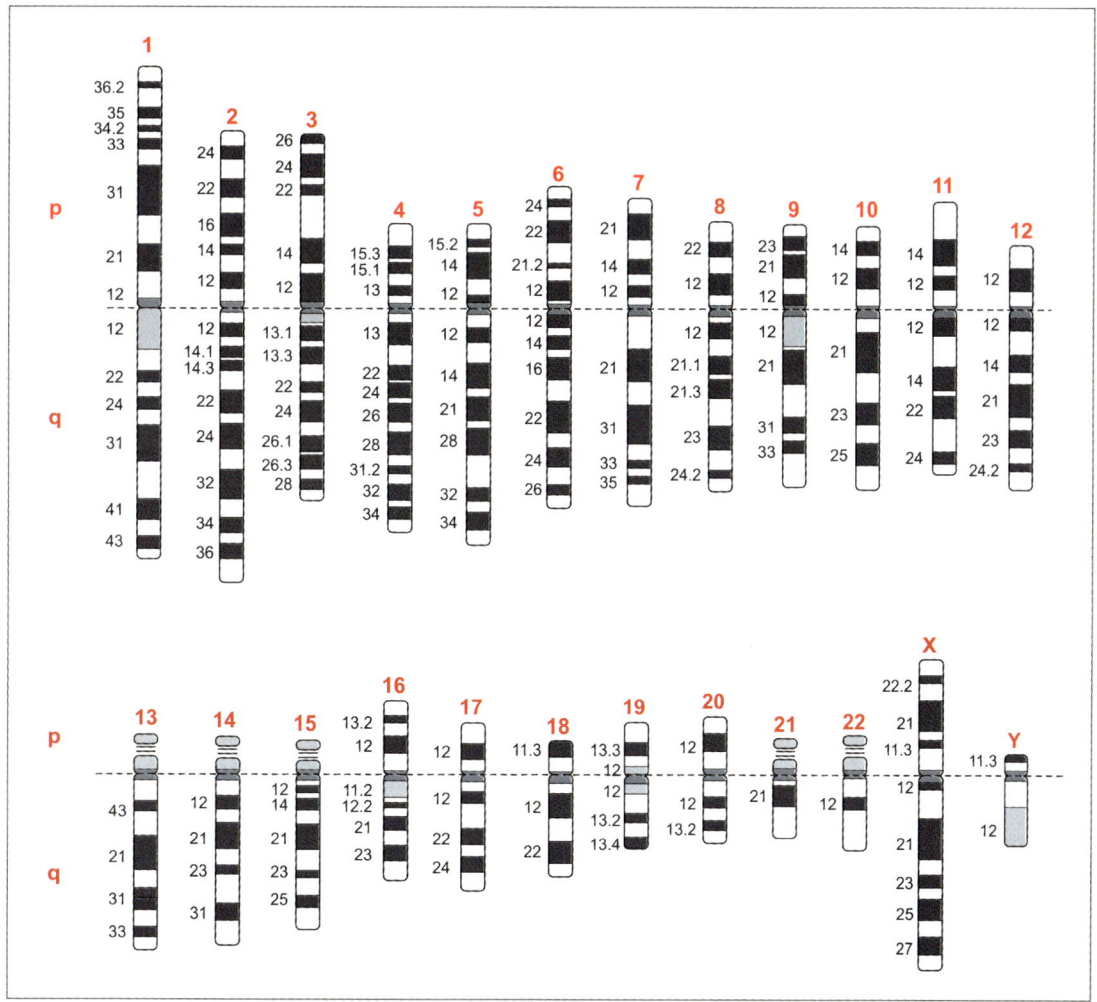

Figure 6.3: Ideogram is a schematic diagrammatic representation of all the 23 chromosomes showing all the bands and sub-bands

marrow, amniotic fluid, chorionic villi samples, skin tissue, products of conception and cord blood. The basic procedure for chromosome preparation from peripheral blood involves the following steps (Figure 6.4).

1. **Culture initiation:** The samples are cultured in Roswell Park Memorial Institute (RPMI-1640) medium along with a mitogen, phytohemagglutinin (PHA) which separates the lymphocytes from the blood.

2. **Harvesting:** The cells are harvested after 72 hours and include three steps:
   a. *Mitotic arrest:* It is usually achieved in the metaphase stage by adding mitotic inhibitors like colchicine or colcemid.
   b. *Hypotonic treatment:* Potassium chloride helps in spreading of chromosomes.
   c. *Fixation:* Methanol and acetic acid (3 : 1) helps to remove the water from the cells and fix the cells permanently.

3. **Metaphase chromosome preparation:** The pellet with metaphase chromosomes are dropped on slides to get good chromosome preparations.

4. **Chromosome banding and staining:** G banding using trypsin and Giemsa is the most commonly used banding technique. The other banding techniques are Q (Quinacrine), R (reverse banding using of acridine orange) and C (constitutive heterochromatin using barium hydroxide). G banding can show 400–500 bands on the haploid set but to get more than 800 bands in prophase or prometaphase stage, methotrexate or thymidine, folic acid or deoxycytidine have to be added in the culture medium.

5. **Chromosome analysis:** It is done under a microscope to rule out chromosomal abnormalities.

Q 10. What are the general principles to write a karyotype report?

Ans. The karyotype results are difficult to interpret. The general principles as per the ISCN guidelines while writing a karyotype with examples are summarized below:

General principles while writing a karyotype (*See* Appendix Table 1)

1. No space to be left in between the characters. *Example:* **46,XX** and **46,XY**

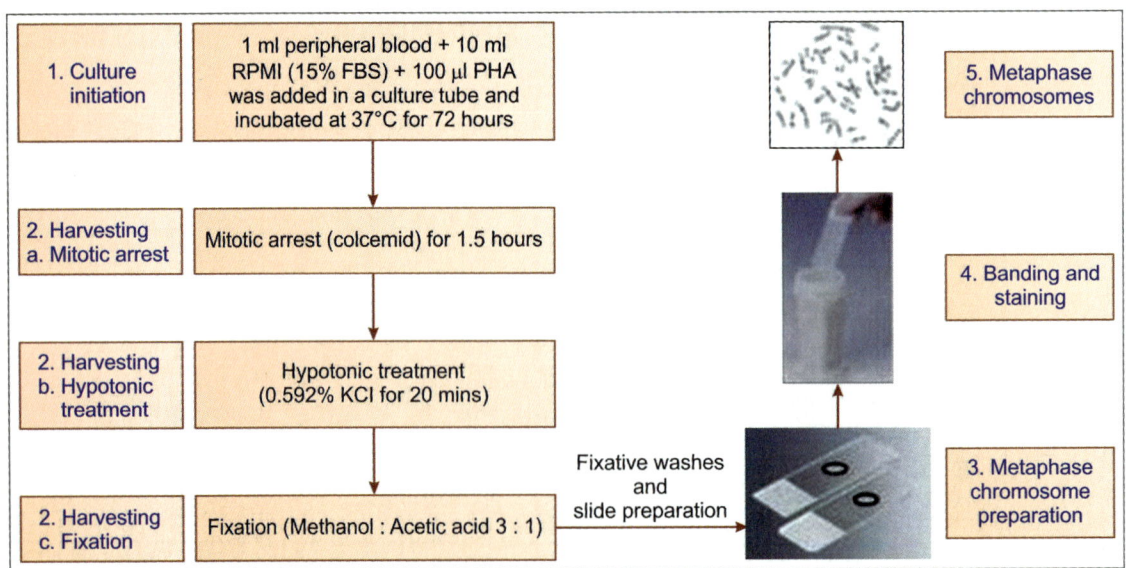

Figure 6.4: The protocol of chromosome preparation from peripheral blood RPMI-1640: Roswell Park Memorial Institute, PHA: Phytohemagglutinin

2. Sex chromosomal abnormalities should be listed first followed by autosomal abnormalities. *Example:* **45,X,+inv(9)**

3. Numerical abnormalities are listed first followed by structural abnormalities. *Example:* **47,XXY,t(2;18)(p12;q11.2)**

4. Chromosomes involved in translocation are written in first bracket; in second bracket the break points on the translocated chromosomes are shown, semicolon separates the translocated chromosomes and the break points. *Example:* **47,XXY,t(2;18) (p12;q11.2)**

5. The break points of the chromosomes are described based on the chromosome nomenclature.
    - The short arm (p) and long arm (q) of each chromosome is divided into regions based on certain landmarks.
    - *The region:* It is area between two landmarks.
    - *Regions:* These are divided into bands and the bands into sub-bands.

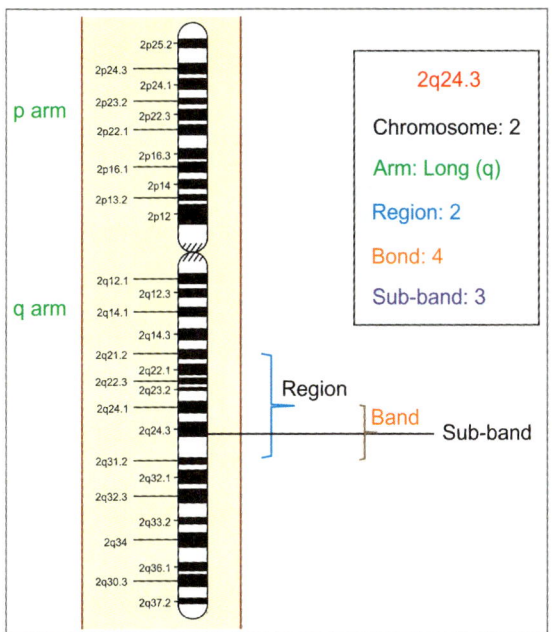

Figure 6.5: The description of regions and bands of chromosome 2

- *A band:* It is part of a chromosome that is lighter or darker in staining intensity (Figure 6.5).

Q 11. How the interpretation of cytogenetic report is done?

Ans. Interpretation of the cytogenetic report:

Report 1

A couple with recurrent miscarriages were analysed and the female karyotype was found to be normal with 46,XX but the male karyotype showed an abnormality with 46,XY,t(2;5)(p23.2;q13) (Figure 6.6).

Interpretation:

- **Female karyotype:** 46,XX is a normal female karyotype with 46 chromosomes along with two X chromosomes.
- **Male karyotype:** 46,XY,t(2;5)(p23.2;q13) is an abnormal male karyotype with a structural aberration. The chromosome number is 46. Here, the translocation happens between short arm of the chromosome 2 at region 2, band 3, sub-band 2 and the long arm of chromosome 5 at region 1, band 3.

Report 2

A 16-year-old referred for short stature revealed a karyotype of mos 45,X[4]/46,XX[16] (Figure 6.7A and B).

Interpretation

Turner-variant karyotype exhibiting mosaicism with two cell lines is abbreviated as mos. The number of cell line 45,X is in 4 cells and 46,XX is in 16 cells.

Q 12. What are the advantages of karyotype?

Ans. Cytogenic test is considered as first line testing for identification of chromosome abnormality. Following are its advantages:

Advantages

1. Chromosomal study can identify the gross anomalies of whole genome at low resolution.

2. All the numerical abnormalities like trisomy, monosomy, triploidy, tetraploidy

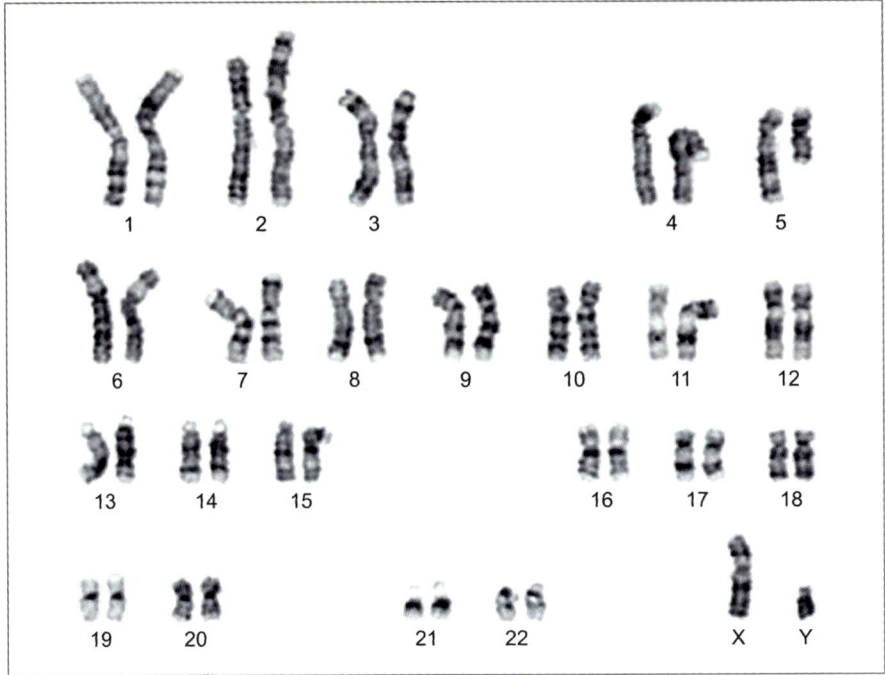

Figure 6.6: The karyogram showing a karyotype of 46,XY,t(2;5)(p23.2;q13)

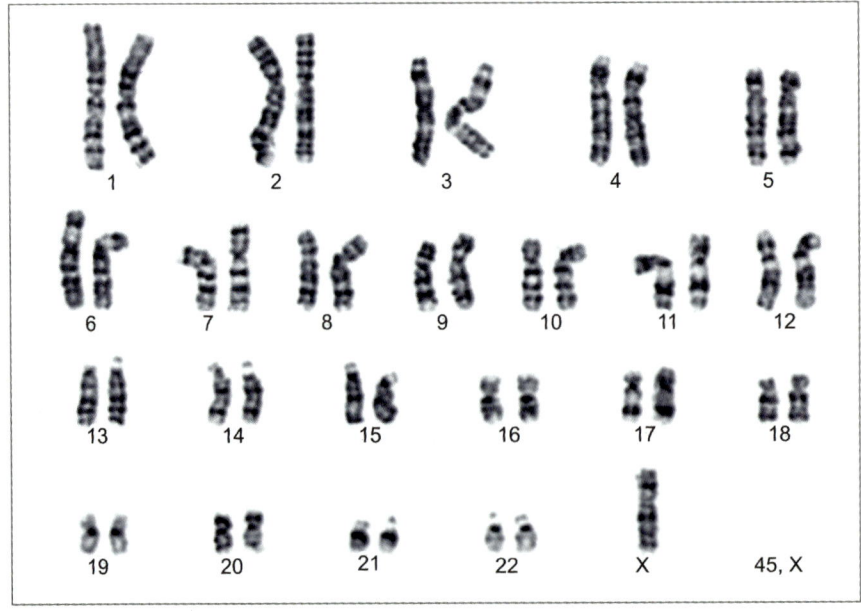

Figure 6.7A: A mosaic karyogram showing a karyotype of 45, X

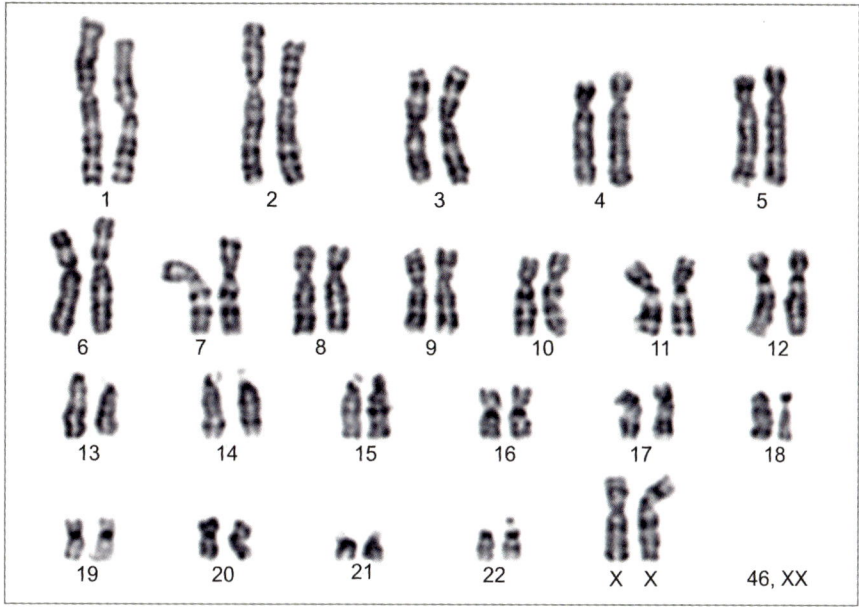

Figure 6.7B: Mosaic karyogram showing a karyotype of 46, XX

and hyperdiploidy and structural variations like inversions, deletions, duplications, ring chromosomes, isochromosomes and trans-locations can be detected (*See* Appendix Table 2).

3. Previous knowledge of any chromosomal anomalies is not required.

4. Chromosomal analysis can be done on fine needle aspirates when dividing cells are present in the tissues.

5. Mosaicism can be best detected by a cyto-genetic study.

6. It is sensitive and specific.

7. Balanced and complex chromosomal re-arrangements involving more than two chromosomes can also be best identified.

Q 13. What are the limitations of karyotype?
Ans. Although, the karyotype is considered as gold standard investigation for chromosomal identification, but there are some limitations also.

Limitations

1. It requires dividing cells and hence, fresh samples are required.

2. *Resolution is limited:* Chromosomal rearrangements lesser than 5–8 Mb, small cryptic rearrangements and subtle abnor-malities during prenatal diagnosis are difficult to identify.

3. Labour intensive, time consuming.

4. Automated technique but still needs skilled personnel and expertise.

5. Sometimes, repeat samples are required in cases with low mitotic index.

6. Mosaicism detection can never be 100% accurate.

7. Maternal cell contamination in prenatal samples occasionally complicates the interpretation of results.

8. Although it can identify the marker chromosomes, but the origin of the marker cannot be determined.

9. When some polymorphic variants are identified, it is necessary to karyotype the parents or to carry out further tests on a repeat sample.

10. Monogenic disorders cannot be identified by karyotype.

Q 14. Explain the principle and procedure of fluorescence *in situ* hybridization (FISH).

Ans. Chromosomal aberrations are a major cause of human genetic diseases. Conventional karyotype can detect both numerical and structural abnormalities (with limited resolution). However, precise identification and characterization of chromosomal abnormalities can only be achieved by advanced molecular cytogenetic techniques which are based mainly on fluorescence *in situ* hybridization (FISH). This is called '*in situ* hybridization' because DNA, intact in the chromosome or interphase gets hybridized. Thus FISH, the invaluable tool in the diagnostic field has enhanced the interpretation of numerical and complex chromosomal rearrangements by bridging the gap between conventional cytogenetics and molecular biology.

Principle

FISH is a cytogenetic technique which uses fluorescent probes that binds only to complementary sequences with high degree of specificity. FISH is based on the principle of complementary hybridization of fluorochrome labeled DNA or RNA probes with normal or abnormal nucleic acid sequences in patient samples on metaphase chromosomes, interphase cells or tissue sections.

Procedure

FISH can be done in the metaphase, interphase or on paraffin blocks involving following steps (Figure 6.8):

a. **DNA and probe denaturation:** Pretreatment with 0.005% of pepsin in 0.01N HCl at 37°C helps to remove extraneous RNA and proteins and enables access of the probes to the DNA sample to fix it on the slide. The target DNA and the probe are denatured to form single strands before hybridization.

b. **Hybridization:** The complementary hybridization of the probe takes place with the target DNA.

c. **Post-hybridization washes and counter staining the chromosomes:** It removes the extra hybridization mixture and unbound probe. After that counter-staining reagents such as DAPI (blue) and/or Propidium

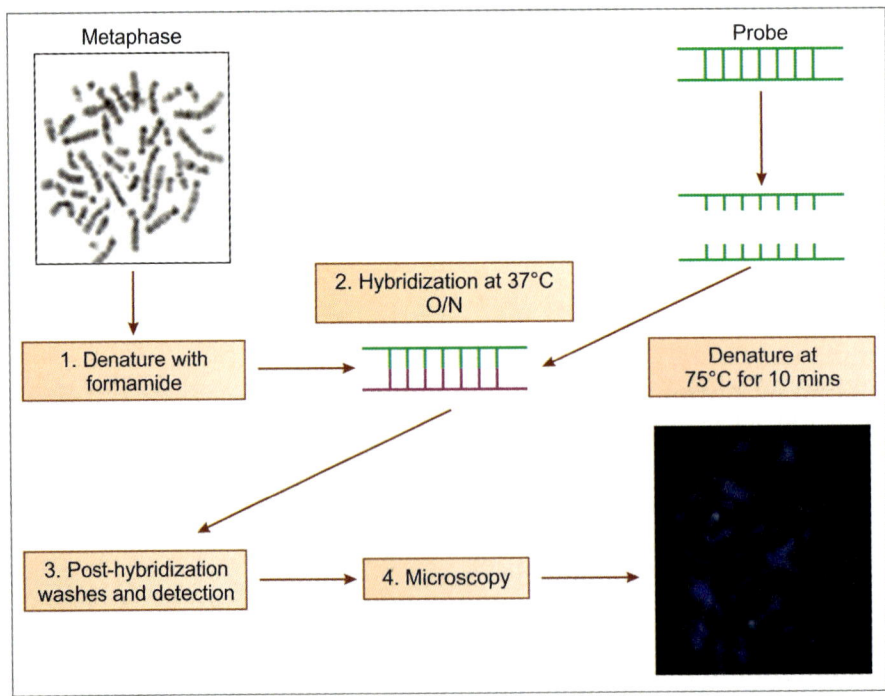

Figure 6.8: FISH protocol

iodide (PI, orange-red) are used along with the antifade solution, which prevents the fading of signals.

d. **Microscopic analysis and digital imaging:** Images are taken with a fluorescence microscope equipped with a CCD (charged coupled device) camera to see the desired DNA, its site and any loss or gain of its part.

Q 15. What are different types of fluorescence *in situ* hybridization (FISH) probes used in clinical practice?

Ans. To identify specific chromosomal micro abnormalities precisely by FISH, there are different types of probes which are given below:

DIFFERENT TYPES OF FISH PROBES
1. **Locus specific probe** is used to analyse specific microdeletion and microduplication in the chromosomes. Example: 7q deletion.
2. **Centromeric probe:** These probes represent repetitive DNA sequence near the centromere and are used to identify numerical abnormalities in the chromosomes (like in trisomies and monosomy of 13,18,21 and X, chromosome).
3. **Whole chromosome paint probe:** These probes are the mixture of probes which paint the different parts of chromosomes and these are used to identify chromosomal translocations and marker chromosomes.
4. **Telomeric probe** is used to identify telomeric regions of chromosomes which are greatly responsible for various intellectual disability disorders in children.

Q 16. Write a note on applications of fluorescence *in situ* hybridization (FISH).

Ans. Clinical applications of FISH

FISH is a very reliable technique to be used in clinical practice. By using different probes based on the clinical indication, FISH is used for following diagnosis:

1. **Cytogenetic test:** FISH is routinely used to identify microdeletion/microduplication syndromes like DiGeorge, William syndrome, etc. to confirm the translocations, complex chromosomal rearrangements and terminal translocations.

2. **Prenatal diagnostics:** Rapid FISH is used to check the aneuploidies in the amniotic fluid for quick result. In case of development of sexual disorders, sex can be determined by using X/Y specific probe. (In India sex determination is not permitted.)

3. **Low level** of mosaicism can be detected.

4. **Preimplantation and fetal DNA analysis** in maternal blood is also possible with FISH.

5. **Intellectual disability:** With telomeric probes, the telomeric regions responsible for unidentified intellectual disabilities can be analysed.

6. **Cancer:** FISH probes recommended as panels is used to detect many types of chromosomal abnormalities in hematological malignancies and on tumor tissues, e.g. acute myeloid leukemia panel, chronic myeloid leukemia panel, etc.

7. **Marker chromosome identification** can be done by FISH.

8. **Break point mapping studies:** FISH technique is extensively used to map the chromosomal break point regions by using bacterial artificial chromosome (BAC) clones.

Q 17. Write a note on advantages and disadvantages of fluorescence *in situ* hybridization (FISH).

Ans. For any technique, there exists advantages and limitations. Although there are several limitations for FISH, still it is considered as the first line investigation for specific chromosomal micro deletion and duplication identification.

Advantages

1. FISH can be performed on metaphases, interphases and paraffin embedded material.

2. FISH is locus specific and can be used to localize the anomaly in a specific tissue or cells.

3. FISH can be done on uncultured cells like amniocytes.
4. It is sensitive and specific with a quick turn-around time and automated system.
5. When conventional cytogenetics has failed to yield results, or when cryptic rearrangements are present, or when the tissue is insufficient, FISH can provide results.

Disadvantages

1. **Target specific:** FISH can only detect deletions or duplications of specifically targeted regions and which are larger than the probe used.
2. **Probe cost:** Probes are commercially available but are limited and very expensive.
3. **Not a screening tool:** It requires prior information of the disorder.
4. **Fluorescence microscopy:** FISH analysis requires expensive fluorescence filters.
5. **Interpretation:** FISH signals fade fast and hence, interpretation may be challenging when analysing suboptimal specimens due to background fluorescence.

Q 18. Write a note on other molecular cytogenetic techniques.

Ans. The fusion of conventional cytogenetics with molecular methodologies emerged as a major field called molecular cytogenetics. It deals with the analysis of genomic alterations using mainly *in situ* hybridization-based technology. Several new emerged techniques are described below (Figure 6.9).

1. **Spectral karyotyping (SKY):** SKY is a new technique of FISH in which chromosomes are visible in distinct colors due to their spectral feature from combination of painted probes and 5 fluorescent dyes. It is used to analyse all the 24 different chromosomes, complex chromosomal rearrangements, the origin of marker chromosomes and terminal translocations.

2. **Array comparative genomic hybridization (aCGH):** aCGH is based on the mechanism of complementary hybridization using small grid probes having known DNA region across the whole genetic material. It

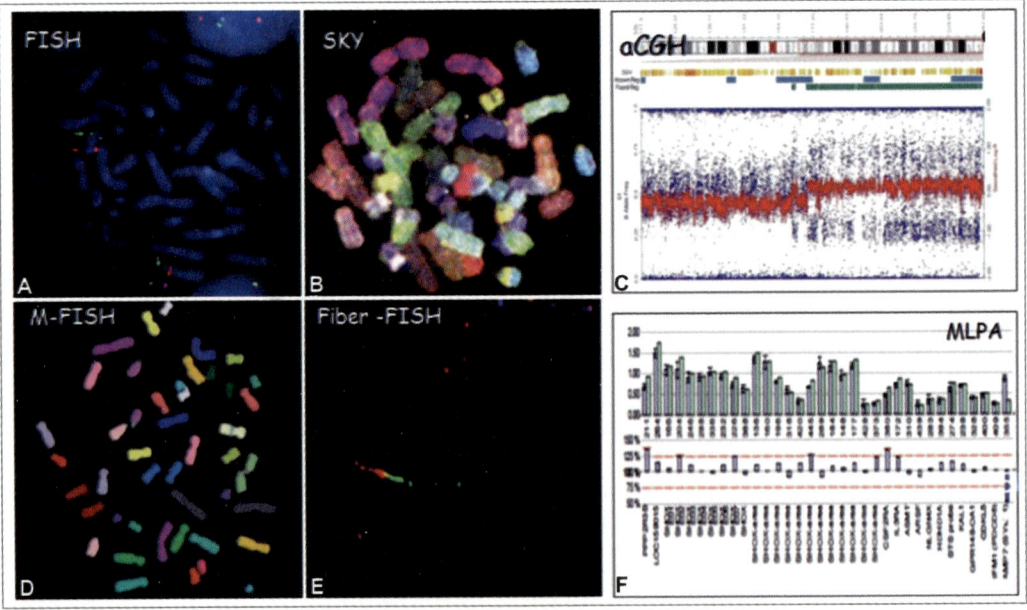

Figure 6.9: : Different types of molecular cytogenetic techniques
(A) FISH showing signals on chromosome15; **(B)** SKY metaphase with 24 different colors; **(C)** aCGH showing a 68 Mb duplication of chromosome 2q31.1-q37.3; **(D)** M-FISH showing ametaphase (*Courtesy*: Spiecher et al., (3)); **(E)** Fiber-FISH with a resolution of approx.1000 bp; **(F)** MLPA showing the SHOX gene probe

especially helps in detecting copy number variations like deletions, duplications and marker chromosomes.

3. **Multiple color FISH (M-FISH):** M-FISH is similar to SKY but the probes are labeled with the combinations of multiple fluorochromes with different fluorescence emission filter. All the 24 multicolored chromosomes are detected by a fluorescence microscope and it does not require additional imaging system.

4. **Fiber FISH:** Here the DNA probes are hybridized to extended chromatin fibers on a microscope slide. It is used for direct visualization of gene duplication and chromosome break points involved in translocation.

5. **Primed *in situ* labeling (PRINS):** Here reannealing of short oligonucleotide primers to target sequences *in situ* occurs. It is followed by elongation and simultaneous labeling of the target sequences with a fluorochrome. The target sequences are examined under a fluorescence microscope. PRINS primarily analyses small gene segment deletion or single copy of gene or aneuploidies.

6. **Multiplex ligation probe amplification (MLPA):** MLPA is a high throughput method developed to determine the copy number variations up to 50 genomic sequences in a single multiplex PCR-based reaction with a single primer pair. It can detect copy number variations.

Q 19. Explain the principle and procedure of chromosomal microarray analysis (CMA).

Ans. Chromosomal microarray (CMA) provides comprehensive genetic testing for most of the common chromosomal abnormalities and other genetic conditions which are not detected by conventional chromosomal analysis. It plays an important role in the detection of copy number variations (CNVs) (as small as 10 kb deletions and duplications in the genetic material).

The microarray resembles small grids having thousands of tiny probes consisting of small pieces of DNA from known locations of the 46 chromosomes. It compares the imbalances of chromosomal material of a control and a test sample.

The DNA microarray that is developed recently, allows simultaneous analysis of several million targets on a miniaturized scale. Short, fluorescently labeled oligonucleotides attached to a glass microscope slide are used to detect hybridization of target DNA under appropriate conditions. These days along with cytogenetic microarray, SNP microarray (array for the detection of polymorphism in population) is combined to identify various single nucleotide polymorphism.

Principle

It is based on the principle of complementary hybridization of DNA. Labeled patient DNA competes with differentially fluorescent labeled normal DNA (control) for hybridizing to all normal human metaphase chromosome (complementary DNA) on the grid. Using fluorescence microscopy and digital image processing, the ratio of the two is measured along the chromosomal axes.

Procedure

The CMA protocol involves the following steps and the detailed procedure is given in Figure 6.10.

Analysis

Computerized softwares are used for digital image analysis. Deviations from the normal ratio of 1 : 0 at certain chromosome regions represent amplification or deletion of genetic material. The test report tells the size, site and the number of lost or amplified bases (called copy number variations: CNVs) and the gene involved in this deleted or amplified region. The CNVs analysed are classified into various variants as shown in Figure 6.11.

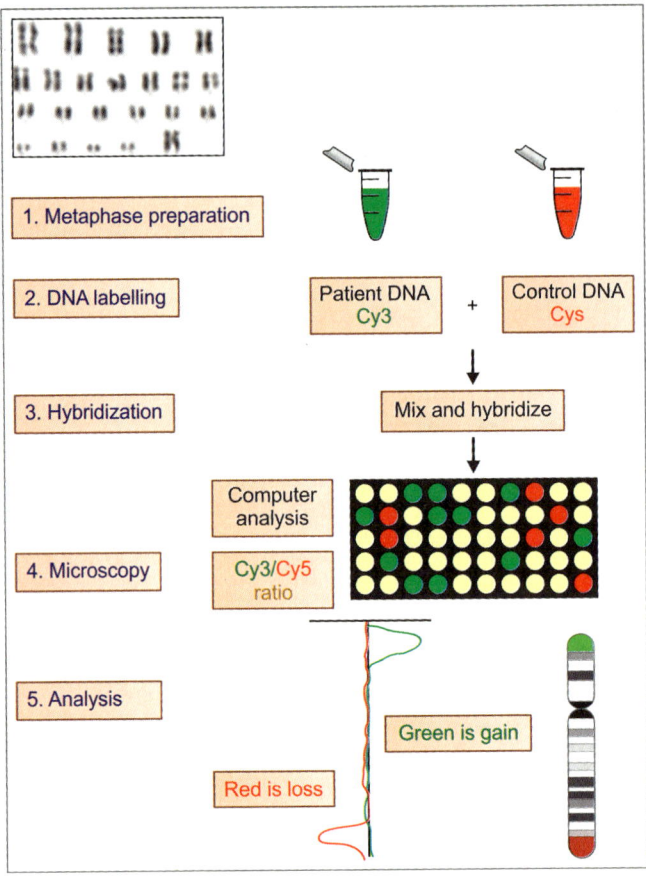

Figure 6.10: The procedural steps involved in CMA

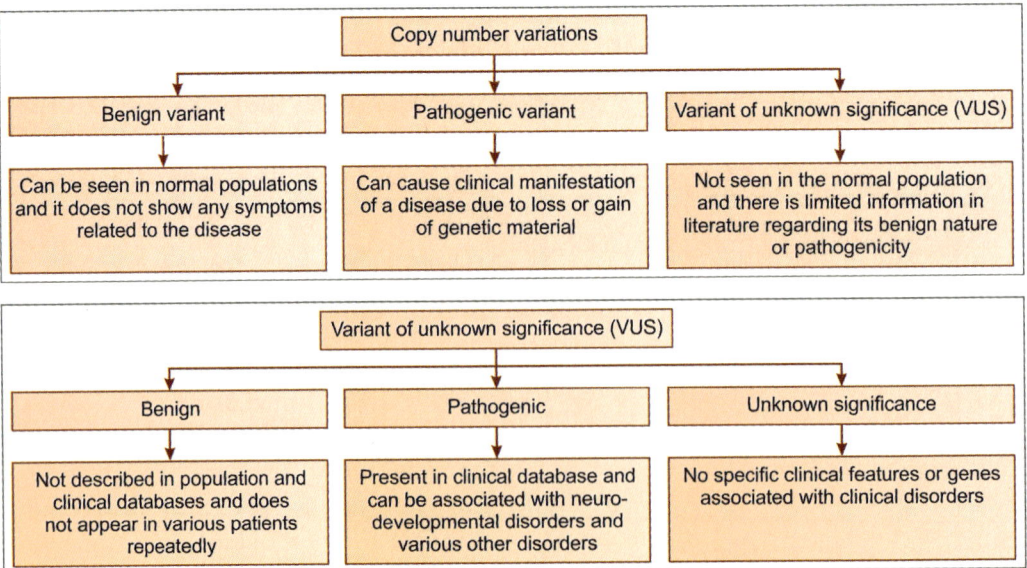

Figure 6.11: Classification of various copy number variants

Q 20. Write the applications of chromosomal microarray analysis (CMA).

Ans. The important basic clinical applications of CMA which can identify various copy number variations at high resolution than conventional cytogenetic tests across the whole genome are mentioned below.

Applications in Clinical Practice

1. The American Congress of Obstetricians and Gynecologists (ACOG) and the Society for Maternal-Fetal Medicine (SMFM) has recommended CMA as a first-level test for genetic analysis in cases with fetal structural anomalies (yield 8–10%).
2. Prenatally, in a structurally normal fetus if the invasive testing is done for any other indication, microarray is also recommended as its yield of detecting copy number variations in structurally normal fetuses is 1.7–2%.
3. CMA is the first line investigation as recommended by American College of Medical Genetics in undiagnosed pediatric patients of dysmorphism, intellectual disability, autism and multiple congenital abnormalities.
4. CMA is used for expression studies to look at the differential expression of thousands of genes at the mRNA level.
5. A combination of the two, SNP–CGH, allows the detection of copy-neutral genetic anomalies, such as uniparental disomy, low level mosaicism, triploidy and marker chromosome.
6. CMA has the ability to analyse DNA from nearly any tissue, including archived tissue or tissue that cannot be cultured.
7. CMA allows detection of cryptic abnormalities that are not identified by standard G-banded chromosome analysis.

Q 21. Write the limitations of chromosomal microarray analysis (CMA).

Ans. Though the chromosomal microarray is widely used in identifying the microstructural abnormalities across the whole genetic material with high efficiency, still there are some limitations which are described as:

Limitations

1. CMA cannot detect balanced chromosomal rearrangements like balanced translocations and inversions.
2. CMA does not provide information about the chromosomal mechanism of a genetic imbalance. For example, if there is a gain of an entire chromosome 13, CMA cannot distinguish between trisomy 13 and an unbalanced Robertsonian translocation, which has relevance for recurrence risk counseling. Therefore, a karyotype needs to be performed.
3. Low-level mosaicism may not be detected by CMA, and some arrays do not detect polyploidy.
4. It will not detect CNVs that are below the level of detection of the probe and that are not represented on the platform.
5. CMA will not detect point mutations within single genes.
6. Cost, lack of proper report interpretation guidelines, lot of new accumulated data and variants of unknown significance are also big concerns.

Q 22. Write the differences between unique features of different cytogenetic tests.

Ans. Chromosomal abnormalities can be detected by several molecular cytogenetic techniques like conventional karyotyping, fluorescence *in situ* hybridization (FISH) and array comparative genomic hybridization (aCGH). The applications, limitations and the chromosomal detection range along with resolution and sensitivity of each test is described in Table 6.1.

MOLECULAR GENETIC ANALYSIS
Aruna Priya Kamireddy ,
T Karthik Bharadwaj, Deepti Saxena

Q 23. What is DNA recombination technology? Write about different tools of recombinant DNA technology used in medicine.

Ans. DNA recombination technology is a DNA-based tool that cuts and joins DNA

TABLE 6.1: Differences between unique features of different cytogenetic tests

Technique	Karyotype	FISH	Array CGH
Principle	G banding technique in the metaphase stage	Complementary hybridization of labeled DNA	Complementary hybridization using small grid probes having known DNA region across the all chromosomes
Advantages	○ Detection of chromosomal numerical, structural rearrangements	○ Detects microdeletion syndromes and aneuploidy, triploidy, insertions, balanced and unbalanced translocation ○ Can be performed in interphase	○ Detects the copy number variations (10–100 kb size), marker chromosomes ○ SNP based array detects loss of heterozygosity region and consanguinity
Limitations	○ Resolution is limited. Lesser than 5–8 Mb cannot be identified. ○ Needs actively dividing cells ○ Laborious ○ Requires expertise ○ Difficulty in identifying telomeric abnormalities	○ Target specific and non-automated ○ Laborious ○ Require skill	○ Cannot detect balanced reciprocal translocations, inversions
Sensitivity & specificity	67.3% and 99% respectively	100% and 100% respectively	○ 100% for aneuploidies ○ 96–98% and 100% overall respectively
Mosaicism	Can be detected	Can detect greater than 10% to 15% (100 cells)	Can detect low level of mosaicism
Maternal cell contamination (MCC)	Can interfere with interpretation of prenatal sample	Rarely interferes with the interpretation	Cannot be identified by aCGH but SNP array can identify
Cost	Low	High	High
Turnaround time	2 weeks	2–3 days	5–7 working days

SNP: Single nucleotide polymorphism.

Note: See Appendix Tables 1 and 2 for ISCN symbols and different chromosomal abnormalities with their karyotype

from two different organisms and then introduced into a host organism to produce new genetic combinations of importance in science, medicine, agriculture and industry. The basis for DNA technology is editing the DNA according to our interest with ultimate goal of replacing the diseased gene to normal gene. The **DNA recombination technology**
tools used at different levels in constructing a recombinant DNA are:

1. **Enzymes (restriction enzymes, polymerases, and ligases):**
   ○ *Restriction enzymes* are the endonucleases of bacterial origin that cut the DNA at specific sites to facilitate the ligation of different nucleic acid strands to result in desired combination.

- *DNA polymerases:* Enzymes that synthesize double stranded DNA using a single stranded DNA template.
- *DNA ligases* join the DNA strands to form hybrids.
- *Taq DNA polymerase:* In polymerase chain reaction
- *Reverse transcriptase:* Converts mRNA to cDNA.

2. **Vectors:** Vehicles that carry genes of interest into the host organism and facilitates its multiplication to increase its copies.
   - Different vectors employed are plasmids, bacteriophages, cosmids, bacterial artificial chromosomes (BACs) and yeast artificial chromosomes (YACs).
3. **Host organism** is the cell in which the recombinant DNA is introduced.
4. **Probes** are small DNA or RNA sequences, complementary to DNA of interest for hybridization.

Q 24. Write a note on therapeutic applications of recombinant DNA technologies.

Ans. Recombinant DNA technology also known as genetic engineering refers to the process of combining DNA segments from two different sources. It has many therapeutic applications.

A. **Production of medications and vaccines:**
   1. *Insulin for diabetes:* Gene of interest is inserted into plasmids which are then incorporated into bacteria to produce insulin
   2. Factors VIII and IX for hemophilia A and B respectively
   3. Growth hormone for growth hormone deficiency
   4. Erythropoietin in anemia
   5. Interferons
   6. Granulocyte colony stimulating factor (G-CSF) and granulocyte monocyte colony stimulating factor (GM-CSF) during chemotherapy and bone marrow transplantation
   7. Monoclonal antibodies

8. Tissue plasminogen activator to dissolve clots in ischemic heart disease
9. Hepatitis B vaccine
10. Antibiotics

B. **Gene therapy** for adenosine deaminase: Severe combined immunodeficiency (ADA- SCID).

Q 25. Write the advantages of recombinant DNA technology.

Ans. **Advantages:**
1. Large-scale production of therapeutic agent
2. Cost reduction.
3. Low chance of immune reaction.
4. Production of desired protein.
5. Low chance of transmission of infections such as human immunodeficiency virus (HIV), hepatitis, etc.

Q 26. What are clinical indications for DNA analysis?

Ans. DNA analysis is done to detect the variants responsible for the phenotype in the proband or to detect other family members who are at risk for that disorder. The clinical indications for DNA analysis are mentioned below:

1. **For accurate disease diagnosis of monogenic disorders:** Beta thalassemia, Friedreich ataxia, Duchenne muscular dystrophy, etc.
2. **To prevent or delay a genetic disease:** Predictive testing in families with hereditary conditions, prenatal diagnosis and preimplantation genetic diagnosis is helpful in preventing the occurrence of disease in future generations.
3. **To know the reason for recurrent pregnancy losses:** Target mutation analysis in the fetal sample and couple carrier screening.
4. **In high-risk pregnancies with positive screening tests:** Amniocentesis followed by target mutation analysis.
5. **In organ transplantation to check host donor complementation:** Donor–recipient genotype match for certain SNPs.
6. **Hereditary cancers** testing.

7. **Precision medicine:** To know the best suit medicine to minimize the side effects of chemotherapy drugs.
8. **Pharmacogenomics:** Targeted therapy for oncology cases.

Q 27. Write the procedure of polymerase chain reaction (PCR).

Ans. Polymerase chain reaction (PCR) is the technique of *in vitro* amplification of a segment of DNA of specific interest or to produce millions of copies of DNA called amplicons, sometimes even a single copy.

Procedure: It is a three-step procedure which requires materials like water, buffer mixture, $MgCl_2$, deoxynucleotide triphosphate (dNTPs), primers and Taq polymerase enzyme (Figure 6.12).

Step 1: Denaturation

- ⊃ The two strands of the DNA get separated into single strand at high temperature (80°C) due to breakage of hydrogen bonds between the complementary DNA strands to facilitate the binding of primers.

Step 2: Annealing

- ⊃ Primers bind to the target DNA sequences and initiate polymerization at 40–70°C temperature which allows the hydrogen bonds to reform, facilitating complementary strands to hybridize.

Step 3: Extension

- ⊃ At **72°C** Taq DNA polymerase binds to the primed single stranded DNA and catalyses replication using the deoxyribonucleoside triphosphates present in the reaction mixture.
- ⊃ Elongation of the amplifying strand happens through extension of the 3'OH group.

These three steps make one complete cycle. It takes 20 to 40 such cycles to synthesize analyzable amount of DNA. The amplified DNA is seen in agarose or polyacrylamide gel electrophoresis and compared with the reference DNA.

Q 28. Write the applications and limitations of polymerase chain reaction (PCR).

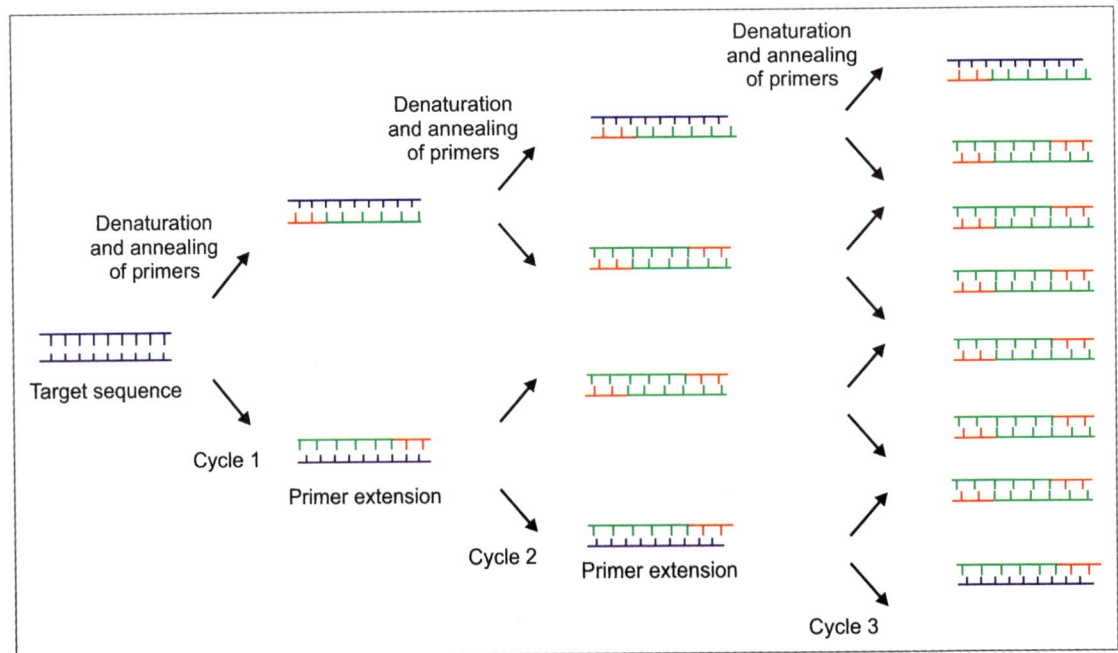

Figure 6.12: PCR amplification procedure

Ans. Applications: PCR is commonly used in biotechnology, microbiology, environmental science, medical science, dentistry, anthropology, food industry, animal and plant research.

➲ The diagnosis and screening of inherited, non-inherited and infectious human diseases.

➲ Identification and characterization of micro-organisms (infections) accurately in rapid time.

➲ PCR-based genetic markers such as STRs (short tandem repeats) and VNTRs (variable numbers of tandem repeats) are used in DNA fingerprint.

➲ Human leucocyte antigen (HLA) matching.

➲ Pharmacogenetics.

Limitations:

1. The DNA polymerase used in the PCR reaction can lead to mutations in the fragment generated.

2. The specificity of the generated PCR product may be altered by nonspecific binding of the primers to other similar sequences on the template DNA.

3. Some prior sequence is usually necessary to design the primers to generate a PCR.

Q 29. Write about the principles of various techniques of DNA analysis and their applications.

Ans.

1. **Nucleic Acid Hybridization**

➲ *Principle:* Nucleic acid hybridization is the formation of a stable duplex between two complementary strands of nucleic acids (DNA or RNA) by means of hydrogen bonding between base pairs. It can be carried out in a solution or with one component immobilized on a gel or, most commonly, on nitrocellulose paper.

➲ *Application:*

■ DNA-DNA hybridization measures the degree of genetic similarity between two organisms.

■ Amplifies the desired part of the genome for disease detection.

■ Fluorescence *in situ* hybridization is utilized in the diagnosis of genetic disorders.

2. **Southern Blot Hybridization**

➲ *Principle:* Southern blotting is a technique that involves the transfer of electrophoresis-separated DNA fragments to a carrier membrane, usually nitrocellulose and the subsequent detection of the target DNA fragment by autoradiography after hybridization with ^{32}P radiolabeled probe.

➲ *Application:*

■ Identifying specific DNA sequence in Fragile X syndrome and determination of the molecular weight and size of repeats

■ Preparation of restriction fragment length polymorphism (RFLP) maps

■ Detection of mutations, deletions or gene rearrangements in DNA

■ Criminal identification and DNA fingerprinting (VNTR)

■ Diagnosis of infectious diseases and prenatal diagnosis

■ Prognosis of cancer.

3. **Restriction Fragment Length Polymorphism (RFLP):** RFLP is enzymatic separation and identification of desired fragments of DNA that uses restriction endonuclease enzymes.

➲ *Principle:* Restriction endonucleases are enzymes that cut lengthy DNA into short pieces. Each restriction endonuclease targets different nucleotide sequence and therefore fragments are separated by electrophoresis.

➲ *Application:*

■ *Mutation analysis*

■ *Carrier testing*

■ *In forensic testing:* Criminal identification, paternity DNA fingerprinting.

■ *Genome mapping:* It is used for the analysis of unique patterns in DNA fragments, called variable number of tandem repeats (VNTRs).

4. **Amplification Refractory Mutation System (ARMS)**

➲ *Principle:* ARMS (allele-specific PCR) is based on the use of sequence-specific modified PCR primers for different alleles that allow amplification of test DNA only when the target allele is contained within the sample. It is a simple method for detecting any mutation involving single base changes or small deletions.

- *Application:*
  - Allele-specific PCR is an accurate method for single-gene disorders having SNPs. Example: Sickle cell anemia, thalassemia, cystic fibrosis
  - Can detect zygosity
  - Detection of HbS, *JAK2* and HIV mutation.

5. RT-qPCR-Real Time PCR

- *Principle:* The amount of the nucleic acid present in the sample is quantified using the fluorescent dye or using the fluorescent labeled oligonucleotides. Instead of looking at bands on a gel at the end of the reaction, the process is monitored in 'real-time'.

- *Application:*
  - Used in gene expression analysis, RNAi validation, microarray validation, pathogen detection, genetic testing and disease research.
  - *Gene expression analysis:* Cancer research (to see treatment response and relapse of disease) and drug research.
  - *Disease diagnosis and management:* Viral quantification.

6. Droplet Digital PCR (ddPCR)

- *Principle:* It is a digital PCR method utilizing a water-oil droplet system which serve the same function as individual test tubes or wells of a PCR. To know the mutation, the fluorescence in each droplet is measured or number of droplets with signal are counted.

- *Application:*
  - *Absolute quantification:* Ideal for target DNA measurements, viral load analysis and microbial quantification.
  - In measuring the acquired or inherited genomic alterations or in noninvasive prenatal testing.

7. Dot Blot Analysis

- *Principle:* Dot blot relies on the principle of binding of mutant sequence with mutant probe and normal sequence with normal probe and carrier with both the normal and mutant probe. It does not provide information regarding the size of the hybridized fragment.

- *Application:*
  - To identify a known protein in a biological sample.
  - Used to detect beta thalassemia mutation in proband and carrier individual.

8. Triplet Repeat Primed PCR (TP-PCR)

- *Principle:* TP-PCR usually uses three primers—one that is fluoresceinated and flanks the repeat region, a second that is complementary to the targeted repeat but carries a nonspecific tail sequence, and a third that is identical to the nonspecific tail sequence.

TP-PCR produces amplicons of increasing length by automated sequencer, which differs by the length of a repeat unit. It is rapid as well as the cost of test is also less.

- *Application:* It is being used for triplet repeat genetic disorders like Fragile X syndrome, myotonic dystrophy, etc.

Q 30. Explain the principle, procedure of multiplex ligation probe amplification (MLPA).

Ans. Multiplex ligation-dependent probe amplification (MLPA) is a variation of the multiplex polymerase chain reactions that permits multiple targets to be amplified with a single primer pair (forward and reverse), in a single reaction. It is in fact the probes that are amplified rather than the target sequences. Each probe set has a stuffer sequence of varying length. MLPA can differentiate sequences differing in a single nucleotide and up to 50 reactions can be multiplexed into a single reaction.

Procedure: (Figure 6.13)

The MLPA reaction can be divided into five major steps:

- **DNA denaturation and hybridization of MLPA probes:** After denaturation, the MLPA probes hybridize to the target sequence.
- **Ligation reaction:** The probes are then ligated using ligase. Probes which are not situated close together are not ligated and are further not amplified in the subsequent reactions.
- **PCR amplification:** With the help of primer pair all the ligated probes are amplified.
- **Capillary electrophoresis:** Separation of amplification products is done by capillary electrophoresis. Fluorescence obtained in the PCR reaction is directly proportional to the amount of target DNA and is used for relative quantification.
- **Data analysis:** Results of capillary electrophoresis are usually analysed using software like Coffalyser or GeneMarker®.

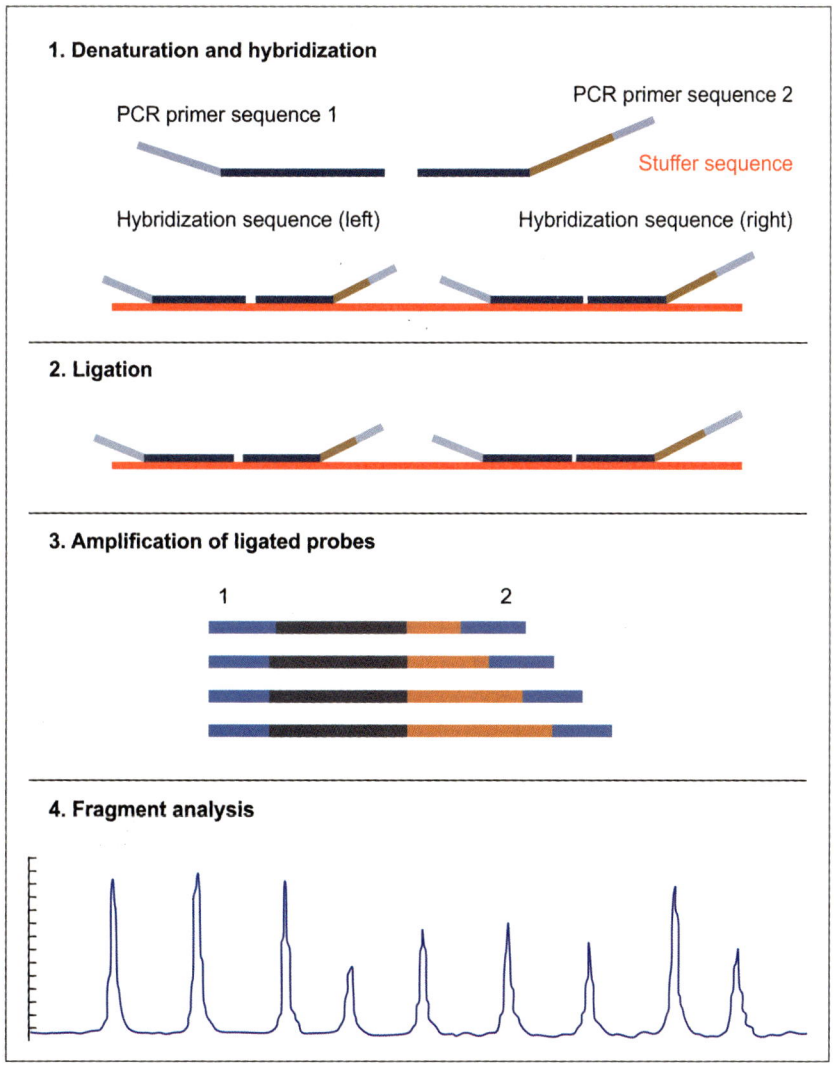

Figure 6.13: Principle of MLPA (*Sourced from* Stichen et al, MRC Holland)

$$\text{Result as mean ratio} = \frac{\text{Normalized peak height of patient}}{\text{Mean of normalized peak height of control}}$$

If > 1.35 duplication

If < 0.65 deletion

Q 31. Write the advantages and disadvantages of multiplex ligation probe amplification (MLPA).

Ans. Advantages:

- It is a robust, cheap and easily reproducible technique.
- It needs very little amount of DNA and does not need culturing of cells.
- Multiple targets and multiple samples can be tested at same time.
- MLPA is method of choice for known common microdeletion gene deletions/ duplications.
- Further modifications in it enables it for RNA quantification and methylation studies.

Disadvantages:

- It requires capillary electrophoresis for fragment resolution and specialized software for analysis.
- It requires prior knowledge of the mutation to design probes, i.e. the technique cannot be used to identify unknown changes.

- It does not tell the difference between size of deletions.
- All MLPA probes currently must be sourced.
- False positive results (deletions) can be obtained due to polymorphisms at the primer binding sites.

Q 32. Explain the clinical applications of multiplex ligation probe amplification (MLPA).

Ans. To detect known microdeletions and microduplications in various genetic disorders with overlapping symptoms.

- **Neurological disorders:** To detect mental retardation without identified cause, neurofibromatosis.
- **Neuromuscular disorders:** To detect deletion in Duchenne muscular dystrophy (70%) (Figure 6.14), spinal muscular atrophy.
- **Prenatal conditions:** To detect rapid aneuploidies.
- **Malignancies:** To detect various cancers like retinoblastoma and familial cancers.
- **Research purpose:** To detect imprinting disorders, mRNA detection

Q 33. Write a short note on principles of Sanger sequencing for DNA analysis.

Ans. DNA sequencing is the method to identify mutation in the single or multiple genes by sequencing of nucleotide base, one by one. Sanger sequencing (Figure 6.15) is the gold standard for sequencing single gene. It is also known as dideoxy sequencing and was

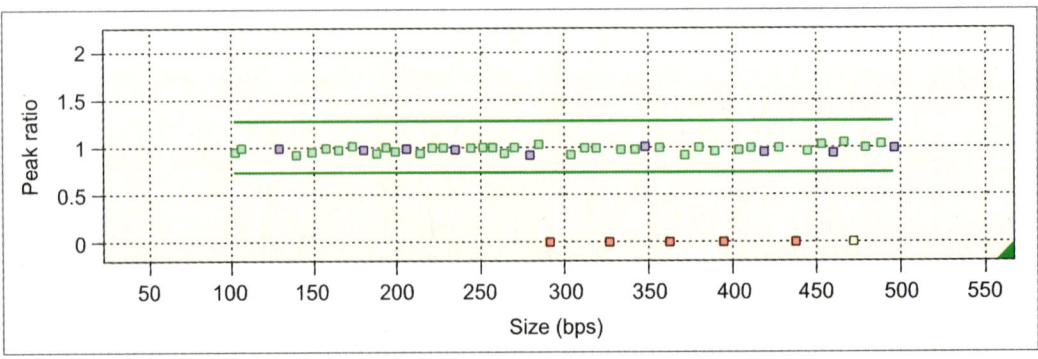

Figure 6.14: : MLPA: Representative picture showing deletion of exons 45–50 in the *DMD* gene

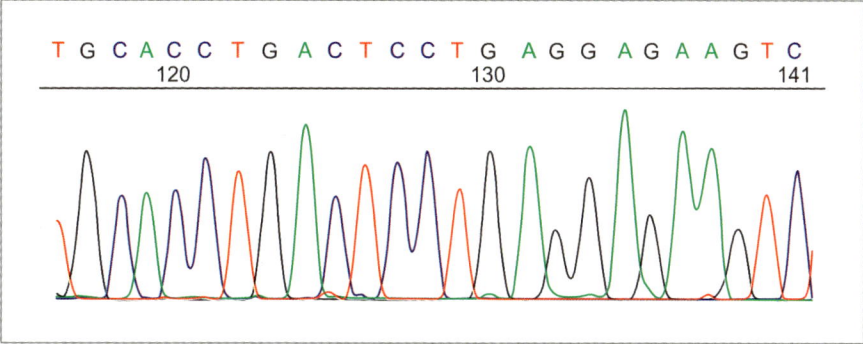

Figure 6.15: Sanger sequencing—electropherogram

invented by Frederick Sanger in 1977. Its steps are as follows:

- First target sequence is amplified by PCR to produce many copies.
- Then, a single primer is used for initiation of DNA synthesis by DNA polymerase.
- Dideoxy nucleotides (ddNTPs) in combination with deoxy nucleotides are supplemented during the sequencing reaction to prevent extension of DNA strand by DNA polymerase.
- These dideoxy nucleotides are fluorescently labeled and the multiple fragments generated by the sequencing reaction are resolved by length using capillary electrophoresis.
- The fluorescent signal indicates the type of nucleotide while the length of the DNA fragment containing it gives an indication of the position of the nucleotide on the target DNA.
- It is the most commonly used method for sequencing short stretches of DNA.

Because of its reliance on electrophoresis, only fragments up to 1 kb can be sequenced at a time.

Q 34. Write a note on principles of next generation sequencing.

Ans. Next generation sequencing (NGS Figure 6.16) is a high throughput; massively parallel sequencing technology where multiple genes/genomic regions are sequenced simultaneously at low cost per base. The development of microchip/microfluidic technologies and high-resolution optics enable great inroads for these technologies in the diagnostic field. Despite the differences in sequencing chemistries of various platforms, the basic steps are common.

Steps:

I. **Template preparation:** The DNA is fragmented into millions of fragments initially and after addition of adapters, these

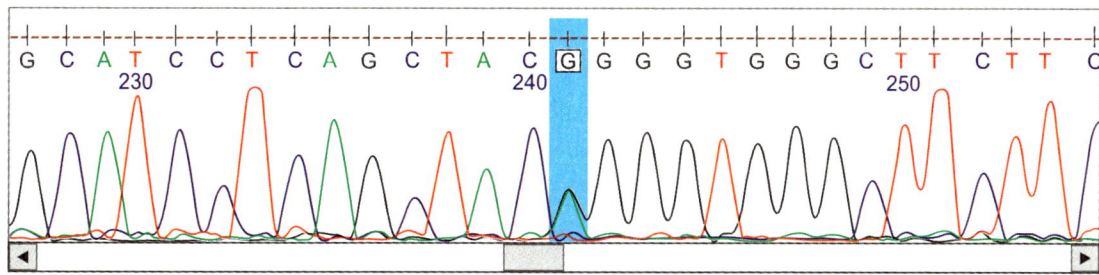

Figure 6.16: Achondroplasia: Common sequence variation: NM_000142: Heterozygous *FGFR3:c.1138G >A(G380R). (Courtesy: Dr Kausik Mandal,* SGPGIMS, Lucknow)

fragments are amplified either on a chip or in an emulsion.

II. **Sequencing and imaging:** These clonally amplified templates are sequenced at one go and the signals obtained during the process are used to generate the sequence of each fragment.

III. **Bioinformatics analysis:** These sequences are bioinformatically identified and aligned to the reference genome and identification of the variations in the genomic sequence of the organism from the reference genome is done. Then the significance of these variations, i.e. their association with causality of the phenotype is inferred from available clinical databases. (*See* Appendix)

Q 35. Write differences between Sanger sequencing and next generation sequencing.

Ans.

Q 36. Write a note on whole genome sequencing, whole exome sequencing and clinical exome sequencing.

Ans. Various platforms for DNA sequencing are:

1. **Whole genome sequencing:** Sequencing of the entire genome of the organism is called whole genome sequencing. Though it gives comprehensive information regarding the genome of the organism, it is expensive and throws up lot of bioinformatic challenges.

2. **Whole exome sequencing and targeted panel testing:** The use of NGS for mendelian disorders became more feasible after the development of exome sequencing and targeted panel testing at low cost. Here, all the coding portions of the genome (~20000 genes) of interest are captured and then sequenced.

The principles of targeted capturing of regions of interest in the genome have

	Sanger sequencing	Next generation sequencing
Throughput	Single locus sequenced at a time	Massive parallel sequencing where multiple loci are sequenced at a go
	One electropherogram (a ladder of DNA sequence) generated per locus	Multiple reads generated for each locus
	Maximum length of sequencing is about 1000 base pairs	Read length ranges from ~50 bp in short read sequencing technologies to few kilobases to even mega bases in third generation sequencing technologies.
Sequencing costs	Low cost per test	Overall, the test is expensive
Diagnostic utilities, accuracy and other technical aspects	Information regarding the sequence of interest needs to be available	No prior information regarding the sequence is necessary
	Specifically designed primers can exclude pseudogenes	Difficult to identify variants in pseudogenes separately
	Cannot detect large heterozygous deletions	Can detect CNV analysis, mosaicism
	Considered gold standard for sequencing	Accuracy has improved over the years, but is still more error prone
	Useful for sequencing specific and small regions/genes of the genome. *Example:* Beta thalassemia, achondroplasia	Useful when multiple areas of the genome have to be explored in one go. *Example:* Retinitis pigmentosa, osteogenesis imperfecta, etc.

been exploited to develop smaller and yet extremely effective panels for more specific genetic testing and for various overlapping phenotypes (*Examples:* Cardiomyopathy panel, muscular dystrophy panels, etc.). These have not only led to the drop in price but has also decreased the unnecessary bioinformatic load seen in nonspecific testing.

3. **Clinical exome sequencing or mendeliome** is one such panel, where about 5000 disease-causing genes responsible for mendelian disorders are captured. However, these targeted sequencing approaches have certain shortcomings like:
   - Non-uniform coverage of the genes
   - Amplification biases
   - Lack of coverage of noncoding regions
   - Need to update the panels frequently due to discovery of new genes, etc.

With decreasing costs of sequencing and improved bioinformatic processing, whole genome sequencing, which is devoid of these limitations is likely to replace the targeted panel testing in the near future.

Q 37. Write a note on advantages and disadvantages of whole genome sequencing compared to whole exome sequencing.

Ans. Advantages of whole genome sequencing (WGS) over exome sequencing:

1. **Entire genome is covered including**
   - Coding areas/exons
   - Untranslated regions and regulatory regions like promoter regions, enhancer and suppressor motifs
   - Non-coding areas/introns/intergenic regions
   - Mitochondrial genome

2. More uniform coverage of clinically important regions is obtained.
3. Copy number variation (CNV) and single nucleotide variant analysis and structural variation analysis especially with betterment in 3rd generation long read sequencing technologies from Oxford Nanopore and PacBio are more accurate.
4. Balanced rearrangements and break points down to the last nucleotide can be identified.
5. Susceptibility to duplicates, PCR errors and capture biases are minimized.
6. More unbiased coverage of the coding regions with lesser false positives.
7. Higher accuracy in predicting repeat expansions.

Disadvantages of WGS over exome sequencing

1. It is still much costlier when compared to exome analysis.
2. As more than 98% of the disease-causing variations are expected to be present in the coding regions of the genome, sequencing the non-coding regions of the genome may not greatly increase the diagnostic rate.
3. Poses significant challenges in bioinformatics analysis, filtering thousands to lakhs of rare variants and long-term data storage.
4. The problems posed by variants of unknown significance and secondary findings.
5. Ethical issues and psychosocial effects of results of tests.
6. It is difficult to prove causality of a possible disease-causing variant identified in non-coding areas with the currently available scientific tools.

At present it may be best suited for research settings rather than for routine diagnosis.

Q 38. What are different methods for detecting copy number variations in the human genome?

Ans.

Methods	Copy number variations	Abnormalities
FISH	Known	o Microdeletion syndromes
Chromosomal microarray	Known/ unknown	o Single nucleotide variations/copy number variations o Intellectual disability, autism and fetuses with multiple malformations
Real-time PCR	Known	o Microdeletion/Microduplications
Quantitative fluorescent PCR	Known	o Rapid aneuploidy detection in prenatal samples
Multiplex ligation-dependent probe amplification (MLPA)	Known	o Common microdeletion syndrome and Duchenne muscular dystrophy
Digital droplet PCR	Known	o Copy number variations
Next generation sequencing (NGS)	Known/ unknown	o Copy number variations single nucleotide variations, break points down to last nucleotide o Noninvasive pregnancy testing

BIBLIOGRAPHY

1. Arsham MS, Barch MJ, Lawce HJ. 2017. The AGT Cytogenetics Laboratory Manual. 4th edition.
2. Bridge JA. Advantages and limitations of cytogenetic, molecular cytogenetic, and molecular diagnostic testing in mesenchymal neoplasms. J OrthopSci (2008) 13:273–282 DOI 10.1007/s00776–007-1215–1.
3. Gardener RJM, Sutherland GR, Shaffer LG. 2012. Chromosome Abnormalities and Genetic Counseling. 4th edition. Oxford University Press.
4. Jordan M, Simons A, Schmid M. 2016. An international system for human cytogenomic nomenclature.
5. Jorde LB, Carey JC, Bamshad MJ. 2009. Medical Genetics, 6th edition.
6. Khan S, Ullah MW, Siddique R, Nabi G, Manan S, Yousaf M, Hou H. Role of Recombinant DNA4.genomic hybridization in obstetrics. ObstetGynecolClin North Am. 2010 Mar;37(1):71–85doi: 10.1016/j.ogc.2010.02.001
7. Usha R Dutta. Precision in chromosome identification with leads in molecular cytogenetics: An illustrated review. Journal of Pediatric Genetics 2014; 3: 1–7.

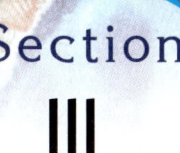

Section III

General Treatment and Prevention of Genetic Disorders

Treatment and Prevention of Genetic Disorders

Deepti Saxena, Prajnya Ranganath, Manisha Goyal, Shreya Tanneru, Suresh Thomas, Komal Uppal

TREATMENT OF GENETIC DISORDERS
DEEPTI SAXENA, PRAJNYA RANGANATH

Q 1. What are various conventional methods currently used for treatment of genetic disorders?

Ans. Treatment of various genetic disorders includes various multidisciplinary strategies, the curative or symptomatic for same, aimed at reducing symptoms and preventing future complications.

A. **Environmental modification** such as lifestyle or dietary changes, avoiding exposure to certain drugs or chemicals can prevent progression of disease. Examples:
   i. Lifestyle and dietary changes for multi-factorial disorders, such as coronary artery disease, hypertension, diabetes, etc.
   ii. Avoiding certain drugs such as prima-quine and fava beans, etc. in glucose-6-phosphate dehydrogenase deficiency (G6PD).
   iii. Cigarette smoking should be avoided in alpha-1 antitrypsin deficiency.
   iv. Barbiturates should be avoided in porphyria.

B. **Medical management:** Genetic disorders with known underlying biochemical defect can be treated by supplementation of various products. *Example:*
   i. *Replacement of end product:* Thyroxine supplementation in case of congenital hypothyroidism, cortisol in congenital adrenal hyperplasia, factor replacement in hemophilia.
   ii. *Enzyme or co-factor replacement therapy:* Supplementation of the deficient enzyme in mucopolysaccharidosis type I, II, Gaucher disease, Fabry disease, etc. or B_6 in homocystinuria.
   iii. *Augmentation of deficient enzyme:* Phenobarbitone can induce the activity of hepatic glucuronyl transferase reducing the levels of unconjugated bilirubin in Crigler-Najjar syndrome type 2.
   iv. *Reducing enzyme activity:* In familial hypercholesterolemia, statins can be given.
   v. *Inhibition of receptors:* Transforming growth factors in Marfan syndrome.
   vi. *Substrate reduction:* Accumulation of a toxic material which cannot be metabolized can be treated by reducing exposure to the substrate. *Example:* In phenylketonuria and galactosemia mental retardation can be prevented by reducing the dietary intake of phenylalanine and galactose respectively.
   vii. *Removal of toxic material:* In Wilson disease, excessive copper is removed by chelating agents, such as penicillamine. In urea cycle defect, sodium benzoate is given to remove ammonia.

viii. *Supportive treatment:* Blood transfusion in thalassemia and other hemoglobino-pathies and pancreatic enzymes in cystic fibrosis.

C. **Surgical management:** Some congenital malformations can be treated surgically like:
   i. Pyloric stenosis, congenital heart disease, cleft lip and palate.
   ii. Reconstructive surgery of virilized external genitalia
   iii. Retinoblastoma, Wilms tumor, etc.
   iv. Prophylactic surgery in case of familial cancer syndromes, such as hereditary breast and ovarian cancer, colorectal cancer, etc.
   v. Plasmapheresis in hereditary hemo-chromatosis to remove extra iron.

D. **Transplantation:** Organ or tissue transplantation from matched donors can provide a permanent alternative source for deficient gene product. For example:
   i. Hematopoietic stem cell transplantation in thalassemia, immunodeficiency syndromes, etc.
   ii. Liver transplantation in metabolic liver diseases.

E. **Gene therapy:** Correction of underlying genetic defect by replacement or modification of defective gene.

F. **Supportive management:** Most genetic disorders need supportive treatment. *Example*:
   i. In Duchenne muscular dystrophy, physiotherapy to prevent joint contractures,
   ii. Vaccination to prevent chest infections,
   iii. Provision of support for schooling, mobility aids may help in improving the quality of life.

G. **Genetic counseling:** It is an integral part of treatment of genetic disorders and includes providing information to the family regarding treatment, prognosis, long-term complications, risk of recurrence, availability of prenatal or presympto-matic diagnosis and treatment to family members.

Q 2. Describe various levels of treatment relevant to genetic diseases with corresponding strategy used at each level.

Ans. The various strategies for treatment of genetic disorders vary according to the underlying disorder and the level at which the available treatment can be targeted (Figure 7.1).

Q 3. Write a note on substrate reduction strategies in the management of various metabolic disorders.

Ans. Substrate reduction strategies:
1. **Dietary restriction:** Accumulation of a toxic molecule can be prevented by reducing its dietary intake. *For example*, reduced intake of phenylalanine in phenylketonuria and galactose in galactosemia.
2. **Reducing endogenous production of substrates:** In amino acidopathies and urea cycle disorders, administration of no-protein, high calorie diet reduces the breakdown of endogenous proteins and prevents the accumulation of toxic metabolites.
3. **Substrate reduction therapy (SRT):** Use of small molecules to reduce the synthesis of molecules that could not be catabolized due to the deficient enzyme. This treatment strategy is particularly useful in disorders with some residual enzyme activity. It can be used as a stand-alone treatment, as adjuvant along with ERT or as maintenance therapy.
   Example: Miglustat in Fabry disease and adult Gaucher disease type 1.
4. **Accelerated removal of substrates:** It can be done by dialysis in urea cycle defect or use of certain drugs such as penicillamine in Wilson disease.

Advantages:
1. Oral treatment is possible.
2. Less chances of immune reaction.

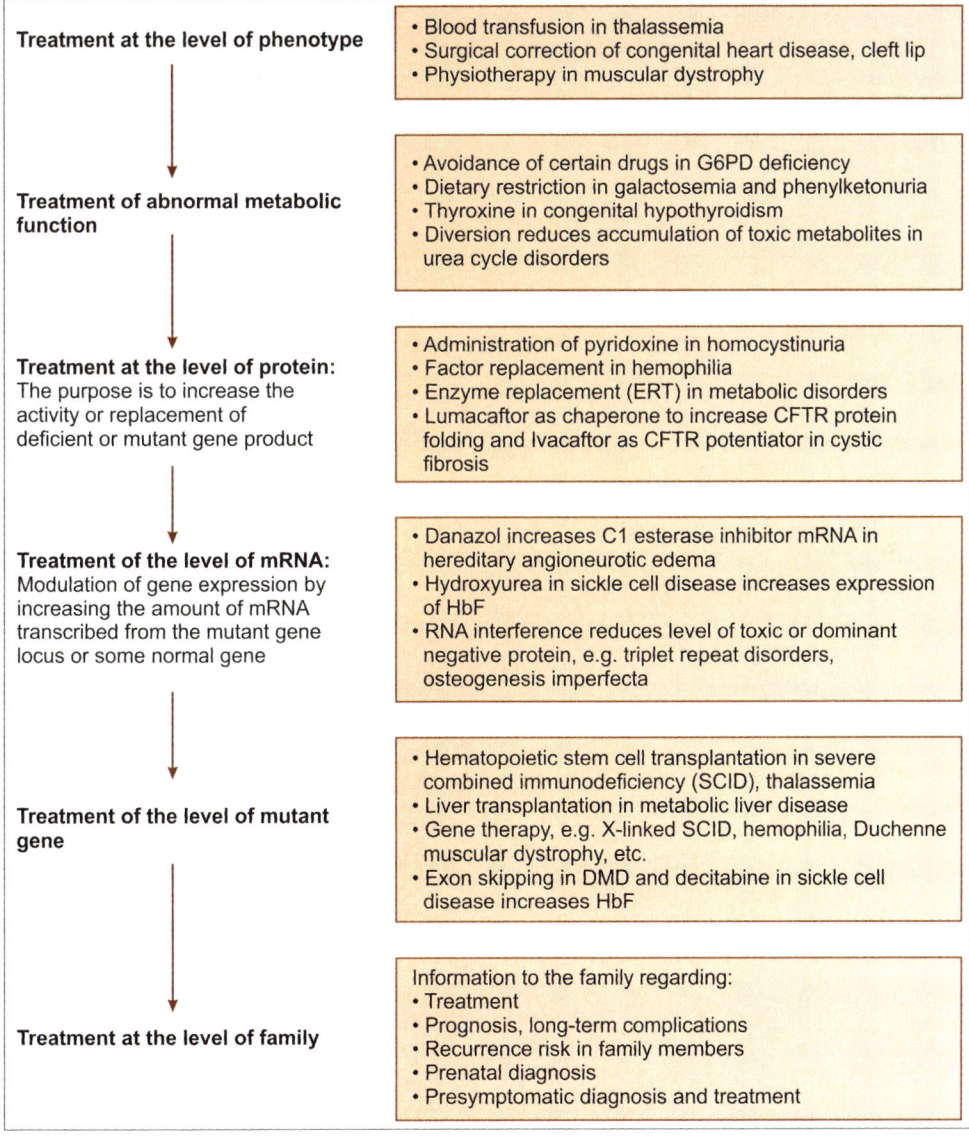

Treatment at the level of phenotype
- Blood transfusion in thalassemia
- Surgical correction of congenital heart disease, cleft lip
- Physiotherapy in muscular dystrophy

Treatment of abnormal metabolic function
- Avoidance of certain drugs in G6PD deficiency
- Dietary restriction in galactosemia and phenylketonuria
- Thyroxine in congenital hypothyroidism
- Diversion reduces accumulation of toxic metabolites in urea cycle disorders

Treatment at the level of protein: The purpose is to increase the activity or replacement of deficient or mutant gene product
- Administration of pyridoxine in homocystinuria
- Factor replacement in hemophilia
- Enzyme replacement (ERT) in metabolic disorders
- Lumacaftor as chaperone to increase CFTR protein folding and Ivacaftor as CFTR potentiator in cystic fibrosis

Treatment of the level of mRNA: Modulation of gene expression by increasing the amount of mRNA transcribed from the mutant gene locus or some normal gene
- Danazol increases C1 esterase inhibitor mRNA in hereditary angioneurotic edema
- Hydroxyurea in sickle cell disease increases expression of HbF
- RNA interference reduces level of toxic or dominant negative protein, e.g. triplet repeat disorders, osteogenesis imperfecta

Treatment of the level of mutant gene
- Hematopoietic stem cell transplantation in severe combined immunodeficiency (SCID), thalassemia
- Liver transplantation in metabolic liver disease
- Gene therapy, e.g. X-linked SCID, hemophilia, Duchenne muscular dystrophy, etc.
- Exon skipping in DMD and decitabine in sickle cell disease increases HbF

Treatment at the level of family
Information to the family regarding:
- Treatment
- Prognosis, long-term complications
- Recurrence risk in family members
- Prenatal diagnosis
- Presymptomatic diagnosis and treatment

Figure 7.1: Various levels of treatment relevant to genetic diseases with corresponding strategy

3. Can cross blood–brain barrier, however clinical effect needs to be validated yet.

Limitations:

1. Adverse events, such as diarrhea, tremors.
2. Less effective than enzyme replacement therapy.

Q 4. Write a brief note on recent therapeutic advances in enzyme replacement therapy (ERT).

Ans. Genetic disorders such as lysosomal storage disorders (LSDs) and severe combined immunodeficiency (SCID) related to adenosine deaminase (ADA) deficiency are caused by deficient or absent production of enzymes in the body, due to mutations in genes coding for these enzymes.

Definition: Enzyme replacement therapy (ERT) is a treatment modality that involves periodic administration of sufficient amounts of the deficient enzyme to act efficiently at the intracellullar sites and to effectively clear the accumulated substrate in the patient and thereby mitigate the manifestations and modify the natural course of the disease. Early treatment is recommended to prevent irreversible damage. However, ERT can be given in later stages also to slow or prevent progression of disease.

Synthesis of recombinant enzymes:

- The enzymes are synthesized using recombinant DNA technology in human-derived fibroblasts, animal cell lines (such as Chinese hamster ovary cells) or plant cells.
- Post-translational modification of the recombinant enzymes through linkage of mannose or mannose-6-phosphate (M6P) residues to the oligosaccharide chains enables their internalization and targeting to the lysosomal compartment.

Diseases for which ERT is available

The lysosomal storage disorders (LSDs) for which ERT is currently available and approved are:

- Gaucher disease (imiglucerase, velaglucerase alfa)
- Pompe disease (alglucosidase alfa)
- Fabry disease (agalsidase alfa and beta), lysosomal acid lipase deficiency (sebelipase alpha).
- Mucopolysaccharidoses (MPS) types I (laronidase), II (idursulfase), IVA (elosulfase alpha) and VI (galsulfase) where the ERT is administered through periodic (once a week or once in 2 weeks) intravenous infusions.
- Late infantile type neuronal ceroid lipofuscinosis (NCL) type 2 (cerliponase alfa), directly administered into the brain through intraventricular infusion.
- ERT is also available for ADA deficiency.

Limitations of ERT

- **Cost is the most important drawback:** Lifelong need for repeated infusions. If ERT is stopped, there is rapid re-accumulation of substrate and worsening of clinical condition.
- Inability to reach the central nervous system and few other tissues due to the blood–brain barrier and lack of the M6P receptor.
- Development of antibodies to the drug.
- Can cause secondary dysregulation of cellular metabolism.
- There is dose-dependent delivery of enzymes depending on the biodistribution to various organs, so high doses are required.

Research is ongoing to develop newer strategies of enzyme replacement to overcome these limitations.

Q 5. **Write the principle and sources of harvesting and storing stem cells. What is the rationale behind stem cell therapy?**

Ans. **Principle of stem cell transplantation:** Stem cells can differentiate into different cell types and can also replicate themselves, referred to as **potency**. It can be used to treat various disorders, such as malignancies, hemoglobinopathies, ophthalmologic conditions, etc. The principle is to ablate the immune system of patient and replace it with stem cells from either the patient (autologous) or from HLA matched donor (allogenic).

They can be classified into various types based on origin:

1. **Embryonic stem cells:** Pleuripotent cells that can differentiate into cells of any of the three germ layers (Figure 7.2).
2. **Fetal stem cells:** Multipotent cells that can differentiate into small number of cell types depending on their origin.
   Example: Hematopoietic, mesenchymal, endothelial, epithelial and neural stem cells.
3. **Umbilical cord stem cells:** Multipotent cells found in cord blood and tissue.
4. **Adult stem cells (somatic stem cells):** Multipotent cells found in various tissues like brain, bone marrow, skeletal muscles, skin, teeth, etc. can be reprogrammed with the use of specific transcription factors to behave as embryonic stem cells, known as **induced pluripotent stem cells (iPSCs)**.

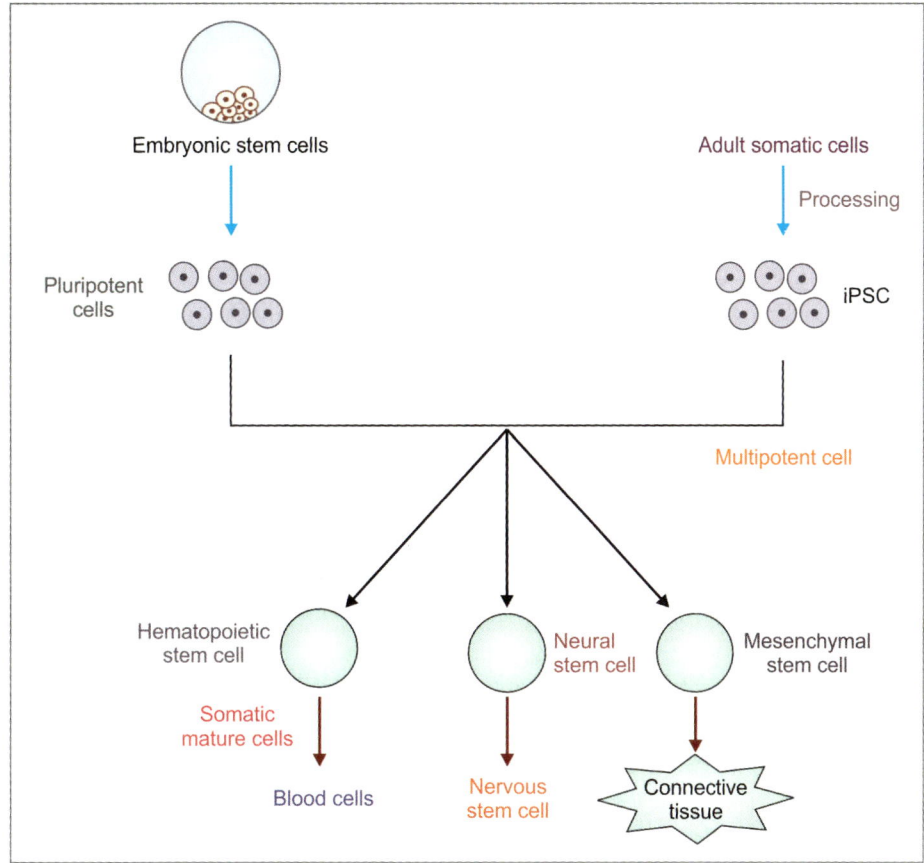

Figure 7.2: Differentiating of embryonic and somatic stem cells into various cell types

Sources of harvesting stem cells are:
1. Bone marrow
2. Peripheral blood
3. Cord blood
4. Stem cell banking

Storage of stem cells

It helps in easy transportation, easy availability of stem cells. They should be cryopreserved as soon as possible after collection. A common cryopreservative used is dimethylsulfoxide. After freezing, they can be stored for a long period of time. Umbilical cord blood stem cells can be stored for prolonged period of time after proper cryopreservation. For this purpose there are now several public and private cord blood banks all-around the world and this is known as **umbilical cord blood banking.** The stored stem cells can be used in stem cell transplantation in unrelated recipients also and act as a large repository for the same. The main advantage is that the search time for appropriate donor is reduced. Also, there are lower chances of GVHD. The main disadvantage of using cord blood stem cells is that there is lesser number of absolute stem cell count. Due to low dose of stem cells, it can cause delayed engraftment.

Rationale of stem cell transplantation:

In this procedure, a person's unhealthy native bone marrow cells are replaced with healthy stem cells. The native stem cells are destroyed using chemotherapy, radiation or a combination of both and healthy donor stem cells are infused. The primary goal of this procedure is to treat an underlying hematological disorder or malignancy. When umbilical cord blood is used as source of stem cells, there is lesser chance of graft versus host disease (GVHD).

Q 6. How is the patient prepared for stem cell therapy?

Ans. Preparation of patient for stem cell therapy:

1. **Selection of donor:** HLA typing is done to select potential donors. Best donors are matched related followed by matched unrelated, cord blood and then haploidentical donors.

2. **Collection of stem cells:** If peripheral blood is used as source of stem cells, then mobilization of stem cells is done initially. Certain medications are used to increase the number of stem cells such as Granulocyte-colony stimulating factor (G-CSF). Chemotherapy can also be used for mobilization of stem cells, known as chemoembolization. Usually stem cells are collected from bone marrow. Multiple aspirations are done from iliac crest under local or general anesthesia.

3. **Conditioning regimen:** It includes adminis-tration of chemotherapy with or without total body radiation. It depends on source of stem cells, indication for transplantation, comorbidities and previous exposure to radiation. Goal is to ablate the recipient's own immune system and bone marrow so that infused stem cells can engraft successfully.

4. **Infusion:** After patient preparation, fresh or cryopreserved donor stem cells are infused intravenously. Quality measures to ensure adequate number of CD34+ cells are performed. Prophylaxis against various infections is also provided.

5. **Monitoring:** Blood counts are monitored daily for engraftment which is defined as 3 consecutive days with neutrophil count more than 0.5×10^9/L.

Q 7. Write the various indications for stem cell transplantation.

Ans. Indications for stem cell transplantation:

1. Regenerative medicine: Spinal cord injury
2. Ischemic cardiomyopathy
3. Musculoskeletal disorders: Mesenchymal stem cells can be used in osteogenesis imperfecta.
4. Retinal disorders
5. Severe combined immune deficiency (SCID) syndrome.
6. Hematological malignancies such as multiple myeloma, leukemia and lymphoma: Hematopoietic stem cells (HSCT)
7. Aplastic anemia: HSCT
8. Hemoglobinopathies such as thalassemia, sickle cell anemia: HSCT
9. Inborn errors of metabolism such as Hurler disease
10. Alpha 1 antitrypsin can be corrected by iPSCs from fibroblast
11. Corneal epithelial (Limbal) stem cell for limbal stem cell deficiency as in corneal infections, trauma, etc.

Q 8. Write about the important compli-cations of stem cell therapy.

Ans. Complications can be divided into three categories as listed below:

A. **Occurring during pre-engraftment period:**
   1. Pancytopenia
   2. Gastrointestinal toxicity
   3. Hepatic sinusoidal obstruction syndrome
   4. *Infections:* Gram-positive and negative bacteria, herpes simplex virus, candi-diasis and invasive aspergillosis

B. **Occurring during early post-engraftment period (0–100 days):**
   1. Acute graft versus host disease (GVHD)
   2. *Infections:* Pneumocystis, cytome-galovirus, common respiratory viruses

C. **Occurring during late post-engraftment period (>100 days):**
   1. Chronic graft versus host disease
   2. Sicca syndrome
   3. Chronic obstructive or restrictive lung diseases

4. Infections

5. Relapse of underlying disorders

6. Increased risk for cardiovascular disorders, metabolic dysfunctions, secondary malignancies, gonadal dysfunction and neuropsychiatric manifestations.

Q 9. Explain gene editing with the help of diagram.

Ans. Genome editing or gene editing refers to the technique of creating a desired sequence alteration in a gene or a genomic region.

Principle of gene editing (Figure 7.3): Double stranded breaks (DSB) in DNA induced by specific nucleases can stimulate the endogenous DNA repair machinery. Breaks in DNA can be repaired by either of the two mechanics: **Homology directed repair (HDR) or non-homologous end joining (NHEJ).** In HDR, repair occurs in a template dependent manner using a homologous sequence. In NHEJ, there is direct joining of cleaved ends. Repair by NHEJ is error-prone and results in insertion or deletion of nucleotides at the site of break. These editing systems are delivered into cells as plasmids through viral vectors or as mRNA transcripts.

Q 10. Write about various strategies that are used for genome editing.

Ans. Various strategies that are being used for genome editing include:

1. **Gene knockout:** NHEJ is more suitable for achieving gene knockout. In Duchenne muscular dystrophy introduction of targeted indels can lead to restoration of reading frame.

2. **Gene deletion:** Deletion of erythroid specific enhancer BCL11A by simultaneous introduction of two DSBs by NHEJ for the treatment of hemoglobinopathies.

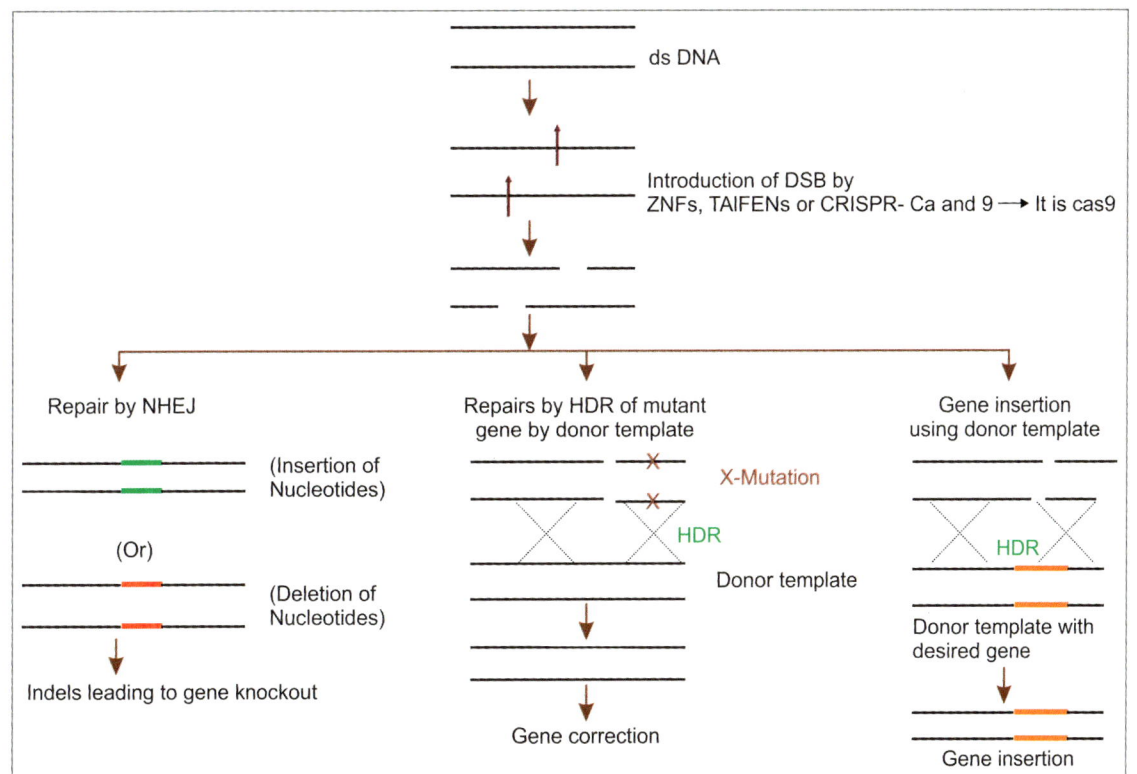

Figure 7.3: Mechanism of gene editing using various nucleases

CRISPR: Cas9 system, transcription activator-like effector nucleases (TALENs), zinc-finger nucleases (ZFNs), homology directed repair (HDR), non-homologous end joining (NHEJ)

3. **Gene correction therapies:** HDR in the presence of a donor template, helps in precise base correction.
   Example: Gene correction in T-cells and CD34+ hematopoietic stem cells in severe combined immunodeficiency.

4. **Gene insertion:** The donor template contains the desired gene insert flanked with sequences homologous to the site of DSB.
   Example: Insertion of missing exons in case of Duchenne muscular dystrophy.

Q 11. Write the various technologies and challenges faced with genome editing.

Ans. **Various technologies** used for genome editing include:

1. Clustered regularly interspaced short palindromic repeats: CRISPR-associated protein 9 (CRISPR-Cas9) system.
2. Transcription activator-like effector nucleases (TALENs)
3. Zinc-finger nucleases (ZFNs)
4. Homing endonucleases or meganucleases.

Challenges with genome editing

- The main challenges include the safe and efficient delivery of genome editing components to the target cells.
- Risk of off-target mutagenesis.
- Long-term regulation of gene function.

Q 12. What are the uses of genome editing?

Ans. **Uses of genome editing:**

Genome editing, especially the CRISPR-Cas9 system, is being extensively researched for various purposes including:

- Assessment of gene expression and gene function
- Therapy for chronic viral infections like human immunodeficiency virus.
- Gene correction therapy for cystic fibrosis and tyrosinemia
- Cell line engineering for understanding molecular targets of drugs
- Genetic modification of organisms to create human disease models, and creation of genetically modified higher yielding plants.

Q 13. Write a note on the types and procedure of gene therapy.

Ans. Gene therapy is a therapeutic modality that involves correction of genetic disorders either by replacing the defective gene with a healthy one, introducing a new gene or by editing a defective gene. It can be of two types:

- **Germline gene therapy:** Changes are introduced directly into germ cells, zygote or early embryo. It is transmissible to the next generation. Due to significant ethical issues, it is not permitted in humans at present.
- **Somatic gene therapy:** 'Transgenes' are introduced in the somatic cells of a patient. The changes are non-heritable so cannot be transmitted to the next generation.

Prerequisites:

1. Corrected gene must be delivered to the target tissue.
2. It must be stably expressed.
3. It must not interfere with function of cells of target tissue.

Procedure

For gene therapy, corrected gene, RNA or oligonucleotides are transferred to patient's cells using a vector, which can be viral or non-viral. When viral vectors are used to transfer DNA into cells, it is known as **transduction.**

Non-viral vectors, e.g. naked DNA, liposomes, nanoparticles, etc. can also be used by electroporation, sonoporation, magnetofection, gene guns, and receptor-mediated gene transfer methods. It is known as **transfection**. They have low efficiency but better safety profile.

Q 14. Write about the various approaches used for gene therapy.

Ans. The main approaches used for gene therapy include:

i. Insertion of the normal copy of the gene into a nonspecific location within the genome to replace the non-functional mutated gene.
ii. Substitution of the abnormal gene with a normal gene.

iii. Repair of the abnormal gene by correcting the mutation

iv. Inactivation or 'knocking-out' of the improperly functioning mutated gene.

There are two approaches of gene therapy (Figure 7.4):

1. *In vitro*: Cells are extracted from the patient, grown in culture and after genetic modification, they are infused back into the patient.

   Example: In case of thalassemia, from hematopoietic stem cells (HPSCs), CD34+ HPSCs are separated and cultured in the presence of growth factors. Lentiviral vector encoding the beta-globin complimentary DNA is inserted into the DNA of HPSCs. The corrected HPSCs are then infused intravenously to engraft in the bone marrow, where they can self-renew as well as differentiate into cells of hematopoietic lineage.

2. *In vivo*: Gene transfer is done within the patient's body. Vectors with transgene are injected either systemically or directly into the target tissue. It requires repeated doses, e.g. in ocular and neurological disorders.

Q 15. Write the limitations of gene therapy.

Ans. Limitations of gene therapy:

1. **Risk of insertional mutagenesis:** Vector inserts in the host DNA and introduces unwanted changes in the DNA which disrupts the normal functioning of these cells. This has been reduced using safer vectors such as lentiviral vectors.

2. **Carcinogenesis:** There is risk of activation of proto-oncogenes due to proviral insertion.

3. There is associated risk of toxicity, immune and inflammatory response to delivery agents.

4. The difficulty of delivering the therapeutic gene to the correct target tissue.

5. The short-lived nature of the therapy as in most cases, does not get passed onto the daughter cells when the original cell divides.

Q 16. Enumerate some diseases that can potentially be treated by gene therapy.

Ans. Disorders that can potentially be treated by gene therapy:

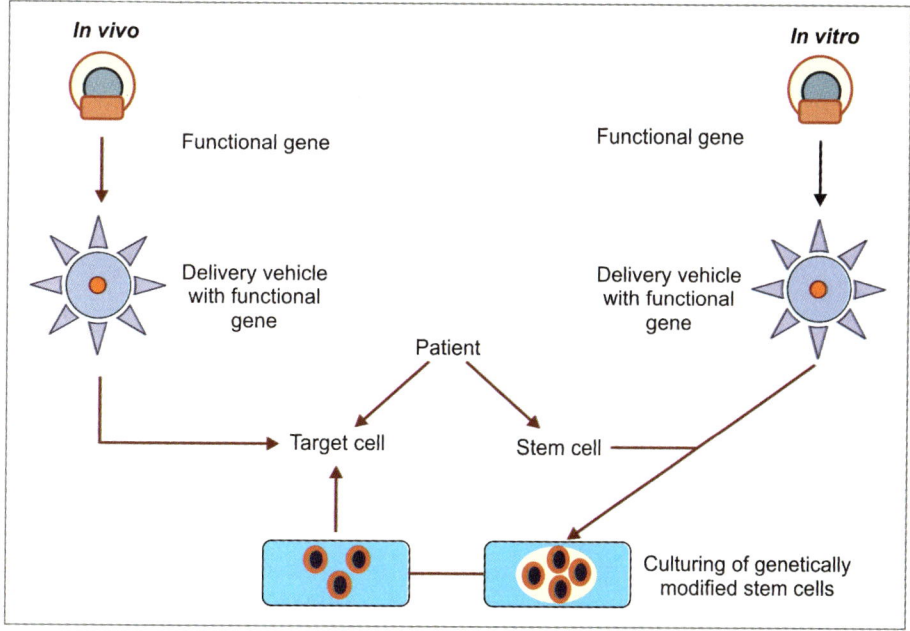

Figure 7.4: Gene therapy

1. **Lipoprotein lipase deficiency:** First disorder for which gene therapy was approved (Glybera).
2. Severe combined immunodeficiency due to adenosine deaminase deficiency
3. **Neuromuscular disorders:** Spinal muscular atrophy (Zolgensma), Duchenne muscular dystrophy
4. **Inherited hematological disorders:** Beta thalassemia, sickle cell disease, hemophilia A and B
5. **Cancer:** Chimeric antigen receptor T cells (CART cells) are most effective in hematological malignancies, mainly B cell-acute lymphoblastic leukemia.
6. **Inherited retinal diseases:** Leber's congenital amaurosis type 2, Luxturna (for RPE65-associated retinopathy), choroideremia.

Q 17. Write a note on the medical prenatal/fetal therapy.

Ans. Fetal therapy includes various interventions given in fetal life either for cure or to alter the natural history of fetal anomaly or disorder. They can be medical or surgical.

Medical treatment includes various medications given to the mother which are then transported to the fetus via placental circulation or amniotic fluid. *For example:*
1. Use of folic acid at a dose of 400 μg/day to prevent neural tube defects.
2. Treatment of fetal arrhythmias with digoxin, sotalol, etc.
3. Replacement of thyroxine 150–600 μg to prevent fetal hypothyroidism.
4. Steroid dexamethasone 20 μg/kg/day in congenital adrenal hyperplasia.
5. Treatment with steroid in case of congenital cystic adenomatoid malformation (CCAM).
6. Biotin in fetal biotinidase deficiency.
7. Fetomaternal alloimmune thrombo-cytopenia can be treated by maternal administration of steroids alone or with intravenous immunoglobulins, or by intrauterine platelet transfusion.

Q 18. Write various prerequisites and ethical considerations for fetal surgery.

Ans. Prerequisites and ethical considerations for fetal surgery:
1. An accurate prenatal diagnosis should be established.
2. The natural history of the disorder should be well defined.
3. It should either be life saving or should prevent serious complications of a disorder.
4. There should not be any associated severe structural anomaly, or no chromosomal or other genetic disorder.
5. Risk of maternal complications and injury to the fetus should be low.

Q 19. Write a note on surgical interventions in prenatal/fetal therapy.

Ans. **Surgical procedures** can be performed under ultrasound guidance with or without fetoscope and by open fetal surgery.
A. **Ultrasound guided procedures:**
   1. *Intrauterine fetal transfusion:* In cases of fetal anemia due to Rh alloimmunization.
   2. *Vesicoamniotic shunting (VAS):* Fetal lower urinary tract obstruction (LUTO) can be treated in selected cases by VAS. In this, a double pigtail catheter is used with one end placed in amniotic sac and other in fetal bladder.
   3. *Thoracoamniotic shunting:* In large fetal pleural effusion and **congenital cystic adenomatoid malformation**, there is mediastinal shift with risk of contralateral pulmonary hypoplasia and fetal hydrops. Placement of shunt is done with one end in the pleural cavity and other in amniotic sac.
   4. *Fetal cardiac intervention:*
      i. In case of severe aortic stenosis, fetal balloon aortoplasty can be done.
      ii. Atrial septostomy using stent across foramen ovale in case of hypoplastic left heart syndrome.
   5. *Selective foeticide:* In complicated monochorionic diamniotic pregnancies, selective termination of one twin can

be done to ensure the survival of the healthy co-twin by bipolar cord coagulation, diathermy, radio frequency ablation or laser.

B. **Fetoscopic procedures:**
1. *Laser photocoagulation in twin-twin transfusion syndrome (TTTS):* Vascular anastomoses between monochorionic diamniotic twins are coagulated using laser between 16 and 26 weeks of pregnancy.
2. *Fetoscopic endoluminal tracheal occlusion (FETO):* In congenital diaphragmatic hernia at 26–29 weeks of gestation, fetal trachea is temporarily occluded to prevent the escape of pulmonary fluid from the lungs. The occlusion increases the pressure in the airways stimulating the alveolar development. After 4–6 weeks the balloon used for tracheal occlusion is removed.
3. *Resection of amniotic band* which lead to formation of constriction bands around digits or cause amputation of limbs.
4. *Laser ablation of chorioangiomas:* Large chorioangiomas can lead to high-output cardiac failure and hydrops in fetus. Laser ablation of feeding vessels can be done to interrupt the blood supply of angioma and reversal of cardiac failure.

C. **Open fetal surgery:**
1. *Open neural tube defects:* In management of myelomeningocele study (MOMS) trial decrease in requirement of postnatal shunt.
2. *Congenital cystic* adenomatoid malformation
3. *Sacrococcygeal teratoma:* Cases with cardiac dysfunction at risk for hydrops can be treated either by open surgery or by laser or radiofrequency ablation.

D. **Fetal stem cell and gene therapy:** Stem cell therapy has been tried on research basis in fetuses with osteogenesis imperfecta.

Q 20. Write about the complications of fetal surgery.

Ans. Complications of fetal surgery:
1. Preterm labor
2. Rupture of membranes
3. Chorioamniotic separation
4. Scar dehiscence
5. Placenta accreta in subsequent pregnancies
6. Requirement of cesarean section for delivery.

PREVENTION OF GENETIC DISORDER
Manisha Goyal, Shreya Tanneru, Suresh Thomas and Komal Uppal

Q 21. Write a note on primary prevention of genetic disorder.

Ans. The care of patients with genetic disorder includes both management and prevention. **Prevention may be primary or secondary.**

Primary Prevention

It is the prevention of genetic disease occurrence or prevention of development of disease complications. It can be done either before marriage or before pregnancy.

A. **Prevention of disease occurrence:**
  ➲ *Pre-marriage preventive measures* are taken where families do not agree for termination of pregnancy and where people do not get married if they are carrier for the disease.
  ➲ In case of X-linked recessive disorders like Duchenne muscular dystrophy and autosomal recessive diseases like beta thalassemia, by doing voluntary carrier screening testing for a high-risk population or family members, considering all the social ethical issues of a country, we can reduce the chances of birth of an affected child.
  ➲ *Pre- and peri-conceptional preventive measures:*
    a. Identify high-risk pregnancy with history of genetic disorders and

counsel them for carrier screening after proper counseling.

b. Supplementation of folic acid 400 µg to women of reproductive age to reduce the risk of development of neural tube defects.

c. Encouraging women to conceive in between 20 and 35 years to reduce the risk of non-hereditary chromosomal abnormalities like Down syndrome in which the association with advanced maternal age offers a basis for prevention.

d. To give rubella immunization and prevention of TORCH infection.

e. Education on prevention of systemic illness like diabetes and thyroid disorders.

f. Avoidance of exposure to teratogens (e.g. alcohol, antiepileptic drugs, chemicals and infectious agents) during pregnancy.

B. **Prevention of development of disease complications:**
  ○ Eye and skin care is advised for patients with albinism to prevent complications.
  ○ Secondary thyroid surveillance and psychosocial support for children with Down syndrome.

Q 22. Write a note on secondary prevention of genetic disorders.

Ans. Secondary preventive measures for **genetic disorders** are taken:

○ To prevent the birth of an affected child by taking preventive measures during pregnancy and by preimplantation genetic diagnosis. It includes prenatal screening and diagnosis and selective termination of pregnancy for untreated genetic disorders and birth defects.

○ To detect treatable genetic disorders so that by early intervention severity of the disease can be controlled.

○ To identify the individuals who are at risk of getting adult onset disease.

Strategies for secondary prevention:

During pregnancy:

○ Identification of pregnant women at risk and suggesting antenatal screening.

○ Ultrasound evaluation at 18–20 weeks for all pregnant women in order to detect fetal defects due to chromosomal abnormalities.

○ Biochemical screening in case of neural tube defect and Down syndrome at 16–18 weeks of gestation.

○ Noninvasive prenatal testing (NIPT) to know common aneuploidies.

○ Invasive procedures such as amniocentesis at 16–18 weeks or chorionic villous sampling at 11–12 weeks in previous chromosomal abnormality, abnormal USG or biochemical screen.

○ Voluntary termination of pregnancy for serious genetic disorders or birth defects.

○ Preimplantation genetic diagnosis to identify genetic defects in embryos to prevent diseases getting passed onto the child.

Postnatal secondary prevention: Newborn screening for metabolic disorders such as phenylketonuria and galactosemia for early identification and intervention.

Adult onset diseases screening testing: For diseases like Huntington disease and familial hypercholesteremia, screening test is done in high-risk person for the purpose of early intervention.

Q 23. Write the difference between prenatal screening testing and prenatal diagnostic testing.

Ans. Differences between prenatal screening test and prenatal diagnostic test.

Prenatal screening test	Prenatal diagnostic test
Prenatal screening is a strategy for the prevention of common genetic disorders and is offered to all pregnant women	Prenatal diagnostic test is used to confirm the existence of a medical condition

It usually involves a simple blood test biochemical screening or imaging, which are noninvasive	It includes invasive procedures. ○ Amniocentesis ○ Chorionic villus sampling (CVS)
It detects pregnant mothers at increased risk of giving birth to a child with a genetic disorder	It diagnoses a child with a genetic disorder during pregnancy
Cost is less	It is costly
It cannot, however, diagnose any of the conditions. For confirmation of positive screening test, confirmatory test should be available	For making a correct prenatal diagnosis, detail examination and all the investigation records of the proband and parents are needed
Possibility of false-positive and false-negative results	Results are confirmatory
Pose no risk to the mother or fetus	Could pose a small risk of miscarriage

Q 24. Write a note on indications for prenatal screening testing.

Ans. Prenatal screening: Prenatal screening is done to identify the fetuses at high-risk to have a congenital abnormality or genetic disorder. Screening tests usually are noninvasive in nature and it includes biochemical screening (first and second trimester, ultrasonography and NIPT) (Tables 7.1 and 7.2).

Indications of prenatal screening:

- Advanced maternal age (greater than 35 years at delivery)
- Presence of birth defects or soft markers on ultrasound
- Past obstetric history of aneuploidy or another genetic disorder.
- A family history of aneuploidy especially if a parent is a balanced Robertsonian translocation carrier.
- To identify neural tube defects.

Q 25. Write a note on indications for prenatal diagnostic testing.

Ans. Prenatal diagnosis includes invasive tests such as CVS after completing 11 weeks,

amniocentesis after 16 weeks or cordocentesis after 18–20 weeks of gestation, to obtain fetal samples for definitive testing to detect genetic disorders with significant morbidity and mortality.

1. **Prenatal chromosomal diagnosis:**
   a. Advanced maternal age >35 years.
   b. Previous child with any chromosomal abnormality like Down syndrome with unbalanced translocation or congenital malformations.
   c. Either partner with balanced chromosomal translocation.
   d. Abnormal USG in pregnancy.
   e. Abnormal maternal serum screening
2. **DNA diagnosis** is done in cases where previous child has a common single gene disorder like thalassemia, cystic fibrosis, DMD, spinal muscular atrophy, etc.
3. **Biochemical diagnosis** for metabolic diseases, such as Gaucher disease, mucopolysaccharidoses, congenital adrenal hyperplasia, etc.
4. **Nongenetic** causes such as maternal infections for positive IgM antibodies, systemic illnesses, teratogen exposure, Rh incompatibility.

Q 26. Write a note on noninvasive prenatal screening techniques.

Ans. Prenatal screening is a strategy for the prevention and detection of common genetic disorders and are being offered to all pregnant women. Generally, this screening testing is noninvasive and confirmatory invasive tests are done to confirm the results of positive screening test. Along with basic screening tests like external examination, fetal heart rate, maternal blood pressure and weight mesurement, specific trimester wise and integrated (combined first and second trimester screening) prenatal screening techniques are done to calculate the risk for common genetic problems (Tables 7.3 and 7.4).

Contingent screening is done in first trimester of pregnancy. Based on the risk level different tests are advised further:

TABLE 7.1: Prenatal screening testing during first trimester

Timing	Investigation	Anomalies tested
First trimester (11 weeks–13 weeks of pregnancy)	o Maternal serum pregnancy-associated plasma protein-A (PAPP-A) o Free beta human chorionic gonadotropin (hCG). o Ultrasonography (USG)	Common aneuploidies such as trisomy 21, 13, and 18. To detect o Gross fetal abnormalities like megacystis, omphalocele, anencephaly, etc. o Aneuploidy screening o Nuchal translucency (NT) measurement o Nasal bone (NB) o Tricuspid regurgitation o Ductal waveform

First-trimester screening provides results earlier than second trimester screening. However, it does not cover screening for NTDs by alpha-fetoprotein (AFP). **Detection rate of first trimester screening for Down syndrome is 85–95% when combined with maternal age and NT/NB with false positive rate of 5%.**

TABLE 7.2: Prenatal screening testing during second trimester

Timing	Investigation	Anomalies tested	Detection rate
Second trimester screening (16–20 weeks)	o **Triple screen:** AFP, hCG, unconjugated estriol (uE3) o **Quadruple screen:** AFP, hCG, uE3, DIA (dimeric inhibin A) o **Pentavalent screen:** AFP, hCG, uE3, DIA, h-hCG (hyperglycosylated-hCG)	o The risk of trisomy 21, 18 o NTD	o **Triple screen:** 65–70% o **DIA detection rate:** 75–80%. o **h-hCG detection rate:** 80%.
	USG targeted anomaly	o Markers for aneuploidy o Neural tube defect can be detected especially if careful attention is paid to the 'lemon' and 'banana' signs which are good pointers to NTDs	

TABLE 7.3: Integrated screening test and NIPT with detection rate

Integerated and other screening tests		Detection rate
Integrated screening	First trimester blood screening + NT ultrasound + second trimester blood screening	94–96%
Serum integrated	First trimester blood screening + second trimester blood screening	85–88%
Noninvasive screening (NIS)/ Noninvasive prenatal testing (NIPT)	Noninvasive screening using cell-free fetal DNA	99% DR with 0.3% FPR

TABLE 7.4: Various screening test results related to specific genetic disease

	First trimester			Second trimester screening screen			
	Nuchal translucency	PAPP-A	Free-β-hCG	uE3	AFP	hCG	Inhibin A
Trisomy 21	↑	↓	↑	↓	↓	↑	↑
Trisomy 18	↑	↓	↓	↓	↓	↓	–
Trisomy 13	↑	↓	↓	↓	↓	↓	–
Neural tube defect	–	–	–	–	↑↑	–	–

- *For low-risk pregnancy:* No further testing
- *Moderate risk:* Quad or pentavalent screening
- *High-risk:* Diagnostic test
- **Noninvasive prenatal test or NIPT:** Cell-free fetal DNA (cffDNA) in the maternal plasma is the latest test done at 9–10 weeks of gestation. Earlier testing may lead to failed result. It remains a screening test though with high sensitivity.
- For trisomy 21, NIPT has a sensitivity and specificity of 99% and 99.92%, respectively.
- For trisomy 18, the reported sensitivity was 96.8% and specificity 99.85%.
- For trisomy 13, they were 92.1 and 99.80% respectively.

Q 27. Write about the indications and procedure of chorionic villi sampling (CVS).

Ans. Prenatal diagnosis is not only important to know whether the fetus is affected with a serious genetic disorder or not in a high-risk pregnancy, but it also helps the family in taking reproductive decisions and gives a chance to provide available prenatal and postnatal treatment. Prenatal diagnosis is done by various tests like chorionic villi sampling, amniocentesis, fetoscopy, cord blood sampling, after 10 weeks by taking X-rays for skeletal dysplasia. The earliest prenatal test done to detect any genetic defect is chorionic villi sampling.

A. **Indications of CVS** based on various tests done on CVS sample (*already described in Q 25*).

B. **Timing:** Ideal time is in between 11 and 13 weeks of gestation. It should not be carried out before 9 weeks in view of the increased risk of limb abnormalities.

C. **Procedure:** Proper counseling and informed written consent about procedure and complications to be done. Ultrasound examination is done to localize placental site, viability of fetus, and gestation. If the placenta is anterior, a transabdominal route is most appropriate while transcervical route is more suited for posterior and low-lying placenta.

1. *Transabdominal CVS (most common) Figure 7.5:* An 18–20 gauge spinal needle is passed through anterior abdominal wall into the substance of the chorion frondosum under continuous ultrasound guidance. With gentle up and down movements with continuous negative pressure villi are aspirated in 20 ml syringe containing 1 ml of nutrient media and examined. It appears as white threaded structures and transferred into the culture media provided by lab.

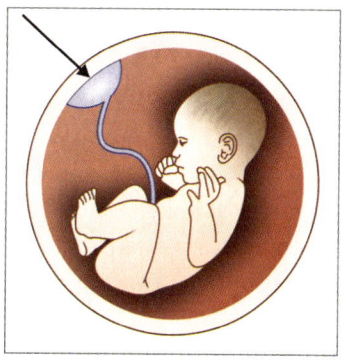

Figure 7.5: Chorionic villus sampling (*Courtesy: Dr Surya Balakrishnan, CCMB, Hyderabad*)

2. *Transcervical route:* After cleaning the vagina, a 1.5 mm plastic cannula with metal obturator is passed through Cervix till internal OS. Cannula tip is visualized on U/S and advanced into the substance of chorion frondosum. Negative pressure is applied to the syringe and villi aspirated. Fetal heart activity is checked at the end of procedure.

D. **Post-procedure care:**
- ⤷ Antibiotics and rest for 2–3 days.
- ⤷ Anti-D is given if mother is Rh negative.

E. **Complications of CVS:** Vaginal bleeding, infection, rupture of membranes, pregnancy loss (1–2%).

Q 28. What are the advantages and limitations of chorionic villus sampling (CVS)?

Ans. **Advantages of CVS**
- ⤷ Option of early termination of pregnancy with more privacy and less mental distress
- ⤷ Procedure of choice for first trimester screen abnormality
- ⤷ Yield DNA from CV tissue is much greater than amniotic fluid
- ⤷ Biochemical or DNA analysis can usually be carried out directly on villi.

Disadvantages of CVS
- ⤷ Difficult cytogenetic analysis
- ⤷ Failure to get sample and culture failure can happen in <1%
- ⤷ Possibility of contamination with maternal cells and the risk of mosaicism
- ⤷ Risk of miscarriage (0.3–0.5%) is estimated to be more when compare with amniocentesis.

Q 29. Describe about the indications and procedure of amniocentesis.

Ans. Though CVS can be done at early period of gestation to know whether the fetus is affected with a serious genetic disorder or not in a high-risk pregnancy, amniocentesis not only detects the abnormalities with more accuracy but also overcome its limitations.

A. **Indications of amniocentesis:** Indications to do amniocentesis for prenatal diagnosis are:
1. Diagnostic indications (described in Q 25)
2. Therapeutic indications:
   - ⤷ To remove excess amniotic fluid, such as in symptomatic polyhydramnios or twin-to-twin transfusion syndrome.

B. **Timing of amniocentesis:**
- ⤷ The ideal recommended time is beyond 15 weeks of gestation.
- ⤷ *Before 15 weeks (i.e. early amniocentesis):* Associated with an increased risk of talipes equinovarus deformity and respiratory complications, culture failure.
- ⤷ At 24 to 32 weeks show a significant decline in cloning efficiency.
- ⤷ *Later procedures:* After 20 weeks, it will be late for termination as termination of pregnancy is legal only till 20 weeks.

C. **Procedure of amniocentesis:** Amniocentesis is done on an outpatient basis. The requisites are as follows (Figure 7.6):

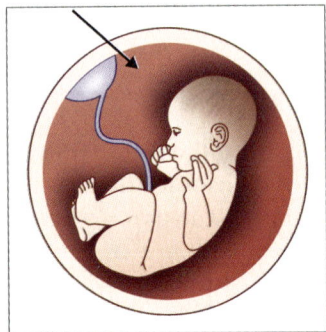

Figure 7.6: Amniocentesis (*Courtesy:* Dr Surya Balakrishnan, CCMB, Hyderabad)

1. Consent from patients and relatives
2. Obstetrical ultrasound to see location for entry of needle
3. Aseptic preparation and ultrasound guided insertion of sterile 22 gauge spinal needle through the abdominal wall into the free pool of amniotic fluid. The stylet is removed and about 10–15 ml of amniotic fluid (AF) is withdrawn after discarding initial drops of fluid.

4. AF fluid is collected in sterile container after proper labeling and transported to the genetic laboratory as early as possible.
5. Post-procedure evaluation of fetal heart
6. Antibiotic prophylaxis for 5 days
7. Following the procedure, the patient is kept under observation for a couple of hours. The patient is advised to take rest for 2 days and immediately report to the hospital if any untoward symptoms like pain in abdomen, bleeding per vagina or watery discharge occur.

Q 30. Describe in brief about the complications and limitations of amniocentesis.

Ans. Complications:

- Failure to obtain sample
- Rupture of membranes and leakage of amniotic fluid
- Fetal injury
- Infection
- Procedure related pregnancy loss (0.1–0.3%).
- Factors that increase pain during procedure include are maternal anxiety, history of menstrual cramps, previous amniocentesis,

and needle insertion into the lower part of the uterus.

Limitations

- A major limitation is that a final result is usually available only after 17 weeks of gestation. It enhances the anxiety of couple during waiting period for a result, particularly when most obstetricians are reluctant to offer a surgical termination late in pregnancy.
- Failure to get sample and culture failure can happen in <1%.

Q 31. Write about various tests which can be done in prenatal diagnosis of fetal sample and their clinical indications.

Ans. Prenatal diagnosis can be done by various tests on prenatal sample taken by various techniques as given in Table 7.5.

Q 32. Write a note on PCPNDT Act, 1994 (Preconception and Prenatal Diagnostic Techniques).

Ans. The Preconception and Prenatal Diagnostic Techniques (PCPNDT) Act aims to stop the female feticide and regulating and banning the practice of sex determination/

TABLE 7.5: Various tests which can be done in prenatal diagnosis of foetal sample and their clinical indications

Technique	Timings	Indication
Chorionic villus sampling	11–13 weeks	o Chromosome analysis (karyotyping) o Molecular genetic diagnosis o Biochemical diagnosis
Amniocentesis fluid or cell	>15 weeks	o Chromosome analysis (cell) o Diagnosis of open neural tube defects (in amniotic fluid) o Molecular genetic diagnosis (cell) o Biochemical diagnosis (cell) o Intrauterine infections (cord blood or amniotic fluid) o Rh isoimmunization—Rh group, hemolysis (cord blood or amniotic fluid)
Cordocentesis	From 16–20 weeks	o Chromosome analysis o Hematological test o Biochemical diagnosis o Infection
Fetal biopsy (skin)	From 20 weeks	o Diagnosis of specific genetic dermatoses

selection and abortion. The PNDT (Prenatal Diagnostic Techniques) Act was passed by the Indian government in 1994 and came into effect on 1st January 1996. Due to the apparent ineffectiveness of this law to improve sex ratios over the years and frequent advances in science, a new law was made in 2003 and became the Preconception and Prenatal Diagnostic Techniques (Prohibition of Sex Selection) Act.

Under this law:
- All centers which have any equipment including ultrasonography machine which can detect sex of fetus have to be registered with the appropriate authorities
- And could warrant punishment if found taking part or being involved in sex determination of fetus.
- Even relatives of pregnant women who ask for sex determination are liable to punishment.

Salient Features of the Act:
- The procedure must be conducted by qualified persons only.
- Every center/institute that offers these tests must be registered.
- Approved applicants will receive (Form B) (certificate of registration) that must be displayed in the center. Renewal request should be sent one month before the expiry of the certificate to the appropriate authority.
- Appropriate form must be filled before conducting a test.
- All the records must be maintained. A complete report of all such tests conducted in a month must be sent to the appropriate authority by 5th day of the subsequent month.
- Any change in the address must be informed to appropriate authority sale of equipment/machines, etc. to anyone who is not registered under the act should be prohibited.

- Notice showing prohibition of sex determination must be displayed in the center.
- A copy of the act and rules must be available in the center/institute.

Q 33. Why is it important to do carrier screening testing for genetic diseases and who should be screened?

Ans. The most effective approach to reduce the burden of genetic diseases is by identifying those at increased risk by implementation of carrier screening testing. A carrier is an asymptomatic person, not aware of their carrier status can pass on the affected gene to his or her child. The aim of carrier screening is to identify asymptomatic carriers so that they are counseled about reproductive risks and options of prenatal diagnosis. Various types of carrier testing that can be done are clinical examination, hematological, biochemical, radiological and DNA-based mutation testing.

Who should be screened?

It is recommended for all couples planning a pregnancy. But because of the financial issues, the test is strongly recommended in the following cases where:
- The couple had a child previously with a genetic disease and child is no more
- One partner is affected by a genetic disease
- There is family history of a genetic disorder on either side
- Couples from ethnic backgrounds with higher prevalence of certain genetic disorders
- Couples are consanguineous
- There is family history of late-onset disorders or autosomal disorders showing reduced penetrance.

Q 34. Write the diseases for which carrier screening test should be done.

Ans. Common diseases where carrier screening should be done:
- **Autosomal Recessive Disorders:** If both partners are found to be carriers of an autosomal recessive condition, they have 25% chance of having an affected child. Example: Beta thalassemia, sickle cell anemia (hematological), metabolic diseases

(biochemical enzyme test), spinal muscular atrophy (mutation analysis), etc.

⊃ **X-linked Recessive Disorders:** If the mother is a carrier for an X-linked disorder, there is 50% chance of males to be affected.
Examples: Duchenne muscular dystrophy (mutation analysis), G6PD deficiency (enzyme analysis), X-linked mental retardation (fragile X syndrome mutation analysis).

⊃ **Autosomal dominant disorders:** Neurofibromatosis (clinical examination and mutation analysis), tuberous sclerosis (MRI brain and ophthalmological examination), Marfan syndrome (2D echocardiography), familial hypercholesterolemia (biochemical test), familial adenomatous polyposis (mutation analysis).

Q 35. Write a note on newborn screening testing and the conditions for which neonatal screening is undertaken.

Ans. Newborn Screening (NBS)

⊃ Newborn screening is the testing of all neonates in the first few days of life for certain congenital disorders or diseases that can cause severe lifelong intellectual or physical disabilities, chronic disease, early mortality if not detected and treated as soon as possible.

⊃ The objective of newborn screening is to detect disorders that are threatening to life or long-term health before they become symptomatic.

⊃ Early diagnosis and initiation of treatment to prevent morbidity and development of intellectual disabilities is the main aim of newborn screening.

⊃ This becomes essential because an affected baby may not exhibit the manifestations of the condition until its too late to initiate treatment. For example, hearing loss if not detected before 6 months of age may lead to permanent hearing and speech impairment. Congenital hypothyroidism if not detected and treated promptly leads to mental retardation and short stature.

NBS is a systematic program including the following elements:

⊃ Counseling and detailed information to public.
⊃ Taking the sample and testing in the laboratory.
⊃ Interpretation of results.
⊃ Avoidance of false results.
⊃ Confirmation of diagnosis in case if screening test is positive.
⊃ Treatment and follow-up.
⊃ Evaluation and monitoring.

What disease to screen?

In 1968, Wilson and Jungner proposed the following criteria for inclusion of a condition in screening:

i. Condition should have an important health problem/frequency.
ii. Test should be acceptable to the population (reliable/simple).
iii. Disease does not manifest at birth/routine examination.
iv. Treatment will prevent mortality and morbidity.
v. Delay in diagnosis will cause irreversible damage.
vi. Screening is cost-effective.

Presently, in our country some of the conditions which are routinely screened are:

⊃ Critical congenital heart disease
⊃ Congenital hypothyroidism
⊃ Congenital adrenal hyperplasia, galactosemia
⊃ Hearing defects, biotinidase deficiency
⊃ Cystic fibrosis, phenylketonuria
⊃ Fatty acid oxidation defects, amino acid disorders
⊃ Organic acidemias, glucose-6-phosphate dehydrogenase deficiency
⊃ Hemoglobinopathies.

The modalities used for newborn screening:

⊃ **Pulse oximetry (the fifth vital sign)** can be used to diagnose some of the critical heart conditions like hypoplastic left heart syndrome, tetralogy of Fallot, total anomalous pulmonary venous connection, transposition of great arteries, patent ductus arteriosus, etc.

- **Hearing assessment**—otoacoustic emissions is the screening test used for hearing assessment. The newborns who test positive are followed up with another test—auditory brainstem response.
- **By Ortolani and Barlow test followed by ultrasound pelvis:** Congenital dislocation of hip.

Tandem Mass Spectrometry

- It includes two types of panel—basic panel (7 diseases) and extended panel (>45 diseases). Various countries have their own different panels for screening depending upon the prevalence and available facilities for the program. Now diseases like Gaucher, Pompe, Fabry, Niemann-Pick disease B and mucopolysaccharidosis I can also be screened by DBS.
- It is usually done between 48 and 72 hrs to 7 days of life (after starting oral feed) by using dried blood spot by heel prick on filter paper circles to screen for various metabolic conditions.
- If sample is taken before 24 hrs of life, results will not be reliable. So repeat sample is must in that case.
- Preterm, babies with intrauterine growth retardation and critically ill babies need repeat testing at 2, 6 and 10 weeks of life and weight should be 1.5 kg.
- Sample should be taken before transfusion of blood if any baby need blood transfusion.
- Filter paper with sample should be reached in the laboratory within 4 hrs at room temperature and can be kept for a long-time at –20°C.

The factors which can affect results of test:
- **Method of collection sample:** Pressing of puncture site, double layer of blood drops, incomplete filling of circle.
- Temperature, moisture and contamination of sample.

- Maternal systemic illness like hypothyroidism, vitamin B_{12} deficiency and maternal drugs like steroids and propylthiouracil.

Positive results from newborn screening should have a confirmatory test performed as quickly as possible. The pediatrician is responsible for ensuring that newborn screening has been completed and that all positive screening results are followed until a diagnosis is confirmed or excluded. In addition, the pediatrician needs to provide guidance counseling and support to families with infants with a false-positive result as well as remain vigilant for development of disease despite a negative screening test (false negative).

The WHO has recommended that genetic services should be introduced in countries with an infant mortality rate (IMR) less than 50. India with an IMR of 40 should introduce newborn screening and genetic services.

In a resource limited setting, the financial condition of the parents and the prevalence of the disease conditions in the general population should be considered before conditions for screening can be chosen.

- All newborns should be screened for hearing defects, congenital dislocation of hip and congenital hypothyroidism.
- Screening for other conditions like glucose-6-phosphate deficiency, hemoglobinopathies can be done in areas of higher incidence.
- Screening for metabolic conditions like phenylketonuria, maple syrup urine diasease, tyrosinemia, alkaptonuria, etc. can be undertaken if there is a significant family history of unexplained death of previous sibling or unexplained intellectual disability/seizures, or in newborns with symptoms and signs suggestive of these conditions.

In a resource rich setting where there is no financial constraint, screening is done for a group of metabolic disorders together using a single test.

PREVENTION (SCREENING AT COMMUNITY LEVEL) OF GENETIC DISORDERS

MANISHA GOYAL, SHREYA TANNERU, SURESH THOMAS AND KOMAL UPPAL

Q 36. What are different criteria which should be applied for starting a population screening program at the community level?

Ans. Population screening is the scrutiny of individuals by doing presymptomatic testing who are at risk of developing a disease to implement early diagnostic and therapeutic intervention. Various population screening programs have been started by the government in various countries like UK related to prenatal care, metabolic diseases and adult onset diseases by considering all the ethical, traditional, social, regional,, financial and technical issues. To start these programs at population level it needs a systematic criteria for its implementation, evaluation, monitoring and quality assurance. The criteria to start a program consists of following aspects:

1. **Disease related aspects:**
   - High incidence and huge burden in the society.
   - Common disease with presymptomatic phase.
   - Ill effects on health.
   - Affordable treatment and preventive measures.
   - Criteria for the treatment of patients.

2. **Diagnostic tests aspects:**
   - Accessible, affordable
   - Noninvasive
   - Accurate and reliable
   - Accurate interpretation skills.

3. **Program aspects:**
   - Fair, honest and equal accessibility.
   - Widely available.
   - Socially, culturally and ethically acceptable.
   - Detailed information and counseling.
   - Informed decision and consent.
   - Voluntary participation.
   - Justifiable, beneficial and harmless.
   - Affordable.
   - Respecting psychosocial aspects.
   - Experienced and skilled manpower.
   - Implementation, evaluation and monitoring of the program.

Q 37. Write a note on diseases for which population carrier screening is needed.

Ans. Population carrier screening is done for autosomal recessive disease so that after knowing the carrier status of a couple they can be counseled regarding the 25% risk of occurrence of the disease in their child and about prenatal testing. The common diseases for which this screening program can be done in various regions are:

- **β Thalassemia:** Carrier screening is done by red blood cell indices and electrophoresis in China and east Asia.
- **α Thalassemia:** Carrier screening is done by red blood cell indices and electrophoresis in Indian communities and Mediterranean regions.
- **Cystic fibrosis:** Common variant identification is done in western Europe regions.
- **Sickle cell disease:** In Afro-Caribbean population screening is done by sickling test and electrophoresis.
- **Tay-Sachs disease:** Ashkenazi Jews population is screened by enzyme hexoaminidase A analysis.

Q 38. Write the positive and negative aspects of population screening?

Ans. Positive effects:
- Systematic program and detailed information of the program gives more and voluntary choices to the population.
- Increase level of knowledge of the public regarding government programs.
- Knowledge of their carrier status leads them to take right reproductive decision.
- Early diagnostic and therapeutic intervention can be done.
- Decrease in incidence of genetic disorders.

Negative effects:

- Involuntary participation causes disbelief among the public.
- Feeling of socially genetic inferiority in carrier positive individual.
- Discrimination at job place and in insurance company.
- Anxiety and guilt in the carrier.
- Low sensitivity and inaccurate interpretation of the result leaves doubtful questions in the minds of public.

Q 39. Write a note on role of fetal autopsy in diagnosing a genetic disorder.

Ans. Fetus is a product of conception, irrespective of the duration of pregnancy. Fetal death is defined as death in the mother's womb. The various causes of fetal malformation and death include genetic causes like chromosomal, single gene disorders, congenital malformation and lethal skeletal dysplasia and nongenetic causes include maternal, fetal and uteroplacental factors.

- Though ultrasound can detect various abnormalities which can cause fetal death, but it has its own limitations in detecting all the abnormalities. It becomes very difficult to counsel the parents about the unexplained fetal death and the abnormal findings in the fetus undetected by ultrasound. So through fetal autopsy including external and internal examination the confirmation of diagnosis of the fetus can be determined with high yield.
- The main objectives of autopsy examination are identification of cause(s) of death, additional findings which were not detected by ultrasound and elucidation of pathogenic mechanism for adverse pregnancy outcomes. Findings at perinatal autopsy can change the clinical diagnosis of cause of death and can provide risk of recurrence and offer prenatal testing in further pregnancy. Adverse obstetric factors causative of fetal death may also be identified by doing autopsy.
- But at present time fetal autopsy is not practiced routinely at many of our health centers. In order to make it a routine procedure, awareness among obstetricians, pediatricians and the public is required.

Q 40. Write a brief note on steps followed in fetal autopsy for diagnosing a genetic disorder.

Ans. Fetal autopsy is not done in all fetuses. It is done in fetuses for whom cause of death is not clear; where genetic cause is suspected for its death, and for those families where the cause for recurrent fetal loss or newborn baby's death has not been detected.

Technique

- Review of complete medical records to obtain the clinical history, with attention to medical and obstetrical history.
- Informed written consent of parents is important before the examination.
- Photographs of fetus.

External examination:

It includes careful observation of eyes, ears, face, limbs, digits, nails, spine, joints, external genitalia, anal opening, skin and all the anthropometric measurements are taken to assess the:
- Gestational age
- Body weight
- Placental weight

Internal examination:

It includes:
- Gross and microscopic examination of major organs like brain, liver, kidney, lungs, heart and the placenta and cord.
- Radiographic studies: Anteroposterior and lateral radiographs of spine, long bones, skull, extremities and pelvis of the fetus should be taken, especially if skeletal dysplasia is suspected.
- In internal examinations, the normal findings according to that particular gestation should always be kept in mind. The thorough examination of fetus can provide a specific diagnosis. But to confirm the diagnosis, genetic tests are needed based on the clinical examination and auxiliary investigation results.

Genetic studies which can be done in a fetal sample:

⊃ **Cytogenetic tests:** It is indicated in the presence of chromosomal abnormalities, malformations, fetal hydrops, intrauterine growth retardation, oligohydramnios or previous fetal loss. These can be done from umbilical cord blood, amniotic fluid, skin tissue or body fluids. Blood should be collected in heparin vial and stored at 2–8°C and should be sent to laboratory within 48 hours.

⊃ **Molecular testing:** DNA-based mutation analysis is done when a monogenic disorder like skeletal dysplasia is suspected and blood should be collected in EDTA vial and can be stored at 2–8°C for short-term and at –20°C for long duration.

⊃ **Specific investigation:** These are done based on suspected diagnosis. For instance, in unknown chromosomal microdeletions and duplications, microarray and in imprinting disorders methylation-based tests can be done.

Q 41. What is the role of a pediatrician in a fetal autopsy for diagnosing a genetic disorder?

Ans. Fetal autopsies performed by an experienced pathologist in conjunction with clinical specialist especially pediatrician could identify the cause of death in a majority of cases. Pediatricians can play an important role in diagnosing a genetic disorder as they can better:

⊃ Identify the cause of death/congenital anomalies which are not picked up in antenatal scan.

⊃ Identify any evidence of genetic disease and allow determination of the likely recurrence risk.

⊃ Provide adequate genetic counseling to the parents.

⊃ Determine the requirement/possibility of additional testing after consultation with a genetic expert.

⊃ Prompt therapy or intervention to prevent a similar outcome in the subsequent pregnancy.

⊃ Contribute to epidemiological studies regarding infant death.

⊃ Remove discrepancy between what clinicians think is the cause of death and findings of a full traditional autopsy.

BIBLIOGRAPHY

1. Baumgarten HD, Flake AW. Fetal Surgery. *Pediatr Clin North Am.* 2019; 66(2):295–308.
2. Bell CJ, et al. Carrier Testing For Severe Childhood Recessive Diseases by NGS. SciTransl Med. 2011 Jan 12;3 (650:65ra4).
3. Concolino D, Deodato F, Parini R. Enzyme replacement therapy: efficacy and limitations. Ital J Pediatr2018; 44: 120. https://doi.org/10.1186/s13052–018-0562–1.
4. Dash P, Puri RD, Kotecha U, Bijarnia S, Lall M, Verma IC. Using noninvasive prenatal testing for aneuploidies in a developing country: Lessons learnt. J Fetal Med. 2014;1:131.
5. Gambello MJ, Li H. Current strategies for the treatment of inborn errors of metabolism. *J Genet Genomics.* 2018; 45(2):61–70. doi:10.1016/j.jgg.2018.02.001.
6. Maeder ML, Gersbach CA. Genome-editing Technologies for Gene and Cell Therapy. *Mol Ther.* 2016;24(3):430–46.
7. National Commission for Protection of Child Rights [homepage on the internet] Pre-Conception & Pre-Natal Diagnostic Techniques Act, 1994.
8. Nawab K, Bhere D, Bommarito A, Mufti M, Naeem A. Stem Cell Therapies: A Way to Promising Cures. *Cureus.* 2019;11(9):e5712.
9. Rimoin D, Pyeritz R, Korf B. Emery and Rimoin's Principles and Practice of Medical Genetics. 7th edition.
10. Steffin DHM, Hsieh EM, Rouce RH. Gene Therapy: Current Applications and Future Possibilities. *Adv Pediatr.* 2019; 66:37–54.
11. Thompson & Thompson, Genetics in Medicine, 8th edition.
12. Yankowitz J, Weiner C. Medical fetal therapy. *BailNieres Clin ObstetGynaecol.* 1995;9(3):553–70.

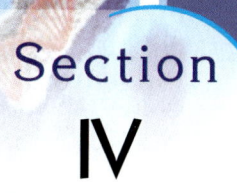

Section

IV

Genetic Counseling, Ethical and Legal Issues in Genetics

- ➲ Genetic Counseling, Ethical and Legal Issues

Genetic Counseling, Ethical and Legal Issues

Aruna Priya Kamireddy, Qurratulain Hasan, Chaitanya A Datar

GENETIC COUNSELING
ARUNA PRIYA KAMIREDDY, QURRATULAIN HASAN

Q 1. What is genetic counseling? Write about its different types.

Ans. Genetic counseling: The communication process of educating the individuals/ families and at-risk individuals for better understanding of their genetic condition by an experienced person. After giving psychosocial support, the details of the genetic disorder are explained and the family is encouraged to make appropriate decision and to plan for reproductive issues in the future, thereby assuring they should receive appropriate support.

Types of Genetic Counseling:

1. **Prenatal counseling**
   a. *Pre-test counseling:*
      ➲ It is recommended to pregnant couples
         ▪ Who is being at high-risk of having a child with genetic problems
         ▪ Who had terminated their previous pregnancy due to abnormal findings.
      ➲ During prenatal genetic counseling, the couple is explained about the risk of genetic disorders their child can have and is also told about the need and all the details of prenatal invasive procedures and available prenatal tests that maybe needed.
   b. *Post-test counseling:*
      ➲ After the confirmation of the disease on prenatal testing, couple is explained about the details of disorder and its prognosis.
      ➲ The decision for continuing or terminating pregnancy is left to the parents.
      ➲ In case of bad obstetric history or if any one parent has some balanced chromosomal aberration, the couple can also be given the option of assisted mode of conception and preimplantation genetic testing.

2. **Postnatal counseling** is important for families with positive family history for serious inherited disease.
   a. *Pre-test counseling:* It is recommended for
      ▪ Couples with two or more pregnancy losses with suspected genetic reasons.
      ▪ Consanguineous couples in order to know their carrier status of familial genetic disorder.
      ▪ To know the etiology of a genetic disorder in an individual in the family.
      ➲ The family is explained about the possibility of genetic disorders in the affected person and is also told about the need and all the details of the available genetic tests to make definitive diagnosis and to assess the recurrence risk of the disease.

b. *Post-test counseling:*
  - After the confirmation of the disease in the proband, the family is explained about the details of disorder, treatment options, inheritance pattern and recurrence risk in the family.
  - All the at-risk individuals are counseled for targeted testing which help them begin surveillance before the disease onset.

Q 2. Write the principles of genetic counseling and steps which are followed during counseling.

Ans. Principles: Following the basic principles of autonomy and privacy, genetic counseling includes three following steps— diagnosis, risk calculation, and communication and support.

1. **Diagnosis:**
   a. *Obtaining detailed medical history* of the consultant and family history from the maternal and paternal side in privacy and with confidentiality.
     - A detailed pedigree is to be constructed.
     - Hidden and wrong information about some relations in the family must always be kept in mind.
   b. *Choice of tests:*
     - Based on the clinical suspicion, right biochemical investigations along with molecular tests also help to make the diagnosis.
     - Relevant knowledge of a disease and its related genomics should be gained from databases to decide the test to be done.
     - Decision regarding proceeding with parental tests if needed should be done carefully as it can create a sense of guilt for the parents.
   c. *Limitations of diagnosis:*
     - Diagnosis of a genetic disease and prenatal tests needs legal permission before performing.

  - Testing for late-onset disorders should normally be postponed until the individual can provide full informed consent.
  - Some of the genetic diseases cannot be identified by available tests.
  - Nonavailability of tests for some diseases should be informed.
  - Information regarding variant of uncertain significance (VUS) in molecular tests which does not provide clue about its association with the pathology and about significant incidental findings should be given to family.

2. **Risk calculation:**
   - Counselors should estimate the quantitative and qualitative risks associated with the observed variants.
   - Risk calculation of VUS may require additional tests to confirm its pathogenicity.

3. **Communication and support:** Communication and body language play a key role in conveying the information.
   - To be done in a positive way considering psychosocial aspects and to avoid the feeling of guilt in the parents.
   - Reassure family about the appropriate support from counselors and other support groups.

Q 3. Write about the clinical indications for genetic counseling.

Ans. Genetic counseling is essential in families with below mentioned history:

1. **Family history:**
   - Family with history of serious genetic conditions like chromosomal structural abnormalities, early deaths due to known or unknown medical conditions, adult-onset health conditions and hereditary cancers.
   - Some couples who would like to have more information about the genetic conditions that occur with higher frequency in their ethnic group.

2. **Pediatric indications:**
   - Children with developmental delays

- Inherited disorder or birth defect and facial dysmorphism
- Abnormal newborn screening results
- Repeated neonatal deaths
- Intellectual and development regression
- Neuromuscular disorders
- Sexual development abnormality
- Chromosomal disorders like Down syndrome or single gene disorders, congenital deafness, skeletal dysplasia, etc.

3. **Reproductive issues:**
- Advanced maternal age
- Multiple pregnancy losses or infant deaths
- Consanguineous couple with family history of genetic conditions
- Positive carrier testing
- Exposure to radiation, medications, illegal drugs, chemicals or infections
- Positive antenatal screening.

Q 4. Write a note on psychosocial aspects of genetic counseling.

Ans. Counseling involves a complex inter-action of social, medical, and psychological factors between the counselor and family.

- A genetic counselor must transform genetic counseling session from a cold clinical encounter into a humanistic approach closer to a psychoeducational experience rather than just a counselor–parent approach.
- The process should be made comfortable by bringing it to a balanced platform by being empathetic and understanding of the emotional, psychosocial, ethical, religious aspects of the proband/families and by sharing the medical information.
- The counselor must help the parents deal with the psychosocial aspects like denial, guilt, hostility, grief, mourning and the psychology of defectiveness before parents make reproductive decisions.
- The psychosocial approach of genetic counseling must improve and enhance both the personal and social functioning of individuals/families by mobilizing their strengths, supporting coping capacities, building self-esteem and linking them to the necessary groups.
- The counselor must help parents in meeting the appropriate social and medical needs of the family.

GENETIC COUNSELING FOR COMMON ISSUES
Aruna Priya Kamireddy, Qurratulain Hasan

Q 5. How will you counsel a parent whose child is affected with chromosomal abnormality or whose child's karyotype is abnormal?

Ans. If a chromosomal abnormality is identified in an affected child after cytogenetic evaluation, then based on the type of anomaly the counseling is provided following all the general rules of counseling and respecting family's psychosocial aspects regarding below mentioned aspects:

- **Etiology:** Common sex chromosomal aneuploidies (45,XO or 47,XXY or 47,XXX) or chromosomal free trisomies (i.e. 13, 18 and 21) result from a meiotic error or non-disjunction.
- **Disease details:** Basic genetics, natural history, clinical features, prognosis and management options.
- **Recurrence risk** for this in subsequent pregnancies is rare (1%) as most chromosomal aneuploidies are the result of random, sporadic nondisjunction.
- **Karyotype**

However, if the karyotype, indicates a Robertsonian translocation or partial deletions or duplications in the child, then parental karyotype is essential to identify if parents are carriers of balanced rearrangements and risk in subsequent pregnancies is high (20–30%) in balanced translocation and they would require prenatal testing. This information can be explained to the parents using visual aids, which will make it easier to understand. If they are religiously or culturally against the termination of pregnancy, pre-implantation genetics can be offered.

Q 6. How will you counsel a couple whose previous child is affected with autosomal dominant disorder?

Ans. Counseling is done following all the general rules of counseling and respecting family's psychosocial aspects.

⊃ Detailed clinical examination of the family, pedigree analysis and molecular testing are three important modalities prior to providing counseling to a couple with autosomal dominant disorder.

⊃ If the reports of a child are indicative of an autosomal dominant disorder, then the variant causative of the disorder will be identified with molecular testing and followed with parents' analysis to assess if it has been inherited or is a *de novo* mutation. Only when a molecular variant associated with the disease is available then family testing and prenatal testing can be offered.

⊃ The details of prenatal procedures such as chorionic villi sampling at 11–13 weeks and amniocentesis at 16–18 weeks, time limit for prenatal testing and other limitations should be conveyed to family.

⊃ Disease details including basic genetics, natural history, clinical features, prognosis, management options, inheritance pattern and recurrence risk of 50% to each offspring must be considered. Recurrence risk will be very low due to *de novo* mutations and will be more than general population in the case of gonadal mosaicism. All these need to be explained to the family.

⊃ It is important to evaluate from the pedigree chart that is the dominant disorder presents in other family members, sometimes it may 'skip a generation'. This implies that it exhibits incomplete penetrance or differential expression. So, the need of molecular testing should be informed to the family.

Q 7. How will you counsel a couple whose first child and a first degree relative both are affected with an autosomal recessive disorder?

Ans. Counseling is done following all the general rules of counseling and respecting family's psychosocial aspects.

⊃ Disease details including basic genetics, natural history, clinical features, prognosis, management options, inheritance pattern and recurrence risk should be explained.

⊃ It must be explained that for a child to be affected with autosomal recessive disorders, both parents have to carriers of the same abnormal gene.

⊃ Many of us carry abnormal genes and it is very unlikely that our partners will also have the same abnormal gene, but this is likely if there is consanguinity or endogamy.

⊃ When both parents are carriers, then the chance of having an affected child is 25%.

⊃ If one parent is a carrier, then there is no chance of producing an affected child.

⊃ If there is an affected first degree relative with such a disorder, then a molecular test should be done ideally in the affected individual and the carrier status of the couple is to be established by targeted molecular testing. Results of the test will indicate whether further prenatal testing during pregnancy and carrier testing of other family members is required or not.

⊃ Carrier screening should be done prior to pregnancy to eliminate anxiety associated with waiting for results when a pregnancy is already established. These tests help in assessing a couple's risk of having a child with a specific disease and help in providing the reproductive options available to them.

⊃ Need for prenatal testing and the details of prenatal procedures such as chorionic villi sampling at 11–13 weeks and amniocentesis at 16–18 weeks and time limit for prenatal testing and other limitations should be conveyed to family.

Q 8. How will you counsel a couple whose first child and a first degree relative both are affected with X-linked recessive disorder?

Ans. Genetic counseling: Parents with an affected male child must be counseled before and after genetic evaluation, although effective counseling is possible only after the genetic defect has been identified. Genetic counseling in an X-linked disease must be sensitively and carefully tailored to address the prevailing psychosocial beliefs and prejudices.

- Disease details including basic genetics, natural history, clinical features, prognosis, management options, inheritance pattern and recurrence risk should be explained.
- Explain the basic concept of two X chromosomes in females and a single one in males, following which the couple needs to be counseled about the father's and mother's contribution of sex chromosomes for developing a male and female child.
- Then a pedigree has to be drawn to assess which side of the family has the affected individual with X-linked recessive disorder. If it is on the paternal side, then they can be reassured. But if it is on the maternal side, then the mother may be classified as an obligate carrier, a potential carrier or a non-carrier. Molecular testing has to be carried out for establishing her status.
- Only once a molecular variant associated with the disease is available, then family testing and prenatal testing can be offered.
- They must also be informed that males are more likely to be affected than females.
- Females being carriers will not manifest an X-linked recessive trait. However, half of the sons of carrier females will be affected and manifest the trait, and half the daughters will be carriers, like the mother.
- All daughters and none of the sons of an affected male will be carriers.
- In an unusual situation, a female may exhibit some characteristics of the phenotype conferred by an X-linked recessive gene.
- All 'at risk' female relatives in the family, aged beyond 18 years, must undergo carrier testing. Care must be taken to avoid gender discrimination and stigmatization of the female carrier.
- In some cases, a child is affected due to a new (*de novo*) mutation or gonadal mosaicism.

Here, the parents are unaffected and other children may or may not be affected.

- Determination of disease recurrence based on fetal sex must be strongly discouraged since it is unreliable, inappropriate and a punishable offence in India respectively. In case of *de novo* mutation, recurrence risk will be very low but in case of gonadal mosaicism it will be more than general population.
- Need for prenatal testing and the details of prenatal procedures such as chorionic villi sampling at 11–13 weeks and amniocentesis at 16–18 weeks and time limit for prenatal testing and other limitations should be conveyed to family.

Q 9. How will you do genetic counseling for a couple whose previous child is dysmorphic and has congenital malformations?

Ans. Counseling should begin with a complete history of the pre- and post-natal period and physical and systemic examination and review of basic investigations and genetic test reports, if available. If not, the first test suggested would be a karyotype or a chromosomal microarray test to confirm the condition. Subsequently, a clinical exome test can be ordered if a karyotype or CMA does not show any results

- Depending on the information received the counseling should be provided regarding etiology, basic genetics, natural history of the disease, prognosis, treatment for their child, inheritance pattern or concern for future children.
- Based on the report, parental genetic tests, i.e. karyotype, microarray or target gene mutation, carrier testing is essential to identify.
- If parents are carriers, in which case risk in subsequent pregnancies is high (25–50% depending upon the mutation) and requiring prenatal testing.
- If they are not carriers of any mutation, then the recurrence risk in next pregnancy will be negligible.

- Counseling at this point is best directed toward explaining the types of genetic tests available for diagnosis, their cost, turnaround time and their uses/shortcomings. This needs to be conveyed to parents with empathy and emotional support.

Q 10. How will you counsel a couple for prenatal screening and prenatal diagnostic testing?

Ans. Genetic counseling is aimed at informing couples about the importance of different screening and diagnostic test options available and supporting couples in their decision-making process. The most important aspects of counseling for prenatal screening and testing are to explain the following:

- Screening tests should be carried out for all pregnancies to identify at-risk ones who can be offered further diagnostic tests to have a healthy baby.
- High-risk indications of screening and diagnostic testing (explained in Chapter 7).
- The difference between a screening and a diagnostic test and the importance of detecting whether the baby is at risk of having genetic disorder or congenital malformation or not.
- Specific period in pregnancy when the test is to be carried out, its relevance and its shortcomings.
- Types of screening tests like
  - Noninvasive monitoring
  - Biochemical evaluation of urine and blood
  - Ultrasound assessment.
- Carrier testing for the couple based on family history and ethnicity should also be indicated in cases such as cystic fibrosis and thalassemia.

Based on the fetal risk indicated in the screening test, diagnostic prenatal testing is offered.

- The couple is counseled about the risks of prenatal diagnosis, accuracy, and limitations of the various modalities, i.e. chorionic villus sampling (CVS) and amniocentesis.

- The time when the testing is permissible, how long the test results would take, what are the options available and legal implications like termination permitted before 20 weeks of gestation must be explained.
- Some couples will choose to continue pregnancies with known fetal abnormalities or genetic disorders. Their autonomy has to be respected and appropriate medical, surgical management support for the baby and psychosocial support to the family should be provided.

Q 11. How will you do genetic counseling for a couple with history of recurrent perinatal loss?

Ans. Both genetic and nongenetic causes should be considered for recurrent perinatal losses. A detailed medical and family history of the couple should be taken and previous investigation records should be seen.

- Many couples are mistakenly convinced that fetal loss has occurred as a result of a preventable factor(s) for which they or their physician are responsible.
- They should be explicitly informed that at least 15% of clinically recognized pregnancies result in fetal loss, and that loss rates increase with increasing maternal age.
- Approximately 50% of abortuses less than 12 weeks of gestation and 20% of abortuses between 13 and 26 weeks of gestation have chromosomal abnormalities and this can be assessed by doing parental testing and the products of conception testing can be planned if needed and appropriate counseling for subsequent pregnancies can be done. Optimally, chromosomal studies should be performed on the abnormal fetus.
- Subsequent counseling regarding prenatal chromosomal studies (CVS, amniocentesis) must be explained in future pregnancies based on the type of result. For example, chance of recurrent loss in a carrier of balanced translocation is 30%.
- Other genetic causes of spontaneous abortion may be single gene variants which

require a carrier screening to establish if this is responsible for recurrent pregnancy losses.

- ⮑ Sometimes MTHFR gene variant in the mother, which elevates homocysteine may be responsible for pregnancy loss. This can be prevented by giving B_6, B_{12} and folic acid supplements prior to pregnancy.
- ⮑ Options like spontaneous conception and amniocentesis at 16 weeks, ovum or sperm donor, adoption or preimplantation genetic diagnosis can also be discussed with the couple if any of the parents is a carrier for mutation.

Q 12. How will you do genetic counseling in special issues of consanguinity, adoption and genetic disorders and disputed paternity?

Ans. **Consanguinity** is defined as relationship by descent from a common ancestor. Couples are concerned if they are closely related or if one of the members of the couple is the product of a consanguineous relationship or has a close relative who is affected. There is no concern as long as the individual is not a carrier of an autosomal recessive genetic disorder. During counseling couple should explain about the following:

- ⮑ Risk of having affected child through first-cousin mating is high compared to the general population for perinatal and childhood death, malformations, and mental retardation.
- ⮑ If there is history of a familial condition, then the carrier status of the couple must be sought.
- ⮑ If both members are heterozygous for a recessive trait, the risk to each offspring for the disease is 25% and they should undergo genetic counseling to understand options for prenatal diagnosis.

Adoption and Genetic Disorders

The American Society of Human Genetics (ASHG) and the American College of Medical Genetics (ACMG) recommend the following:

- ⮑ All genetic testing of newborns and children in the adoption process should be consistent with the tests performed on all children of a similar age for the purposes of diagnosis or of identifying appropriate prevention strategies.
- ⮑ Primary justification for genetic testing of any child is a timely medical benefit to the child.
- ⮑ Genetic testing should be limited to testing for conditions that manifest themselves during childhood or for which preventive measures or therapies may be undertaken during childhood.
- ⮑ In the adoption process, newborns and children should not be tested for the purpose of detecting genetic variation susceptibility to physical and neuropsychiatric traits or adult onset disorders.

Disputed Paternity

In genetics, a disputed paternity event may occur when someone who is presumed to be an individual's father is not in fact the biological father. This presumption may be on the part of the individual, the couple, or the physician. Where there is uncertainty, the most reliable technique for establishing paternity is DNA fingerprinting. This is medically relevant during interpreting the genetic test reports, during genetic screening or testing for hereditary illnesses and to assess the risk of hereditary disorder in the future generation. But where it is not medically relevant, generally non-paternity is not disclosed as it can affect the family relations.

ETHICS IN GENETICS

Chaitanya A Datar

Q 13. Write a note on fundamental ethical principles of medical genetics.

Ans. Ethics is one of the most important tenets of practicing genetic medicine. Ethical principles are broadly divided into the following:

A. **Beneficence:** Doing good for the patient
B. **Respect for individual autonomy:** Safeguard right to medical care, free of coercion.

C. **Justice:** Ensuring all individuals are treated equally and fairly.

A. **Beneficence and non-maleficence:**
- Prenatal testing for non-lethal or potentially treatable conditions or for gender determination is discouraged, e.g. biotinidase deficiency.
- Pre-symptomatic screening of minor individuals for late onset conditions (non-treatable) or cancers.
- Testing in minor individuals for carrier status of autosomal or X-linked recessive conditions.
- Newborn screening for non-treatable conditions.
- Reporting of secondary findings especially pertaining to cancer and other non-treatable conditions. It is necessary to take proper consent from patients in this regard.

B. **Respect for individual autonomy**
- *Non-directive:* Provide options to the patients and do not lead patients to take decisions, e.g. in case a condition has a guarded outcome, this may be informed to the family, but the decision regarding discontinuation of pregnancy must be left to the family.
- *Non-coercive:* Never force the patient/family to take decision against their wishes. Their wish must be respected, e.g. despite counseling regarding the outcomes, the couple may want to continue with pregnancy with a child having Down syndrome.
- *Non-stigmatizing:* Do not blame any individual or family in the process of counseling. This is true especially for cases with recurrent pregnancy loss or carriers of X-linked conditions or genetic mutations/aberrations.
- *Non-disclosure/privacy of counseling details:*
  - Reports of the patients and raw genetic data should not be revealed to a third party without taking a consent from the patient/relative.

- Private mutations detected may be uploaded to the databases or discussed in literature without identifying the patient.
- The stored DNA of the patients must not be considered for testing for research purposes or otherwise, without an explicit consent from the patient/relatives.

C. **Justice**
- Providing genetic information to health/life insurance providers or to employers may cause discrimination. Hence, this must be done only after taking consent of patient/relative.
- No discrimination based on gender, caste, creed, religion or economic progress, etc.
- The patient pictures should not be published or displayed without consent.
- Decision to initiate treatments/therapies in a neonate or child rests on the parents. However, enrolment of a minor for clinical trials pertaining to gene therapy is a matter of considerable debate.

Q 14. Write a short note on ethical dilemmas in prenatal diagnosis.

Ans. Prenatal diagnosis involves testing the fetus to detect potentially lethal and significantly morbid genetic disorders *in utero*. The ethical considerations while doing a prenatal diagnosis will be as follows:
- The decision to consider testing the fetus and taking further actions should be with informed consent after detailed counseling.
- **Revealing the gender or considering sex selection** is a crime in India according to PCPNDT.
- **Termination of pregnancy** for non-critical conditions is not allowed beyond 20 weeks of pregnancy. In the current scenario, termination of pregnancy for critical cases diagnosed beyond 20 weeks can still be considered up to 24 weeks after medicolegal intervention.
- Direct empiric testing on the fetal sample alone is strongly discouraged in the absence of a specific diagnosis in the index child.

- Decision regarding prenatal diagnosis and subsequent termination for conditions with a mild phenotype (e.g. delta-beta-thalassemia) or for conditions which can be managed postnatally (e.g. galactosemia) and for non-lethal conditions (e.g. albinism) is a matter of debate, and may be left to the choice of the couple.
- Decision regarding undergoing prenatal testing for a genetic trait for some communities where they consider that trait to be normal for their community is also an ethical concern.
- Preimplantation genetic test for research on embryo or fetus and three-parent baby for mitochondrial disorders is also a big ethical issue.
- Preimplantation testing for HLA matching bone marrow for survival of the affected sibling can affect the psychology of donor baby later on.
- Any prenatal testing or termination of pregnancy in the following conditions is strongly discouraged:
  - Eugenics, i.e. for achieving ideal physical attributes
  - To rule out carrier state of disorders
  - Disorders with adult onset, e.g. Huntington disease
  - Cancer predispositions.

Q 15. Write briefly on ethical issues in carrier detection testing in asymptomatic childhood.

Ans. Carrier detection testing to detect the carrier status of an individual for autosomal recessive and X-linked recessive disorders is not recommended in asymptomatic child due to some ethical issues.
- Carrier screening should be voluntary and pre-test consent should be taken.
- It should be done after 18 years of age as before this age, child cannot give their informed consent.
- It can have psychosocial implications on the child.
- It can be done only in treatable conditions like familial hypercholesterolemia.

- Parents and other family members attitude towards asymptomatic carrier child can be different after knowing child's status.
- Carrier screening should not be considered in minors, except in cases where the girl is a potential donor for a bone marrow transplantation for the sibling affected with an X-linked condition, e.g. X-linked adrenoleukodystrophy.
- Disclosure of genetic information should not be done to anyone without family's consent.

Q 16. Write on ethical issues in predictive testing in asymptomatic childhood.

Ans. Predictive testing in asymptomatic children is done to conduct genetic investigations in asymptomatic or otherwise healthy children for specific disorders when there has been a positive family history or sometimes prospectively to know if the child suffers from any genetic/metabolic condition. Rarely, it may be considered to determine genetic attributes to be able to pursue specific goals, e.g. to pursue a career in sports. However, there are many ethical issues which need consideration before these tests are planned in children.
- Testing for untreatable disorders in minors without their consent may be considered unethical and must be discouraged.
- Such predictive testing may be considered for conditions where early, accessible and affordable treatments can be offered to the patients, e.g. in female carriers of Fabry disease, surveillance for renal and heart disease and certain therapeutic options may be considered when these organs are relatively unaffected. Newborn screening is also helpful for some treatable metabolic disorders.
- Confidentiality of genetic reports should be always maintained.
- There is likely to be social discrimination and rejection of insurance claims based on these results.

Q 17. Write a note on ethical issues in doing newborn screening.

Ans. Newborn screening (NBS) is the presymptomatic testing of the newborn for potentially treatable disorders between 48 hours of life till 28 days, but ideally in the first week of life. The following are ethical issues in doing newborn screening.

ᴐ **Cost of testing:** Being a paid program, NBS is not accessible to all. Only patients who can afford can undertake the advanced NBS test. This leads to discrimination.

ᴐ **Cost of treatment:** For congenital hypothyroidism, congenital adrenal hyperplasia, galactosemia, G6PD deficiency and biotinidase deficiency, the treatment is not so expensive, and outcomes are generally excellent when detected and treated early. However, for most other conditions, the treatment is expensive and lifelong and is not covered under government programs/ schemes. For lysosomal storage disorders the treatment by enzyme replacement therapy is expensive and inaccessible to most of the patients.

ᴐ **Consent** for newborn screening is given by the guardians. So, taking a non-critical decision to consider presymptomatic testing may be a matter of debate among ethicists.

ᴐ **Insurance:** If a child is diagnosed to have an inborn metabolic error, they are not likely to be insured even for common illnesses and surgeries.

ᴐ **Insecurity of sample and data:** Surety of DNA sample and data that these are not being used for any other purpose is also a big ethical concern.

Q 18. Write a note on ethical issues in doing population screening program.

Ans.

ᴐ **Consent for voluntary participation:** After counseling regarding population screening programs, participation should be voluntary ensuring autonomy and informed decision.

ᴐ **Insurance:** If a person is diagnosed to have a genetic disorder, they are not likely to be insured even for common illnesses and surgeries.

ᴐ **Insecurity of sample and data:** Surety of DNA sample and data that these are not being used for any purpose is also a big ethical concern.

ᴐ **Stigmatization:** After knowing the carrier status, individuals could have feelings of genetic inferiority.

ᴐ **Confidentiality:** Ensuring the confidentiality of genetic information should always be kept in mind.

ᴐ **Employment discrimination:** Based on the positive report, individuals can face discrimination at their workplace.

Q 19. What are ethical dilemmas in stem cell therapy?

Ans. Stem cell therapy is a ray of hope for mitigation or cure of some of the genetic conditions such as beta thalassemia, X-linked adrenoleukodystrophy, etc. However, there are many ethical issues that need to be taken into consideration while availing these therapies.

ᴐ Injection of multipotent/pluripotent/ differentiated mesenchymal stem cells obtained from a matured donor are preferred over the embryonic stem cells (multipotent) or induced pluripotent stem cells. The ethical concern of destruction of viable human embryos in embryonic stem cell processing has caused a ban on embryonic stem cell therapy.

ᴐ Use of embryonic stem cells will exploit the right of embryo and can lead to human cloning issues.

ᴐ Case selection for stem cell therapy must be considered in a presymptomatic stage.

ᴐ Obtaining a suitable donor is a frequent challenge.

ᴐ Subjecting the unaffected donor to an invasive procedure to obtain these stem cells is also an ethical issue.

ᴐ Balance the risks of death from the underlying genetic disease versus the mortality arising out of the transplantation procedure or the subsequent immunosuppression is a critical challenge which must be discussed while counseling the family.

Q 20. What are ethical dilemmas in gene therapy?

Ans. Gene therapy includes replacing, suppressing or editing a gene to modify its function in order to mitigate or cure an underlying genetic disease.

- ∋ Germ line gene therapy is ethically unacceptable and has been banned in most countries worldwide to avoid transmission of desirable genes to next generation.
- ∋ Gene therapy should not be used to enhance basic traits such as height, athletic ability and must not be used for eugenics.

BIBLIOGRAPHY

1. Emery & Rimoin's Principles & Practice of Medical genetics, 7th edition.
2. Thompson & Thompson, Genetics in Medicine, 8th edition.
3. Yang M, Kim JW. Principles of genetic counseling in the era of next-generation sequencing. Annals of laboratory medicine. 2018 Jul 1;38(4):291–5.

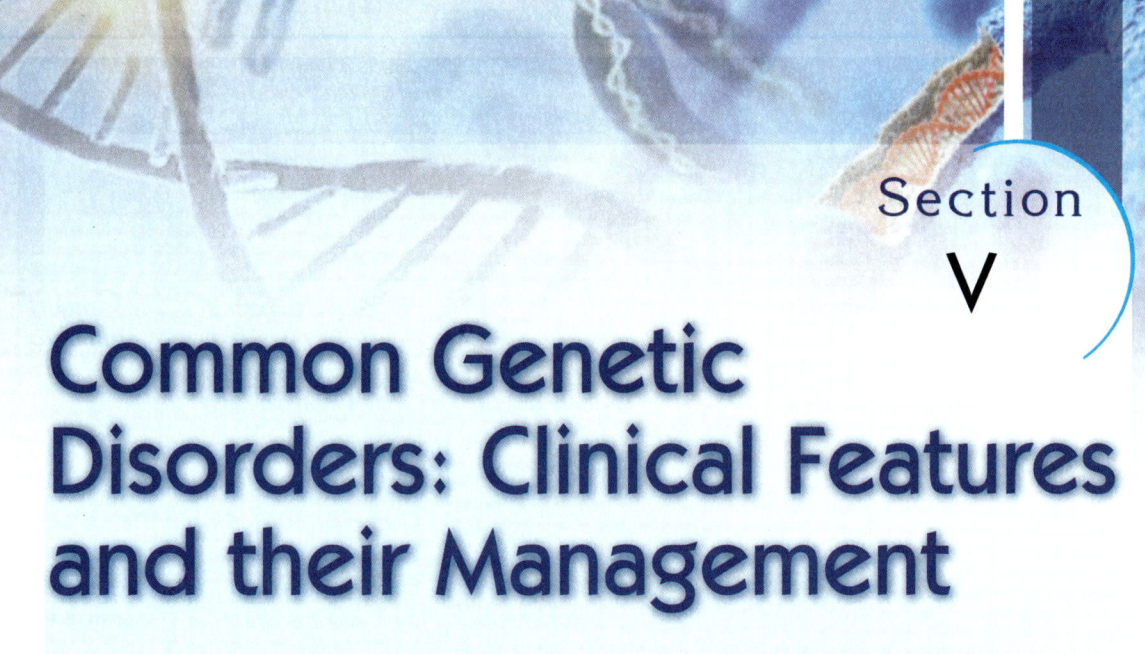

Section V

Common Genetic Disorders: Clinical Features and their Management

Common Chromosomal Disorders

Suvarna Ghanashammagar, Gayatri R Iyer, Priyanka Srivastava

Q 1. Discuss the genetic basis, risk factors and mechanism of Down syndrome.

Ans. Down syndrome is the most common genetic cause of moderate intellectual disability due to trisomy 21 with the incidence of 1 : 850 live births. It presents with specific facial dysmorphic features and various systemic developmental abnormalities.

Genetic basis:

- 95% of Down syndrome cases are due to an extra copy of chromosome 21, called trisomy 21.
- <5% of Down syndrome occurs because of Robertsonian translocation between acrocentric chromosomes 13, 14, 15, 22 and chromosome 21 which leads to triple dose of genes on chromosome 21q (Chapter 3, Figures 3.5 b, 3.6 a, 3.6 b, 3.6 c).
- 1% of cases are due to mosaicism. This has milder clinical features than rest of the two types.
- Partial trisomy of 21q chromosome is also responsible for Down syndrome features in very few patients depending upon the increase of gene dosage in the triplicate region of the chromosome.

Mechanism:

- The trisomy 21 occurs due to nondisjunction of one of the pair of homologous chromosomes during anaphase of meiosis I and less often it can be because of failure of separation of sister chromatids in meiosis II (Chapter 3, Figures 3.2 and 3.3).
- Increase in gene dosage due to trisomy alters the chromatin modification and the gene expression at the level of mRNA and noncoding RNA, causing variable features in Down syndrome.

Risk factors for birth of a baby with Down syndrome:

1. Increased maternal age (>35 years)
2. With increased ovarian age, increased meiotic errors lead to aneuploidies; in which Down syndrome is the most common.
3. The risk of having a child with Down syndrome:
   - 1/1,300 for a 25-year-old woman
   - the risk increases to 1/365 at age 35
   - the risk increases to 1/30 at age 45.

Q 2. Discuss the clinical features and complications of Down syndrome.

Ans. Clinical features of Down syndrome (Figure 9.1)

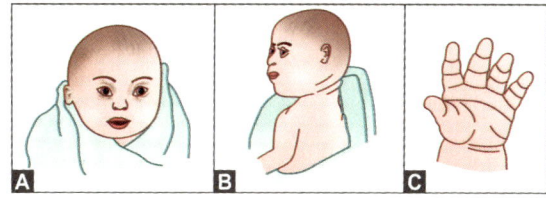

Figure 9.1: : Clinical features of Down syndrome: A. Flat facies, hypertelorism, up-slanting palpebral fissures; B. Flat occiput, flat nasal bridge; C. Simian crease on palm

Hall's criteria are the diagnostic criteria useful in neonatal age which are as follows:

Central nervous system	o Hypotonia o Developmental delay o Poor Moro's reflex
Dysmorphism	o Brachycephaly with flat occiput o Flat facies o Upward slanted palpebral fissures o Epicanthal folds o Speckled irises o Mild microcephaly o Flat nasal bridge o Protruding tongue o Small low set ears
Cardiovascular system	o Endocardial cushion defects o Ventricular septal defects o Atrial septal defects o Patent ductus arteriosus
Gastrointestinal	o Duodenal atresia o Annular pancreas o Tracheoesophageal fistula o Hirschsprung disease o Imperforate anus
Musculoskeletal	o Joint hyperlaxity o Short neck o Redundant skin o Short 5th digit with clinodactyly o Single transverse palmar crease o Wide gap between 1st and 2nd toe o Pelvic dysplasia
Cutaneous	o Cutis marmorata

Complications of Down Syndrome:

Neuropsychiatric	o Autism spectrum disorders o Behavioral disorders o Alzheimer disease in later age
Sensory	o Hearing loss o Refractive errors o Cataract o Squint o Glaucoma
Cardiopulmonary	o Acquired mitral, tricuspid or aortic valve regurgitation o Obstructive sleep apnea

Musculoskeletal	o Atlantoaxial instability o Hip dysplasia o Slipped capital femoral epiphyses o Recurrent joint dislocation
Endocrine	o Congenital or acquired hypothyroidism o Hyperthyroidism o Diabetes mellitus o Male infertility o Obesity
Hematological	o Transient myeloproliferative syndrome o Acute lymphocytic leukemia o Acute myelogenous leukemia o Immunodeficiency
Gastrointestinal	o Celiac disease (3.6–13.8% of children) o Delayed tooth eruption
Cutaneous	o Hyperkeratosis o Seborrheic dermatitis

Q 3. How will you diagnose Down syndrome? Discuss the early stimulation and management in Down syndrome.

Ans.

I. **Diagnosis of Down syndrome** can be done by Karyotype (Figure 9.2)

   Auxiliary investigations: (Figure 9.2a)

II. **Early stimulation of Down syndrome:**

   - The aim of early stimulation therapy and behavioral therapy is to enhance independence in later life of the child by giving training in different relevant areas of development to the child and the parents.
   - It includes speech therapy, physiotherapy, and occupational therapy.
   - An early intervention program reduces costs of rehabilitation and special schools and reduces the parental stress and frustration.

III. **Management of Down syndrome** involves surveillance for complications and their appropriate treatment along with early intervention. Time frame for screening is shown in Table 9.1.

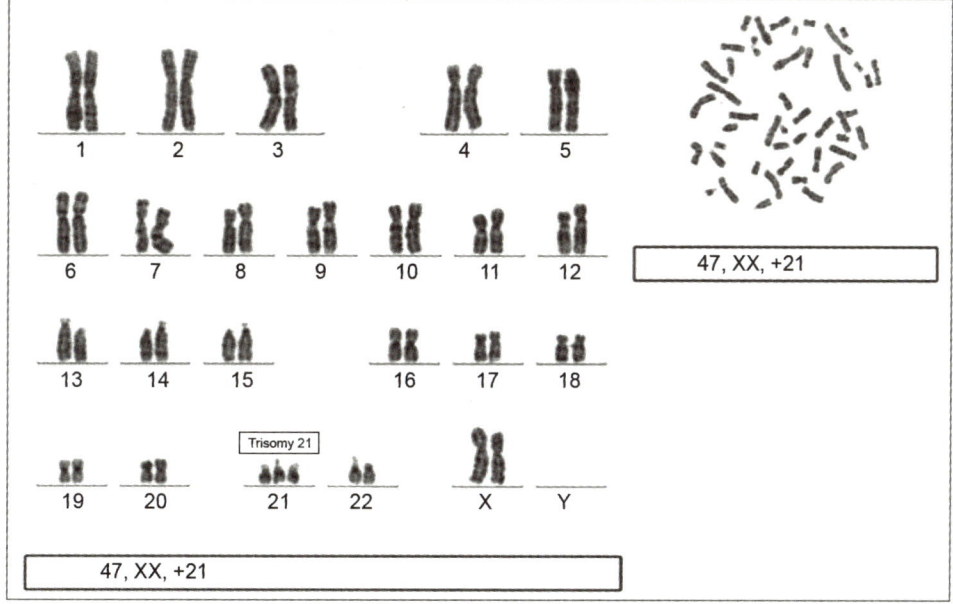

Figure 9.2: Karyotype showing trisomy 21

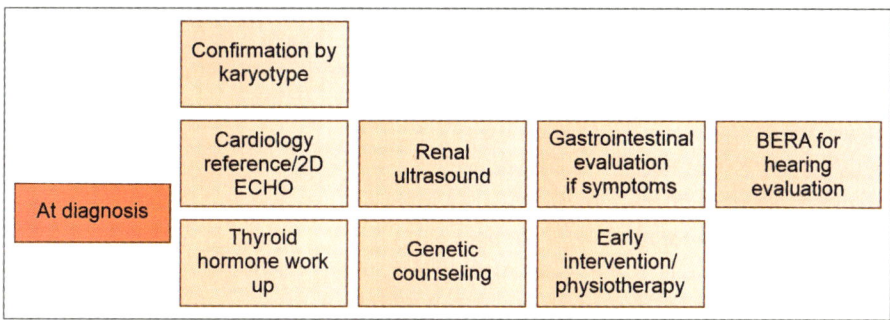

Figure 9.2a: Karyotype showing trisomy 21

Q 4. Mention the recent therapeutic trials for Down syndrome.

Ans. The recent therapeutic trials for Down syndrome:

- Pharmacological trials of donepezil, galantamine, memantine and rivastigmine on cognitive decline are going on.
- **Chromosomal silencing:** Silencing the whole extra chromosome especially DYRK1A locus of chromosome 21 in induced pleuripotent stem cells emerged as to evolve trisomy into disomy but it was noted that the extra chromosome was reactivated.
- **Role of megavitamins:** High dose vitamin A and folinic acid, vitamin C and nutritional therapies in improving cognition to decrease the oxidative stress.

Q 5. What is the recurrence risk in the sibling and other family members of a child who is affected with Down syndrome?

Ans. The risk of Down syndrome with trisomy 21 is 1% in next pregnancy.

- In Robertsonian translocation, risk depends on the translocation and the parental carrier status of translocation, as t(14:21)

TABLE 9.1: Time frame for screening

System	Methods	Age: 0–1 year	Age: 1–5 years	After 5 years	Treatment
Growth	Anthropometry	At least twice in first year	Annually	Every two years	Ensure optimal diet and physical exercise
Hearing evaluation	OAE/BERA	Same	Same	Same	Standard treatment and follow-up as indicated
Eye examination	Clinical examination	Same	Same	Same	Same
Thyroid profile	Serum TSH, FT3, FT4	Same	Same	Same	Same
Hematological problems	CBC, peripheral smear	Same	Same	same	Same
Dental problems	Examination	Same	Same	Same	Same

has recurrence risk of 5–7% if father is carrier and is 10–15% if mother is carrier. t(21:21) has recurrence risk of 100% in future pregnancies.

Q 6. How will you do genetic counseling in a couple whose previous child is affected with Down syndrome? or Discuss prenatal management for this couple for a subsequent pregnancy.

Ans. Genetic counseling and prenatal management: After confirmation of the diagnosis, following all general principles of counseling and respecting psychosocial aspects of the family, family should be counseled about the following:

- Details of the disease like etiology, basic genetics of the disease, natural history, prognosis, management options, and the recurrence risk in future generation.
- If translocation is identified in the previous affected child, then parental karyotype to identify balanced rearrangements, prenatal screening (biochemical and ultrasound, noninvasive prenatal testing) and diagnostic test karyotype, FISH or QF-PCR via chorionic villous sampling (11–13 weeks) or amniocentesis (16–18 weeks) should be advised.

- Family should be informed about the details of prenatal procedure and prenatal test.
- If the result of prenatal diagnosis suggests presence of Down syndrome, the decision regarding continuation or termination of pregnancy should be left to the couple.

Q 7. Describe the genetic basis, karyotype picture and clinical features of Edward syndrome and Patau syndrome.

Ans.

Edward syndrome (trisomy 18)	Patau syndrome (trisomy 13)
Genetic basis	
o Almost 95% cases of Edward syndrome are due to trisomy 18 (Figure 9.3).	o 80% of the cases of Patau syndrome are due to trisomy 13 (Figure 9.4).
o Maternal advanced age is the risk factor for trisomy.	o Maternal advanced age is the risk factor.
o Very few cases of Edward syndrome are due to mosaicism and an isochromosome for 18q.	o Very few cases of Patau syndrome are due to Robertsonian translocation between chromosome 13 and another chromosome.
	o Few cases are due to mosaicism.

Contd.

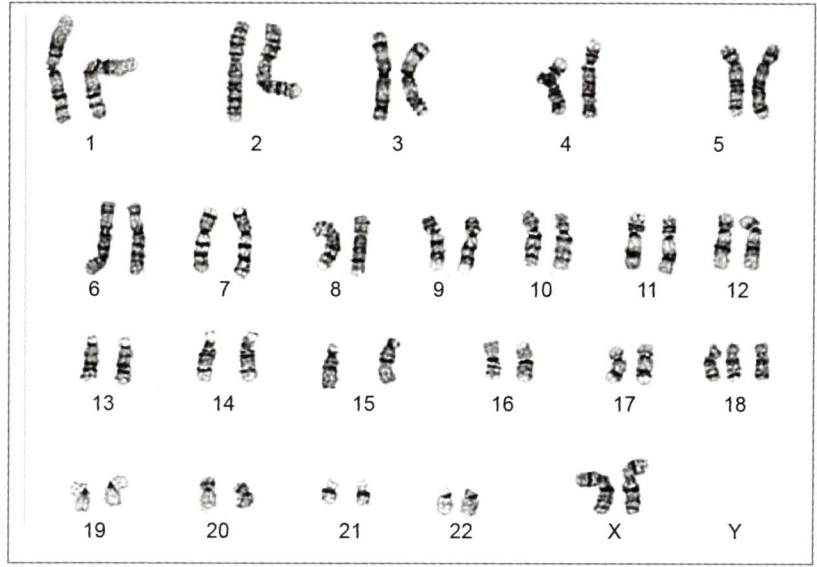

Figure 9.3: Karyotype showing trisomy of chromosome 18

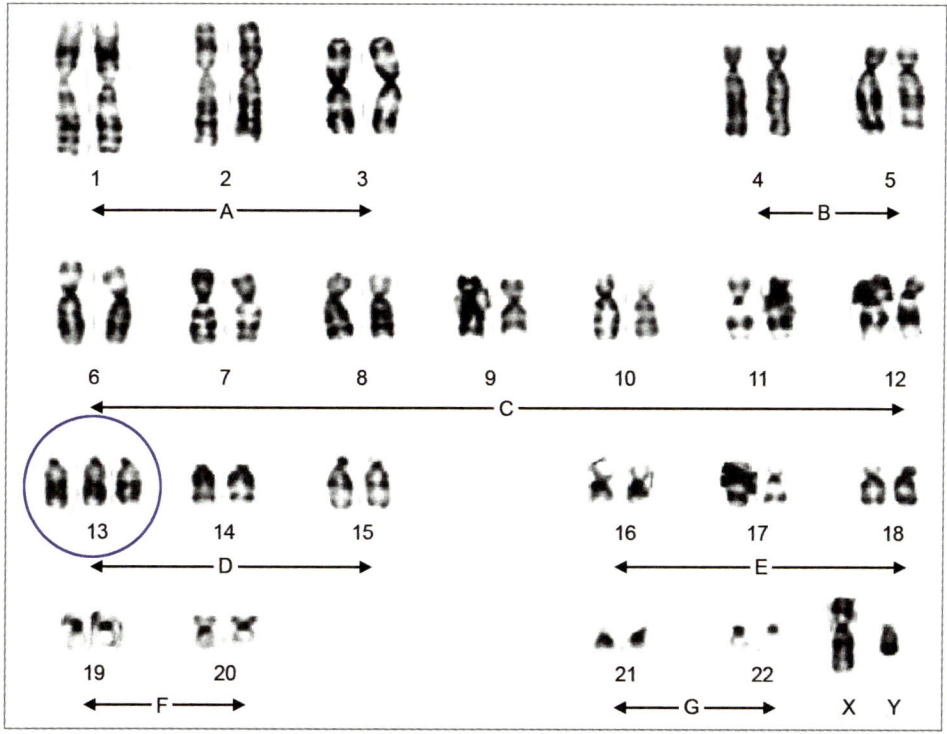

Figure 9.4: Karyotype showing trisomy 13

Edward syndrome (trisomy 18)	Patau syndrome (trisomy 13)
Clinical features (Figures 9.5 and 9.6)	
○ Growth retardation ○ Clenched fists with overlapping digits (index finger over 3rd, 5th over 4th) ○ Radial limb defects, rocker bottom feet, hypoplastic nails, heart defects. ○ Exomphalos, inguinal or abdominal hernias, meningomyelocele ○ Micrognathia, prominent occiput ○ Cryptorchidism, hypertonia ○ Death in infancy.	○ Microcephaly ○ Holoprosencephaly (cyclopia), anophthalmia/ microphthalmia, ○ Hypoplastic ribs, hypoplastic nails ○ Midline cleft lip ○ Scalp defects ○ Heart defects ○ Renal abnormalities ○ Post-axial polydactyly ○ Death in neonatal life.

Karyotype	Description (frequency %)
45,X	Monosomy for X chromosome (50%)
45,X/46,XX and 45,X/46, XY	Mosaic for Turner syndrome (20%)
46,X,i(Xq)	Isochromosome for long arm of X chromosome or iso X (20%)
46,X,r(X)	Ring chromosome X (5%)
46,X,del(Xp)	Deletion of short arm of X chromosome (5%)
46,X,t (X, autosome no.)	X autosome translocation
46,X,i(Yq)	Isochromosome Y chromosome
46,X,t(X,Y)	X, Y translocation

Q 8. What is a contiguous or microdeletion syndrome? Give examples.

Ans. When two or more genes are deleted in continuity in microdeletion syndrome, it is called contiguous gene deletion syndrome.

Phenotype can be very distinctive depending on number of genes deleted. With availability of chromosomal microarray, microduplications involving similar regions are also identified and those contiguous gene duplications also have similar phenotype.

Sex Chromosome Abnormalities:

⊃ In Duchenne muscular dystrophy, child can be having retinitis pigmentosa (RP) also due to deletion of gene responsible for RP located near to Xp21.

⊃ 4p deletion, 5p deletion, 22q11.2 deletion, etc. (*See* **appendix Tables 3 and 4**)

Q 9. Describe the etiology, genetic basis of Turner syndrome.

Ans. Turner syndrome is a numerical sex chromosome abnormality that occurs in females with incidence of 1:5000–1:10000. The various genotype abnormalities which can lead to Turner syndrome are:

Mechanism:

⊃ As with trisomy, monosomy can result from nondisjunction in meiosis (Chapter 3, Figures 3.2 and 3.3).

⊃ If one gamete receives two copies of a homologous chromosome (disomy), the other corresponding daughter gamete will have no copy of the same chromosome (nullisomy).

⊃ Monosomy can also be caused by loss of a chromosome as it moves to the pole of the cell during anaphase, an event known as anaphase lag.

⊃ Loss of SHOX gene located at X chromosome is responsible for short stature and other skeletal abnormalities.

⊃ The candidate gene for causing impairment in cognitive and behavior disorder has not been identified but it can be either due to possibility of imprinting defects (retaining of maternal X chromosome causes more impairment in cognition) or structural X chromosomal abnormalities.

Q 10. Describe the clinical features of Turner syndrome.

Ans.   Clinical features (Figure 9.7)

⊃ **Prenatal manifestations:** Generalized edema (hydrops) or swelling localized to the neck (nuchal cyst or thickened nuchal pad)

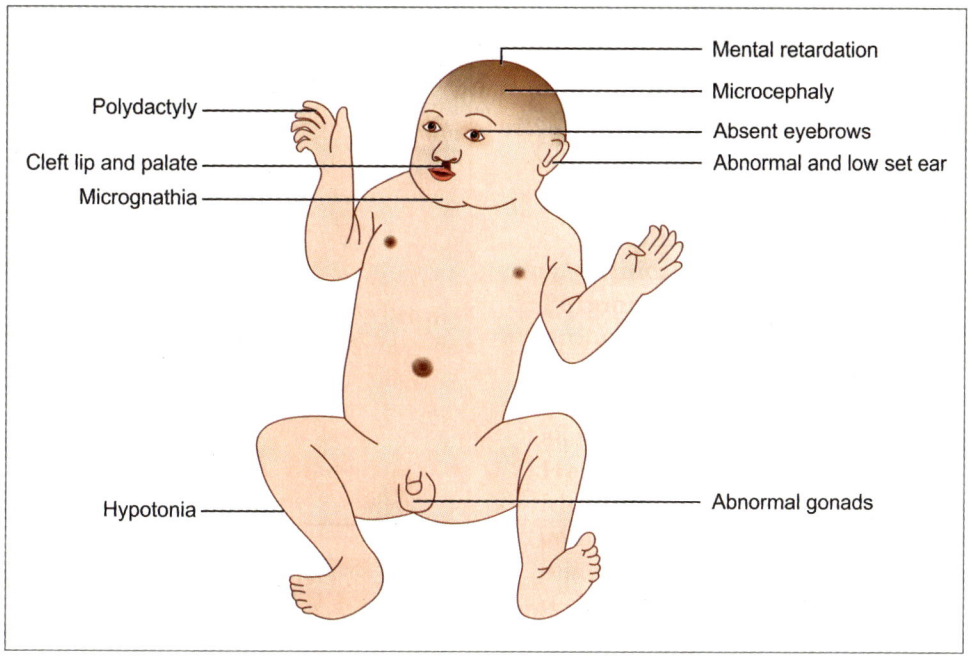

Figure 9.5: Clinical features of Patau syndrome
(*Source:* https://twitter.com/AAPAstudents/status/1075451188328448000/photo/1)

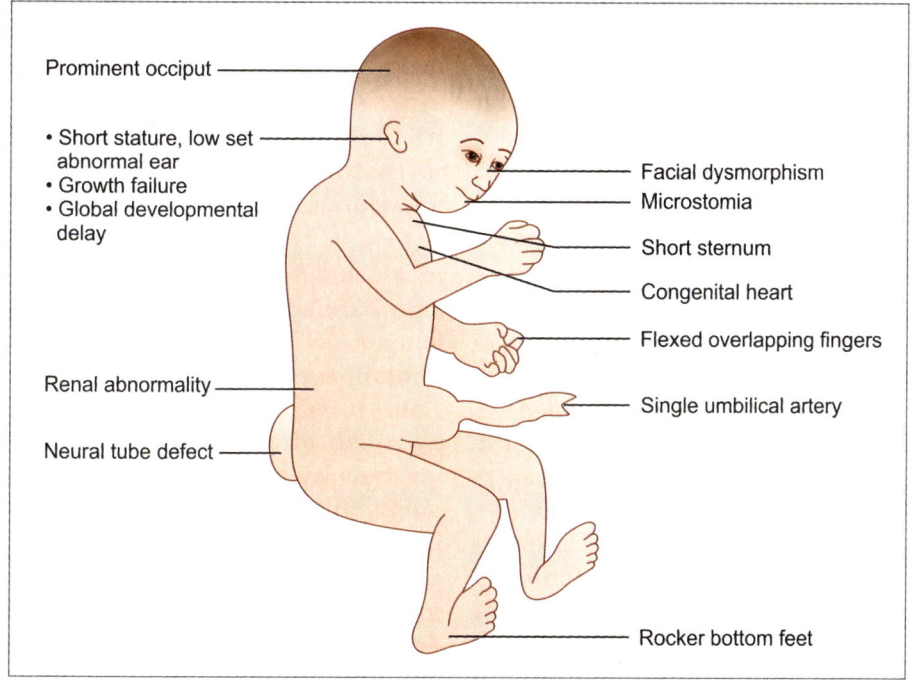

Figure 9.6: Clinical features of Edward syndrome
(*Source:* https://www.google.com/imgres?imgurl=https://i.pinimg.com/originals/20/84/07/20840795b08013a
924 c6cfaa6af02790.jpg&imgrefurl=https://www.pinterest.com/pin/135319163783883772/&docid=eXIx
4t7a2_VMvM&tbnid=M7cXHgD6aztOaM&vet=1&w=448&h=346&hl=en-GB&source=sh/x/im)

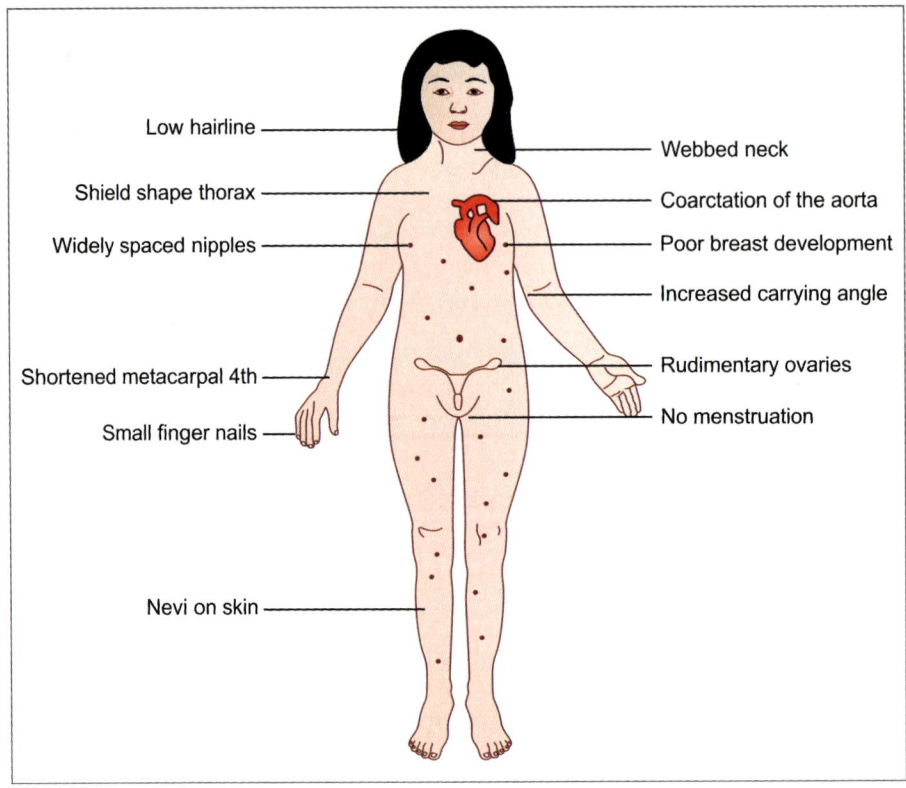

Figure 9.7: Turner syndrome: Clinical features
(*Source*: https://pedclerk.bsd.uchicago.edu/page/turner-syndrome)

⊃ **At birth:** Edematous extremities, neck webbing and low posterior hairline.

⊃ **After infancy:**

System	Clinical features
General dysmorphism	○ Short stature the average adult height is 145 cm ○ Webbed neck ○ Low posterior hairline ○ Lymphedema ○ Short fourth metacarpals ○ Increased carrying angles at the elbows (cubitus valgus) ○ Widely spaced nipples, shield shape chest.
Reproductive system	○ Hypoplastic uterus ○ Gonadal dysgenesis, gonadoblastoma ○ Primary amenorrhea ○ Infertility.

Cardiovascular	○ Bicuspid aortic valves ○ Coarctation of the aorta ○ Pulmonary venous abnormalities.
Renal system	○ Renal aplasia or hypoplasia ○ Horseshoe shaped kidney.
Skin	○ Pigmentary nevi ○ Lymphedema of hands and feet ○ Alopecia.
Ophthalmology	○ Myopia ○ Ptosis ○ Strabismus.
Autoimmune	○ Thyroiditis ○ Celiac disease ○ Inflammatory bowel disease.
Hearing deficit	—
Intelligence	○ Normal ○ However, higher cognitive behavior deficit may be present.

Q 11. How will you diagnose Turner syndrome?

Ans. Diagnosis can be done by:

⮞ Clinical examination

⮞ Investigations like full blood count, renal function test, liver function test, X-ray of left hand and wrist for bone age, blood sugar levels, growth hormone and insulin like growth factor, Estradiol (low in Turner), FSH and LH (high), chest X-ray and serum calcium, phosphorus and vitamin D levels.

⮞ Conventional karyotyping (Figure 9.8).

Auxiliary Investigations: (Figure 9.8a)

Q 12. How will you do management of Turner syndrome?

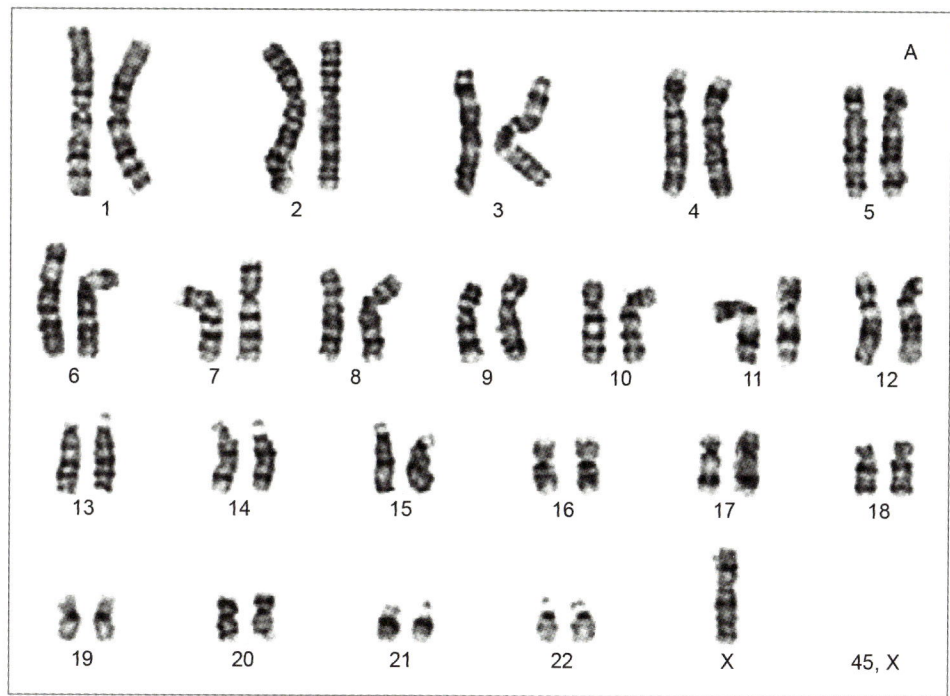

Figure 9.8: Karyotype showing monosomy X

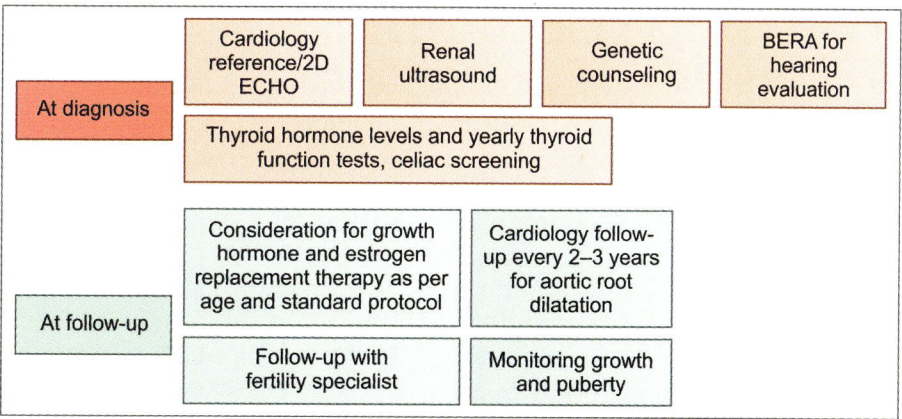

Figure 9.8a: Auxiliary investigations

Ans. Management:

- **Growth hormone therapy:** It is started usually at 2–5 years of age.
- **Estrogen replacement therapy** should be initiated at adolescence for the development of secondary sexual characteristics and long-term prevention of osteoporosis.
- **Progesterone therapy:** Two years after starting of estrogen therapy to start menstrual cycle.
- Calcium supplements due to decreased estrogen.
- **Fertility and family planning issues:**
  a. Although most of the females with TS are infertile but a few can achieve spontaneous pregnancy due to functional ovaries. Those who have spontaneous menstrual cycles and ovulate normally should plan early pregnancy or they can have option of oocyte or embryo cryopreservation. They should be informed about the risk of miscarriage, chromosomal abnormalities in the offspring and to get prenatal screening or diagnostic genetic testing.
  b. Women without functional ovaries can have option of:
     - Oocyte or embryo donation
     - Adoption
     - Embryo cryopreservation
     - Cryopreservation of ovarian tissue and immature oocytes, obtained before regression of the ovaries in early childhood, is currently under intensive investigation.

Q 13. What is the recurrence risk of Turner syndrome?

Ans. Recurrence risk: As Turner syndrome occurs due to a random event so the recurrence risk is low. In rare cases, Turner syndrome may be caused by inherited partial deletion of the X-chromosome. So, genetic testing of an affected fetus or child can be done to identify the type of abnormality and it will help to estimate the risk of recurrence in next pregnancy.

Q 14. Describe the genetic basis of Klinefelter syndrome.

Ans. Genetic basis: It is the most common sex chromosome aneuploidy in males, with incidence of 0.1% in general population.

Karyotype abnormalities in Klinefelter syndrome:

- 47,XXY karyotype (80–85% of patients)
- Mosaics 46,XY/47,XXY (15% of patients)
- Other abnormalities include 46,XX/47,XXY; 46,XX/46,XY/47,XXY; 46,XY/48,XXXY; 45,X/46,XY/47,XXY
- Rare structural abnormalities of the X chromosome.

Mechanism:

- Non-disjunction in gametogenesis occurs either in the first or second meiotic division or at both.
- Error is maternal origin in 54% of cases and paternal in 46%.
- Usually, the extra X chromosome undergoes X inactivation but genes on pseudo-autosomal regions remain activate. This triple dose of genes on XXY chromosomes is responsible for the clinical symptoms.

Q 15. Describe the clinical features of Klinefelter syndrome.

Ans. Clinical features and complications: (Figure 9.9)

- Tall and eunuchoid habitus, long legs, disproportionate to the arms
- Small testes, hypogonadism, delayed secondary sexual characteristics
- Gynecomastia (80%)
- Infertility
- Low IQ, learning difficulties, deficits in executive function
- Central obesity, metabolic syndrome, varicose veins, and cancer of the breast.

Q 16. How will you diagnosis and manage Klinefelter syndrome? What is the recurrence risk of Klinefelter syndrome?

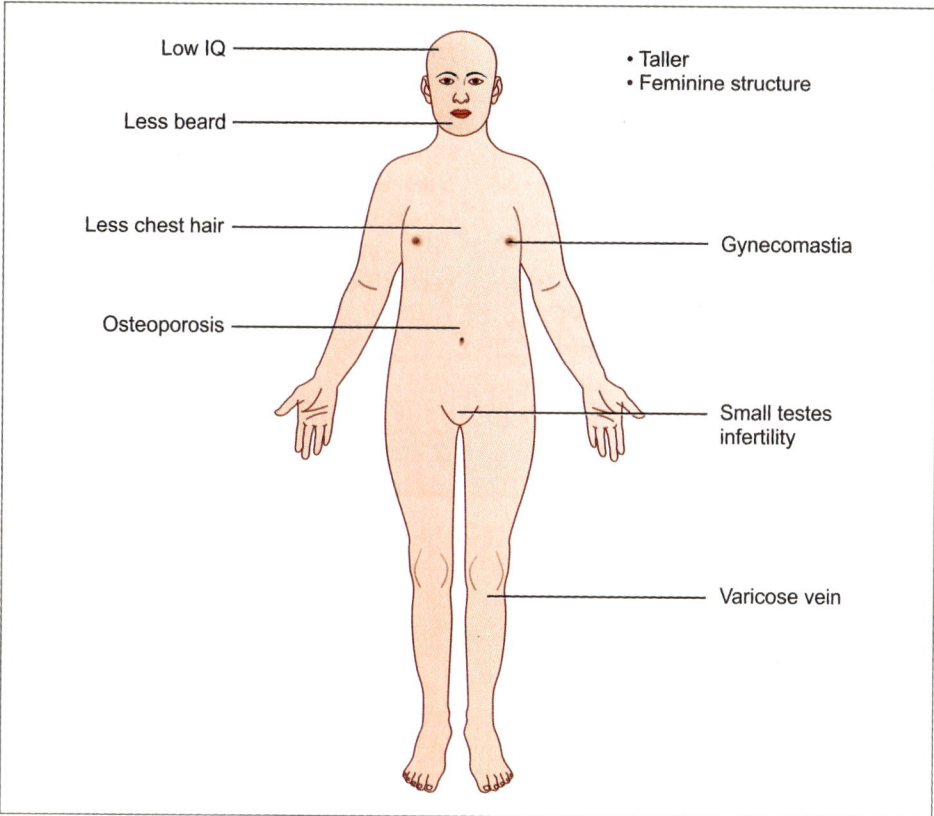

Low IQ

Less beard

Less chest hair

Osteoporosis

• Taller
• Feminine structure

Gynecomastia

Small testes
infertility

Varicose vein

Figure 9.9: Clinical features of Klinefelter syndrome (*Source of human body outline*: DLPNG.com)

Ans.

1. **Diagnosis**
   - Usually, these patients are referred for evaluation of hypogonadism or infertility.
   - Follicle stimulating hormone > leutinizing hormone, low testosterone, low inhibin B, increased anti-mullerian hormone.
   - Confirmation of diagnosis is done by karyotyping (Figure 9.10).

2. **Management:**
   - Testosterone therapy in adolescent age for development of secondary sexual characteristics
   - Mastectomy in gynecomastia to reduce chance of breast cancer
   - Psychosocial support.

3. **Recurrence risk:** As Klinefelter syndrome is a sporadic chromosomal process. The recurrence risk is not increased above that of the general population.

Q 17. How will you do genetic counseling and prenatal management for subsequent pregnancy in chromosomal aneuploidies?

Ans. Genetic counseling: (*See* Chapter 8)

Prenatal management:
   - Routine antenatal biochemical screening or cell free DNA and ultrasonography and anomaly scan of fetus will be done.
   - Aneuploidies can be detected prenatally by amniocentesis and cytogenetic amniotic fluid testing after informing the details of prenatal procedure and prenatal test to the family.

If test comes positive, the reproductive decision should be left up to the family.

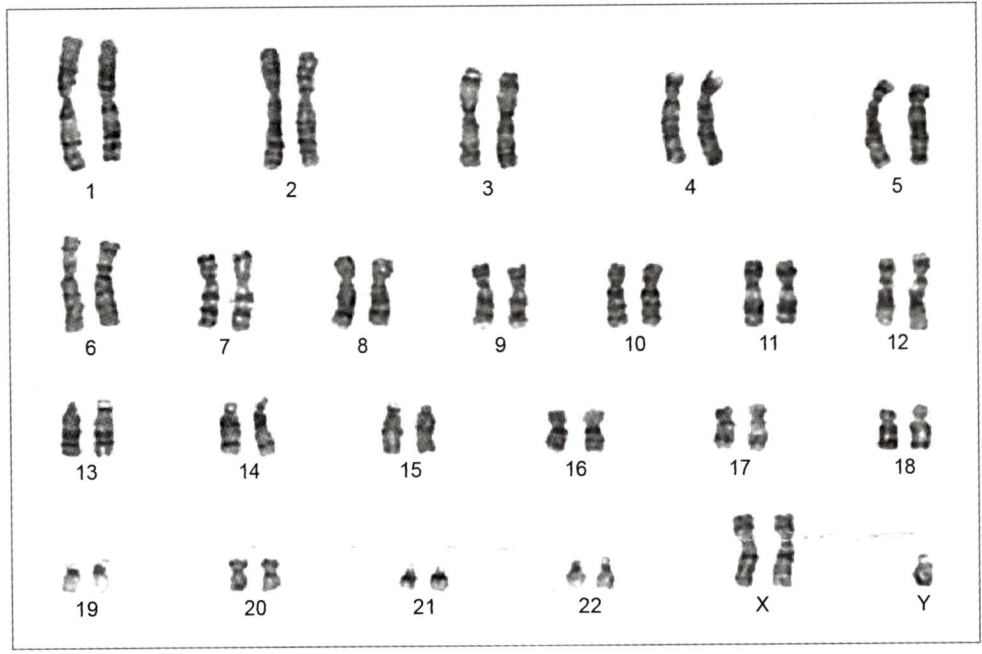

Figure 9.10: Karyotype in Klinefelter syndrome

Q 18. Describe the clinical features of other sex chromosome abnormalities.

Ans.

Karyotype	Clinical Features
47,XXX (1:1000 females)	o Females o Tall o Normal to low IQ, learning difficulties o Severity increases with no. of X chromosomes (48XXXX) o No medical or sexual problem.
47,XYY (1:1000 males)	o Males o Tall o Low IQ, language delay, learning difficulties o No other medical or sexual problem
46,XX males (1:20,000 males) XX males inherit one X chromosome from	o Male phenotype o Small testes, undescended testes, a small phallus
mother and other X from father with SRY region translocated on X chromosome.	o No evidence of ovarian or Mullerian structures (present in 46, XX ovotesticular) o Hypospadias in few o Infertility.
46,XY female (1:20,000 males) Most of the cases are due to mutations in SRY region, sex determining region on Y chromosome.	o Female phenotype or ambiguous genitalia o With non-functional gonads o With or without uterus o No puberty o Need removal of the streak gonads and hormonal replacement therapy.
Mosaic forms (45,X/46,XY; 45,X/46,XX; 46,XY/47,XXY)	o May have normal sexual development o 45,X/46,XY may be associated with the Turner phenotype o Ambiguous genitalia o Risk of gonadoblastoma o May be seen in normal males as well.

Q 19. Describe the genetic basis of Prader-Willi syndrome.

Ans. Genetics:

i. Prader-Willi syndrome (PWS) is an imprinting disorder caused due to chromosomal aberrations like deletion (≈70%), duplication, translocation or mutations on the paternal chromosome 15q11–13 regions.

ii. The 15q11–13 region is PWS critical region with multiple genes exclusively expressed from the father like SNRPN, SNORD116 cluster and silenced from the mother.

iii. PWS can also arise due to maternal uniparental disomy of chromosome 15 (≈ 20–30%).

iv. In 1–3% of PWS, there is an imprinting center defect; resulting in abnormal female DNA methylation during spermatogenesis on the paternal chromosome (paternal imprinting defect).

Q 20. Describe the clinical features and complications of Prader-Willi syndrome.

Ans. Clinical features: (Figure 9.11)

- **Prenatally:** Oligohydramnios, decreased fetal movements, small for gestational age.
- **Postnatally:** Severe hypotonia, poor suck, feeding difficulties and undescended testis in males.
- **Infancy:** Child becomes hyperphagic, increased incidence of hypothyroidism and diabetes, mild to moderate intellectual disability, behavioral abnormalities, dysmorphic appearance, strabismus, truncal obesity, short stature.

Q 21. How will you diagnose and manage Prader-Willi syndrome?

Ans. Diagnosis (Figure 9.11a)

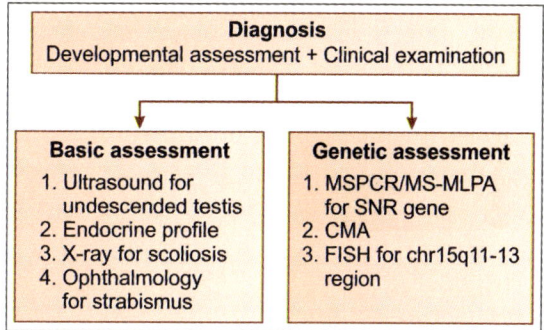

Figure 9.11a: Diagnosis and investigations in PWS: Methylation specific polymerase chain reaction (MSPCR sensitivity of 99%). of SNRPN gene, methylation specific multiple ligation probe dependent amplification (MSMLPA), fluorescent *in situ* hybridization (FISH) sensitive as 50–75%.

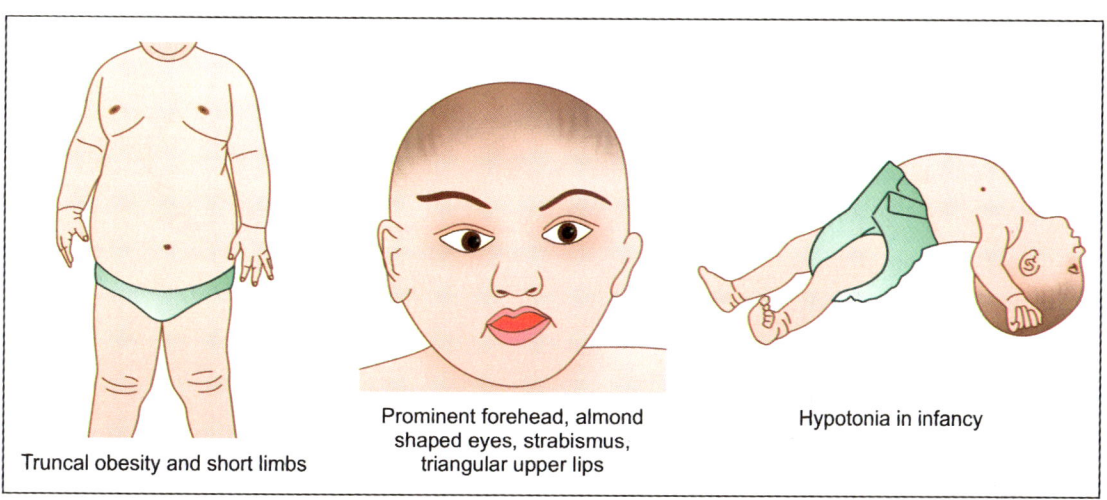

Truncal obesity and short limbs

Prominent forehead, almond shaped eyes, strabismus, triangular upper lips

Hypotonia in infancy

Figure 9.11: Features of Prader-Willi syndrome

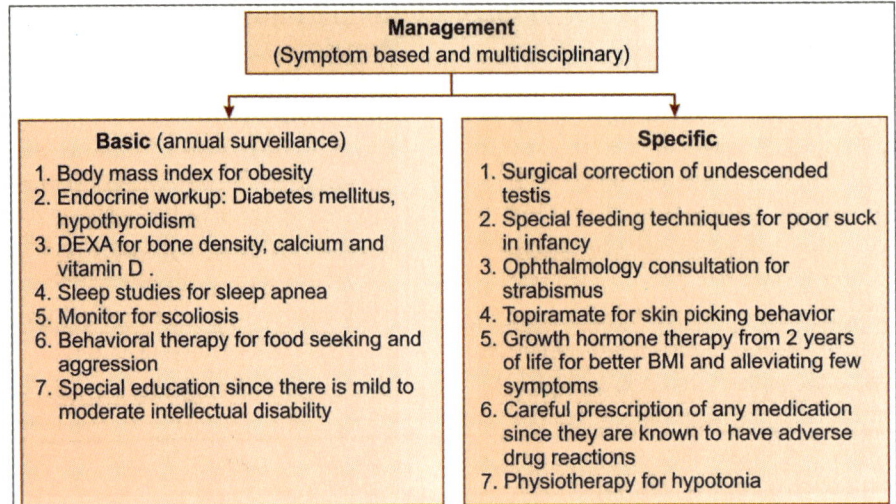

Management
(Symptom based and multidisciplinary)

Basic (annual surveillance)	**Specific**
1. Body mass index for obesity	1. Surgical correction of undescended
2. Endocrine workup: Diabetes mellitus,	testis
hypothyroidism	2. Special feeding techniques for poor suck
3. DEXA for bone density, calcium and	in infancy
vitamin D .	3. Ophthalmology consultation for
4. Sleep studies for sleep apnea	strabismus
5. Monitor for scoliosis	4. Topiramate for skin picking behavior
6. Behavioral therapy for food seeking and	5. Growth hormone therapy from 2 years
aggression	of life for better BMI and alleviating few
7. Special education since there is mild to	symptoms
moderate intellectual disability	6. Careful prescription of any medication
	since they are known to have adverse
	drug reactions
	7. Physiotherapy for hypotonia

Q 22. What is the recurrence risk of Prader-Willi syndrome?

Ans. Recurrence risk:

➲ It is essential to detect the type of mutation to accurately predict the recurrence risk in PWS.

➲ The recurrence risk in subsequent pregnancy is less than 1% in most cases.

➲ The recurrence risk is 50% if the father harbors the same deletion as the proband.

➲ If there is a parental chromosomal translocation, the recurrence risk can be 25–50%.

➲ Maternal UPD carries recurrence risk of 25–30%.

➲ Fetuses conceived by assisted reproductive techniques are at higher risk of developing imprinting disorders.

Q 23. Describe the genetic basis of Angelman syndrome.

Ans. Genetics:

i. Angelman syndrome (AS) is an imprinting disorder caused due to chromosomal aberrations like deletion, duplication (70%) translocation or mutations on the maternal chromosome 15q11–13 regions.

ii. The 15q11–13 region is AS critical region with UBE3A gene exclusively expressed from the mother and silenced in the father. Imprinting defect, or UBE3A sequence variations on the maternal chromosome 15 (10% of cases) can cause AS.

iii. AS can also arise due to paternal uniparental disomy of chromosome 15 (7%).

iv. In 2–4% of AS, there is an imprinting center defect; resulting in abnormal male DNA methylation during oogenesis on the maternal chromosome (maternal imprinting defect).

v. In 10% of cases, cause of etiology is unknown

Q 24. Describe the clinical features of Angelman syndrome.

Ans. Clinical features: (Figure 9.12)

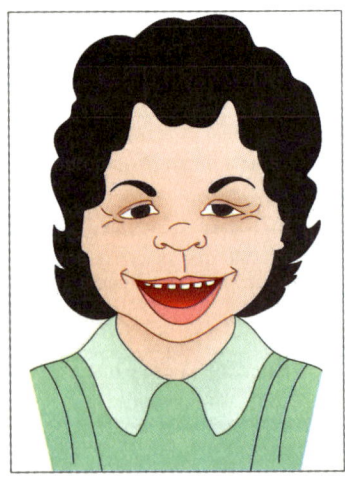

Figure 9.12: Features of AS: Sunken nasal bridge, puffiness around eyes, long philthrum, small widely spaced teeth, prominent lower lip, micrognathia

- Microcephaly
- Moderate to severe intellectual disability
- Gait ataxia
- Speech impairment
- Autistic behavior
- Widely spaced teeth
- Drooling
- Happy demeanor
- Inappropriate laughter
- Seizures.

Q 25. How will you diagnose Angelman syndrome and manage it?

Ans. Diagnosis and investigations in AS:

Q 26. What is the recurrence risk in AS?

Ans. Recurrence risk: It is essential to detect the molecular class of mutation to accurately predict the recurrence risk in AS.

- Fetuses conceived by assisted reproductive techniques are at higher risk of developing imprinting disorders.
- The recurrence risk in subsequent pregnancy is less than 1% in most cases (UBE3A sequence variation, UPD or deletion).
- The recurrence risk is 50% if the mother harbors the same deletion or mutation as the proband or if there is an imprinting defect.

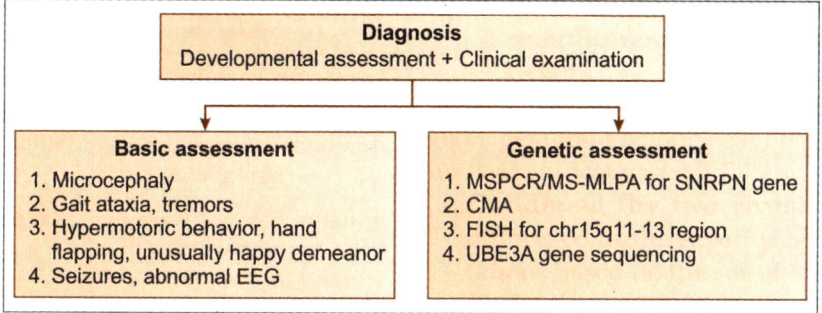

Methylation specific polymerase chain reaction (MSPCR sensitivity of 80%) of SNRPN gene, methylation specific multiple ligation probe dependent amplification (MSMLPA), fluorescent *in situ* hybridization (FISH) sensitive as 10%.

- If there is a parental chromosomal translocation the recurrence risk can be 25–50% which is observed in 1% of AS cases.

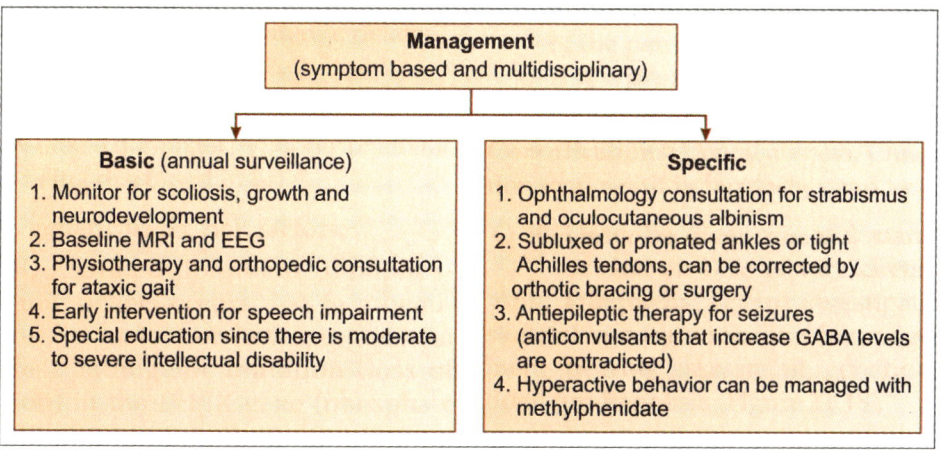

Q 27. Describe the genetic basis of Beckwith-Wiedemann syndrome.

Ans. Genetics: Beckwith-Wiedemann syndrome (BWS) is an imprinting disorder caused due to chromosomal aberrations (<1–3%) like deletion, duplication (paternal), translocation on the chromosome 11p15 region.

- The 11p15 region has two imprinting control regions 1 and 2 (ICR1 and ICR2). The ICR1 hypermethylation (5%) or ICR2 hypomethylation can cause BWS (55%).
- BWS can be caused by CDKN1C sequence variations (10%).
- BWS can also arise due to pat UPD 11 (20%).
- In 10% of cases, cause of etiology is unknown.

Q 28. Write the clinical features and complications of Beckwith-Wiedemann syndrome.

Ans. Clinical features (Figure 9.13)

- Polyhydramnios
- Large for gestational age
- Hypoglycemia
- Segmental hypertrophy
- Macrosomia
- Macroglossia
- Cleft lip and palate

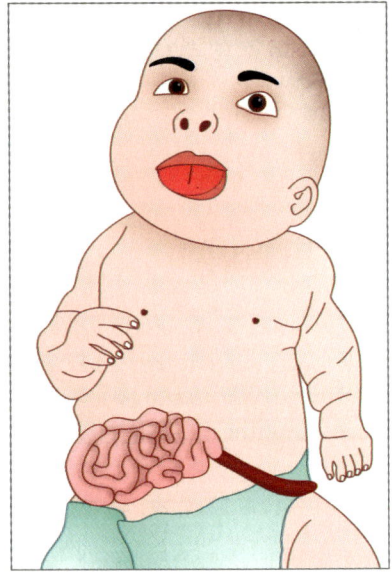

Figure 9.13: Features of BWS: Nevus flammeus, exophthalmos, macroglossia, ear creases, hemihypertophy, omphalocele

- Renal tumors
- Wilms' tumor
- Liver tumors
- Organomegaly
- Ear pits.

Q 29. How will you diagnose and manage Beckwith-Wiedemann syndrome?

Ans. Diagnosis and investigations in BWS:

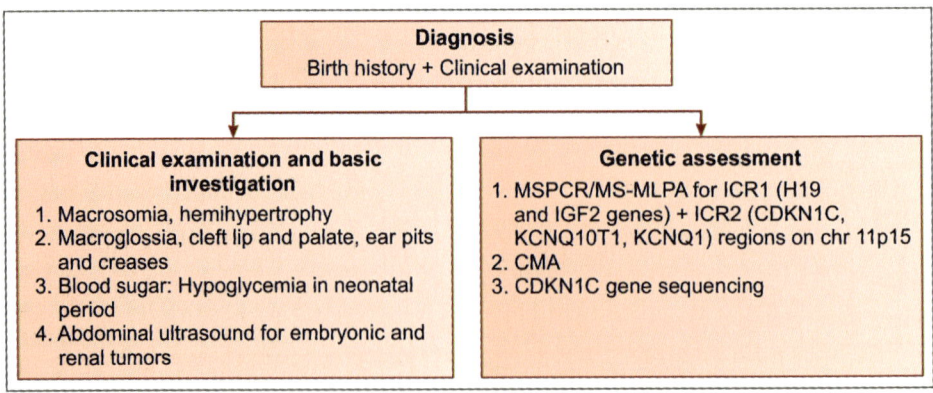

Methylation specific polymerase chain reaction (MSPCR) gene, methylation specific multiple ligation probe dependent amplification (MSMLPA), cytogenetic microarray (CMA).

- SRS can be caused due to imprinting defect, IGF2, CDKN1C, PLAG1, HMGA2 gene sequence variations (10%).
- It can also arise due to maternal uniparental disomy of chromosome 7 (10%).

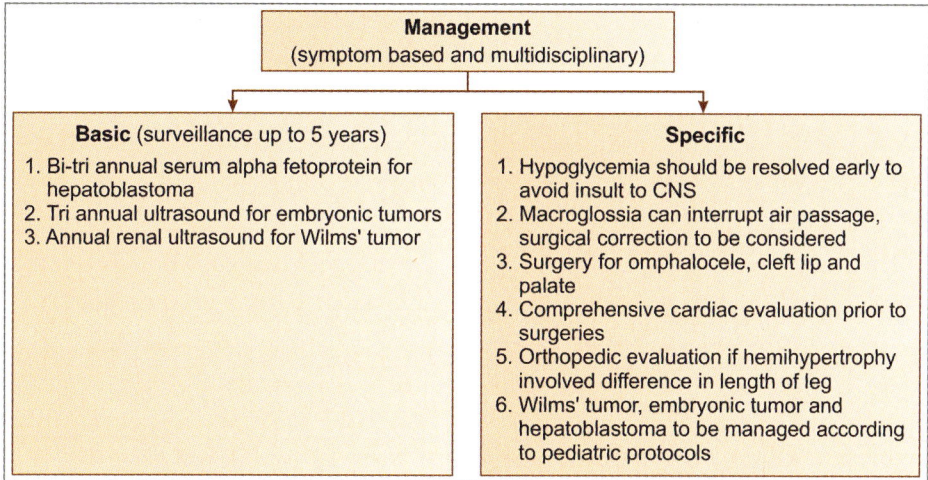

Management
(symptom based and multidisciplinary)

Basic (surveillance up to 5 years)	Specific
1. Bi-tri annual serum alpha fetoprotein for hepatoblastoma 2. Tri annual ultrasound for embryonic tumors 3. Annual renal ultrasound for Wilms' tumor	1. Hypoglycemia should be resolved early to avoid insult to CNS 2. Macroglossia can interrupt air passage, surgical correction to be considered 3. Surgery for omphalocele, cleft lip and palate 4. Comprehensive cardiac evaluation prior to surgeries 5. Orthopedic evaluation if hemihypertrophy involved difference in length of leg 6. Wilms' tumor, embryonic tumor and hepatoblastoma to be managed according to pediatric protocols

Q 30. What is recurrence risk of Beckwith-Wiedemann syndrome?

Ans. Recurrence risk: It is essential to detect the molecular class of mutation to accurately predict the recurrence risk in BWS.

- The recurrence risk in subsequent pregnancies is less than 1% in most cases.
- Fetuses conceived by assisted reproductive techniques are at higher risk of developing imprinting disorders.
- The recurrence risk is 50% if the parent harbors the same deletion/duplication as the proband or if the mother also has the variation in CDKNIC gene.
- If there is a parental chromosomal translocation, the recurrence risk can be 25–50% which is observed in 1% of BWS cases.

Q 31. Describe the genetic basis of Silver-Russell syndrome.

Ans. Genetics: Silver-Russell syndrome (SRS) is heterogeneous imprinting disorder caused due to chromosomal aberrations (1–2%) like deletion, duplication (maternal), translocation on the chromosome 11p15 region.

- The ICR1 (present on the chromosome 11p15 region) hypomethylation (35–50%) or mat UPD 11 can cause SRS.

Q 32. What are the clinical features of Silver-Russell syndrome?

Ans. Clinical features: (Figure 9.14)

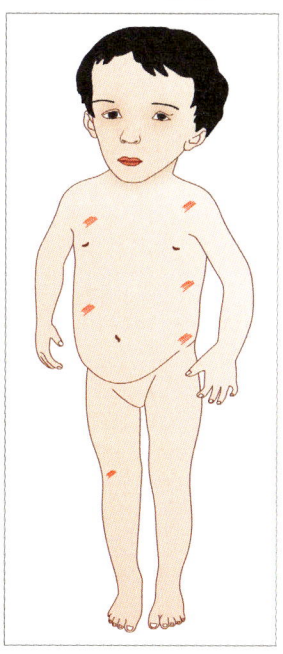

Figure 9.14: : Features of SRS: Pseudohydrocephaly, frontal bossing, triangular face, downturned angles of mouth, micrognathia, hemihypertrophy, café au lait spots, short stature

⊃ Oligohydramnios
⊃ Severe growth restriction during gestation
⊃ Apparent macrocephaly
⊃ Segmental hypertrophy
⊃ Frontal bossing triangular facies
⊃ Clinodactyly
⊃ Feeding difficulties, postnatal growth failure
⊃ Short stature
⊃ Cafe au lait spots.

Q 33. How will you diagnose and manage Silver-Russell syndrome?

Ans. Diagnosis and investigations in SRS:

Q 34. What is the recurrence risk of Silver-Russell syndrome?

Ans. Recurrence risk

⊃ It is essential to detect the molecular class of mutation to accurately predict the recurrence risk in SRS.
⊃ The recurrence risk in subsequent pregnancies is less than 1% in most cases.
⊃ Fetuses conceived by assisted reproductive techniques are at higher risk of developing imprinting disorders.
⊃ The recurrence risk is 50% if the parent harbors the same deletion/duplication or gene sequence variation as the proband.

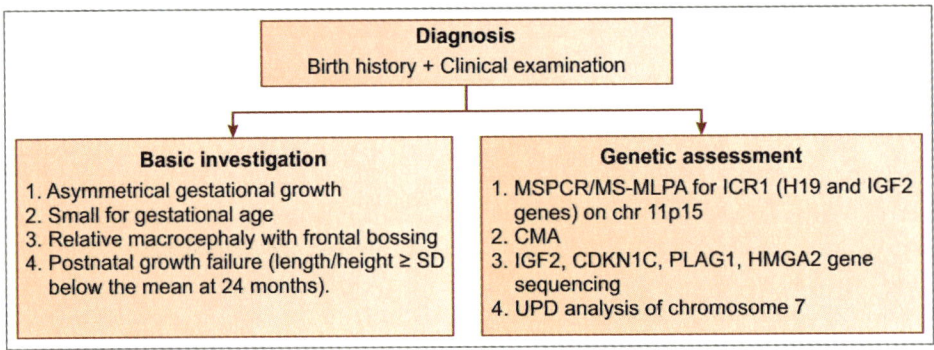

Methylation specific polymerase chain reaction (MSPCR) gene, methylation specific multiple ligation probe dependent amplification (MSMLPA), cytogenetic microarrays (CMA).

⊃ If there is a parental chromosomal translocation, the recurrence risk can be 25–50% which is observed in 1% of SRS cases.

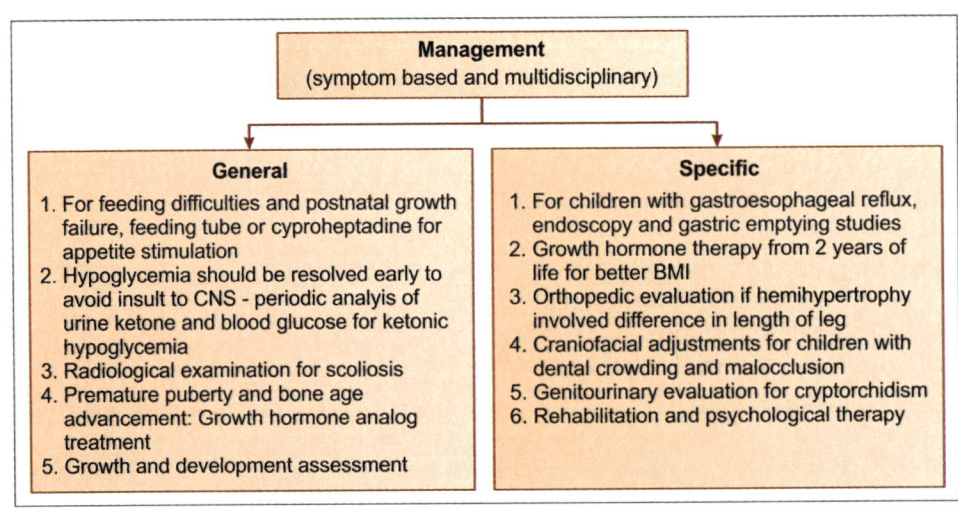

Q 35. How will you do genetic counseling and prenatal management for subsequent pregnancies in genomic imprinting disorders?

Ans. Genetic counseling: Following all the general principles of counseling and respecting the psychosocial aspects of family, discuss the following with families during counseling:

- Need of genetic testing in the proband and parents, details of the disease, management options, the recurrence risk in future generation and prenatal testing.
- Prenatal diagnosis for identified mutation by chorionic villi sampling at 11–13 weeks or amniocentesis at 16–18 weeks can be offered to know whether fetus is affected or not.

Before prenatal testing, family should be informed regarding:

- Prenatal procedure and prenatal test details
- Likely benefits of early diagnosis
- Appropriate support and preparedness if the result returns positive.

Q 36. Write a brief note on chromosomal breakage syndrome.

Ans. Chromosomal breakage syndromes (chromosomal instability syndromes) typically have autosomal recessive mode of inheritance.

Various causes of chromosomal breakage syndrome:

1. **Loss of DNA repair:** Nucleotide excision repair
2. Inter strand crosslinks
3. Genomic instability
4. Nucleotide change
5. Double stranded DNA breaks
6. Increase exchange between sister chromatids

The following chromosome instability syndromes are known:

Syndromes	Chromosomal locations and genes involved	Phenotypes	Cancer predisposition
Ataxia telangiectasia	o 11q23 o ATM	o Ataxia o Respiratory infections o Eye and skin telangiectasia o Immunodeficiency o Hematological malignancies o Premature aging o Radiation sensitivity	Yes
Ataxia telangiectasia-like disorder	o 11q21 o Mre11	o Cerebellar degeneration o Radiation sensitivity	Yes
Bloom's syndrome	o 15q26.1 o NLM	o Immunodeficiency (IgA and IgG decreased) o Photosensitive skin o Premature aging	Yes
Fanconi anemia	o Multiple o FANC-A, B, C, D1, D2, E, F, G, I, J, L, M, N, O, P, Q, R, S and T	o Radial ray defect, short stature o Bone-marrow failure (aplastic anemia) o Congenital renal and cardiac abnormalities o Cutaneous pigmentation	Yes

Contd.

Syndromes	Chromosomal locations and genes involved	Phenotypes	Cancer pre-disposition
Nijmegen breakage syndrome	o 8q21.3 o NBS1	o Microcephaly o Facial dysmorphism o Intellectual disability o Immunodeficiency o Radiation sensitivity o Non-Hodgkin's lymphoma o Brain tumors	Yes
Xeroderma pigmentosum	o 6p21.1 o POLH	o Affects eyes and areas of skin exposed to the sun	Yes

BIBLIOGRAPHY

1. Agarwal Gupta N, Kabra M. Diagnosis and management of Down syndrome. Indian J Pediatr. 2014;81(6):560–7. doi:10.1007/s12098–013-1249–7
2. Emery's elements of Medical Genetics, 15th edition.
3. Nelson's Textbook of Pediatrics, 21st edition.
4. Turner syndrome. Genetics Home Reference. January, 2012;http://ghr.nlm.nih.gov/condition/turner- syndrome.

Multifactorial Disorders

Ami Shah, Chaitanya A Datar, Komal Uppal

Q 1. What is meant by genetic susceptibility?

Ans. Genetic susceptibility:

- Genetic susceptibility is the increased chance of developing a particular disease due to the presence of one or more gene variations and/or a family history that indicates increased risk of the disease.
- These genetic changes contribute to the development of a disease but do not directly cause it. Thus, some individuals with a particular genetic variation may get the disease while others may not.
- Genetic susceptibility plays a major role in multifactorial congenital malformations where the disease liability results from genetic susceptibility and environmental triggering factors. If both components, genetic and environmental, exceed a certain threshold, the malformation appears.
- This also explains why clinical and etiologic heterogeneity of congenital malformations cannot always be explained by a single genetic/environmental factor.

Q 2. How can monozygotic (MZ) and dizygotic (DZ) twins prove a genetic susceptibility to common multifactorial inherited diseases?

Ans. Disorders resulting from a combination of both genetic and environmental factors are known to have multifactorial inheritance.

- To demonstrate genetic susceptibility in multifactorial diseases, it is important to compare individuals sharing similar genes but having different environments.
- Twin studies which compare monozygotic and dizygotic twins, helps to investigate both genetic and environmental factors.
- Monozygotic twins share both their genes and environment, whereas dizygotic twins share a common environment but only 50% of their genes (like other siblings).
- When twins share a disease or trait, they are said to be concordant, and discordant if only one of the twins is affected. Concordance rates in monozygotic and dizygotic twins can help in identifying genetic susceptibility.
- If a trait or disease is entirely genetic, 100% of MZ twins and 50% of DZ twins should be concordant for the trait. If a trait does not have a genetic component, there should be no difference in concordance rates between MZ and DZ twins.
- Thus, all phenotypic dissimilarity can be attributed to differing environmental factors in monozygotic twins but in dizygotic twins it can result from differences in genetic and/or environmental factors.
- Normally both set of twins share a common environment; studies on identical twins reared separately would also throw additional light on genetic susceptibility.
- Correlation coefficient is a measure of the association of a continuous trait between two relatives and suggests genetic susceptibility. In twin studies, a correlation coefficient

of 1 in monozygotic twins would mean a trait was entirely determined by genes. A correlation coefficient of 0 means there is no similarity between monozygotic twin pairs for the trait in question.

- Important to note that rare events like chromosome nondisjunction or a new mutation in one of the twins and epigenetics are exceptions to above deductions.
- This way twin studies give an insight into various etiological and clinical factors of multifactorial disorders which play an important role in formulation of preventive and curative therapies.

Q 3. Write about the mechanism of genetic susceptibility in causing multifactorial congenital malformations like holoprosencephaly and neural tube defect.

Ans. Holoprosencephaly is a structural brain anomaly occurs due to incomplete division of prosencephalon. Normally, prosencephalon gets divided into telencephalon and diencephalon leading to further brain structures formation. Due to this abnormal brain development, lobar, alobar or semilobar holoprosencephaly can occur. It can occur due to various genetic (chromosomal trisomy 13 or 22q11 deletion or SHH gene disorders) or non-genetic factors (maternal diabetes mellitus).

Neural tube defect: Like spina bifida, anencephaly, encephalocele, meningocele or myelomeningocele occur due to failure of closure of neural tube during first 21 days of gestation. It can occur due to:

- Various genetic syndromes (chromosomal trisomy 13, 18 or Meckel-Gruber syndrome, MTHR methylene tetrahydrofolate reductase mutation)
- Isolated malformation
- Can be due to non-genetic factors (low socioeconomic level, multipara mother, sodium valproate).

Q 4. How does modified environment reduce *the incidence of* congenital malformations in children?

Ans. Modifying the environmental factors in multifactorial disorders may help to mitigate the severity or rarely prevent its occurrence altogether. Prevention of certain congenital malformations such as neural tube defects, cleft lip, and palate and congenital heart disease by modification in the environment in the first 3 months of pregnancy when organogenesis takes place is given in Table 10.1.

TABLE 10.1: Modified environment to reduce the incidence of congenital malformations	
Modification of environmental risk factors	*Prevention of congenital malformations*
No smoking, drinking alcohol or taking certain "street" drugs during pregnancy	o Congenital heart defect o Microcephaly
o Consumption of 400–800 µg of folic acid along with multivitamins (B_{12} in particular) periconceptionally. o MTHFR gene polymorphisms may need higher doses of folic acid and other B complex vitamins.	o Neural tube defect (incidence reduces by 50–75%) o Cleft lip and palate o Congenital heart disease
Avoid isotretinoin or valproate or older drug thalidomide 3–6 months before and during pregnancy.	o Cardiac defect o Limb defect o Ear defect o Holoprosencephaly o Eye defect
Obesity control or having controlled diabetes before and during pregnancy.	o Cardiac defect o Holoprosencephaly o Neural tube defect o Skeletal defects
Intrauterine infections and phenylalanine restricted diet in maternal phenylketonuria.	o Microcephaly o Ear defect o Eye defect o Cardiac defect
Radiations and chemicals.	o Microcephaly o Neuronal migration o Eye defects defects

Q 5. What is the empiric recurrence risk for common multifactorial disorders.

Ans. The inheritance patterns of multifactorial disorders are complex, and the recurrence risks are difficult to predict for the following reasons:

- They do not follow a classical Mendelian inheritance pattern.
- In many cases the gene/s involved have not been characterized or the interaction between these disorders is not known.
- The mode, degree, impact and interaction of the environmental factors are largely unknown.

For these reasons, prenatal diagnosis is not possible for most of the multifactorial disorders. The follow-up for ruling out recurrence is based on antenatal ultrasound scans and rarely by using markers such as alpha-fetoprotein (AFP) in the maternal serum.

The empiric recurrence risk for common multifactorial disorders **(Tables 10.2 to 10.4) depends upon various factors as:**

- When associated with known syndromes or as an isolated monogenic disorder, the recurrence risk depends on the specific inheritance pattern.
- In a suspected multifactorial inheritance, the empiric recurrence risk that another child of the same parents will be affected by a multifactorial congenital disorder or the risk to a child of a single affected parent is small ~5%.
- The risk of recurrence increases if more than one family member is affected. *Example:* Risk increases to 10% if there are two affected siblings.
- When three or more affected siblings are present, possibility of monogenic disorder should be investigated.
- Similarly, the recurrence risk will reduce with increasing distance in relation to the proband risk is 2% in presence of an affected second degree relative.
- Occurrence/recurrence of multifactorial disorders are discussed only for the purpose of genetic counseling:

TABLE 10.2: The empiric recurrence risk for common multifactorial disorders

Type of multifactorial disorder	Sibs affected	Parents affected	Empiric risk of recurrence (in %)
Neural tube defects	0	0	0.3
	1	1or 2	10–40
	1 or 2	0	5–10
Cleft lip-palate	0	0	0.1
	1 or 2	0	3–10
	1	1 or 2	10–14
Congenital hip dislocation	2	Unaffected	6
	1	Affected	12
Pyloric stenosis	2	Unaffected	2 (male), 10 (female)
	1	Affected	4 (male) 17 (female)
Schizo-phrenia	2	Unaffected	10
	1	Affected	14
Autism	2	Unaffected	2–3
	1	Affected	5
Epilepsy	2	Unaffected	5
	1	Affected	5
Congenital hearing loss	2	Unaffected	10–15
	1	Affected	5–10
Diabetes mellitus type 1 (depending on common DR haplo-type)	1	Unaffected	1–17
	0	Affected	3–5
Diabetes mellitus type 2	0	Affected mother	40
	0	Both affected	70

TABLE 10.3: The empiric risk of recurrence in common congenital heart disease

Type of congenital heart disease	Empiric risk of recurre-nce in siblings (in %)
Ventricular septal defect	4
Patent ductus arteriosus	3
Atrial septal defect	3

TABLE 10.4: Coronary artery disease	
Proband	*Increased risk in other close family members (relative to general population)*
Male	2.5–3 fold
Female	7–11.4 fold

Q 6. Write a note on genetics of diabetes mellitus 1 (DM 1).

Ans. **Diabetes mellitus 1:** It is a multifactorial disease caused by both genetic and non-genetic factors. Monozygotic twins which show concordance rate for diabetes 40% not 100% shows involvement of environmental factors in its etiology. The environmental factors like food, viral infections and some medicines stimulate the production of antibodies against islet β cells and show the association between these factors and immune system in a genetically susceptible person. By knowing the genetics of diabetes mellitus 1 by genetic testing exact risk of recurrence cannot be predicted but the empirical risk and gene susceptibility can be identified. Empirical risk of DM 1 to siblings is given in Table 10.2.

Genetics

HLA (human leucocyte antigen) 30–50% association: More than 200 genes are known in association with DM 1. Following are the common ones which are discovered:

- HLA1 (A, B, C) and HLA 11{(DR3, DR4-95%), DQ8, DQA1, DQB2,DP}
- DQB1* 0303: Protective haplotype.
- DQB1 where aspartic acid provides protection.

Non-HLA association: Genome wide studies show about 50 different loci in the genome which can increase the risk for DM1. Some of these are:

- INS VNTR, PTPN22, IL10, IL19, IL20, IL27, IL2RA, IFIHI, cytotoxic T-lymphocyte associated protein (CTLA-4), CD 25: Associated with autoimmune diseases by

activating immune system especially T-cells, inflammatory cytokines and interferones.
- AIRE (autoimmune regulator responsible for immune self-tolerance), Fox P3 (IPEX syndrome), STAT3 (polyautoimmune syndrome).
- Common genetic syndromes and disorders associated with DM I: Down syndrome, Turner syndrome, Bardet-Biedl syndrome, Alstrom syndrome, Wolfram syndrome, Huntington disease, Friedreich ataxia, etc.
- By knowing the genetic susceptibility, various preventive measures can be taken to prevent occurrence of DM 1. For example, oral insulin trials for children with HLA DR3/DR4-DQ8 alleles and affected close first degree relatives, are being studied for preventive trials.

Q 7. Write a note on genetics of diabetes mellitus 2 (DM 2).

Ans. **Genetics of DM 2**

- Approximately 70 genes are associated with DM 2 identified by gene wide association studies (GWAS) in various populations like Europeans and Asians.
- KCNJ11, KCNQ1, PPARG, HNF1A, HNF1B, HNF4A, WFS1, TCF7L2, FTO, CAPN10 and other genes identified by GWAS and associated with obesity are the most common genes related with DM 2.
- Mutations in these genes disturb the insulin and insulin receptor function and along with environmental factors like obesity and epigenetics changes, results in DM 2.
- Knowing these variants in the genes can help in assessing the risk and delaying the development of diabetes by modifying environmental factors and by changing the lifestyle.
- Knowledge of the genetics has a great role in pharmacogenetics in prescribing the right drug with right doses and with less adverse effects. For example, KCNJ11 has an important role in effecting the efficacy of sulfonylureas.

Q 8. Write a note on genetics of maturity onset diabetes of the young (MODY).

Ans. MODY is autosomal dominant (AD) monogenic non-insulin dependent diabetes mellitus. It is caused by 14 genes but the common ones are:

MODY 1: Hepatocyte nuclear factor HNF-4-α gene, HNF-1A, 1B.

MODY 2: Glucokinase gene. Associated with DM 1, 2 and pregnancy associated DM.

MODY 3: Hepatic transcription factor-1

MODY 4: Insulin promoter factor gene

MODY 5: Hepatic transcription factor 2 gene.

As it is AD in pattern so there is risk of 50% to develop MODY in close relatives. By knowing the genetic variant it can help in assessing the risk and can help in planning the treatment and surveillance of other organs (kidney involvement in HNF1B mutation). By modifying environmental factors and by changing the lifestyle the development of diabetes can be delayed.

Q 9. Write a note on genetics of coronary artery disease (CAD).

Ans. CAD is a multifactorial disease caused by various predisposing environmental factors like lack of physical activity, fat rich diet and medicines and genetic susceptibility. The various genes causing CAD discovered are associated with lipid metabolism, inflammatory and blood vessel wall changes leading to atherosclerosis and result in myocardial infarction. These genes along with environmental factors increase the risk for CAD in close relatives. The risk of CAD in siblings is shown in Table 10.4. Various genes causing CAD are as follows:

- ⇒ MEF2A (transcriptional factor) non-lipid gene causes myocardial infarction by abnormal endothelial development.
- ⇒ **Prolonged QT interval:** KCNQ1, KCNH2, SCN5A
- ⇒ **Single gene mutations affecting lipid metabolism:** LDLR gene in familial hypercholesterolemia, PCSK9, Apo B 100, CYP7A1, ARH, ABCA1, USF1, ApoE.
- ⇒ **Cytokine genes:** LTA, LGALS2 (Lymohotoxin-alfa and regulatory genes).
- ⇒ Lipoxygenase activating protein gene ALOX5AP
- ⇒ *CDKN2A, CDKN2B, ANRIL, PDE4D:* Related with inflammation in blood vessels and atherosclerosis.
- ⇒ Various other new genes identified by GWAS and other molecular technologies help in early diagnosis and can help in delay onset of disease by lifestyle changes and various target therapy like PCSK 9 inhibitors for decreasing the level of cholesterol can be tried.

Q 10. Write a note on genetics of hypertension.

Ans. Hypertension when blood pressure in adults raised above 130/80 mmHg, can be asymptomatic or can present as stroke, heart failure, renal problems or retinopathy. It can be essential where no cause is known (95%) or can be secondary to underlying renal, blood vessel, fluid and electrolyte or endocrine abnormality. It is a multifactorial disease involving various genetic and non-genetic factors like ethnicity, high intake of sodium, alcohol, lack of exercise, smoking, stress, obesity and diabetes mellitus. Among the genetic factors it involves:

1. **Genetic syndromes:**
   - ⇒ Liddle syndrome due to mutation in epithelial sodium channel.
   - ⇒ Autosomal dominant hyperaldosteronism: Mutation in 11β-hydroxylase and aldosterone synthase enzyme.
   - ⇒ Pseudohypoaldosteronism (CUL3)
   - ⇒ Primary hyperaldosteronism (ATPA1)
   - ⇒ Congenital adrenal hyperplasia (CYP21A2)
   - ⇒ Paragangliomas, pheochromocytomas. (RET, VHL, SDHA, B, C, D)
2. **Polymorphism in genes:** GWAS has discovered more than 100 genetic mutations responsible for essential hypertension. The common one is:
   - ⇒ Renin angiotensin (AGT), angiotensin converting enzyme (ACE), ACE II receptor genes.
   - ⇒ Susceptible genes for blood vessel integrity (PDE1A, HRH1)

○ UMOD gene at loop of Henle, NPPB natriuretic peptide, ATP2B1, STK39, GRK4, SLC4A5 salt sensitivity genes, MTHFR, CLCN6, etc.

3. Epigenetics changes

Molecular technologies can help in early diagnosis of these susceptible genes which help in assessing the risk of disease in close relatives. Early diagnosis helps in delay onset of disease by making changes in lifestyle and various target therapeutic drugs.

Q 11. Write about the epidemiology of autistic spectrum disorders.

Ans. Definition: Autism is a developmental disorder characterized by impairments in social skills, communication skills and restrictive/repetitive patterns of behavior.

The severity may vary from mild to severe and this could be variably associated with attention deficit and hyperactivity, intellectual impairment or other neurological findings including seizures, tone abnormalities, etc.

The term autism spectrum disorder (ASD) is nowadays preferred as it encompasses many other conditions such as pervasive developmental disorder not otherwise specified (PDD-NOS), Asperger syndrome, etc.

Epidemiology: ASD has a high prevalence with an estimated 1 in every 1000 children in the US. Though the exact incidence in India is unknown, it is predicted to be high.

Q 12. What are the diagnostic criteria of autistic spectrum disorders?

Ans. Diagnostic criteria: The features of ASD may be observed by parents anytime between 1 and 2 years, but a formal diagnosis is usually done much later.

There are no blood-based tests or markers to diagnose this condition. Clinicians follow the DSMV criteria for the diagnosis of ASD which is based on the following two areas:

1. Social communication and interaction:
○ Unable to interact socially/emotionally.
○ Difficulty in establishing or maintaining conversations.
○ No sharing of attention or emotions with others.
○ Lack of interest in other people, difficulties in pretend play and unable to engage in age-appropriate social activities.
○ Abnormal eye contact or facial expressions.
○ Language delay and unable to use sign language.

2. **Restricted and repetitive behavior:** Two of the four symptoms need to be present in early childhood and need to be functionally impairing:
○ Stereotyped or repetitive speech, motor movements, etc.
○ Excessive adherence to routines, ritualized patterns of behavior, or excessive resistance to change.
○ Highly restricted interests.
○ Compulsive behavior.
○ Hyper- or hypo-sensitivity to sensory input.

Q 13. What is the recurrence risk of autism?

Ans. Recurrence risks:

Autism case	Recurrence risk (in future pregnancies of parents) (in %)
With identified genetic cause	
Chromosomal microdeletion or microduplication—absent in parents	1–3
De novo genetic variant/s for common conditions absent in parents	1–3
Fragile X syndrome (mother is a carrier)	50 (males)
With no identified cause	
Previous male child with autism	1–3
Previous female child with autism	3–5

Q 14. Write the etiology and genetic basis of autism.

Ans. Autism is multifactorial in origin. Various gene-gene and/or a gene-environment interaction, environmental factors may be acting either *in utero* or in early infancy to modify the brain circuits or may be acting at an epigenetic level. It has higher male preponderance with male : female ratio being 4 : 1.

Etiology and genetic basis:

- The **genetic cause** may be identified in about 25% cases, known as syndromic autism.
- Chromosomal microdeletions / microduplications, e.g. Dup15q syndrome, deletions in the 16p11.2 region. Chromosomal microarray must be considered as first-line studies in cases with autism to detect these deletions / duplications.
- Defined single gene conditions (detected in ~3–5% ASD cases), e.g. fragile X syndrome (*FMR1*), tuberous sclerosis (*TSC1* and *TSC2*), Rett syndrome (*MECP2*), and neurofibromatosis (*NF1*). TP-PCR for fragile X syndrome and NGS/Sanger-based testing to identify the mutations for the relevant gene/s should be done.
- *De novo* **single gene variants:** With the advent of NextGen sequencing techniques, many *de novo* single gene variants account for a significant proportion of cases and show phenotypic heterogeneity and variable penetrance.
- **Heritability:** Non-classical monozygotic twins show 92% and dizygotic twins show 10% concordance for autism.
- **Idiopathic autism:** In the remaining cases, the cause is obscure.

BIBLIOGRAPHY

1. Emery & Rimoin's Principles & Practice of Medical Genetics, 7th edition.

2. Thompson & Thompson, Genetics in Medicine, 8th edition.

Common Monogenic Disorders

Shruti Bajaj, Mounika Endrakanti, Neerja Gupta, Gayatri N, Kausik Mandal

CONNECTIVE TISSUE DISORDER
SHRUTI BAJAJ

Q 1. Describe the etiology, genetic basis of Marfan syndrome.

Ans. Etiology and genetic basis:

- Marfan syndrome (MFS) occurs due to a heterozygous mutation in one of the alleles of the fibrillin-1 *(FBN1)* gene (chromosome 15q21.1)
- *FBN1* gene encodes for the protein fibrillin-1, an extracellular matrix protein, plays a crucial role in the formation of microfibrils in elastic and non-elastic tissues for the structural integrity of the ocular, cardiovascular and the skeletal structures.
- Abnormal fibrillin leads to increase in transforming growth factor beta (TGF beta) which leads to pulmonary and vascular pathological changes.
- Three-fourths of all mutations are inherited from an affected parent, while one-fourth of them occur *de novo.*
- Missense mutations show dominant negative effect (abnormal fibril in hinders the formation of normal microfibrillin). So, haplo insufficiency is also responsible for the pathology of disease.

Q 2. Describe the clinical features and complications of Marfan syndrome (MFS).

Ans. Clinical features and complications: (Figure 11.1)

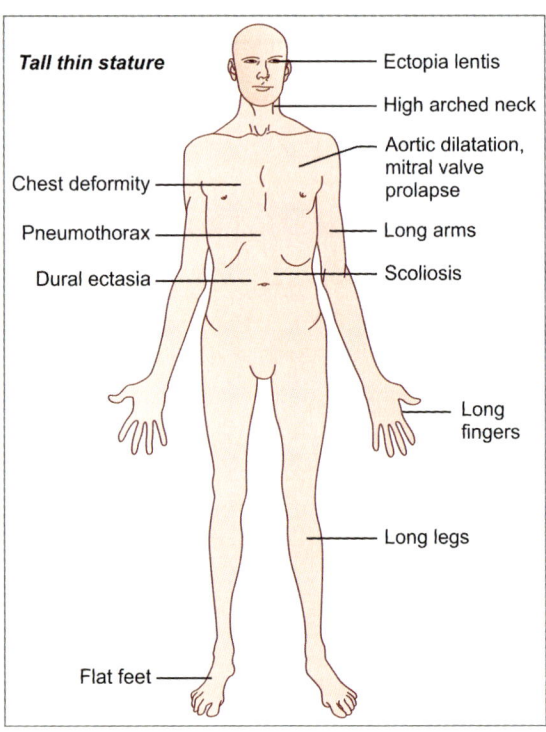

Labels: Tall thin stature; Chest deformity; Pneumothorax; Dural ectasia; Flat feet; Ectopia lentis; High arched neck; Aortic dilatation, mitral valve prolapse; Long arms; Scoliosis; Long fingers; Long legs

Figure 11.1: Marfan syndrome features
(*Source of human body outline*: DLPNG.com)

1. MFS depicts significant pleiotropism and clinical variability.
2. The cardinal systems involved in MS include the skeletal, ocular and cardiovascular systems.
   a. **Skeletal and growth:** Disproportionate tall stature (upper segment: lower segment<0.85), dolichostenomelia, i.e.

arm span: height >1.05, kyphoscoliosis, pectus excavatum or carinatum, joint hypermobility, joint contractures, arachnodactyly (positive wrist and/or thumb sign), genu recurvatum, protrusion acetabuli (appreciated radiologically), pes planus.

b. **Ocular:** Ectopialentis (superotemporal dislocation), myopia, corneal flatness, glaucoma and cataract.

c. **Cardiovascular:** Aortic root dilatation, aortic dissection, aneurysm of the ascending aorta, pulmonary artery dilatation, aortic regurgitation, mitral regurgitation, mitral valve prolapsed.

d. **Facies:** Dolichocephaly, long and narrow face, deep-set eyes, downslanting palpebral fissures, malar hypoplasia, microretrognathia, high-arched palate, dental crowding.

e. **Others:** Spontaneous pneumothorax, recurrent hernias, striae distensae, decreased subcutaneous fat, retinal detachment.

Q 3. How will you diagnose Marfan syndrome?

Ans. Diagnosis: (Figure 11.2)

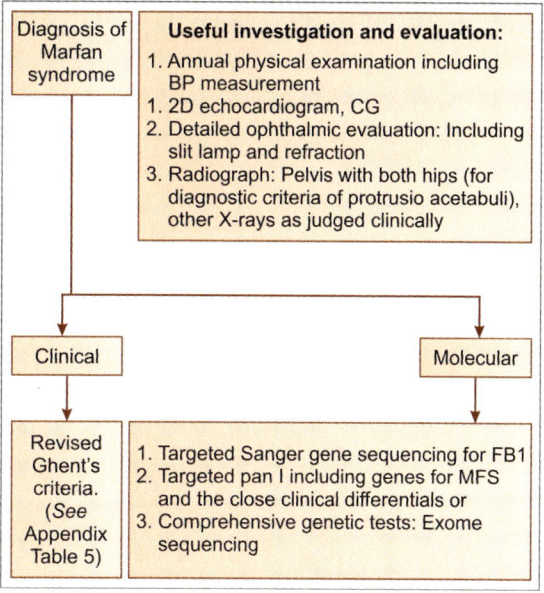

Figure 11.2: : Diagnosis of MFS. BP: Blood pressure, ECG: Electrocardiography

Q 4. How will you do management of Marfan syndrome? Write about the inheritance pattern, recurrence risk and genetic counseling of Marfan syndrome.

Ans. Management: (Figure 11.3)

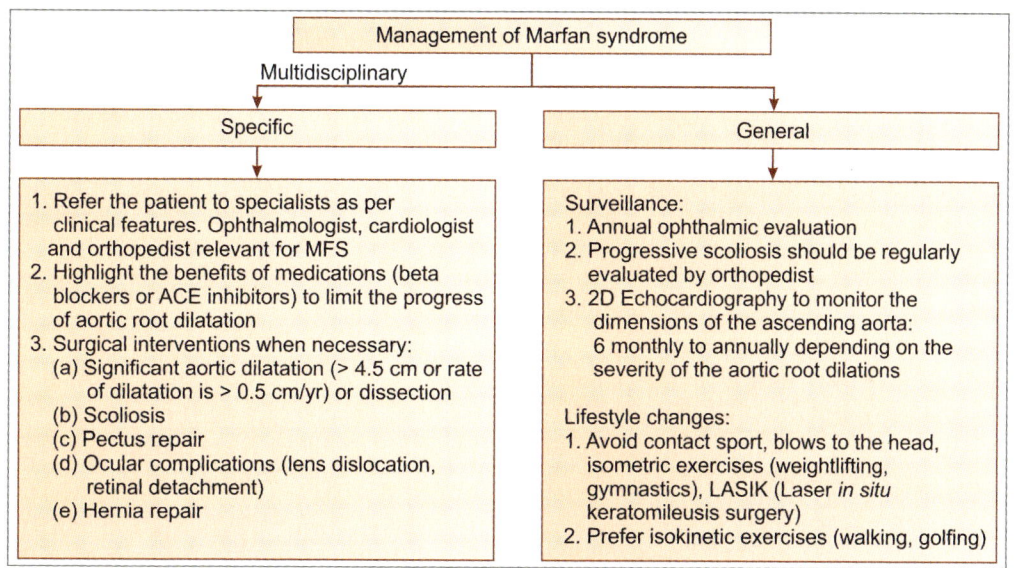

Figure 11.3: Management of Marfan syndrome

Inheritance Pattern, Recurrence Risk and Genetic Counseling (Figure 11.4)

Genetic counseling: Regarding details of the disease like natural history, prognosis, management options, inheritance pattern, recurrence risk in future generation.

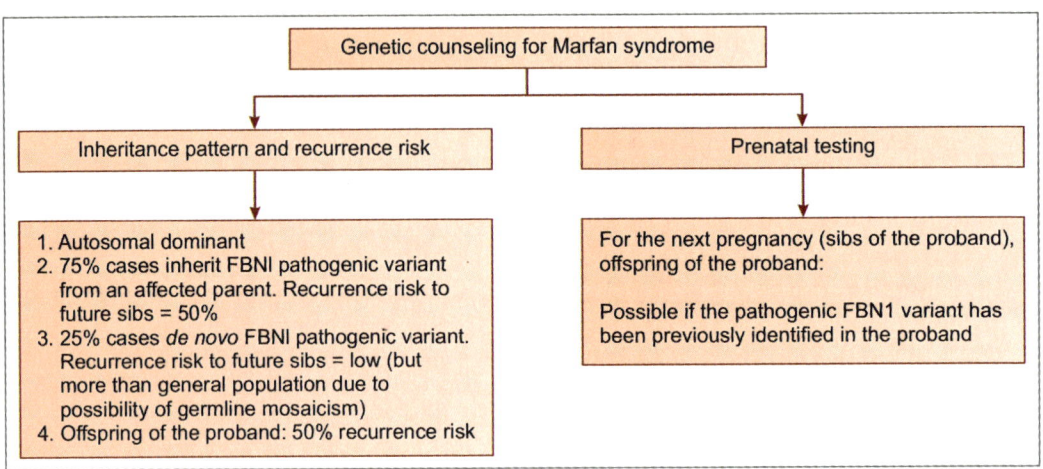

Figure 11.4: Recurrence risk and genetic counseling of Marfan syndrome

Q 5. Write differential diagnosis for Marfan syndrome.

Ans:

Name of condition	Genetic basis	Features resembling MFS	Features differing from MFS
Loeys-Dietz syndrome	Autosomal dominant (TGFBR1, TGFBR2)	o Pectus excavatum or carinatum, scoliosis, arachnodactyly, positive thumb and wrist sign o MVP o Joint hypermobility and contractures o Myopia o Dilatation of the aortic root	o Absent ectopia lentis o Typical craniofacial involvement o Vascular aneurysm/dissection of any medium-large artery o Bruisability, dystrophic scars o Overgrowth affecting digits o Organ ruptures, viz spleen, bowel
Congenital contractual arachno-dactyly	Autosomal dominant (FNB2)	o Arachnodactyly, mild elbow contractures o Mild dilatation of aorta	o Crumpled ears o Scoliosis
Ehlers-Danlos syndrome	o **Classic type—** autosomal dominant (COL5A1, COL5A2) o **Kyphoscoliotic type—** Autosomal recessive (PLOD1)	o Joint hypermobility o Progressive scoliosis o Dilatation of the aortic root	o Hyperlaxity, soft velvety skin and easy bruisability, dystrophic scars o Predominant neonatal hypotonia (kyphoscoliotic type)

Contd.

Name of condition	Genetic basis	Features resembling MFS	Features differing from MFS
	o **Vascular type—** Autosomal dominant (COL3A1)		o Characteristic facies and organ ruptures (EDS vascular type) o Vascular aneurysm/dissection of any medium–large artery
Homo Cystinuria	o Autosomal recessive (CBS) o Cystathionine β-synthase deficiency	o EL o Severe myopia o Skeletal manifestations o Asthenic lean habitus (marfanoid) o MVP o Hernias	o Dislocation of lensis inferotemporal o Intellectual disability o Thromboembolism
Stickler syndrome	o Autosomal dominant (COL2A1, COL11A1, A2) o Autosomal recessive (COL9A)	o Myopia, retinal detachment o Scoliosis o Joint laxity o MVP	o Hearing loss o Midface hypoplasia, flat nasal bridge, micro/retrognathia o Cleft palate o Precocious arthritis
Fragile-X syndrome	o Trinucleotide repeat expansion (CGG repeats > 200)	o Joint hypermobility o Pectus excavatum, scoliosis o MVP, aortic root dilatation o Inguinal hernia	o Intellectual disability o Behavioral abnormalities o Macroorchidism o Large head, long face

Abbreviations: MFS—Marfan syndrome; EL—Ectopialentis; MVP—Mitral valve prolapse

NEUROCUTANEOUS DISORDERS
Shruti Bajaj

Q 6. Describe the etiology, genetic basis for neurofibromatosis type 1 and neurofibromatosis 2 (NF1 and NF2).

Ans. Etiology and genetic basis: NF1

1. **NF1** is an autosomal dominant neurocutaneous disorder with incidence of 1:3500 occur due to heterozygous mutations in the NF1 gene (chromosome 17q11.2).
2. NF1 gene produces neurofibromin 1 protein for normal tumor suppression and downregulation of the RAS pathway.
3. **NF1 mutations** like deletions, duplications, insertion and point mutation cause loss of function of gene.

a. In half of the cases, the pathogenic mutation is inherited from an affected parent
b. Remaining half occurs as *de novo* (80% paternal in origin).
c. In case more than two children affected, there is possibility of gonadal mosaicism.

4. NF1 has complete penetrance by adulthood (i.e. by adulthood, essentially 100% of the individuals with NF1 will manifest the disease in some form or the other).
5. Although completely penetrant, even then NF1 has extreme intrafamilial and interfamilial clinical variability.

Etiology and genetic basis: NF2

1. It is autosomal dominant due to heterozygous mutations in the NF2 gene (chromosome 22q12) with incidence of 1:35000.

2. NF2 gene produces neurofibromin 2 protein for normal tumor suppression.

3. Deletion and point mutation responsible for loss of function of gene.

4. Deletion manifests as mild form and point mutation causes severe form of disease.

Q 7. Describe the clinical features and complications of neurofibromatosis type 1 (NF1).

Ans. Clinical features and complications of neurofibromatosis type 1 (NF1): NF1 is one of the classic examples of a pleiotropic disorder, age-dependent penetrance and clinical variability (Table 11.1). Sometimes clinical features manifest only in one part of the body due to somatic mosaicism and is called segmental neurofibromatosis. Patients with large deletions can present with great severity.

TABLE 11.1: Clinical features and complications of NF1

System	Manifestation
Cutaneous	o Café au lait macules (present at birth, increase in number with time) o Freckles in the axialle, groins and intertriginous areas o Dermal neurofibromas o Plexiform neurofibromas o Rarely hemangiomas and juvenile xanthogranulomas
Ocular	o Lisch nodules: Asymptomatic, usually not evident before 5 years age
	o Optic nerve glioma (present < 6 years age): Loss of vision, proptosis, strabismus.
Peripheral neurofibromas	o Benign
Skeletal	o Short stature o Macrocephaly o Scoliosis o Congenital pseudoarthrosis of the tibia o Sphenoid wing dysplasia
Endocrine	o Precocious puberty o Hypogonadism and delayed puberty o Hypopituitarism
Cardiovascular	o Vasculopathy o Hypertension (any age) o Hypertrophic cardiomyopathy
Neuro-psychiatric	o Normal intelligence (for most) o Intellectual disability (6–7%) and learning disability o Behavioral abnormalities o Seizures
Tumors/malignancies	o Neurofibromas, astrocytoma, other CNS tumors o Rhabdomyosarcoma, pheochromocytoma o Malignant peripheral nerve sheath tumors (adolescence, adulthood) o Myeloid leukemia, myelodysplastic syndromes o Breast cancer (present before 50 years of age usually)
Life expectancy	o 8–15 years lesser than the general population

Q 8. Write age dependent clinical features of NF1.
Ans.

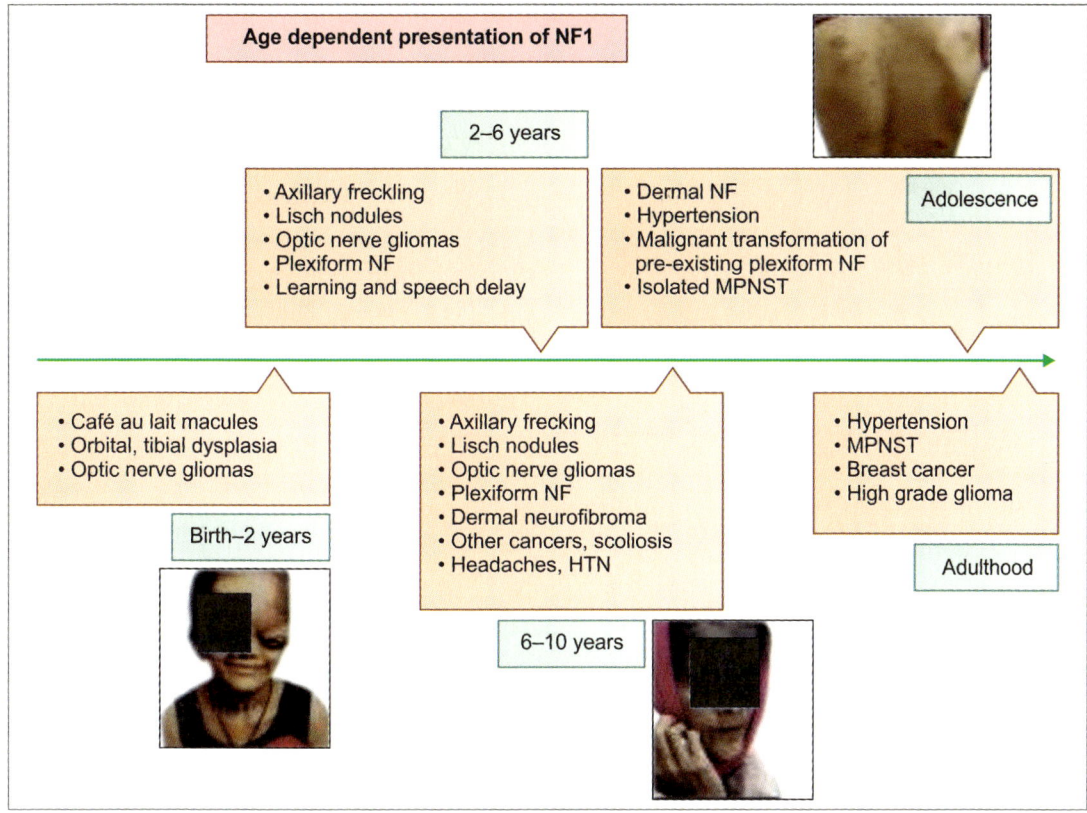

Age dependent presentation of NF1

2–6 years

• Axillary freckling
• Lisch nodules
• Optic nerve gliomas
• Plexiform NF
• Learning and speech delay

• Dermal NF
• Hypertension
• Malignant transformation of
  pre-existing plexiform NF
• Isolated MPNST

Adolescence

• Café au lait macules
• Orbital, tibial dysplasia
• Optic nerve gliomas

Birth–2 years

• Axillary frecking
• Lisch nodules
• Optic nerve gliomas
• Plexiform NF
• Dermal neurofibroma
• Other cancers, scoliosis
• Headaches, HTN

6–10 years

• Hypertension
• MPNST
• Breast cancer
• High grade glioma

Adulthood

Figure 11.5: Clinical features of NF1 have an age-dependent penetrance
MPNST: Malignant peripheral nerve sheath tumors; HTN: Hypertension

Q 9. Describe clinical features and compli-cations of neurofibromatosis 2 (NF2).
Ans. Clinical features of NF2: It usually develops around puberty or adolescence.
1. **Bilateral acoustic neuromas/vestibular schwannomas:** Gait disturbance, dizziness, facial weakness, numbness, tinnitus/progressive hearing loss.
2. **Ophthalmological:** Juvenile posterior subcapsular cataracts.
3. **Central nervous system tumors:** Meningiomas, neurofibromas, low grade gliomas, schwannomas.

4. **Cutaneous manifestations:** Café au lait macules (fewer than those in NF1)
5. **Peripheral nervous system:** Mononeuropathy in childhood (persistent facial palsy, hand-foot drop).

Q 10. Write the diagnosis and management for neurofibromatosis type 1 (NF1).
Ans. Diagnosis and management: (Figures 11.6 and 11.7).
The clinical criteria for the diagnosis of NF1 is sensitive after eight years of age.

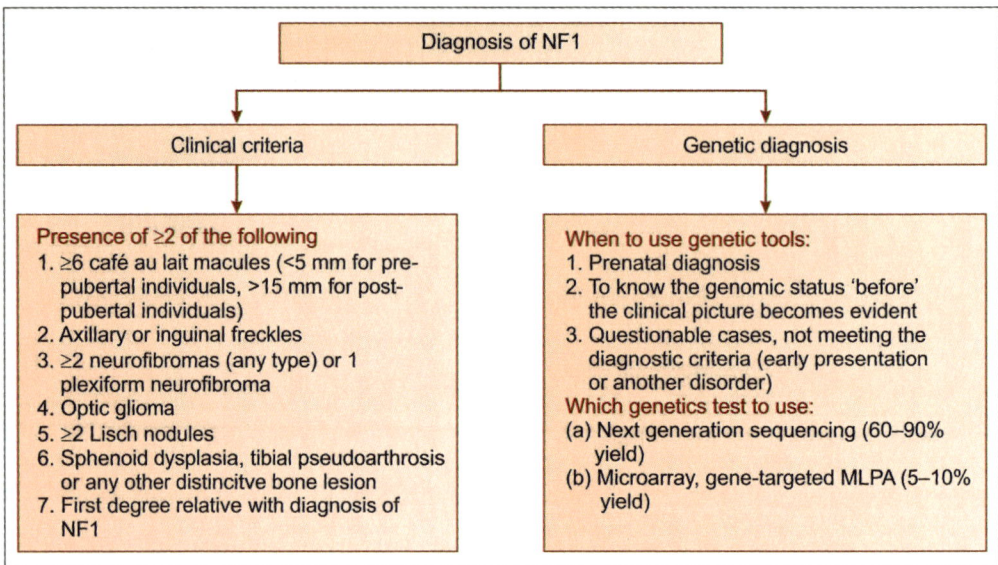

Figure 11.6: Diagnosis of NF1. MLPA: Multiplex ligated probe amplification

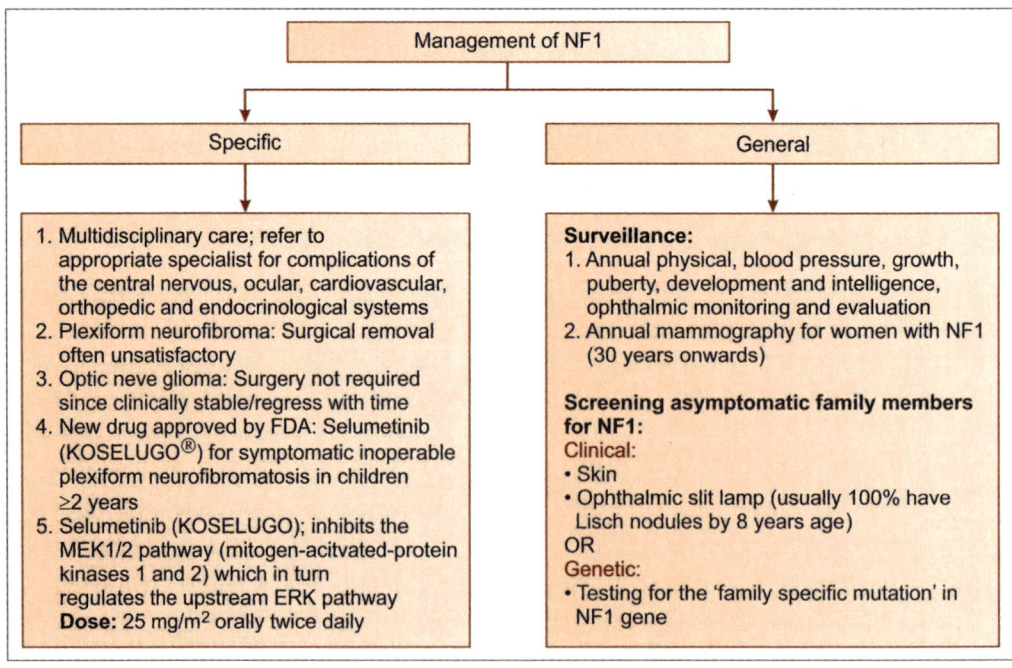

Figure 11.7: : Management of NF1

Q 11. Write differential diagnosis for neurofibromatosis type 1 (NF1).
Ans. Differential diagnosis of NF1

Name of the condition	Genetic basis	Features resembling NF1	Features differing from NF1
Legius syndrome	Autosomal dominant (AD) (*SPRED1*)	o Multiple café au lait spots o Freckling o Macrocephaly o Learning disability	o No neurofibromas and Lisch nodules o Dysmorphic features present (not clear)
Constitutional mismatch repair deficiency (CMMRD)	Autosomal recessive (*MLH1, MSH2, MSH6, PMS2*)	o Cutaneous manifestation o Clinical criteria	o Blood cancer, brain tumors o Family history of cancers/Lynch syndrome o Usually consanguineous parents
NF2	AD (*NF2*)	o Café au lait spots	o Bilateral acoustic neuromas o Meningiomas o Subcapsular cataracts
Noonan syndrome with multiple lentigines (NSML)	AD (*PTPN11, RAF1, BRAF, MAP2K1*)	o Lentigines o Pulmonary stenosis o Cardiomyopathy o Short stature	o Facial dysmorphism o Deafness
McCune-Albright syndrome (MAS)	Postembryonic somatic activating mutation of *GNAS*	Large café au lait spots Polyostotic fibrous dysplasia (FD)	Distribution and margins of café au lait spots differ from NF1 (large, usually do not cross the midline, have irregular margins) Fibrous dysplasia
Multiple café au lait spots	AD (*SPRED1*)	Only multiple café au lait spots in the family members	Other features of NF1 absent
AD : Autosomal dominant			

Q 12. Describe the etiology and genetic basis for tuberous sclerosis.

Ans. Etiology and genetic basis:

1. Autosomal dominant inheritance.
2. Tuberous sclerosis complex (TSC) occurs due to heterozygous mutation in either *TSC1* (chromosome 9q34) or *TSC2* (chromosome 16q13.3) genes.
3. *TSC1* and *TSC2* genes coding for hamartin and tuberin respectively. 'Loss of function' mutations in *TSC1* or *TSC2* result in reduced functioning of the tuberin-hamartin complex (AKT/mTOR signalling pathway regulator); causing a loss of the inhibitory influence on of the cell cycles; resulting in uncontrolled cell growth and proliferation.

4. Incidence of
   ○ *De novo* mutations (80%) in *TSC2>>>> TSC1*
   ○ Familial mutations (20%) in *TSC2 = TSC1*
   ○ Overall incidence of mutations in *TSC2>>TSC1*
   ○ In rare instances germline **mosaicism** can be present in either of the parents.
5. TSC shows complete penetrance and extreme clinical variability.

Q 13. What are the clinical features and complications for tuberous sclerosis?

Ans. Clinical features and complications: TSC is another example of a pleiotropic disorder, age-dependent penetrance and clinical variability.

The classical Vogt triad of seizures, intellectual disability and facial angiofibromas is present in hardly 30% of the patients.

System	Manifestation
Cutaneous (80–95%)	o Hypopigmented macules (ash-leaf spots) (90%) o Facial angiofibroma (malar region of the face involved typically) (75%) o Shagreen patch (lower back involved typically) (50%) o Periungual and subungual fibromas (usually develop >15 years of age) o Confetti skin lesions (numerous 1 to 3 mm hypopigmented macules)
Brain	o Subependymal nodules (SEN) (80%), cortical dysplasia (90%), subependymal giant cell astrocytoma (SEGA) (5–15%) o Seizures (80%) o Developmental delay and intellectual disability
Neuro-psychiatric (TSC-associated-neuro-psychiatric disorder/ TAND) (90%)	o Autism spectrum disorder (may resemble non-syndromic autism) o Attention deficit hyperactivity disorder o Learning disability, cognitive impairment o Emotional problems, self-injurious behavior

Contd.

System	Manifestation
Kidneys (80%)	o Renal cysts, renal cell carcinoma o Benign and malignant angio-myolipomas
Heart	o Cardiac rhabdomyomas (50–65%) can be present from the fetal period. Usually regress within the first three years of life. Can cause outflow tract obstruction and arrhythmias.
Lungs	o Lymphangioleiomyomatosis (LAM) in 30–40% of women and incidence increases with age. Present with dyspnea, hemoptysis pneumothorax, respiratory failure and death.
Ocular	o Retinal hamartomas o Asymptomatic, can progress to exudative retinal detachment and neovascular glaucoma.
Others	o Neuroendocrine tumors: Pituitary/parathyroid/pancreatic adenomas.
Life expectancy	o Lesser than general population o Central nervous system tumors, followed by renal disease—major cause of morbidity and mortality.

SEN: Subependymal nodules (80%)
LAM: Lymphangioleiomyomatosis
SEGA: Subependymal giant cell astrocytoma

Q 14. How will you diagnose a case of tuberous sclerosis?

Ans. Diagnosis: (Figures 11.8 and 11.9)

Diagnostic criteria for TSC

Clinical diagnosis:
2 Major features or
1 Major + ≥1 minor features

OR

Genetic diagnosis:
Identification of heterozygous
pathogenic variant in TSC1/TSC2 gene

Major criteria:
- Angiofibromas (≥3) or fibrous cephalic plaque
- Cardiac rhabdomyoma
- Cortical dysplasias, including tubers and cerebral white matter migration lines
- Hypomelanotic macules (3 to >5 mm in diameter)
- LAM
- Multiple retinal nodular hamartomas
- Renal angiomyolipoma
- Shagreen patch
- SEGA
- SENs
- Ungual fibromas (≥2)

1. Genetic testing[+] for TSC1/TSC2 variants by:
(a) Targeted TSC1,TSC2 gene sequencing and gene-specific deletion-duplication analysis
OR
(b) Multi-gene panel sequencing

SEN: Subependymal nodules (80%)
LAM: Lymphangioleiomyomatosis
SEGA: Subependymal giant cell astrocytoma

Minor criteria:
- Confetti skin lesions
- Dental enamel pits (>3)
- Intraoral fibromas (≥2)
- Multiple renal cysts
- Retinal achromic patch
- Nonrenal hamartomas

Figure 11.8: : Diagnostic criteria of tuberous sclerosis

Investigation useful following the diagnosis of TSC

Recommended work-up following the diagnosis:
1. Blood tests: Renal function tests
2. MRI brain
3. Renal ultrasound and MRI abdomen
4. EEG, ECG
5. Baseline PFT for asymptomatic patients at-risk for LAM (especially in females ≥18 years)
6. Baseline clinical evaluations: Detailed examination, blood pressure, growth and department, ophthalmic, neurobehavioral (for TAND)

Evaluation of asymptomatic at-risk relatives*
Molecular:
Check for the family-specific mutation causing TSC
OR
Clinical:
Detailed skin evaluation (including Wood's lamp)
Ophthalmic evaluation
Cranial MRI
Renal ultrasound or MRI abdomen

Recommended surveillance following the diagnosis:
Annual: Renal functions tests, MRI brain and MRI abdomen, 2D Echo, ophthalmic, clinical and neuropsychiatric assessment
3–5 yearly: ECG
Asymptomatic patients at risk of LAM: 5–10 yearly high resolution HRCT and periodic PFT
Periodic EEG: Frequency decided clinically

* Due to clinical variability the other affected family members (including parents and siblings) may seem to be unaffected/ mildly affected clinically. Early confirmation of diagnosis in these at-risk individuals, helps targeted screening for associated comorbidities and limiting the complications

Figure 11.9: : Evaluation of tuberous sclerosis
MRI—Magnetic resonance imaging; EEG—Electroencephalogram; ECG—Electrocardiogram; PFT—Pulmonary function test; 2D-ECHO—Echocardiography; HRCT—High resolution computed tomography; TAND—TSC-associated-neuropsychiatric disorder; LAM—Lymphangioleiomyomatosis

Q 15. Write the management of tuberous sclerosis.

Ans. Management: (Figure 11.10)

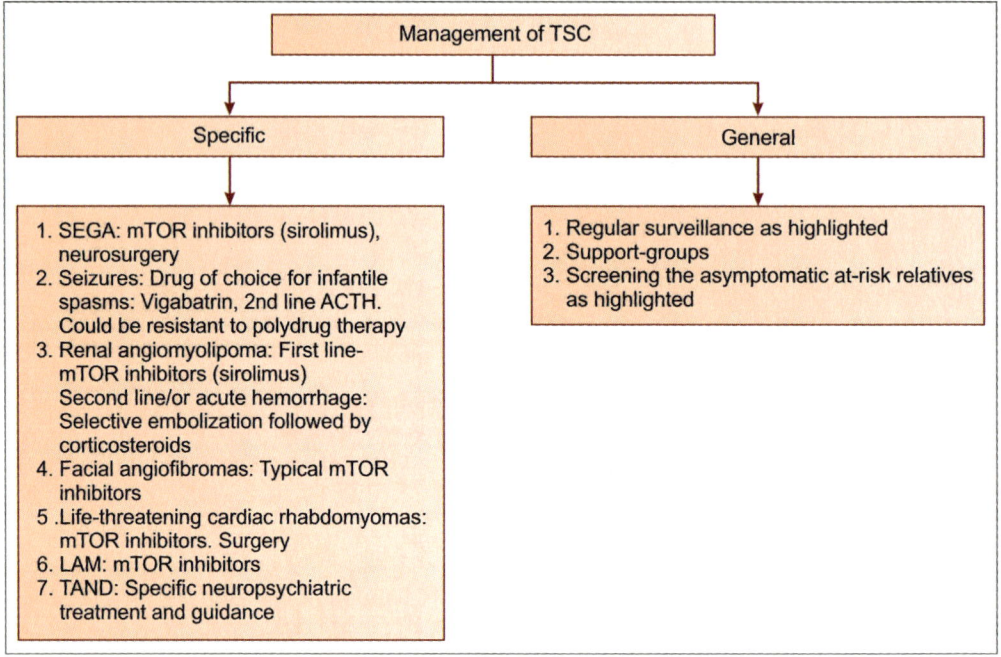

Figure 11.10: Management for tuberous sclerosis
TAND—TSC-associated-neuropsychiatric disorder; ACTH—Adrenocorticotrophic hormone;
LAM— Lymphangioleiomyomatosis

Q 16. Write the inheritance pattern, recurrence risk, prenatal management and genetic counseling for subsequent pregnancy for neurocutaneous disorders (neurofibromatosis NF1 and tuberous sclerosis TSC).

Ans. Inheritance pattern: Autosomal dominant inheritance.

Recurrence risk, prenatal management and genetic counseling

Recurrence risk

Parental status	Risk of recurrence
One parent having NF1 or TSC and other parent normal	50% chance of normal child, 50% chance of child with NF1 or TSC
Both parents normal, one child with NF1 or TSC	Less than 1–2% chance of recurrence of NFI or TSC in every subsequent pregnancy (risk is very low, but more than the general population due to the possibility of germline mosaicism)

Prenatal management

With a previously affected parent or sibling, diagnosed of NF1 or TSC genetically (i.e. genetic mutation confirmed)	Check for the targeted NF1 or TSC mutation in the fetal DNA obtained through amniocentesis or chorion villous biopsy
Isolated cardiac rhabdomyoma in a fetus on antenatal scans, the risk of developing TSC is 75–80%, even in the absence of any family history of TSC	Provide option of testing for TSC1/TSC2 genes in the fetus after discussion of the pros and cons of testing

RESPIRATORY DISORDERS
SHRUTI BAJAJ

Q 17. Describe the etiology and genetic basis of cystic fibrosis (CF).

Ans. Etiology and genetic basis:

- Autosomal recessive disease seen in all races but originated in North European population.

- Biallelic pathogenic mutations in the *CFTR* gene (chromosome 7q31.2) that encodes for cystic fibrosis transmembrane conductance regulator (CFTR).

- **Role of CFTR:** *CFTR* mutations results in qualitative and quantitative defects in the normal functioning of the CFTR channel in the epithelial lining of the respiratory, biliary and pancreatic tracts, sweat ducts and intestines. This results in defective release of chloride ions, increased viscosity of the secretions, obstruction and plugging of the tracts and resultant dysfunction at the organ level.

- **Mutational spectrum:** Over 2000 different mutations (missense, frameshift, splice-site, nonsense and deletions) classified in five different categories (I–V) have been described in CF. Globally ΔF508 (same as p.Phe508del) is the commonest mutation in almost 90% of the cases. The frequency of ΔF508 in the Indian subcontinent is between 19 and 34%. The other common mutations described in India include 1161delC, c.3849+10 kb C>T and p.S549N, G542X, G551D, IVS8–6(5T), R117H.

Q 18. Describe the clinical features and complications of cystic fibrosis (CF).

Ans. Clinical features:

1. **Pulmonary:** Chronic productive cough, bronchiolitis, asthma, respiratory tract infections (*Pseudomonas aeruginosa*, staphylococcal, atypical mycobacterial, allergic bronchopulmonary aspergillosis)

2. **Hepatobiliary and gastrointestinal:** Meconium ileus, prolonged neonatal jaundice, fat-soluble vitamin deficiencies, biliary cirrhosis and portal hypertension, rectal prolapsed.

3. **Exocrine pancreas:** Pancreatic insufficiency, recurrent pancreatitis

4. **Reproductive tract:** Male infertility, bilateral absence of vas deferens

5. **Sinuses:** Sinusitis, nasal polyposis, sleep disturbances

6. **Skin:** Acrodermatitis enteropathica

7. **Other:** Osteoporosis and arthropathy, pseudotumor cerebri, hypochloremic hyponatremic alkalosis, renal calculi.

Complications

- Pulmonary exacerbations, intercurrent infections, progressing lung failure bronchiectasis, hemoptysis, pneumothorax
- Chronic rhinosinusitis
- Distal intestinal obstruction syndrome
- Cystic fibrosis-related diabetes mellitus, liver disease.

The clinical manifestations in cystic fibrosis depend upon the age (Figure 11.11), type of mutation (allelic heterogeneity), various modifying factors like transforming growth factors and environmental factors.

Q 19. Write the age-related presentations of cystic fibrosis.

Ans. Age-related presentations of cystic fibrosis. (Figure 11.11)

Prenatal: Hyperechogenic bowel, meconium peritonitis, bowel dilatation, absent gallbladder

↓

Infancy and childhood: Exocrine pancreatic insufficiency (85–90% of newborns), Meconium ileus (10% of newborns), recurrent respiratory symptoms, (may mimic asthma, pneumonias), failure to thrive, rectal prolapse, dehydration, DIOS, ABPA, sinusitis, nasal polyps

↓

Adulthood: Chronic lung diseases, recurrent respiratory symptoms, hemoptysis, pneumothorax, sinusitis, nasal polyps, ABPA, diabetes millitus, infertility, delayed puberty, cystic fibrosis related liver diseases (30% of adults), DIOS osteoporosis

Figure 11.11: Age-related clinical presentation of cystic fibrosis
DIOS—Distal intestinal obstruction syndrome; ABPA—Allergic bronchopulmonary aspergillosis

Q 20. How will you diagnosis cystic fibrosis (CF)?

Ans. Diagnosis (Figure 11.12)

Q 21. How will you do management for cystic fibrosis?

Ans. Management of CF typically involves multidisciplinary and ongoing care (Table 11.2):

Q 22. Write the inheritance pattern, recurrence risk, genetic counseling and prenatal management for subsequent pregnancy for cystic fibrosis.

Ans. Inheritance pattern: Autosomal recessive inheritance (Figure 11.12).

Recurrence risk

Sibs of the proband: Both parents of the proband are asymptomatic carriers. The risk to their subsequent pregnancy can be:

- 25% risk of recurrence in every subsequent pregnancy.
- 50% risk of being a carrier.
- 25% chance of being normal.

Genetic counseling: Discuss the following with families:

Details of the disease like basic genetics, natural history, prognosis, management options, inheritance pattern, recurrence risk in future generation, carrier screening of parents and other relative at risk and prenatal testing.

Before prenatal testing family should be informed regarding:

- Prenatal procedure and prenatal test details.
- Likely benefits of early diagnosis and preparedness if the result returns positive.

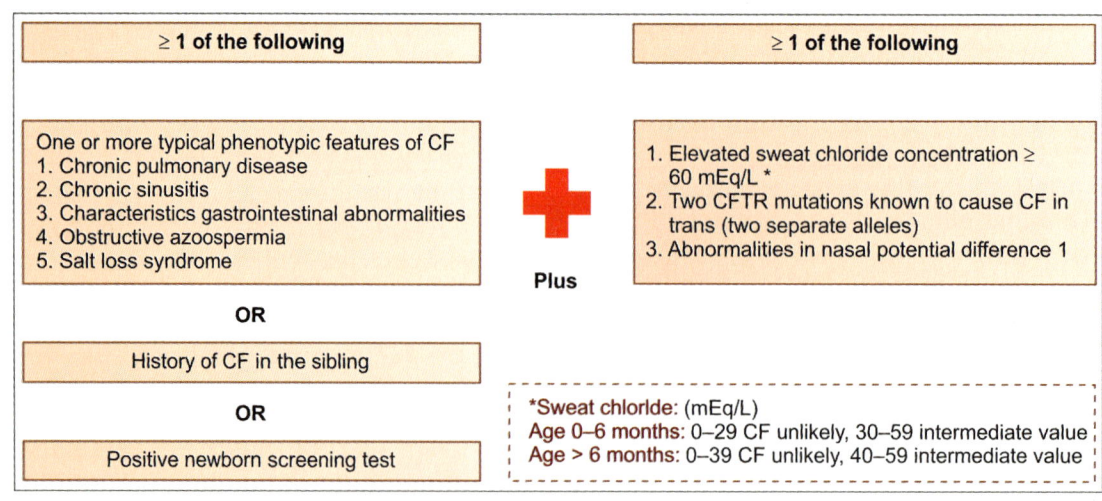

≥ 1 of the following	≥ 1 of the following
One or more typical phenotypic features of CF 1. Chronic pulmonary disease 2. Chronic sinusitis 3. Characteristics gastrointestinal abnormalities 4. Obstructive azoospermia 5. Salt loss syndrome	1. Elevated sweat chloride concentration ≥ 60 mEq/L * 2. Two CFTR mutations known to cause CF in trans (two separate alleles) 3. Abnormalities in nasal potential difference 1

Plus

OR

History of CF in the sibling

OR

Positive newborn screening test

*Sweat chloride: (mEq/L)
Age 0–6 months: 0–29 CF unlikely, 30–59 intermediate value
Age > 6 months: 0–39 CF unlikely, 40–59 intermediate value

Figure 11.12: Diagnosis of cystic fibrosis

TABLE 11.2: Management of clinical manifestations of CF

Manifestation	Management
Pulmonary	

1. Respiratory tract infections	**Airway clearance by**
	○ Physiotherapy and postural drainage
	○ Nebulization of one of the following
	  ♦ Human recombinant dornase alpha (DNase α) ≥ 6 years (Dose: Single daily aerosol, 2.5 mg)
	  ♦ N-acetylcysteine solution (5–10%) followed by β_2-agonist agents
	  ♦ Hypertonic saline (7%) 2–4 times a day
	
	Preventive strategies
	○ Annual influenza vaccine
	○ MMR, varicella, conjugate pneumococcal vaccines, HiB
	
	Prophylactic antibiotics:
	a. Nebulized tobramycin/colistin/gentamycin: Intermittent therapy
	  Examples: Inhaled tobramycin (300 mg twice daily, alternate months, for 6 months)
	b. Oral ciprofloxacin/azithromycin/amoxiclav: Continuous or intermittent therapies. The dose may be 2–3 times the amount recommended for routine minor infections.
	  Examples: Oral ciprofloxacin (20–30 mg per kg per day in 2–3 divided doses), oral clindamycin (10–30 mg per kg per day in 3–4 divided doses), oral azithromycin (10 mg per kg per day on day 1 followed by 5 mg per kg per day from day 2–5), Intravenous amikacin (15–30 mg per kg per day) in 2–3 divided doses
	Treatment of the infections as per culture reports using appropriate antibiotics. Duration of therapy usually ≥ 2 weeks

2. Allergic bronchopulmonary aspergillosis	Oral corticosteroids
3. Reversible airway obstruction	Inhaled bronchodilators and inhaled/short-course oral steroids
CFTR modulator therapy ○ Ivacaftor for ≥ 2 years who have at least one CF mutation p.Gly551Asp ○ Ivacaftor/lumecaftor combination for ≥ 12 years patients who are homozygous for p.Phe508del (F508) ○ Challenges: High cost and low ease of availability. ○ Lung or heart-lung transplantation in severe/end stage respiratory failure.	
Gastrointestinal	
1. Exocrine pancreatic insufficiency	○ PERT ○ Fat soluble vitamins ○ High-calorie, high-fat nutritional support
2. GERD	○ Prokinetic agents ○ H2 receptor blockers or PPI
3. Meconium ileus	○ Enemas ○ Surgery (with/without intestinal resection)

Contd.

TABLE 11.2: Management of clinical manifestations of CF *(Contd.)*	
Manifestation	*Management*
4. Rectal prolapsed	o PERT, rarely surgery
5. Fatty liver disease, cirrhosis	o Ursodeoxycholic acid o Severe disease, progressive hepatic dysfunction: Liver transplant
6. Distal intestinal obstruction syndrome	o Bowel cleansing agents o PERT
Others	
1. Polyps, sinusitis	o Topical steroids o Antibiotics o Surgery if needed
2. Cystic fibrosis—related diabetes	o Insulin o Diet management o Rarely OHA
3. Osteopenia	o Vitamin D o Bisphosphonates o Weight-bearing exercises
4. Bilateral absence of vas deferens	o Microscopic sperm aspiration or artificial insemination using donor sperm o Artificial reproductive techniques
PERT—Pancreatic enzyme replacement therapy; PPI—Proton pump inhibitors GERD—Gastroesophageal reflux disease; OHA—Oral hypoglycemic agents	

Prenatal Management (Figure 11.13).

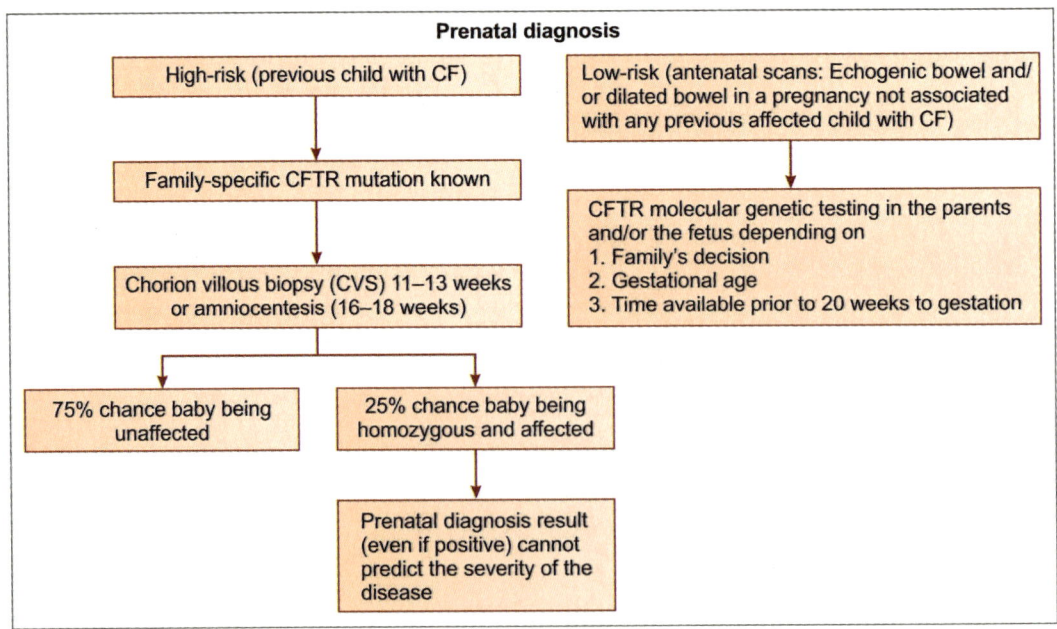

Figure 11.13: Prenatal management for subsequent pregnancy

Q 23. Explain the need of newborn screening (NBS) for cystic fibrosis in current health scenario in India.

Ans. Some of the countries like USA, Canada, Australia, New Zealand, Europe have started NBS for CF based on the burden of the disease and the criteria for a screening program. To start it in India, we must understand the techniques and pros and cons of the disease as below.

Newborn screening for CF

Techniques for CF NBS: Two methods
1. Immunoreactive trypsinogen (IRT): A precursor of trypsin, due to pancreatic dysfunction in CF gets elevated in infants with CF.
2. DNA-based analysis for CFTR mutations (DNA)

Two Protocols:
1. IRT/DNA: Initial positive IRT is followed by DNA testing on the baby's blood.
2. IRT/IRT/DNA: One positive IRT is followed by another IRT analysis after two weeks, if repeat positive, then DNA testing is done.

Positive NBS for CF (IRT/DNA or IRT/IRT/DNA) mandatory to do sweat chloride in the child to establish the diagnosis of CF.

Pros	Cons
1. Early diagnosis of CF associated with overall improved clinical outcomes.	1. In India, cystic fibrosis is considered rare. Estimated prevalence: 1/43,321 to 1/100,323.
2. Early diagnosis of CF allows early initiation of active surveillance and timely identification of complications.	o Logistic challenges: availability and access to IRT, especially DNA based tests, and the access to its rational interpretation.

In India, we would need more studies and logistics prior to including CF NBS universally on a nationwide scale. Test can be offered on a case-base to high-risk infants.

SKELETAL DISORDERS
Shruti Bajaj, Mounika Endrakanti, Neerja Gupta

Q 24. Describe the etiology, genetic basis, risk factors of achondroplasia.

Ans. Etiology and genetic basis:
1. Autosomal dominant inheritance with incidence of 1:15,000–1:40,000.
2. Achondroplasia occurs due to heterozygous mutation in *FGFR3* gene on chromosome 4, coding for fibroblast growth factor receptor 3. The normal function of FGFR3 receptor is to inhibit and coordinate the chondrocyte proliferation and differentiation at the growth plate, thus acting as a 'negative regulator' of bone growth.
3. The commonest mutation causing achondroplasia (98% of the cases) is c.1138G>A (same as p.Gly380Arg) which causes substitution of glycine by arginine, a 'gain of function' mutation, resulting in excess of 'negative signalling' and downregulation of bone growth by the FGFR3 receptor; leading to abnormal and deficient endochondral development of the bones.
4. The mutation occurs *de novo* in 80% of the cases (both parents unaffected) which always originates in the unaffected father's gametes, while in 20% they are inherited from an affected parent.
5. Instances of two unaffected parents having more than one child with achondroplasia, can be explained by the presence of gonadal mosaicism in either of the parents.

Risk factors: Advanced paternal age (>35 years) responsible for positive selection and clonally expansion of the mutant spermatogonia.

Q 25. Describe the clinical features and complications of achondroplasia.

Ans. Clinical features (Figure 11.14)

Clinical features	
Clinical	*Radiological*
o Short stature; short-trunk type o Rhizomelic (proximal) shortening of the long bones o Macrocephaly, delayed closure of anterior fontanel o Small chest o Thoracolumbar kyphosis, lumbar lordosis o Trident hands, brachydactyly o Genu varum, hypermobile hip and knee joints o Limited elbow extension o Normal intelligence o Delay in motor milestones, hypotonia language delayed, middle ear dysfunction o Abdominal type obesity	o Infancy: Oval radiolucent proximal femur o Short robust tubular long bones with metaphyseal abnormalities o Progressive caudal narrowing of the lumbosacral interpediculate distance o Trident pelvis, flat and round iliac bones, squared superior iliac margins o Short narrow chest o Large calvarium with reduced size of the base of the skull, narrowing of foramen magnum
Complications:	
Causative feature resulting in complications	*Related complications*
o Narrowing of the craniovertebral junction	o Sudden infant death (related to central apnea, compression of the cord) o Hydrocephalus
o Impingement of the spinal cord by the stenotic bone of the spinal canal	o Spinal cord stenosis (chronic back pain, exercise-induced claudication, weakness of the lower limbs, incontinence)
o Midface retrusion, resulting in smaller airway size, airway malacia	o Obstructive sleep apnea
o Small chest, decreased compliance of the chest	o Restrictive lung disease
o Recurrent otitis media	o Impaired hearing
o Neurological and cervicomedullary complications o Cardiovascular disease o Higher risk of accidents	o Overall mortality rate is increased in adults. Life expectancy reduced by 10 years overall

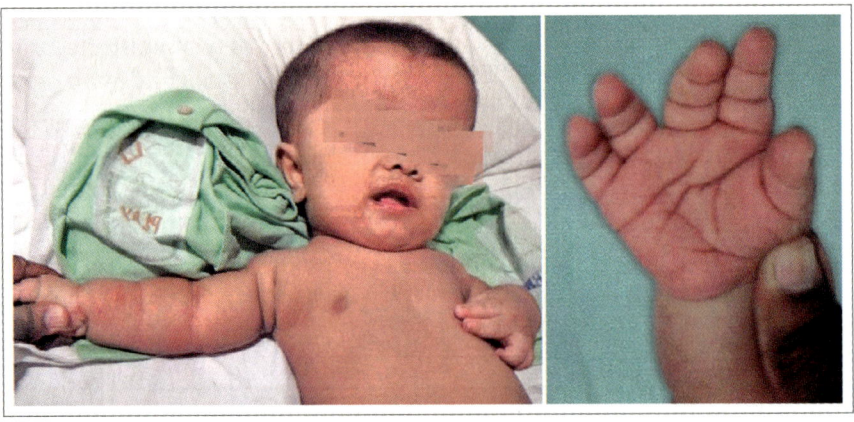

Figure 11.14: Achondroplasia: Prominent forehead, rhizomelia, trident hand in a child. (*Courtesy:* Dr Kausik Mandal, SGPGI, Lucknow)

Q 26. How will you diagnose and do management of achondroplasia?

Ans. **Diagnosis:** (Figures 11.15 and 11.16a to c)

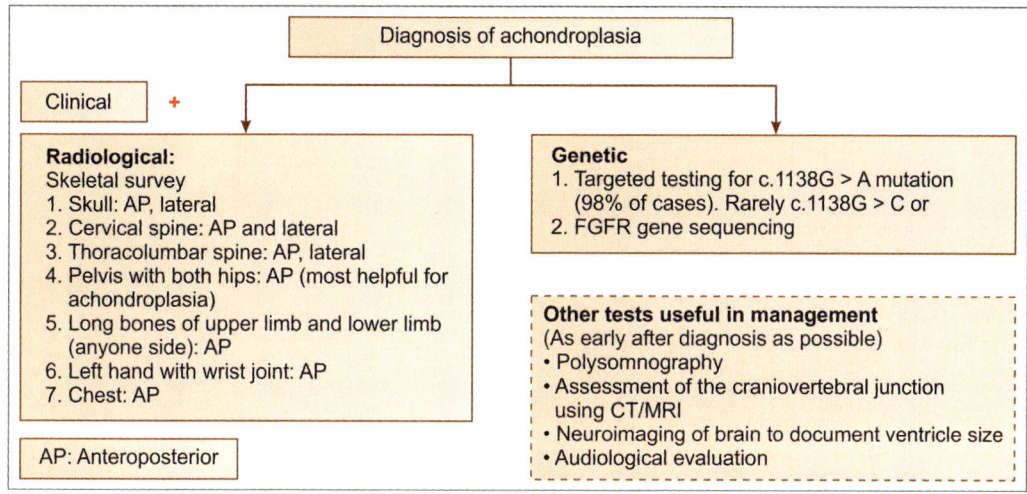

Figure 11.15: Diagnosis of achondroplasia

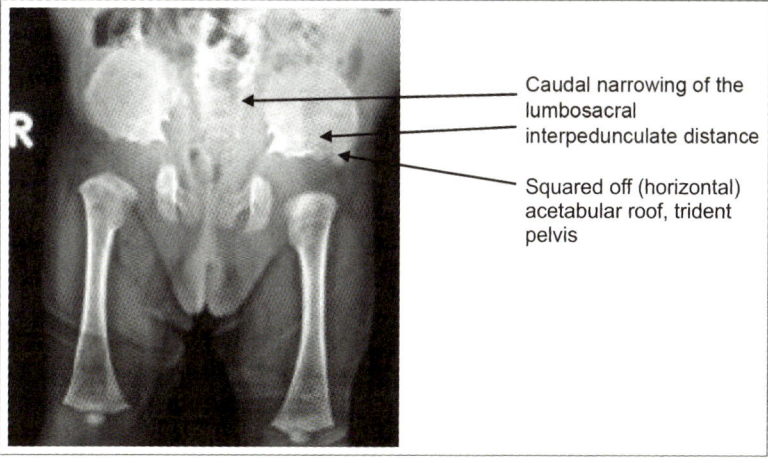

Figure 11.16a: X-ray pelvis with both hips, anteroposterior view. Note trident pelvis, squared off acetabular roof, rounded iliac wings with lack of flaring, short and robust femurs. Progressive narrowing of the lumbosacral interpedunculate distances

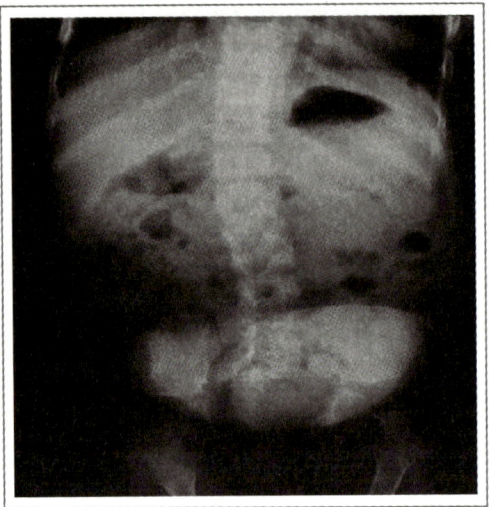

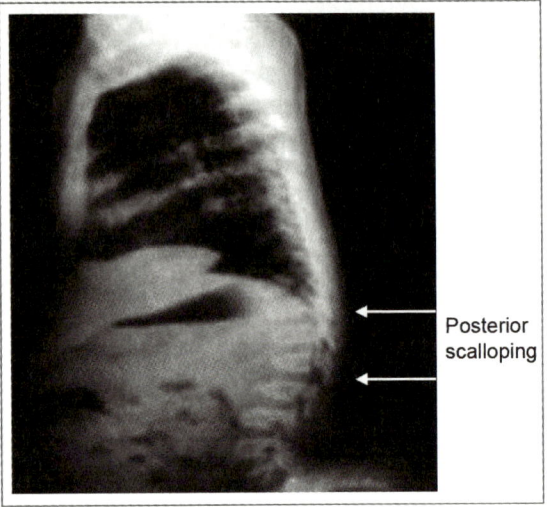

Figure 11.16b: X-ray thoracolumbar spine: anteroposterior view. Note scoliosis and progressive caudal narrowing (rather than the normal widening) of the lumbosacral interpediculate distance

Figure 11.16c: X-ray spine, lateral view. Note increased lumbosacral angle (due to lordosis), relatively flattened lumbar vertebrae. The posterior aspect of the lumbar vertebral bodies appears concave (posterior scalloping)

Management (Figure 11.17)

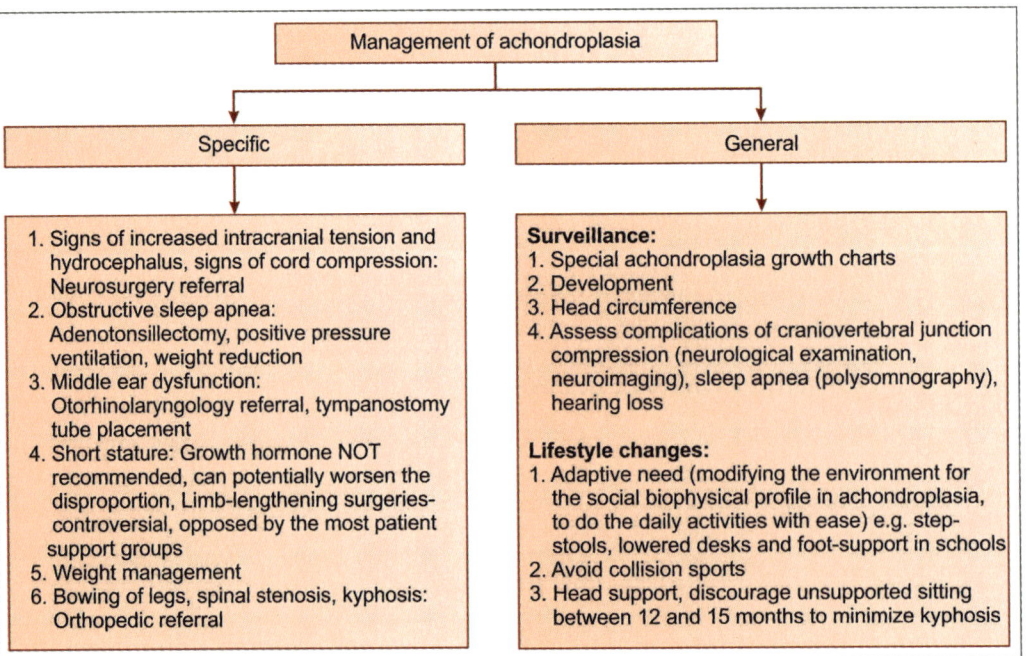

Figure 11.17: Management of achondroplasia

Q 27. What is the inheritance pattern and recurrence risk in the next child of a couple whose previous child is affected with achondroplasia?

Ans. Inheritance pattern: Autosomal dominant inheritance.

RECURRENCE RISK	
Parental status	*Risk of recurrence*
Both parents having achondroplasia	○ 25% chance of normal child ○ 50% chance of child with achondroplasia ○ 25% chance of severe/ lethal homozygous achondroplasia
One parent having achondroplasia and other parent normal	○ 50% chance of normal child ○ 50% chance of child with achondroplasia
Both parents normal, one child with achondroplasia	○ Less than 1% chance of recurrence in every subsequent pregnancy (risk is very low, but more than the general population)

Q 28. Describe the etiology, genetic basis of vitamin D resistant rickets (VDDR).

Ans. VDDR can be classified into various types:

1. Hereditary VDDR: X-linked dominant, autosomal dominant, autosomal recessive or idiopathic hypophosphatemic rickets.
2. VDDR of renal origin
3. Oncogenic VDDR

Here, X-linked dominant hypophosphatemic rickets is being discussed in brief.

Etiology, genetic basis, risk factors:

1. VDRR, X-linked dominant hypophosphatemic rickets occurs due to a hemizygous (in males) or heterozygous (in females) pathogenic mutation (loss of function) in the *PHEX* gene (phosphate regulating neutral endopeptidase) located on chromosome Xp22.2–22.1.
2. About 300 different mutations like missense, nonsense, indels, deletions and duplications can occur in *PHEX* gene.
3. **Pathogenesis:** *PHEX* mutation causes increased fibroblast growth factors (FGF23) levels which result in downregulation of renal phosphate resorption and renal phosphate wasting. FGF23 also impairs 1-alpha-hydroxylase activity and reduces levels of activated vitamin D, i.e. 1,25(OH)2 vitamin D or calcitriol which results in poor bone mineralization.

Q 29. Describe the clinical features and complications of vitamin D resistant rickets.

Ans. Clinical features: VDDR is nearly 100% penetrant by one year of age and shows marked clinical variability.

1. **Childhood (by two years):** There is no difference in the severity of the manifestations based on the sex of the patient.
   Skeletal:
   - Genuvarus and genuvalgus
   - Hypotonia and delayed motor milestones
   - Craniosynostosis and dolichocephaly
   - Delayed dentition.
2. **Adulthood presentations:**
   - ***Skeletal:*** Mild-moderate short stature (short-limb), enthesopathy, deformities, joint pains, impaired mobility.
   - ***Sensorineural hearing loss:*** Probably due to increased osteosclerosis and thickening of the petrous bones.
   - ***Asymptomatic:*** Isolated laboratory abnormality (hypophosphatemia).

Complications: Dental abscess, Chiari formation (can result in headaches and vertigo).

Q 30. Describe diagnosis and management of vitamin D resistant rickets.

Ans. Diagnosis: Useful investigations like skeletal survey, including bone age assessment, hearing assessment, genetic tests are done for diagnosis (Figure 11.18).

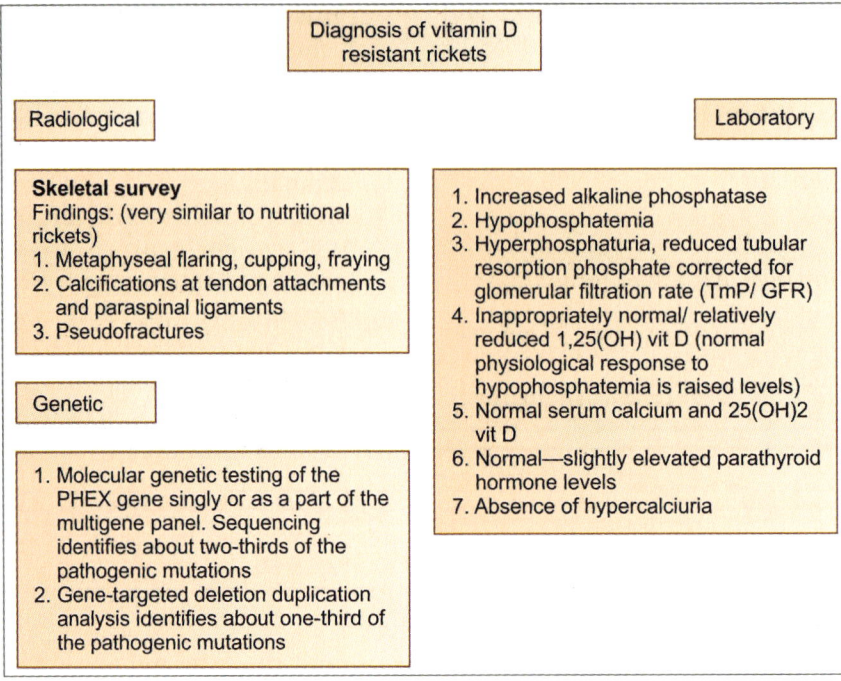

Figure 11.18: Diagnosis of vitamin D resistant rickets

Management (Figure 11.19)

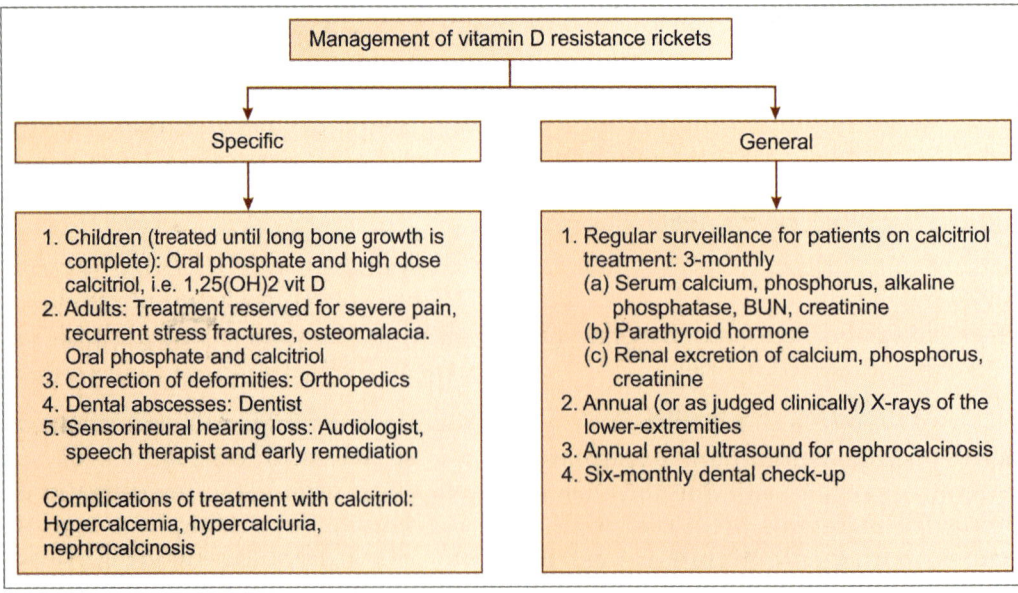

Figure 11.19: Management of vitamin D resistant rickets

Important Notes (Figure 11.19)

- **Dose of phosphorus** varies based on age and severity of manifestations. 20–60 mg per kilogram body weight per day of element phosphorus, in 4–6 divided doses. Early treatment associated with better clinical outcomes.

- **Dose of active vitamin D i.e. 1,25(OH)2 vitamin D** varies from patient to patient. Single oral dose titrated based on biochemical values of alkaline phosphatase, parathyroid hormone and urine calcium.

- **New FDA approval (2018):** Subcutaneous injection of Burosomab (0.4 mg per kilogram body weight) every 14 days in children over one-year age and adolescents in the following situations: Complications of conventional therapy, severe bone disease unresponsive to conventional therapy. *Mechanism:* Fully human IgG1 monoclonal antibody neutralizing FGF23.

Q 31. What is the inheritance pattern and recurrence risk in the next child of a couple whose previous child is affected with vitamin D resistant rickets?

Ans. **Inheritance pattern:** X-linked dominant.

Recurrence risk to sibs of the proband depends upon the genetic status of the parents.

RECURRENCE RISK	
Parental status	*Risk of recurrence*
Father of proband has pathogenic PHEX variant and has passed it to the proband.	○ 100% risk of recurrence in all the daughters ○ 0% risk of recurrence in the sons
Mother of proband has pathogenic PHEX variant and has passed it to the proband.	○ 50% chance of normal child ○ 50% chance of child with VDRR. The severity of the phenotype may vary within the same family
Neither of the parents have the PHEX mutation, proband represents a simplex case (single occurrence in the family).	○ <1% risk of recurrence (risk is very low, but more than the general population, due to the possibility of germline mosaicism)

Q 32. Describe the etiology, and genetic basis of osteogenesis imperfecta.

Ans. Osteogenesis imperfecta (OI), also called brittle bone disease, is a common connective tissue disorder characterized by decreased bone density, bone deformities and increased propensity to fractures, with approximate incidence of about 1 in 20,000 live births.

Etiology: Type I collagen fibers, the major constituent of extracellular matrix of the skin and bone is defective in about 85–90% of individuals with OI. Genetic defects in proteins interacting with type I collagen contribute to the remaining 10–15% cases.

Genetic basis: OI resulting from defective type I collagen result from pathogenic variants in *COL1A1* and *COL1A2* genes and are inherited in autosomal dominant manner. Autosomal recessive, though less common is also described. They result from null mutations of genes coding for proteins involved in collagen propyl 3-hydroxylation, collagen trafficking, collagen folding and mineralization and X-linked forms also exist though less common.

Q 33. Write the clinical features and complications of common types of osteogenesis imperfecta.

Ans. **Types of OI:** OI has a broad spectrum of clinical presentation ranging from mild forms usually diagnosed in adulthood to lethal perinatal forms. Broadly, OI was classified according to Sillence classification into OI type I–IV based on clinical and radiological criteria. The other types of OI, named subsequently as OI V–XI, are described based on the histopathology and molecular genetic defects.

Clinical features and distinguishing points for common types of OI and genes associated with them are described.

OI type	Presen-tation	Genetic defect	Mode of inheritance	Distinguishing clinical features	Radiological features
OI type 1	Mild non-deforming OI	COL1A1> COL1A2	Autosomal dominant with variable expressivity	○ Blue sclera ○ Dentinogenesis imperfecta (DI) may be absent (OI type IA) or present (OI type IB) ○ Recurrent fractures in childhood, improves after puberty ○ Straight long bones ○ Early onset sensory neural hearing loss ○ Short stature	○ Generalized osteopenia ○ Scoliosis ○ Wormian bones
OI type II	Severe lethal form, perinatal lethal OI	Genetically hetero-genous COL1A1 COL1A2> LE PRE1, CRTAP, PP1B	Autosomal dominant, autosomal recessive	○ Multiple long bone and rib fractures ○ Externally rotated abducted thighs ○ Disproportionately large skull	○ Small thorax with short beaded ribs ○ Short long bones with multiple fractures
				○ Blue sclera ○ Micromelia ○ Neuronal migration defects ○ Respiratory failure at birth	○ Broad rectangular femur ○ Flattened vertebrae ○ Hypoplastic pelvis ○ Flattening of acetabular roof
OI type III	Severe non-lethal form, progressive deforming OI	Genetically hetero-zygous COL1A1, COL1A2, LEPRE1, CRTAP, PP1B, FKBP10, SERPINH1	Autosomal recessive, autosomal dominant	○ Neonatal or infantile presentation with multiple fractures ○ Progressive deformities of long bones and spine ○ Extreme short stature ○ Blue/normal sclera ○ Variable DI and hearing loss	○ Severe osteopenia ○ Kyphoscoliosis and vertebral compression fractures ○ Popcorn metaphysis
OI type IV	Moderate severity OI	COL1A1, COL1A2	Autosomal dominant	○ Recurrent bone fractures with variable age of onset and osteoporosis without blue sclera or early onset deafness ○ Bowing of limbs ○ Variable DI	○ Generalized osteopenia ○ Vertebral compression fractures ○ Fewer fractures than type III

Contd.

OI type	Presen-tation	Genetic defect	Mode of inheritance	Distinguishing clinical features	Radiological features
OI type V	Moderate to severe OI with	*IFITM5*	Autosomal dominant	○ Recurrent fractures ○ Severity like OI type IV ○ Restricted pronation and supination ○ Ligamentous laxity ○ Normal sclera ○ No DI	○ Hyperplastic callus ○ Radiodense metaphyseal band
OI type VI	Progressive deforming OI with bone	*SERPINF1*	Autosomal recessive	○ Recurrent bone fractures ○ Blue sclera ○ Short stature ○ Bowing of limbs ○ Clinical severity similar to OI type IV	○ Osteopenia ○ Wormian bones ○ Flattened vertebra ○ Delayed bone age
OI type VII	Moderately severe to lethal OI	*CRTAP*	Autosomal recessive	○ Multiple fractures at birth ○ Decrease frequency of fractures postpuberty ○ Normal hearing ○ No DI ○ Clinical severity similar to OI type II and III	○ Osteopenia ○ Rhizomelia ○ Vertebral
OI type VIII	Moderately severe to lethal OI	*P3H1*	Autosomal recessive	○ Multiple fractures at birth ○ Disproportionate short stature ○ White sclera ○ Proptosis ○ No DI ○ Clinical severity similar to OI type II and III	○ Severe osteopenia ○ Wormian bones ○ Vertebral compression fractures ○ Platy spondyly ○ Normal bone age
OI type IX	Moderately severe to lethal OI	PPIB	Autosomal recessive	○ Multiple fractures at birth ○ Short limb dwarfism ○ Bowing of limbs ○ White to gray sclera	○ Scoliosis ○ Kyphosis
OI type X	Severe deforming OI	SERPINH1	Autosomal recessive	○ Multiple bone fractures ○ Relative macrocephaly with midface hypoplasia ○ Blue sclera ○ Bowing of legs ○ Joint laxity ○ Dentinogenesis imperfecta	○ Generalized osteopenia ○ Platyspondyly ○ Vertebral compression fractures

Contd.

OI type	Presentation	Genetic defect	Mode of inheritance	Distinguishing clinical features	Radiological features
OI type XI	Moderately deforming OI	FKBP10	Autosomal recessive	o Brachycephaly, triangular face o Joint laxity o Bowing of limbs o Short stature o Dentinogenesis imperfecta	o Osteopenia o Wedge shaped/biconcave vertebrae o Kyphoscoliosis o Vertebral compression fractures

Complications:

- Cardiopulmonary complications—recurrent pneumonia and worsening pulmonary function due to restrictive lung disease.
- Neurological complications—basilar invagination and brainstem compression.

Q 34. How will you diagnosis and do management of osteogenesis imperfecta?

Ans. Diagnosis:

- It is based on clinical features.
- **Biochemical:** Serum concentrations of calcium, phosphorus and alkaline phosphatase are usually normal.
- **Radiological findings** of characteristic transverse fractures, vertebral compression fractures and Wormian bones and decreased bone density on X-rays and bone densitometry by DEXA (dual energy X-ray absorptiometry), support the clinical diagnosis.
- **Molecular genetic testing** to identify pathogenic variants helps in definitive diagnosis of OI.

Management:

Aim: Treatment of OI aims at reduction of further fractures and optimization of functional outcome. It involves multidisciplinary management.

Medical management:

- **Bisphosphonate therapy:** They act by inhibiting bone resorption by osteoclasts and allowing osteoblast activity, thereby promoting bone formation and result in improved bone density, final adult height and decrease in fracture. Commonly used bisphosphonates include intravenous pamidronate as 3-day infusions (9 mg/kg/year) every three months or intravenous zolendronate as a single dose (0.1 mg/kg/year) 6 monthly infusion.
- **Calcium supplementation and vitamin D supplementation** as per recommended daily allowance.

Orthopedic management:

- Fracture management includes cast application and splinting.
- Corrective surgeries for deformity may need osteotomy and intramedullary rod placement surgeries.

Follow-up: Regular follow-up to monitor the following:

- Hearing evaluation.
- Bone mineral density by dual energy X-ray absorptiometry (DEXA) scan at least yearly (height-based bone density standards are available for older children)
- Pulmonary function testing annually
- X-ray lumbar spine to monitor for vertebral compression fractures annually.

Recent therapeutic advances under trial: Recombinant parathyroid hormone, anti-RANK-ligand monoclonal antibody, antisclerostin antibody, cathepsin K antibody, transforming growth factors and stem cell therapy.

Q 35. Write the recurrence risk of osteo-genesis imperfecta.

Ans. Recurrence risk:

- Autosomal dominant forms of OI is about 50% when either of the parents is affected.
- Autosomal recessive forms have a risk of recurrence of about 25% if both parents are carriers.
- In unaffected parents with gonadal mosaicism, recurrence risk of OI in next offspring is about 1–3%.

Q 36. How will you do genetic counseling and prenatal management for next pregnancy for skeletal disorders?

Ans. Genetic counseling:

- Details of the disease like natural history, basic genetics, prognosis, management options, inheritance pattern, recurrence risk in future generation should be explained to the family.
- Discuss the reasons and likely benefits, as perceived by the family, for the prenatal diagnosis. The decision to terminate an affected fetus or continue pregnancy needs to be respected. Families could opt for prenatal diagnosis only to be 'prepared' and plan the surveillance and management earlier, thus limiting the complications.

Prenatal management:

- Antenatal USG helps in detecting the presence of fractures and short/long bones early as 15–18 weeks of gestation and helps in prenatal diagnosis of OI type II and type III though milder forms of OI can be missed.
- In prenatal period, target molecular gene testing is performed on fetal DNA obtained by either amniocentesis or chorionic villus sampling. In cases where the diagnosis of the proband is not known or for a fetus suspected to have OI based on ultrasound findings, a panel testing or exome sequencing can be offered for prenatal molecular diagnosis. Detailed ultrasound of the fetus showing phenotypic characterization of achondroplasia, targeted FGFR3 variant analysis for achondroplasia can be done.

Q 37. Write the genetic basis, diagnosis and characteristic features of various radial ray defects syndromes.

Ans. Radial ray defects are characterized by defective formation of radial ray components—thumb and radius either unilaterally or bilaterally. Of these, syndromic forms account to about two-thirds of cases. The various radial ray defect syndromes and their genetic basis and characteristic clinical features include as follows.

Radial ray defect syndrome	Genetic basis	Diagnosis	Characteristic features

Holt-Oram syndrome	○ Autosomal dominant
	○ Reduced penetrance
	○ *TBX5* gene coding for transcription factor TBX5
	○ Phenotypic heterogeneity is seen (all carriers of *TBX5* mutation do not have the phenotype)
		○ Clinical
		○ Confirmation by targeted gene sequencing (*TBX5* mutation absent in about 15%)
			○ **Preaxial radial ray defects:** Thumb anomaly (absent/bifid/triphalangeal thumb) with asymmetric hypoplastic to absent radius
			○ **Ostium secundum atrial septal defect (OS-ASD)**
			○ **Other features:**
			  • Ventricular septal defect (VSD), patent ductus arteriosus and hypoplastic left heart syndrome
			  • Asymmetric radial-ulnar anomalies
			  • Pectus excavatum or carinatum, thoracic scoliosis and vertebral anomalies

Contd.

Radial ray defect syndrome	Genetic basis	Diagnosis	Characteristic features
Duane radial ray syndrome (Okihiro syndrome)	o Autosomal dominant o Haploinsufficiency of *SALL4* gene which codes for a transcription factor	o Targeted gene sequencing/next generation sequencing	o Duane eye anomaly (limited eye abduction) o Renal malformations o Ventral septal defect o Radial ray defect o Phenotypic overlap with Holt-Oram syndrome
Townes-Brocks syndrome (TBS)	o Autosomal dominant o Mutations in transcription factor gene *SALL1*	o Clinical o Targeted gene sequencing next generation sequencing	**Presence of two or more of the following clinical features is diagnostic:** o Anorectal malformation o Bifid thumb, preaxial polydactyly. o External ear malformation with SNHL o Family history of TBS in a relative **Other features:** o Genitourinary anomalies—renal hypoplasia/dysplasia
Fanconi anemia (FA)	o Autosomal recessive disorder due to defective DNA cross-linking repair due to mutations in *FANCA, FANCB, FANCC, FANCD1, FANCD2, FANCE, FANCF, FANCG, FANCI, FANCJ, FANCL AND FANCN* genes o Phenotypic variability is marked	o Chromosomal hypersensitivity to cross linking agents like mitomycin C, diepoxybutane which induce chromosomal breakage is diagnostic o Targeted gene sequencing/panel testing by next generation sequencing	**Congenital abnormalities include:** o **Skeletal:** Radial ray defects (thumb and radial hypoplasia are most common; hip dislocation and rib anomalies, scoliosis) o Skin hypo/hyperpigmentation o Short stature o Cardiac malformations o Renal anomalies o Hypospadias, undescended testis o **Hematologic abnormalities:** Bone marrow failure, increased risk of leukemia and solid tumors
Thrombocytopenia with absent radius (TAR) syndrome	o Autosomal recessive inheritance o Inherited or *de novo* microdeletion of 1q21.2or o Single nucleotide polymorphisms in 5'UTR region or intron 1 of the gene RBM8A (RNA binding motif protein 8A) important for exon-junction complex	o Clinical o Moecular test o CMA and *RBM8A* gene	o Absence of the radii in both forearm in the presence of bilateral thumbs and thrombocytopenia is diagnostic. **Additional features include:** o Ulnar or humeral anomalies and phocomelia in most severe cases o Lower limb involvement is variable (40–47%) and includes patellar/hip dislocation, absent fibula. o Thrombocytopenia o Intracranial bleed and cardiac malformation are a common cause of death.

Contd.

Radial ray defect syndrome	Genetic basis	Diagnosis	Characteristic features
			Other features: ○ Tetralogy of Fallot, ASD,VSD ○ Horseshoe kidney ○ Cleft palate ○ Forehead capillary hemangioma ○ Delayed motor development, seizures and absent corpus callosum ○ Cow milk intolerance
VACTERL association	Usually isolated cases No specific chromosomal region or gene is implicated	○ Clinical ○ **Chromosomal microarray:** *De novo* deletions and duplications have been described mostly in sporadic cases, e.g. dup(1)(q41), del(13)(q31.2), del(17)(p13.3), etc. ○ **Next generation sequencing:** Many candidate gene mutations have been identified in cases with VACTERL association. e.g. *HOXD13, FGF8, DLL3. TRAP1, FOXF1*	**Presence of three out of seven defects below is considered diagnostic.** ○ V : Vertebral anomalies ○ A : Anal atresia ○ C : Cardiovascular anomalies (tetralogy of Fallot,VSD) ○ T : Tracheoesophageal fistula ○ E : Esophageal atresia ○ R : Renal anomalies (renal aplasia/dysplasia/ectopia) ○ L : Limb anomalies (preaxial-radial aplasia/hypoplasia; thumb hypoplasia, polydactyly) **Other features include:** Prenatal or postnatal growth retardation Choanal atresia, laryngeal stenosis Neural tube defects

NEUROMUSCULAR DISORDERS
GAYATRI N

Q 38. Describe the etiology and genetic basis of Duchenne muscular dystrophy and Becker muscular dystrophy.

Ans. Muscular dystrophies are inherited disorders that causes progressive muscle weakness and atrophy due to mutations in the genes that cause complete lack or decrease of proteins, essential for muscle cell stability, and structure and function of muscle. Duchenne muscular dystrophy (DMD), Becker muscular dystrophy (BMD) are grouped under the category of dystrophinopathies which are X-linked muscular disorders.

Etiology and Genetic basis:

- Duchenne muscular dystrophy, Becker muscular dystrophy are caused by mutation in the DMD gene on Xp21 locus, which spans around 2.4 Mb with 79 exons, and codes for dystrophin (Figure 11.20a).
- Dystrophin is a muscle membrane protein complex that links the cytoskeleton with membrane proteins and proteins in the extracellular matrix.
- **Deletions and duplications:** 60–70% of cases of DMD and BDM are due to deletions and duplications of exon(s) at hot spot in first 20 or 45–53 exons in DMD gene, during maternal meiotic division.
- **Sequence variants:** The remaining 20–30% of cases are due to sequence variants

(nonsense, missense and splice site variants) and small indels (insertions/deletions) in paternal meiotic division.

- Pathogenic variants in DMD gene lead to lack of dystrophin expression which leads to degeneration of muscle cell.
- The pathogenic deletions and duplications of exons, nonsense variants, some splicing variants alter the reading frame of the gene (out-of-frame) resulting in severely truncated dystrophin protein. So DMD is more severe and rapidly progressive when compared to BMD (Figure 11.20b).
- In few cases pathogenic variants do not alter the reading frame but are located in protein-binding domains resulting in DMD phenotype.
- **In BMD, pathogenic variants do not alter reading frame of the gene (in-frame) resulting in** partially functioning dystrophin protein.

Structure of DMD gene:

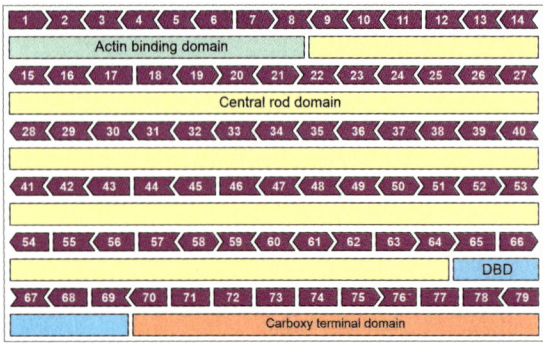

Figure 11.20a: Dystroglycan binding domain (DBD)

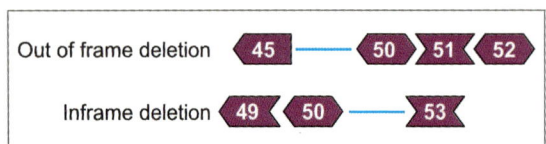

Figure 11.20b: Mechanism of DMD gene mutation

Q 39. Describe the clinical features and complications of Duchenne muscular dystrophy and Becker muscular dystrophy.

Ans. Duchenne muscular dystrophy (DMD): (Figure 11.21)

- DMD is an X-linked recessive disorder with incidence of 1:3500 in affected males.

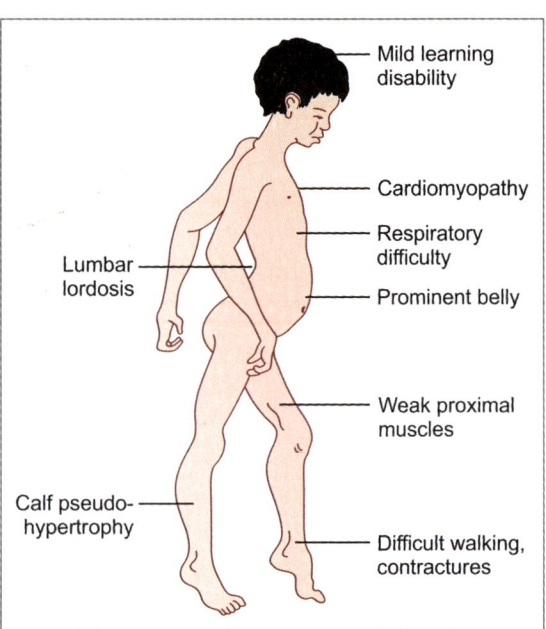

Figure 11.21 : Clinical features of Duchenne muscular dystrophy

- It usually presents in early childhood with delayed motor milestones, symmetrical proximal muscle weakness causing waddling gait, frequent falls, difficulty climbing stairs, and standing up from a sitting position.
- It is a rapidly progressive disorder and the affected children are wheelchair dependent by 13 years of age.
- Dilated cardiomyopathy is the cause of death in most cases.

Becker muscular dystrophy:

- It is characterized by late onset symmetrical proximal muscle weakness with onset of symptoms after late teens and wheelchair dependency after 16 years of age. Some of them remain ambulatory even after 30 years and 40 years.
- Dilated cardiomyopathy is the most common cause of death in BMD.

- Some patients with DMD present with atypical presentation like asymptomatic with raised creatine phosphokinase (CPK) and transaminase, low IQ and autism.
- As DMD and BMD are X-linked recessive disorders, female carriers are usually asymptomatic. There are rare instances where female carriers are symptomatic.

The reasons for symptomatic female carriers could be due to the following:
- Skewed X chromosome inactivation
- Presence of only one X chromosome as in Turner syndrome with DMD gene mutation on single X chromosome
- Phenotypic female with 46,XY as seen in androgen insensitivity syndrome with DMD gene mutation on the X chromosome
- Uniparental disomy of X chromosome carrying the DMD gene mutation
- Balanced X-autosome translocation with a break point in DMD gene.

Complications:
- Progressive dilated cardiomyopathy and cardiac failure
- Respiratory complications
- Contractures
- Scoliosis of spine.

Q 40. Differential diagnosis for Duchenne muscular dystrophy.

Ans.

	Duchenne muscular dystrophy	*Becker muscular dystrophy*	*Limb girdle muscular dystrophy*	*Spinal muscular atrophy*	*Emery-Dreifuss muscular dystrophy*
Pattern of Inheritance	X-linked	X-linked	AD/AR	AR	X-linked/AD/AR
Gene	DMD	DMD	Many genes	SMN1	EMD, FHL1 LMNA
Age of onset	Early childhood	Late childhood	Late childhood to adulthood	Prenatal to early childhood to adulthood	Early childhood to late onset
Progression	Fast	Slow	Slow	Fast/slow	Fast/slow
Muscle group involved	Proximal muscles of lower limbs followed by upper limbs	Proximal muscles of lower limbs followed by upper limbs	Proximal muscles of upper and lower limbs	Proximal muscle of lower limbs	Humero-peroneal muscles and later extends to the pelvic girdle muscles
Contractures	-	-	-	+/-	+

Contd.

	Duchenne muscular dystrophy	Becker muscular dystrophy	Limb girdle muscular dystrophy	Spinal muscular atrophy	Emery-Dreifuss muscular dystrophy
Cardiac involvement	Dilated cardio-myopathy	Dilated cardio-myopathy	Dilated cardio-myopathy	No cardiac involvement	Cardiac arrhythmias
Tone	Hypotonia	Hypotonia	Hypotonia	Hypotonia with weakness	Hypotonia
Reflexes	N/diminished	N/diminished	N/diminished	Diminished/Absent	Diminished
CPK	Elevated (10 times the normal)	Elevated (10 times the normal)	Elevated above 1000 U/L	Normal or mildly elevated	Normal to moderately elevated
ENMG	Primary muscle disease	Primary muscle disease	Primary muscle disease	Neurogenic disorder	Primary muscle disease

AD: Autosomal dominant; AR: Autosomal recessive; CPK: Creatine phosphokinase; ENMG: Electroneuromyography; N: Normal

Q 41. What is the recurrence risk in siblings and other family members of a child who is affected with Duchenne muscular dystrophy?

Ans.

RECURRENCE RISK IN SIBLINGS

- Duchenne muscular dystrophy is inherited in an X-linked recessive manner.
- The risk to the siblings of a proband depends on the carrier status of the mother.
  - Heterozygous carrier mother has 50% chance of transmitting the DMD pathogenic variant in each conception, i.e. 50% recurrence risk to male siblings to be affected with the disease and 50% risk to female siblings to be carriers.
  - If the mother is not a carrier for pathogenic variant in the DMD gene, then the recurrence risk for the siblings of proband ranges from 5–15% due to the phenomenon of gonadal mosaicism.

RECURRENCE RISK IN OTHER FAMILY MEMBERS

- Carrier testing for at-risk females through targeted mutation analysis is recommended if the pathogenic variant in DMD gene is identified in the affected child and if the mother of the affected child is a carrier for the same variant.
- The risk to offspring of at-risk relatives depends on their carrier status for DMD.

Q 42. How will you diagnose and manage Duchenne muscular dystrophy and Becker muscular dystrophy?

Ans. Diagnosis:

- **History and clinical examination,** signs of calf muscle hypertrophy and positive Gower's sign.
- Raised serum creatine kinase (CPK) to more than 10 times the normal value.
- Confirmation of the diagnosis of DMD and BMD is by multiplex ligation dependent probe amplification (MLPA) to detect hemizygous deletions and duplications in DMD gene.
- In MLPA negative cases clinical exome sequencing/multigene panel testing for muscular dystrophies detects sequence variants, small indels in DMD gene.
- **Muscle biopsy:** Histopathological examination, immunohistochemistry (IHC) and immunoblotting (IB) is done in atypical presentation or where new diagnostic techniques are not available. Its results are confirmed by genetic analysis.

Management of DMD: Treatment is multidisciplinary—supportive and specific. Though there is no definitive cure for DMD, early identification helps to prevent complications and prolong life.

Supportive treatment	Specific treatment
o **Regular physiotherapy** to maintain muscle function and prevent contractures, weight control. o **Screening for dilated cardiomyopathy** by 2D ECHO and ECG (electrocardiogram) at the time of diagnosis and annually thereafter. Female carriers are screened in their teens or before/during conception. o Single dose of pneumococcal vaccine and annual influenza vaccine for children at 6 months of age and older. o **Lung function testing** should begin around age 9 or 10 years and should be repeated if lung function worsens. o **Bone density** should be maintained with calcium supplements to reduce risk of fractures.	o **Deflazacortin** a dose of 0.9 mg/kg/day is the primary treatment for DMD and is started in boys who are over the age of five years. o **Glucocorticoids** significantly increase strength, muscle function. o **Recent treatment:** Various new therapies are under trial for the treatment of DMD (discussed in Recent Advances chapter). o **Prognosis:** Though the treatment slows the progression of disease, prognosis is poor for DMD with death in their late teens as a result of respiratory infections or cardiomyopathy.

Management of BMD: No specific treatment is available for Becker muscular dystrophy.

- Regular physiotherapy helps in maintaining muscle function and in preventing joint contractures.
- Corticosteroids, started before physical disability, can help slow down the muscle dysfunction and is beneficial in delaying the onset of cardiomyopathy and scoliosis, prolongs survival.
- Surgery is sometimes recommended to treat contractures or scoliosis.

Q 43. Describe the etiology and genetic basis of spinal muscular atrophy.

Ans. Etiology and genetic basis: Spinal muscular atrophy (SMA) is an autosomal recessive genetic disorder with incidence of 1:1000 live births, characterized by progressive symmetrical proximal muscle weakness and atrophy due to irreversible loss of the anterior horn cells in the spinal cord and can manifest from prenatal period to adulthood.

- 95–98% cases are caused by deletion of exon 7 and/or exon 8 in the SMN1 gene.
- 2–5% cases are caused by sequence variants in SMN1 gene.
- Two almost identical SMN genes (SMN1 and SMN2) are present on chromosome 5q13.
- Normally, the coding sequence of SMN2 gene differs from that of SMN1 gene by a single nucleotide C to T at six position in exon 7, which results in alternative splicing of exon 7 of SMN2 and production of reduced amount of functional SMN2 protein (Figure 11.22).

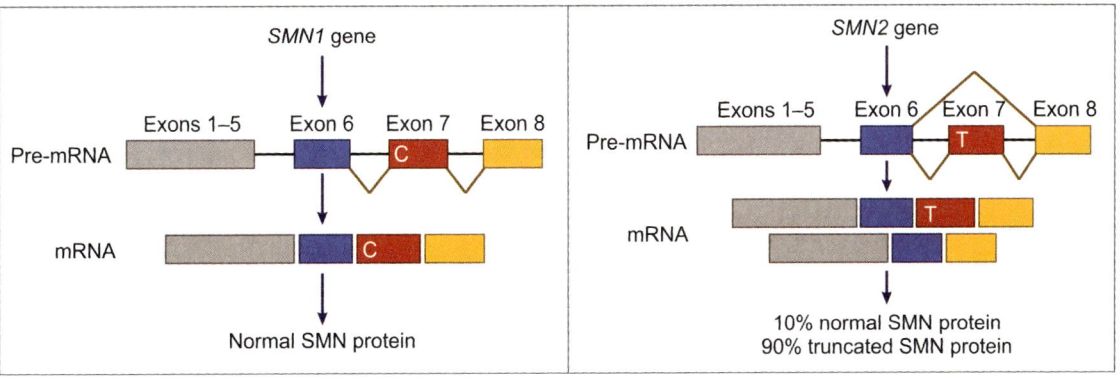

Figure 11.22: Depicts the splicing of SMN1 and SMN2 pre-mRNA to mRNA

- The phenotype of SMA is due to mutations in SMN1 gene and severity is often based on SMN2 copy number which varies from 1–4.
- The greater the number of SMN2 copies, lesser the severity of the disease.
- Most SMA type I patients have two copies of SMN2, while most type II patients have three copies of SMN2. Types III and IV generally have three or four copies of SMN2.

Q 44. Describe the clinical features and complications of spinal muscular atrophy.

Ans. Clinical features depend on the type of SMA (Figure: 11.23).

- **SMA0:** Onset is in the prenatal period, floppy infant, facial weakness, respiratory distress, arthrogryposis with survival less than 6 months.

- **SMA 1:** Onset at <6 months. Difficulty in sucking and swallowing, lack of head control, facial weakness may or may not be present.
- **SMA 2:** Onset at 6–18 months. The child attains head control and roll over but will not attain independent sitting and standing. Fasciculations of tongue are seen in most of them.
- **SMA 3:** Onset at >18 months. Loss of attained motor skills like difficulty in walking, running and climbing stairs, fasciculations of tongue are present.
- **SMA 4:** Seen in adulthood. Presents with proximal muscle weakness and fatigue.

Complications:

- Growth failure
- **Gastrointestinal:** Bulbar dysfunction and gastroesophageal reflux

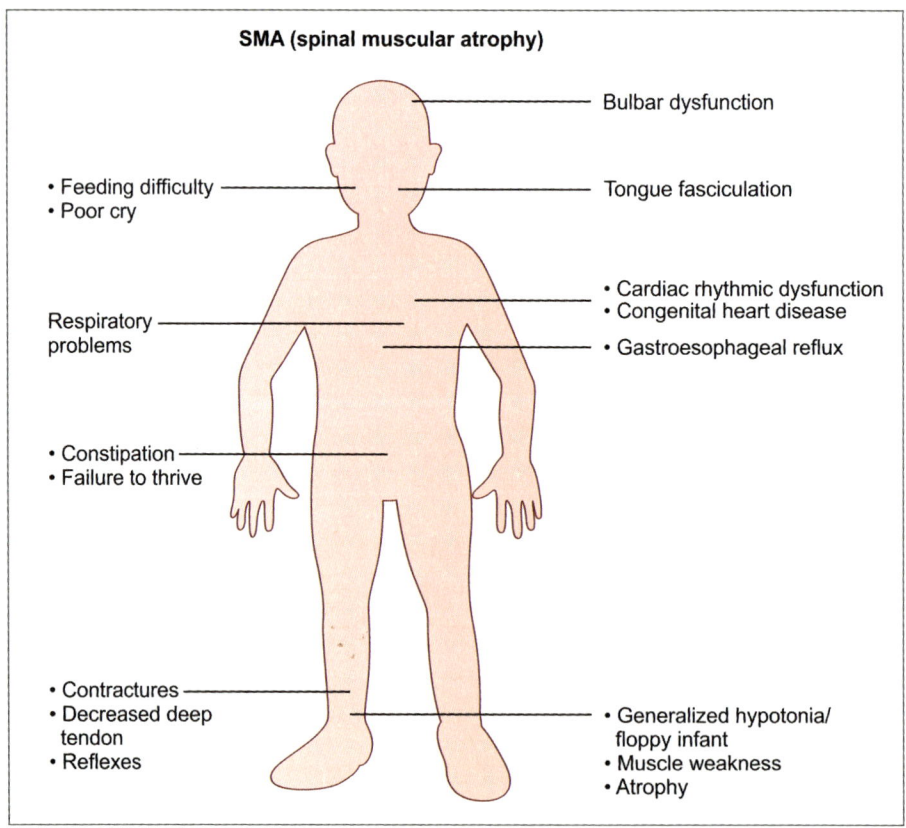

Figure 11.23: Clinical features of spinal muscular atrophy. (*Source of Human body outline*: docformats.com)

◌ **Skeletal:** Joint contractures, scoliosis
◌ **Respiratory:** Recurrent pneumonia, respiratory failure.

Q 45. What is the recurrence risk in siblings and other family members of a child who is affected with spinal muscular atrophy?

Ans. Recurrence risk:
◌ As SMA is autosomal recessive disorder, there is 25% chance of recurrence of the disease in siblings of the index child.
◌ Carrier testing for at-risk relatives is recommended.
◌ In the other family members only if the parents are carriers for SMA, there is 25% recurrence risk of SMA in their offspring.
◌ If only one of the parents is a carrier or if both parents are normal, then there is no recurrence risk in their offspring.

Q 46. How will you diagnose and manage spinal muscular atrophy?

Ans.

A. Diagnosis:

◌ **Clinical features and signs** like motor developmental delay, hypotonia with absent reflexes, tongue fasciculations.
◌ **Creatinine kinase** is normal or mildly elevated.
◌ **Electromyography** shows denervation, fibrillation and fasciculations. It is not done nowadays due to available molecular testing.
◌ **Muscle biopsy** shows muscle fiber atrophy with hypertrophic regions.
◌ **Molecular genetic testing:**
  ▪ PCR-RFLP: For homozygous deletion of exon 7/8, does not detect heterozygous deletion.
  ▪ Multiplex ligation dependent probe amplification (MLPA) of SMN1 gene which shows homozygous deletion of exon 7 and/or 8 in SMN1gene.

▪ In cases with strong suspicion of SMA with MLPA showing heterozygous deletion of exon 7 and/or 8 in SMN1 gene, SMN1 gene sequencing has to be done to look for sequence variant in the second copy of SMN1 gene.

B. Management by multidisciplinary approach can be supportive or specific.

Supportive treatment	Specific treatment
○ Monitoring for the growth, feeding and respiratory insufficiency. ○ Regular physiotherapy improves motor skills ○ Contractures or scoliosis treatment. ○ **Support groups:** to provide psychological and financial support and to give information about new interventions for the disease	○ **Nusinersen (Spinraza),** an SMN2 directed antisense oligonucleotide, is an US FDA approved drug for SMA. ♦ It is administered intrathecally. ♦ Recommended dosage is 12 mg per administration. ♦ Initiated as 4 loading doses with first three loading doses administered at 14 days interval and fourth loading dose 30 days after the third dose. ♦ Maintenance dose is administered once every 4 months thereafter. ♦ The long-term effect of the drug is unclear. ○ Various therapeutic interventions to increase SMN2 expression and gene therapy are under trial (discussed in Recent Advances Chapter 23).

Q 47. Differential diagnosis for spinal muscular atrophy.
Ans. Table 11.3

TABLE 11.3: Differential diagnosis for 0 SMA type

Disorder with pattern of Inheritance		Facial weakness	Respiratory distress	Muscle weakness	Contractures	Hypotonia	Reflexes
Neurogenic disorders	○ SMA type 0(AR)	−	+	+	+/−	Peripheral	Absent
	○ SMARD1(AR)	−	+	+	−	Peripheral	Absent
Muscular disorders	○ Congenital myopathies (AR/ AD/X-linked)	+	+/−	+	−	Peripheral	Diminished/ normal
	○ Congenital muscular dystrophy (AR)	+	+/−	+	+/−	Peripheral	Diminished/ normal
	○ Congenital myotonic dystrophy (AD)	+	+/−	+	+/−	Peripheral	Diminished/ normal
	○ Congenital myasthenic syndrome (AR/AD)	+	+/−	+	+/−	Peripheral	Diminished/ normal
Dysmorphic syndromes	○ Prader-Willi syndrome (15q11.2 microdeletion) (AD)	−	+/−	−	−	Central	Normal
Inborn errors of metabolism	○ Pompe disease (AR)	−	+/−	+	−	Central and Peripheral	Normal/ diminished
	○ Metabolic myopathies (AR)	−	+/−	+	−	Peripheral	Diminished
	○ Zellweger spectrum disorders (AR)	−	+/−	−	−	Central	Normal/ diminished

AD: Autosomal dominant; AR: Autosomal recessive; SMARD1: Spinal muscular atrophy with respiratory distress

The other differential diagnosis for type 0 SMA includes X-linked infantile SMA with arthrogryposis (XL-SMA), SMA due to mitochondrial dysfunction, SMA with pontocerebellar hypoplasia (SMA-PCH) (Tables 11.4 and 11.5).

TABLE 11.4: Differential diagnosis for SMA type 3

Abnormality	SMA type 3	Duchenne muscular dystrophy
Cardiac involvement	Not involved	Dilated cardiomyopathy
Tone	Hypotonia	Hypotonia
Reflexes	Absent/diminished	Diminished/normal
CPK	Normal/mildly elevated	Increased 10 times the normal
ENMG	s/o neurogenic disorder	s/o muscular disorder
Gene	SMN1	DMD
Pattern of inheritance	Autosomal recessive	X-linked recessive

TABLE 11.5: Differential diagnosis for adult onset SMA			
Abnormality	Adult onset SMA	Spinal and bulbar muscular atrophy	Amyotrophic lateral sclerosis
Hypogonadism	-	+	-
Tone	Hypotonia	Hypotonia	Hypotonia, initially, later hypertonia
Reflexes	Absent/diminished	Absent/diminished	Normal/exaggerated
Gene	SMNI	AR	Many genes
Pattern of inheritance	Autosomal recessive	X-linked recessive	Autosomal dominant/autosomal recessive X-linked

Q 48. Describe the etiology and genetic basis of myotonic dystrophy type 1, congenital myotonic dystrophy.

Ans. Myotonic dystrophy type 1 (DM 1): It is a multisystem genetic disorder that affects skeletal and smooth muscle, central nervous system, eyes, heart, endocrine system. Clinical features vary from mild to severe with overlapping phenotypes based on type of DM 1.

Etiology and genetic basis of myotonic dystrophy type 1 (*see* Figure 16.1, Chapter 16)

- It is an autosomal dominant trinucleotide repeat disorder.
- It is caused by expansion of a CTG trinucleotide in the 3′ region of DMPK gene.
- Clinical manifestations occur due to gain of function owing to the presence of more CUG RNA binding protein.
- There are 5–34 CTG repeats in 3′ region of DMPK gene in normal individuals.
- Alleles with 35–49 CTG repeats are called premutation alleles. Individuals with premutation alleles do not have symptoms, but their offsprings are at increased risk of inheriting a repeat size >49. This is because if CTG repeats are greater than 34 they are unstable and may expand further during maternal meiosis (during paternal meiosis small expansion happens) and the offspring of these individuals may inherit expanded repeats. This results in increased disease severity and early age of onset of

the disease in successive generations due to anticipation.
- Alleles with >50 CTG repeats are called full-penetrance alleles. These alleles are associated with disease manifestations.

Q 49. Describe the clinical features and complications of myotonic dystrophy type 1 and congenital myotonic dystrophy.

Ans.

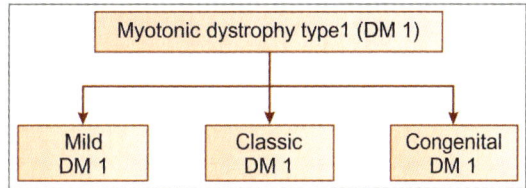

Clinical features: Clinical features vary based in the type of the myotonic dystrophy type 1 (Figure 11.24).

1. **Mild DM 1:** These individuals usually present with mild myotonia and cataract. The CTG repeat size is approximately between 50 and 150.

2. **Classic DM 1:**
   - *Neuromuscular:* Distal muscle weakness in the form of handgrip myotonia, gait disturbance and foot drop, facial muscle weakness (hatchet appearance), mild intellectual disability. Handgrip myotonia and muscle strength may improve with repeated contraction of muscles. This is called warm-up phenomenon.

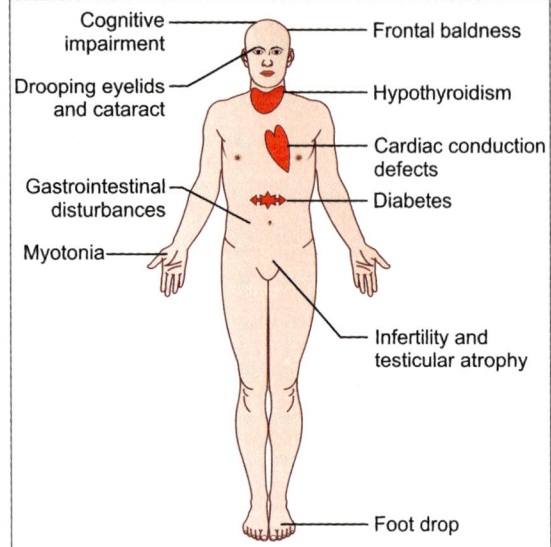

Figure 11.24: Clinical features of myotonic dystrophy type 1

- ○ *Ophthalmological:* Drooping of eyelids, cataract.
- ○ *Cardiac:* Cardiac arrythmias.
- ○ *Gastrointestinal:* Dysphagia, constipation or diarrhea, gallstones.
- ○ *Endocrine abnormalities:* Thyroid dysfunction, diabetes mellitus, hyperinsulinism, infertility. The age of onset is between 20 and 30 years. The CTG repeat size is approximately between 100 and 1000.
- ○ *Other:* Baldness, respiratory failure, neuropsychiatric manifestations.
3. **Congenital DM 1:** This type is manifested in the neonatal and infantile period with following clinical features:
   - ○ *Muscular:* Severe generalized weakness, facial weakness (V-shaped lip), hypotonia, sometimes contractures, respiratory distress, feeding difficulty.
   - ○ *Neurological:* Developmental delay and intellectual disability.
   - ○ *Antenatal:* History of decreased fetal movements and polyhydramnios are the findings. The CTG repeat size is more than 1000.

Complications
i. Respiratory insufficiency
ii. Life-threatening arrhythmias
iii. Hypersomnia and sleep apnea
iv. Psychiatric disturbances like anxiety and depression.

Q 50. How will you diagnose and manage myotonic dystrophy type I?

Ans. Diagnosis: Presumptive diagnosis is based on classic clinical features of the disease.

- ○ **Basic investigations:**
   i. Elevated creatine kinase.
   ii. Liver function test raised in 50%.
   iii. Myotonic discharges in electroneuromyography.
   iv. IQ assessment.
   v. Ophthalmology evaluation.
   vi. Electrocardiogram (ECG).
   vii. Thyroid profile and blood sugar evaluation.
   viii. Neuroimaging shows cerebral atrophy and white matter changes.
- ○ **Confirmation of diagnosis by:**
   i. *Southern blotting* can detect copy number repeats and size of repeats. But due to more time consumption, the other sensitive and more specific technique triplet repeat PCR (TP-PCR) is done.
   ii. *Molecular genetic testing* using TP-PCR of DMPK gene.
   iii. *Muscle biopsy* shows muscle fiber fibrosis and atrophy.

Management is multidisciplinary: Treatment can be general supportive and specific.

General management	Specific management
○ Regular physiotherapy	○ Tab. Mexiletine 150–200 mg, 3 times a day for myotonia
○ Surgery for cataract	
○ For thyroid dysfunction and diabetes	○ Noninvasive ventilation for sleep apnea
	○ Tricyclic antidepressant for depression
○ Cardiologist consultation for cardiac arrhythmias	○ Gene therapy is under trials at present

Support groups provide psychosocial and financial support and give new information regarding management to patients and their families.

Surveillance

⊃ Measurement of fasting serum glucose and HbA1c annually
 ▪ ECG annually to detect asymptomatic cardiac conduction defects
 ▪ Ophthalmology examination every two years

Q 51. Describe the etiology, genetic basis, clinical features of myotonic dystrophy 2.

Ans. Myotonic dystrophy type 2 (DM 2): Onset of the disease is usually between 30 and 40 years.

Etiology and genetic basis:

⊃ Caused by expansion of a CCTG repeat ranging from approximately 75 to more than 10,000 within a complex repeat motif, (TG)n(TCTG)n(CCTG) in CNBP gene.
⊃ Normal number of CCTG repeats is ≤30 without any interruptions or 11–26 CCTG repeats with GCTC or TCTG interruptions.
⊃ Alleles with approximately 30–54 CCTG repeats are called premutation alleles. Individuals with premutation alleles do not manifest symptoms of disease.
⊃ Alleles with approximately 55–74 CCTG repeats are either premutation alleles or pathogenic.
⊃ Alleles with 75–11,000 CCTG repeats are pathogenic and associated with disease.
⊃ Anticipation is not seen in DM 2.

Clinical features:

⊃ **Muscular weakness:** Myotonia and axial, proximal muscle weakness with neck flexors being involved first followed by hip flexors, extensors and myalgia. Facial muscle weakness and weakness of ankle dorsiflexors. (Figure 11.25)
⊃ **Eye:** Cataracts
⊃ **Cardiac:** Cardiac conduction defects

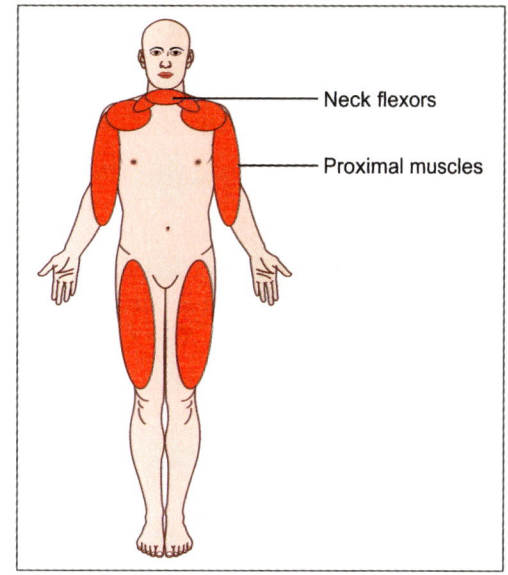

Figure 11.25: Muscle involvement in DM 2

⊃ **Gastrointestinal:** Dysphagia, constipation or diarrhea
⊃ **Endocrine abnormalities** like thyroid dysfunction, diabetes mellitus.

Q 52. How will you diagnose and manage myotonic dystrophy 2?

Ans. Diagnosis: The diagnosis of DM 2 is made by classic clinical features. The presence of expansion of CCTG repeat >75 in CNBP gene in triplet repeat PCR.

General management	Specific management
○ Regular physiotherapy ○ Surgery for cataract ○ Treatment for thyroid dysfunction and diabetes ○ Cardiologist consultation for cardiac arrhythmias	○ Tab. Mexiletine 150–200 mg, 3 times a day for myotonia ○ NSAIDs or gabapentin or tricyclic antidepressants for myalgia ○ Noninvasive ventilation for sleep apnea ○ Tricyclic antidepressant for depression

Surveillance: Similar to DM 1.

Q 53. What is the recurrence risk of myotonic dystrophy 1 and 2?

Ans. Recurrence risk: Myotonic dystrophy type 1 and 2 is inherited in an autosomal dominant manner. The recurrence risk to offspring is 50%.

Q 54. How will you do genetic counseling of the parent of a child who is affected with neuromuscular disorder?

Ans. Genetic counseling: Considering all the general principles of genetic counseling and psychosocial aspects, the following is discussed with families:

➲ Details of the disease like etiology, genetic basis, natural history, prognosis, management options, inheritance pattern, recurrence risk in future generation.
➲ Details of prenatal procedure and testing for target mutation analysis if needed.
➲ Likely benefits of early diagnosis and preparedness if the result returns positive.
➲ If the test comes positive, parents can take reproductive decision by their own.

Q 55. How will you do prenatal management for subsequent pregnancies in a couple whose first child is affected for neuro-muscular disorder?

Ans. Prenatal management: In view of recurrence risk of neuromuscular in a couple whose first child is affected, prenatal testing for targeted gene mutation (DMD gene in DMD, MLPA of SMN1 gene, testing of DMPK gene by triplet repeat PCR, testing of CNBP gene by triplet repeat PCR) analysis is recommended in each conception of couple.

Prenatal testing can be done either at 11–13 weeks of gestation by chorionic villus sampling or through amniocentesis after 16 completed weeks of gestation. Explain the limitations of procedure include risk of miscarriage associated with the procedure.

BLOOD DISORDER
KAUSIK MANDAL

Q 56. Describe the etiology, genetic basis, clinical features and complications of hemophilia A and hemophilia B.

Ans. Hemophilia essentially is a bleeding disorder due to deficiency of clotting factor activity. There are two major varieties, hemophilia A and B due to deficiency of factor VIII and IX respectively.

	Hemophilia A	Hemophilia B
Etiology	o Deficiency in factor VIII clotting activity	o Deficiency in factor IX clotting activity
Genetic basis	o X-linked recessive, mutation in F8 gene at Xq28 o One-sixth of all mutations is inversion of intron 22 occurring in males during spermatogenesis due to no crossover of Xq with homologous chromosome. o 5% include deletions more common in females o Rest are frameshift, missense and non-sense mutations more commonly occurring in males during spermatogenesis.	o X-linked recessive, mutation in F9 gene at X27.1 o 96% cases point mutations, deletions and insertions occur o A rare mutation in Leydon specific region (LSR) at promoter, but symptoms due to mutation resolves during puberty due to presence of androgen sensitive element in LSR.
Clinical features and complications	**Severe hemophilia A:** o Usually diagnosed within first two years of life o Males are affected more with incidence of 1:5000	**Severe hemophilia B:** o Usually diagnosed within first two years of life o Males are affected more

Contd.

	Hemophilia A	Hemophilia B
	o 30% of females with factor level below 40% can be at risk of bleeding o Bleeding from minor mouth injuries o Large 'goose eggs' from minor head bumps o Spontaneous joint bleeds or deep-muscle hematomas o Prolonged bleeding following minor injuries, surgery, etc. **Complications:** o Develops joint contractures and at times life-threatening bleeding like intracranial hemorrhage o Infections like HIV, hepatitis B and C from plasma derived factors. o Inhibitor development against factors VIII.	o 30% of females with factor level below 40% can be at risk of bleeding o Spontaneous joint bleeds or deep-muscle bleeds o Prolonged bleeding following minor injuries, surgery, etc. **Complications:** o Same as hemophilia A.
Moderate hemophilia A and B	o Prolonged or delayed oozing after relatively minor trauma o Usually diagnosed before age 5 to 6 years	
Mild hemophilia A and B	o Abnormal bleeding with surgery or tooth extractions o Often not diagnosed until later in life	

Q 57. Write on diagnosis and management, inheritance pattern, recurrence risk, genetic counseling and prenatal management for subsequent pregnancy for hemophilia A and hemophilia B.

Ans. **Diagnosis and management of hemophilia A and hemophilia B**

	Hemophilia A	Hemophilia B
Diagnosis	**Basic:** o Complete blood count: Anemia o Platelet count: Normal o Liver function test, prothrombin time: Normal and activated prothrombin time: Increased o Coagulation factor o HIV, hepatitis B, C screening o Orthopedic consultation for joint examination.	**Basic:** o Similar to hemophilia A.
	Specific: Low factor VIII clotting activity in the presence of a normal, functional von Willebrand factor level: o Severe hemophilia A:<1% factor VIII o Moderate hemophilia A: 1–5% factor VIII o Mild hemophilia A: 6–40% factor VIII	**Specific:** Low factor IX clotting activity: o Severe hemophilia B:<1% factor IX o Moderate hemophilia B: 1–5% factor IX o Mild hemophilia B:>5–40% factor IX

Contd.

	Hemophilia A	Hemophilia B
	Molecular genetic testing: Identification of a hemizygous F8 pathogenic variant in a male proband: ○ Intron 22 inversion is present in around 50% of severe hemophilia A. ○ Intron 1 inversion and various forms of sequence variations are present in the rest. ○ If inversion is not identified, sequence analysis and deletion and duplication testing is done. ○ For female carrier, molecular testing is done to detect carrier status as factor VIII levels are not reliable.	**Molecular genetic testing:** Identification of a hemizygous F9 pathogenic variant in a male proband: ○ Almost all are sequence variations and Sanger sequencing is done for mutation identification. ○ For female carrier, molecular testing is done to detect carrier status as factor VIII levels are not reliable.
Management of hemo-philia A and B	Referral to a hemophilia treatment center (HTC): ○ Intravenous infusion of factor VIII in hemophilia A and IX concentrate in hemophilia B is most effective when infused within one hour of the onset of bleeding ○ Training to facilitate home infusions ○ Immune tolerance therapy to remove inhibitors to factors VIII and IX. ○ Mild disease: Intravenous or nasal desmopressin acetate in hemophilia A ○ Immunization should be given subcutaneously not intramuscular. **Prophylaxis:** Alternate day infusion of factor VIII or IX in severe cases to maintain factor level activity above 1%. **Surveillance:** Periodic evaluation of hemophilia patient based on the severity. **Testing of inhibitors to factor** depends upon the duration and clinical response to the treatment. **Recent treatment under trial for hemophilia A:** Bypass factor VIII, long-acting coagulation factors, non-replacement therapy like Emicizumab and gene therapy are under clinical trials.	
Inheritance pattern of hemophilia A and B	○ X-linked recessive. ○ Around 30% heterozygous females have clotting factor VIII activity less than 40% can be symptomatic.	
Recurrence risk	○ 50% male offspring can be affected when the female is a carrier	
Genetic counseling and prenatal management of hemo-philia A and B	○ Explanation of the disorder and its inheritance pattern ○ Mutation testing in proband, mother of the proband, female relatives and their children at risk and prenatal testing by chorionic villi sampling and amniocentesis.	

BIBLIOGRAPHY

1. GeneReviews® [Internet]. Seattle (WA): University of Washington, Seattle; 1993 [cited 2020 Jun 26]. Available from:http://www.ncbi.nlm.nih.gov/books/NBK1295/

2. Kliegman R. Nelson textbook of pediatrics. 21st ed. Philadelphia, PA: Elsevier;2016.

3. Kresak JL, Walsh M. Neurofibromatosis: a review of NF1, NF2 and Schwannomatosis. J Pediatr Genet 2016;5:98–104.

4. Kumar P, Goyal JP. Positive newborn screening for cystic fibrosis, what to do next? Indian JPediatr 2019;86:1147.

5. Randle S. Tuberous sclerosis complex: genetics, clinical features, and diagnosis. In: Up-to-date, Firth H, Pappo A, Patterson MC, Dashe J (Eds), Up-to-date, Waltham, MA. (Accessed on June 01, 2020).

6. Rimion DL, Pyeritz RE, Korf BR. Emery and Rimoin's Principles and Practice of Medical Genetics, 7th ed. San Diego: Academic Press; 2013.

Hemoglobin and Hemoglobinopathies

Meenakshi Bothra Gupta, Seema Kapoor

Q 1. Explain the incidence, etiology, genetic basis and pathophysiology of beta thalassemia.

Ans. Beta thalassemia: Hemoglobin is a tetrameric protein composed of two pairs of globin chains (usually alpha and beta globins), each with its own heme group. The human hemoglobins are encoded by two gene clusters: **α-like** globin genes present on chromosome 16 and β-like globin genes on chromosome 11 (Figure 12.1). Normally an individual inherits two β-globin genes and 2-α globin genes from each parent, i.e. normal adult hemoglobin is $\alpha_2 \beta_2$, depending upon whether the genetic defects or deletion lies in transmission of α or β globin chain gene, thalassemias are classified into α and β-thalassemias. Patients with β-thalassemias have impaired production of β chains. Beta thalassemias may occur as heterozygous (minor) or homozygous state (major).

The overall prevalence of β-thalassemia in India is 3–4% with an estimate that around 10,000–12,000 children are born every year with β-thalassemia major. The prevalence of β-thalassemia trait in some ethnic groups is> 9–10%.

More than 80 mutations have now been found to be responsible for β-thalassemia following various mechanisms like: (Figure 12.1)
1. Mutation at the promoter site at TATA box.
2. Splicing site mutations involving 5'GT or 3'AG intronic nucleotides.
3. Abnormal capping and polyadenylation defects leading to defective RNA.
4. Nonsense, missense and frameshift mutations.
5. Some synonymous mutations in the exons leading to abnormal splicing.

Few common mutations accounting for 80–90% of the mutant alleles. 92+5 G>C (IVS-1–5)

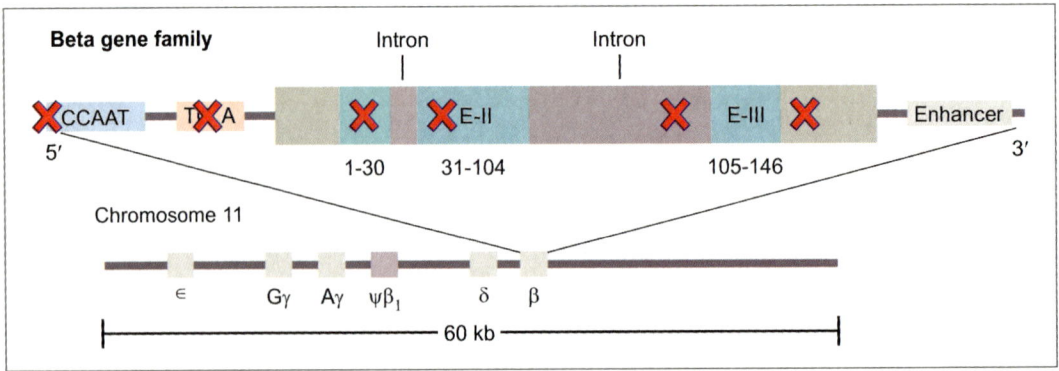

Figure 12.1:: : Beta globin gene structure cluster and different mutation sites—**X** represents β gene mutation sites

is the most common reported mutation in most of the regions followed by deletion 619 bp. Other common mutations include IVS 1–5(G-C), IVS1–1(G-T),Fr8/9 (+G), Fr41/42(-TTCT), c.79G>A (p.E27K), c.47G>A (p.Trp16Ter).

Various modifying factors like combination of alpha-beta, delta-beta, triplication of alpha chains, persistence of fetal hemoglobin, unstable beta chains, etc. cause variability in severity of the disease.

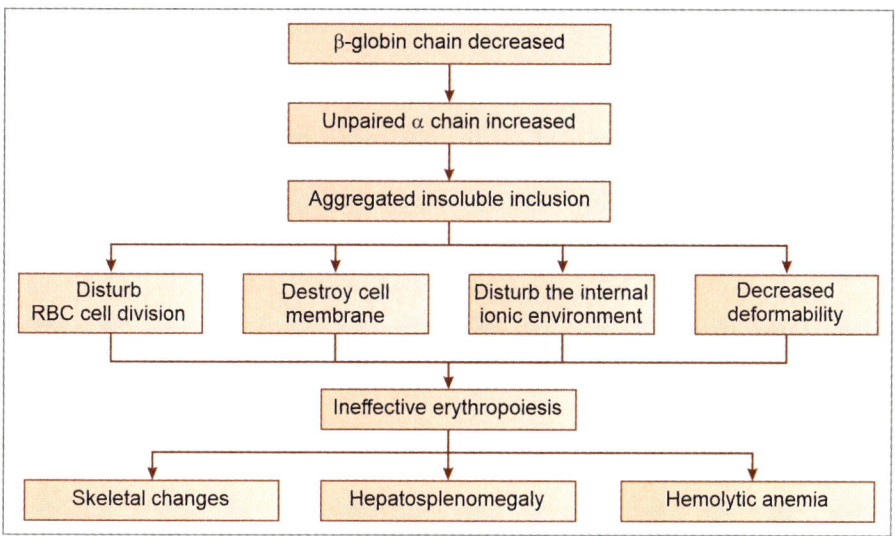

Figure 12.2: Pathophysiology of β-thalassemia

Q 2. Write the clinical features and complications, diagnosis and management of beta-thalassemias.

Ans. β-thalassemias can be classified into:

- Thalassemia minor or β-thalassemia carrier or β-thalassemia trait.(β^+/β^N, β^0/β^N)
- Thalassemia intermedia β^{++}/β^+, β^{++}/β^{++}.
- Thalassemia major or Cooley's anemia or Mediterranean anemia. ($\beta^+/\beta^+\beta^{++}/\beta^0$ $\beta^+/\beta^0\beta^0/\beta^0$)

Clinical features (Figure 12.3)

- Anemia is mild in thalassemia minor and it increases in severity from intermedia to major forms.
- Children develop pallor, jaundice, feeding problems, growth restriction and hepatosplenomegaly.
- Ineffective erythropoiesis and compensated erythroid hyperplasia produce maxillary marrow hyperplasia and frontal bossing leading to characteristic 'hemolytic facies'.

Complications

- Skeletal deformities like genu valgum and pathological fractures of long bones and vertebrae may occur early due to cortical invasion by erythroid elements.
- Thalassemia patients on chronic transfusion are susceptible for acquiring blood-borne infections (hepatitis B, C, human immunodeficiency virus) apart from developing iron overload.
- Complications arising from iron overload are cirrhosis, endocrine dysfunction (glucose intolerance, hypogonadism, hypothyroidism, hypoparathyroidism) and cardiomyopathy.
- Susceptibility to infection and improper transfusion of blood may lead to even death in severe cases.
- Massive splenomegaly leading to pancytopenia.
- Vascular thrombotic episodes.
- Gallbladder stones, leg ulcers.

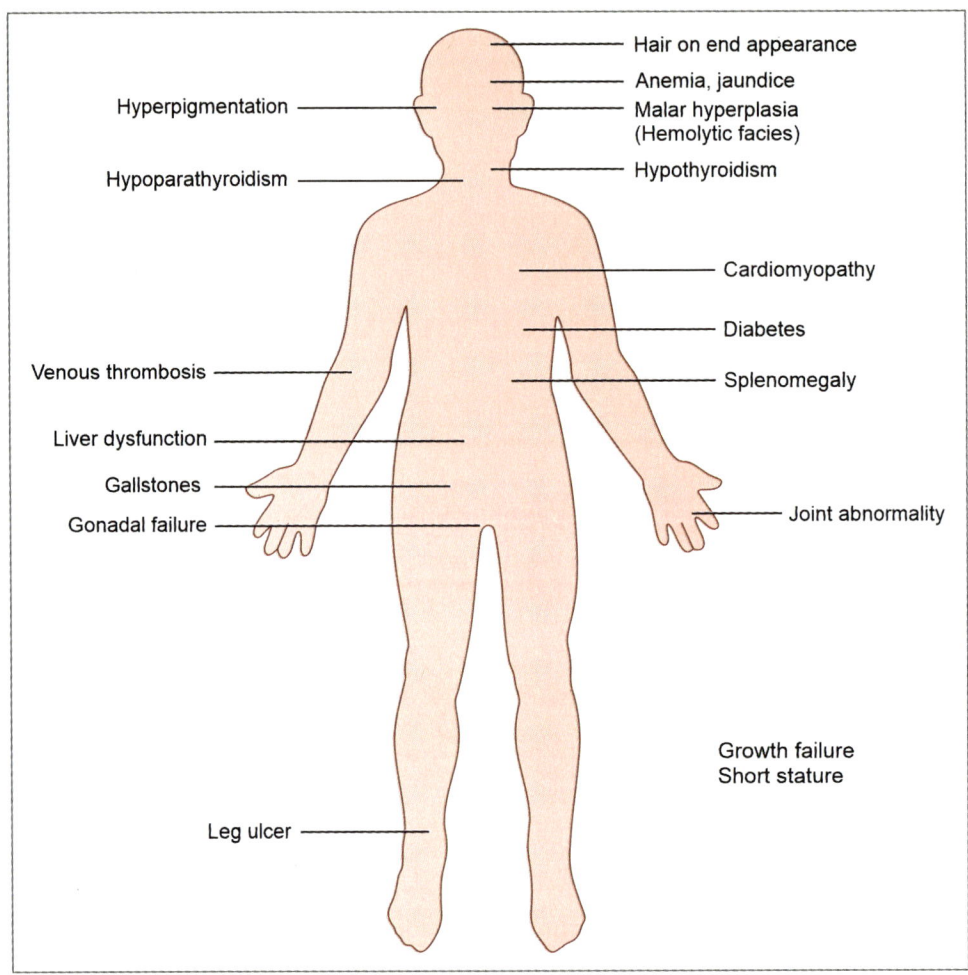

Hair on end appearance

Anemia, jaundice

Hyperpigmentation

Malar hyperplasia
(Hemolytic facies)

Hypoparathyroidism

Hypothyroidism

Cardiomyopathy

Diabetes

Venous thrombosis

Splenomegaly

Liver dysfunction

Gallstones

Gonadal failure

Joint abnormality

Growth failure
Short stature

Leg ulcer

Figure 12.3: Clinical features and complications of beta-thalassemia
(*Source of human body outline*: DLPNG.com)

Q 3. Write the diagnosis and management of beta thalassemias.

Ans. **Diagnosis** is based on:

1. Clinical features
2. Laboratory investigations
   ⊃ **Complete blood picture:**

Thalassemia type	Hemoglobin (g/dl)	Mean corpuscular volume (MCV) & mean corpuscular hemoglobin (MCH)	Peripheral smear	Hemoglobin electrophoresis
Thalassemia minor	11–12 g/dl	Reduced	Microcytosis, hypochromia	HbA2>3.4%,
Thalassemia intermedia	7–10 g/dl	50–80 fl 16–24 pg	Microcytosis, hypochromia, anisocytosis, poikilocytosis	HbA2 (2–5%) HbF (70–90%)
Thalassemia major	<7 g/dl	<70 fl <20 pg	Microcytosis, hypo-chromia, anisocytosis, poikilocytosis	HbA2 (2–5%) HbF (95–98%)

- ➲ **Molecular genetic testing of HBB gene.**
- ➲ **Other auxiliary investigations:**
  - a. *Osmotic fragility test*: Decreased
  - b. *Urinary urobilinogen:* Increased (Ehrlich test)
  - c. *Stool examination:* Dark stools, increased stercobilinogen.
  - d. *Radiological changes:* Seen after 1 year
    - ➲ X-ray of skull shows "hair on end appearance"
    - ➲ Generalized skeletal osteoporosis

Q 4. Write the management of beta thalassemias.

Ans.

MANAGEMENT

The management of thalassemia is guided by the severity of anemia, suppression of excessive erythropoiesis and prevention of excess iron overload. It includes:

○ **Blood transfusion:**
- Severe anemia with hemoglobin <7 g% for more than 2 weeks is widely accepted as an indication to start blood transfusion.
- The goal should be aimed to maintain a pretransfusion Hb level of 9 to 10 g/dl
- And a post-transfusion Hb level of 13 to 14 g/dl to prevent growth impairment, organ damage and bone deformities.
- The frequency of transfusion is usually every 3 to 4 weeks.

○ **Splenectomy:**
- Patients with thalassemia intermedia may survive without chronic transfusion but the development of hypersplenism may require splenectomy and folic acid supplementation.
- Vaccination against capsulated organisms like *Streptococcus pneumoniae*, *Hemophilus influenzae* and Neisseria's.
- Penicillin prophylaxis oral penicillin (125 mg twice daily for children up to 2 years 250 mg twice daily for children 2 years and above)
- And aspirin after splenectomy required in such individuals.

○ **Iron chelation:**
- Patients who receive regular blood transfusion may develop hemosiderosis.

- Serum ferritin, liver biopsy and imaging modalities like magnetic resonance imaging and biosusceptometry can measure iron overload in the body.
- These individuals may develop iron overload from increased gastrointestinal absorption of iron even without transfusion
- And therefore chelation therapy is started when the serum ferritin concentration exceeds 300 ng/ml.
- Iron chelating agents like deferoxamine (parenteral use), deferasirox (oral use) or combination of drugs may be used.

○ **Bone marrow transplantation (BMT):** BMT remains the only definitive cure currently available for patients with thalassemia. However, the major limitation of allogenic BMT is the lack of a human leukocyte antigen-identical sibling donor and the very high cost. Cord blood transplantation is another option where with a low risk of graft versus host disease.

Recent advances in management (*see* Chapter 23):

Surveillance:
- ➲ Monthly growth and development assessment.
- ➲ Adverse effects of iron overload and chelation therapy monthly.
- ➲ Liver function test, hepatitis B, C and alpha fetoprotein once in three months.
- ➲ Annual ophthalmological, cardiac, hormonal, skeletal assessment (bone density).

Q 5. Explain the alpha-globin gene structure cluster with the help of a diagram and describe the etiology and genetic basis of alpha-thalassemia.

Ans. **Alpha-thalassemia:** The α-globin-gene HBA1 and HBA2 cluster (Figure 12.4) is located on the short arm of chromosome 16. It is responsible for production of alpha and zeta globin chains, which are combined with the beta, epsilon, gamma or delta globins to form hemoglobin. It also contains two pseudogenes, HBD, HS 40 regulatory region and X, Y and Z homologous region,

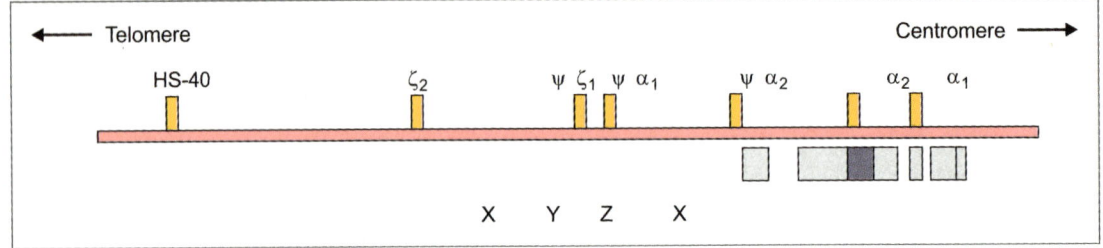

Figure 12.4: Alpha-globin gene structure cluster

responsible for unbalanced chromosomal rearrangements during meiosis due to deletion and duplications in this region.

Etiology and genetic basis:

- Most common mutations leading to alpha thalassemia are deletions of *HBA1* and *HBA2* genes.
- Some of the non-deletional mutations either due to single base substitution or insertion leads to missense, nonsense or frameshift mutation causing abnormal transcription, splicing and translation process.

Mutation in the alpha globin gene leads to decreased production of alpha globin chains, that results in α-thalassemia. Decreased production of alpha-globin chains results in a relative excess of gamma-globin chains in fetuses and newborns and of beta-globin chains in children and adults. Beta-globin chains are capable of forming tetramers (β_4), which can precipitate on and damage the red cell membrane.

Normally, there are four α-globin genes, and the severity of α-thalassemia depends on how many α-globin genes are affected (Figure 12.5):

- Persons who inherit 3 normal alpha-globin genes **(-α/αα)** are referred to clinically as silent carriers.
- Inheritance of 2 normal alpha-globin genes through either heterozygosity for alpha thalassemia (αα/--) or homozygosity **(-α/-α)** results in the development of alpha thalassemia trait.
- Inheritance of only one out of the four normal alpha-globin genes **(-α/--)** leads

to HbH disease, or alpha-thalassemia intermedia.

- Deletion of all four α-globin genes leads to the most severe form of α-thalassemia, i.e. hydrops fetalis (Hb Barts).

Chromosome 16		Functional gene
	Normal	4
	Silent carrier	3
	α thal trait *cis*	2
	α thal trait *trans*	2
	HbH	1
	Hydrops fetalis	0

Figure 12.5: Deletions of HbA1 and HbA2 in alpha-thalassemia

Q 6. Explain the clinical features and complications of alpha-thalassemia.

Ans. Clinical features and complications: The severity of the clinical manifestations in alpha thalassemia is proportional to the number of α-globin genes that are deleted, as mentioned in previous question.

- **Silent carrier state:** These individuals are completely asymptomatic but may have slight microcytosis.
- **α-Thalassemia trait:** The clinical picture is similar to β-thalassemia minor including minimal or no anemia and microcytosis.
- **Hemoglobin H (HbH) disease:** HbH has an extremely high affinity for oxygen and therefore leads to tissue hypoxia disproportionate to the level of hemoglobin. HbH might also precipitate and form intracellular inclusions that promote hemolysis in the spleen, resulting in a moderately severe anemia, splenomegaly, mild jaundice, osteoporosis and gallstones.
- **Hydrops fetalis:** The fetus shows severe pallor, generalized edema, pleural and pericardial effusion, and massive hepatosplenomegaly. It is usually lethal *in utero*, without transfusions.

Q 7. How will you diagnose and do management for alpha thalassemia?

Ans.

DIAGNOSIS
○ Ultrasound can show features of hydrops fetalis prenatally.
○ Hb: HbH: 9–11gm/dl, Hb Barts: 3–8 gm/dl
○ In milder varieties, peripheral smear may show hypochromia and microcytosis.
○ In moderate to severe subtypes, significant anemia along with reticulocytosis is seen.
○ In HbH disease, brilliant crassly blue stain shows HbH inclusion bodies.
○ Hb electrophoresis is not very useful to diagnose alpha thalassemia syndromes, but it can be useful in quantitating and identifying different hemoglobin types. Hemoglobin Bart's is elevated at birth in patients with alpha thalassemia. • With HbH disease, 20–40% of total hemoglobin is Hb Bart's.

• With alpha-thalassemia trait, Hb Bart's accounts for 5–15% of total hemoglobin.
• In silent carriers, however, the percentage is only 1–2%,
○ Molecular genetic testing of HBA1 and HBA2 gene.

MANAGEMENT
○ In asymptomatic cases, no treatment is required.
○ In severe cases: There is a lifelong dependence on blood transfusions for survival, with the associated risk of iron overload.
○ Iron chelation therapy with iron load monitoring. Hb Barts: Intrauterine blood transfusion splenectomy with massive splenomegaly.
○ Medical or surgical treatment for gallstones and leg ulcers. Hematopoietic stem cell transplantation can be curative.
○ Growth and development assessment.
○ The recurrence risk assessment, genetic counseling and prenatal management for subsequent pregnancy.

Q 8. Describe the etiology, genetic basis and pathophysiology of sickle cell disease.
Ans. Sickle cell disease:

Etiology: Sickle cell disease is a hereditary structural hemoglobinopathy caused by a point mutation in β-globin gene that leads to a novel property in the protein and causes synthesis of an abnormal sickle hemoglobin (HbS). This leads to tissue damage and clinical features due to ischemia (Figure 12.6).

Genetic basis: It is an autosomal recessive disease due to a point mutation in the 6th codon of the beta globin chain gene *HBB*. As a result of this, there is replacement of a glutamate residue with a valine residue (9 GAG-GTG). Individuals who are heterozygous for HbS usually remain asymptomatic. Those who are homozygous for this condition, may manifest varied clinical features. The various modifier genes like BCL11A and MYB inhibitors of gamma chains can lead to more severe disease due to low level of HbF.

Pathophysiology of sickle cell disease:

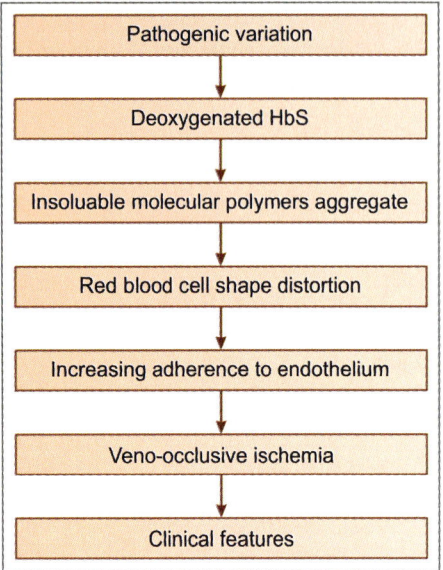

Figure 12.6: Pathophysiology of sickle cell disease

Ans.

CLINICAL FEATURES OF SICKLE CELL DISEASE (FIGURE 12.7)
○ Varying degrees of anemia, jaundice can cause chronic hypoxia in individuals with sickle cell disease.
○ Generalized impairment of growth and development.
○ There is increased susceptibility to infection with encapsulated organisms like *Streptococcus pneumonia*, *Neisseria meningitidis*, *Hemophilus influenzae* due to altered splenic function. Osteomyelitis can occur due to *Staphylococcus aureus* or *salmonella*.
○ Neurological: Stroke, cerebral infarcts or hemorrhage.
○ **Others:** Cardiomyopathy, cholelithiasis and complications due to iron overload in heart, lungs, pituitary, testes, liver and pancreas.

Q 9. Describe the clinical features and complications of sickle cell disease.

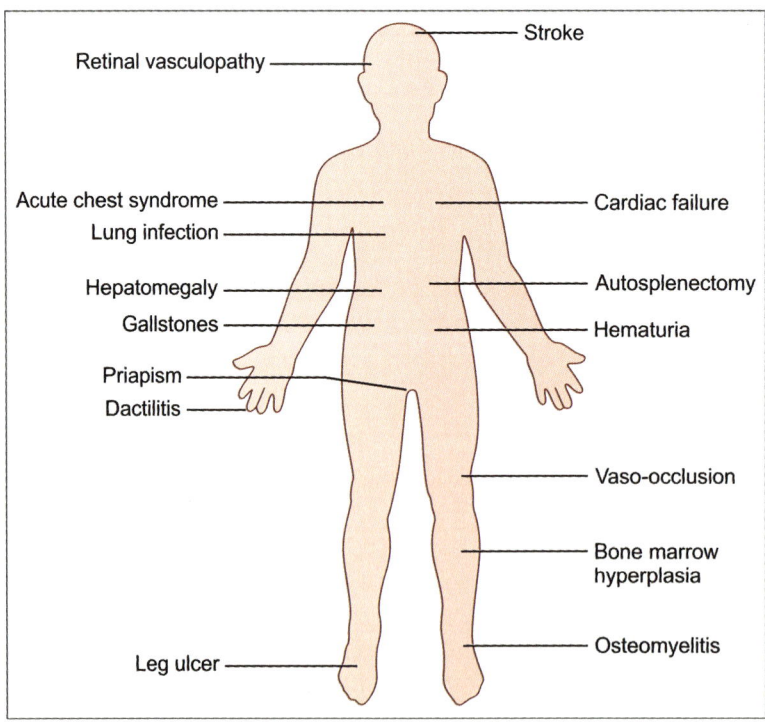

Figure 12.7: : Clinical features and complications of sickle cell disease
(*Source of human body outline*: DLPNG.com)

Symptoms in sickle cell trait:

⤵ Asymptomatic

⤵ During stress conditions like dehydration and exercise, increased risk of thromboembolism leading to pulmonary embolism, stroke, leg ulcers, renal disease, splenic infarcts.

⤵ Renal medullary carcinoma.

COMPLICATIONS

The disease course may be complicated by a variety of "crises" including:

○ **Vaso-occlusive crises:** Episodes of hypoxic injury and infarction cause severe pain in the affected regions like bones, lungs, liver, brain, spleen, and penis. Infection, dehydration, and acidosis can act as triggers for this. It may manifest as the **hand-foot syndrome** or dactylitis of the bones of hands or feet, or both. Disorders related to vascular obstruction, include priapism, stroke, pulmonary and systemic hypertension and retinopathy, which might even cause blindness.

○ **Acute chest syndrome is** a vaso-occlusive crisis involving the lungs, which typically presents with fever, cough, chest pain, and pulmonary infiltrates.

○ **Sequestration crises** occur due to massive entrapment of sickle red cells in spleen, resulting in rapid splenic enlargement, hypovolemia and sometimes shock.

○ **Aplastic crises** may result from the infection of red cell progenitors by parvovirus B19, which causes a transient cessation of erythropoiesis and a sudden worsening of the anemia.

Q 10. How will you make a diagnosis and do management for sickle cell disease?
Ans.

DIAGNOSIS

○ By the clinical features of hemolytic anemia.

○ Blood counts and peripheral smear (PS): Normocytic normochromic anemia, sickled RBCs associated with reticulocytosis, Howell-Jolly bodies.

○ Sickling of RBC, if not readily visible on the PS, can be induced by mixing a blood sample with an oxygen consuming reagent, such as metabisulfite, which induces sickling of red cells if HbS is present.

○ Hyperbilirubinemia.

○ Hemoglobin electrophoresis or HPLC is also used to demonstrate the presence of HbS and HbF.

○ Other abnormal S/C ($\beta^s\beta^c$): HbA2 < 3.6, $\beta^s\beta^+$ or $\beta^s\beta^0$ HbA2>3.6

○ Molecular genetic testing of HBB gene.

MANAGEMENT

○ **Pain management:** Hydration, massage, anti-inflammatory ketorolac, ibuprofen and analgesics.

○ **Fever and infections:** Culture sensitive antibiotics.

○ **Acute chest syndrome:** Chest X-ray, pulmonary function test, oxygen, blood transfusion.

○ **Aplastic crisis and splenic sequestration:** Hematocrit and reticulocyte monitoring and blood transfusion.

○ **Pulmonary hypertension:** Oxygen, transfusion, hydroxyurea.

○ **Stroke:** Blood counts, reticulocyte monitoring, magnetic resonance imaging of brain, exchange transfusion, chronic transfusion hydroxyurea.

○ **Priapism:** Hydration, analgesics and aspiration and irrigation.

○ **Supportive:** Immunization, folic acid, iron chelation therapy.

○ **Recent advances in treatment** (*see* Chapter 23)

SURVEILLANCE

○ Growth and development assessment.

○ Blood counts and reticulocytes, lactate dehydrogenase.

○ Vitamin D, renal and liver function test, iron load assessment.

○ Transcranial Doppler, chest X-ray, electrocardiogram, 2D ECHO, pulmonary function test

Q 11. Explain the recurrence risk, genetic counseling and prenatal management for subsequent pregnancy for hemolytic anemia.

Ans. Recurrence risk: As hemolytic anemia shows autosomal recessive inheritance, if both the parents are found to have the trait, each of the next offspring will have a 1/4 chance of having alpha thalassemia.

Genetic counseling and prenatal management: Considering all the general principles and psychosocial issues of counseling, family is explained about the details of disease.

Both pre- and post-test counseling are important particularly for prenatal diagnosis to eliminate the irrational fears among people particularly in respect of stigmatization. It also helps the couples at risk to take the right decision for future reproductive choices to avoid the birth of another child with the disease. The family should be given all the available options including prenatal diagnosis.

In areas where β-thalassemia and sickle cell disease are endemic, ideally, the pregnant lady should undergo HPLC or Hb electrophoresis.

If both, the woman and her partner are found to have thalassemia or sickle cell trait, the couple should be offered prenatal diagnosis. Prenatal diagnosis is possible by analysis of fetal DNA obtained by chorionic villous biopsy or amniocentesis.

Couples having a fetus with hydrops fetalis should be offered prenatal diagnosis for homozygous α^0-thalassemia. It usually carries a poor prognosis, and the couple should be counseled accordingly.

Couples, for whom termination of pregnancy is unacceptable due to cultural or religious reasons, can be given an option of preimplantation diagnosis or artificial insemination with a donor who is not a carrier of hemolytic anemia or another hemoglobinopathy or even adoption of a child.

Q 12. Describe the genetic basis and clinical features of other different hemoglobin variants and their combinations.

Ans. Hemoglobin variants occur when genetic changes in the globin genes cause alterations in the amino acids that make up the globin protein. These changes may affect the structure of the hemoglobin, its behavior, its production rate, and/or its stability.

Hb variant combinations	Genetic basis	Clinical features
Hb constant spring	Sense mutations in alpha chain causes change from a stop codon to other codes for an amino acid, e.g. hemoglobin constant spring alpha 142 UAA (Stop codon) to CAA (Gln) leading to elongation of amino acid chain causing mRNA unstable and further leads to degradation of RBCs.	Symptoms of hemoglobin H disease.
Hereditary persistence of fetal hemoglobin (HPFH)	Expression of g-globin genes at the same level in adult life as in fetal life due to large deletion in α, β, γ promoter region.	Asymptomatic
HbSC	Co-inheritance of 1 *HbS* and 1 *HbC* genes HbS→point mutation in 6th codon of beta globin chain → replacement of glutamate with valine HbC→substitution of glutamic acid with lysine at 6th position of β-globin chain	○ Milder phenotype than full-blown sickle cell disease. ○ Splenomegaly and mild anemia may be seen. ○ A proliferative retinopathy may lead to progressive loss of vision.

Contd.

Hb variant combinations	Genetic basis	Clinical features
HbSE	Co-inheritance of 1 *HbS* & 1 *HbE* genes ○ *HbS* → as stated above ○ *HbE* → point mutation leading to replacement of glutamic acid by lysine at position 26 of β chain	May remain asymptomatic or have sickling-related complications including acute chest syndrome, vaso-occlusive crisis and recurrent infections.
HbDE	○ *HbD* → derived from a point mutation in the beta-globin gene in the 1st base of the 121 codons (GAA → CAA) with the substitution of glutamine for glutamic acid (Glu>Gln) in the beta globin chain ○ HbE → as stated above	○ HbD disease does not typically cause clinical symptoms. ○ Occasionally, it can cause mild hemolytic anemia and mild splenomegaly.
HbD--Beta Thal	*HbD* → as stated above Beta Thal → due to impaired production of β chains	HbD: Punjab becomes significant when it is co-inherited with HbS or β thalassemia.
HbDS	HbD → as stated above *HbS* → as stated above	May cause mild hemolytic anemia and mild splenomegaly
E-Beta Thal	*HbE* → as stated above Beta Thal → due to impaired production of β chains	Heterogenous disease with a phenotype ranging from mild anemia to the most severe forms of β-thalassemia major
Beta-Delta Thal	Decrease in both beta and delta globin chain production due to deletion of delta and beta globin genes or due to nucleotide substitutions in promoter region of Aγ and β-globin gene	Usually remains asymptomatic
Hb Lepore thalassemia	Fusion of δβ globin chains. Homozygotes have only HbF and Hb Lepore.	○ Asymptomatic ○ Silent stroke.

Q 13. Write the various preventive strategies which can be taken at community health level to prevent thalassemia.

Ans. Strategies to prevent thalassemia at community health level include:

1. **Educating** health professionals, school and college students, pregnant women and the population about thalassemia is an effective strategy to spread awareness about it. Mass media may be used to have a significant impact on the general population.

2. **Screening pregnant ladies and newborns for thalassemia:** Both pre- and post-test counseling for targeted group (like consanguineous couple, positive family history of disease) or universal screening for thalassemia should be done wherever feasible.

3. **Establishing prenatal diagnosis facilities:** Complete blood counts during the first antenatal visit of every pregnant woman, an estimation of HbA2 and HbF with reduced mean corpuscular volume (MCV) and mean corpuscular hemoglobin (MCH) values and the carrier testing of couples at risk, prenatal diagnosis and counseling in different regions of the country is important.

4. **Data on the prevalence** of β thalassemia carriers does not estimate the true burden of the disease. The extremely variable prevalence even within small geographic

regions and very high frequencies of carriers in some communities highlights the need for micro mapping in every state.

5. **Training and capacity building:** At least one center in the government setup in every state with experience obstetricians and sonologists, trained auxiliary workers and genetic counselors would be required.

Q 14. Explain the need of newborn screening for hemoglobinopathies in current health scenario.

Ans. India has a huge burden of hemoglobino-pathies with an estimated average prevalence of β-thalassemia carriers about 3–4%. Several ethnic groups have a much higher prevalence (4–17%).

Of the 10,000 to 12,000 thalassemic children born annually in India, very few are optimally managed mainly in urban regions. It has been estimated that 2 million units of packed red cells would be needed for transfusion of thalassemia patients in the country.

Allogeneic stem cell transplant, which is the only curative treatment available for these diseases is currently unaffordable for the majority of families, due to its exorbitant cost and due to very few centers only in the urban setting offering transplant. The chance of a successful transplant is around 90% in patients with good risk features while the outcome is still challenging for high-risk patients. Thus, prevention of the birth of an affected child is a feasible and realist option.

To prevent the birth of babies with thalassemia, mass population screening with special focus on pregnant ladies and their spouses with appropriate genetic coun-seling and offering prenatal diagnosis and termination of pregnancy if the fetus is found to be affected by thalassemia. Universal screening of neonates would help in detecting babies affected by hemoglobinopathies in the pre-symptomatic stage and planning appropriate timely management for them. It will also help in initiating cascade screening to identify other family members who are carriers for the disease, so that further birth of affected babies can be prevented by timely genetic counseling and prenatal diagnosis and management.

BIBLIOGRAPHY

1. Aggarwal R, Prakash A, Aggarwal M. Thala-ssemia: An overview. J Sci Soc 2014; 41:3–6.
2. Daniel E Sabath. Molecular Diagnosis of Thalassemias and Hemoglobinopathies: An ACLPS Critical Review, American Journal of Clinical Pathology, Volume 148, Issue 1, July 2017, Pages 6–15
3. Emery & Rimoin's Principles & Practice of Medical Genetics, 7th edition.
4. Nelson's Textbook of Pediatrics, 21th Edition.
5. Thompson & Thompson, Genetics in Medicine, 8th Edition.
6. Zhang J, Li P, Yang Y, et al. Molecular epidemiology, pathogenicity, and structural analysis of hemoglobin variants in the Yunnan province population of Southwestern China. Sci Rep 9, 8264 (2019).

Congenital Malformations and Dysmorphism

Kausik Mandal, Ami Shah

Q 1. What is the incidence of structural congenital abnormalities? What do you mean by major and minor congenital anomalies and normal variant?

Ans. Congenital anomalies vary substantially in severity involving cardiovascular, nervous system, gastrointestinal, urogenital and skeletal system. Some of these are associated with 80–85% of spontaneous abortion, 25% of stillbirth, or death in 25% of early infancy. **These can be major and minor congenital anomalies and normal variant.**

1. **Major anomalies** are those which affect an infant's life expectancy, health status, physical or social functioning. Worldwide, around 3–5% of all live born infants have a major congenital anomaly. Examples of major congenital anomalies are:
   - Cleft palate with cleft lip
   - Craniorachischisis
   - Encephalocele
   - Exomphalos/omphalocele
   - Gastroschisis
2. **Minor anomalies** are those with little or no impact on health or short-term or long-term function. A single minor anomaly is found in around 14% newborns. With 2–3 minor anomalies, risk of having a major anomaly increases to 10–20%. Examples of minor congenital anomalies are single palmar crease and clinodactyly, accessory nipples, preauricular tags, etc.

3. **Normal variants** are those which though might look different but are within ± 2SD of standards for that age, sex and race.

Q 2. Explain: Malformations, dysplasia, deformations and disruptions.

Ans. Mechanism of congenital malformations during embryonic life are (Figure 13.1)

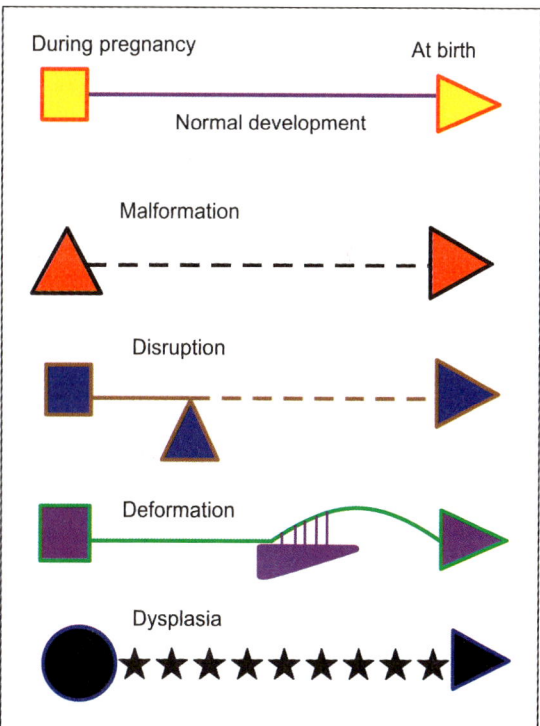

Figure 13.1: Different mechanisms of congenital malformations during development

A. **Malformation** (primary or intrinsic abnormality) signifies that fetal growth and development did not proceed normally due to underlying genetic, epigenetic, or environmental factors that altered the development of a particular structure. It can affect single structure or multiple structures. *Example:* Cleft lip, various chromosomal and monogenic syndromes.

B. **Disruption** is an anomaly where a normally growing fetal structure is found to have its growth arrested due to something which disrupts the process. The common example is amniotic band disruption, where a digit or extremity may be growing normally but then growth is disrupted due to amniotic band at the end of that extremity, result in missing fingers, toes, or hands and feet (Figure 13.2).

C. **Deformation** Abnormal external force on the fetus during *in utero* development results in abnormal growth or formation of the fetal structure. For example, in fetuses that grow in a uterine environment where there is oligohydramnios, the fetus may have a flattened face due to compression of the face against the uterine wall.

D. **Dysplasia** is a generalized anomaly related to an underlying tissue dysplasia where the intrinsic cellular architecture of a tissue is not normally maintained throughout growth and development. Many of the skeletal syndromes are due to dysplasia in the developing bone and cartilage.

Q 3. Explain: Syndrome, association and sequence.

Ans.

A. **A syndrome** is a well-characterized constellation of major and minor anomalies that occur together in a predictable fashion presumably due to a single underlying etiology. For example, Down syndrome (due to trisomy 21) and Turner syndrome.

B. **An association** is a group of anomalies that occur more frequently together than would be expected by chance alone and do not have a predictable pattern of recognition and/or a suspected unified underlying etiology. VACTERL or VATER associated with various anomalies of vertebra, anorectal region, cardiac, tracheoesophageal renal, limbs, etc. is a common example.

C. **A sequence** is a group of related anomalies that generally stem from a single initial major insult that alters the development of related tissues or structures. Example: Potter's sequence where newborn is often characterized by flattened abnormal facial features and deformations of the hands and

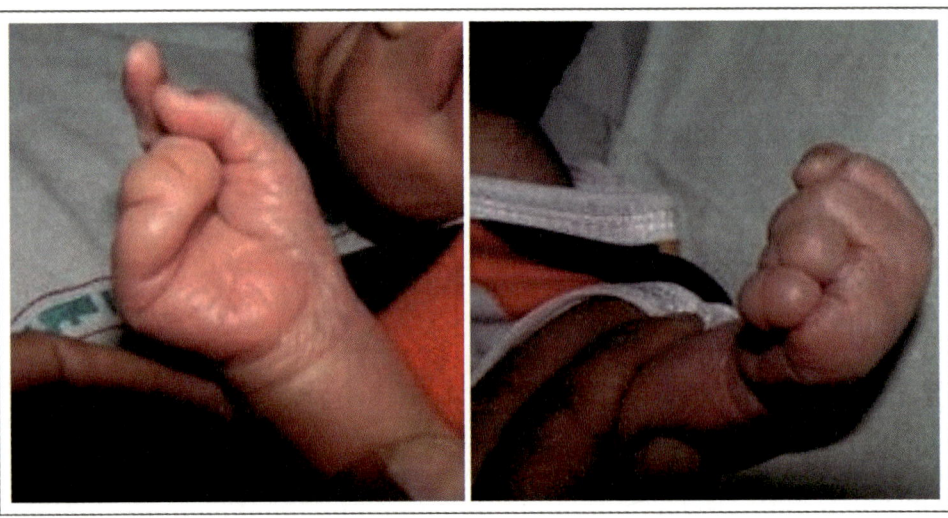

Figure 13.2: Amniotic band disruption: Note the constriction bands, amputation and pseudosyndactyly

feet along with poor lung development, secondary to oligohydramnios.

Q 4. Describe the etiology, genetic basis and risk factors for dysmorphism and congenital malformation.

Ans. The etiology and genetic basis of dysmorphism and congenital anomalies are extremely diverse. It includes genetic, environmental and idiopathic factors.

A. **Genetic factors constitute** 30–40% of etiology and include:

➲ *Chromosomal abnormalities:* Various chromosomal numerical anomalies like trisomy or monosomy and structural anomalies like deletion or translocation are responsible for 6% of the congenital malformation. It can be either due to overdose, less dose of genes or abnormal interaction of various pathways involved in development.

➲ *Single gene disorders* constitute 7–10% of the etiology for congenital malformations. It can cause either isolated involvement of single system like cardiovascular or renal system or can cause multiple abnormalities involving multiple systems of the body which give rise to specific patterns of malformations. Common examples are achondroplasia, Apert syndrome, Hutchison-Gilford progeria, etc. Here, the mutations are generally at very specific positions.

➲ *Congenital anomalies due to multiple genes:* The genes generally work in a common pathway. The anomalies are generally similar but varies in their patterns. Common examples are Bardet-Biedl syndrome, Meckel-Gruber syndrome, cardiofaciocutaneous syndrome, etc.

➲ *Multifactorial causes* are responsible for 20–30% of malformations. Various malformations occur due to interaction of environmental factors and susceptible genes. Example: Congenital heart disease, cleft lip and palate, holoprosencephaly, etc.

B. **Environmental factors:**

➲ *Folic acid deficiency* leads to genesis of malformations of the central nervous system and causes neural tube defect.

➲ *Teratogens* like lithium (Ebstein anomaly), phenytoin (heart abnormality, cleft palate), retinoids (ear and eye abnormality), valproic acid (neural tube defect, limb abnormality, facial dysmorphism), etc.

➲ *Intrauterine infections:* Congenital rubella (congenital heart disease and deafness), toxoplasma (hydrocephalus, chorioretinitis and deafness), cytomegalovirus (chorioretinitis and deafness, microcephaly).

➲ *Systemic maternal illness:* Phenylketonuria (microcephaly, congenital heart disease) and diabetes mellitus (congenital heart disease, holoprosencephaly, vertebral deformity).

➲ *Radiation* exposure causes microcephaly, malignancy and eye abnormality.

➲ *Chemicals:* Fetal alcohol syndrome (microcephaly, low IQ, facial dysmorphism), thalidomide (limb defect).

C. **Idiopathic:** In 50% of cases, cause has not been found.

Q 5. Describe the various phenotypic features associated with dysmorphism and congenital malformation.

Ans. Phenotypic features associated with dysmorphism and congenital malformation:

➲ Some of the congenital malformations are associated with typical dysmorphic faces 'gestalt of the syndrome' like in case of Down syndrome, William syndrome, Noonan syndrome, etc.

➲ Some are associated with nonspecific dysmorphic features.

➲ Congenital malformation can be associated with

▪ *Abnormal anthropometric measurements:* Short stature, microcephaly, macrocephaly.

- *Skin abnormalities:* Hypo or hyper-pigmentation
- *Skeletal abnormalities:* Polysyndactyly, joint contractures.
- *Genital abnormalities:* Small phallus or ambiguous genitalia and imperforate anus.

 ⊃ Developmental delay, low IQ, behavior disorders, growth and development failure.

 ⊃ Systemic abnormalities of major system can be congenital heart disease, anencephaly, structural brain defect, neural tube defect, cleft lip or palate, diaphragmatic hernia, reduction of limbs, renal dysplasia or polycystic kidney.

Q 6. How will you diagnose and will do management of a child with congenital malformation and dysmorphism?

Ans. Diagnosis:

A. **Clinical history, general head to toe examination includes:**

 ⊃ Anthropometry and facial measurements.

 ⊃ Dysmorphic features examination.

 ⊃ Skeletal system and extremities examination, ophthalmological and hearing assessment.

 ⊃ Genital and skin examination

 ⊃ Systemic examination includes cardiovascular, neurology, abdomen and respiratory system.

 ⊃ Photograph of the patient and the parent should be taken.

B. **Basic investigations:**

 ⊃ Complete blood counts

 ⊃ Liver function test

 ⊃ Renal function test.

C. **Imaging investigations:**

 ⊃ Skeletal survey (mentioned in achondroplasia answer)

 ⊃ *X-ray of hand and wrist:* For bone age assessment

 ⊃ *Magnetic resonance imaging brain:* For seizures and microcephaly

 ⊃ *Computer tomography brain:* For TORCH abnormalities

 ⊃ *Ultrasound abdomen:* To see organ abnormalities.

D. **Dysmorphology databases** can be referred if no cause is found based on clinical and laboratory findings **(See Appendix).**

E. **Genetic testing:** Confirmation of genetic disorders by diagnostic genetic testing are necessary for management, prognostication, and prenatal diagnosis to prevent recurrences in future pregnancies.

 ⊃ *Karyotype:* To identify chromosomal numerical and structural defects.

 ⊃ *Fluorescent in situ hybridization (FISH), multiplex ligation dependent probe amplification (MLPA):* For microdeletion syndrome.

 ⊃ *Biochemical testing:* For metabolic disorders like peroxisomal disorders.

 ⊃ *Sanger sequencing:* To identify target gene defect.

 ⊃ *Chromosomal analysis:* To detect CNVs (copy number variations/deletions and duplications) throughout the genome and is done to detect etiology of unidentified malformation with or without intellectual disability.

 ⊃ *Next generation sequencing (NGS) based clinical exome or whole exome* are often necessary to delineate the genetic cause underlying the malformation.

Management: A multidisciplinary approach for symptomatic and supportive treatment is essential for appropriate management. The goal of the treatment is to lessen the morbidity due to disabilities and to improve the quality of life of the individual suffering from disorder.

A. **Supportive care:**

 ⊃ Control of seizures, feeding problems, etc.

 ⊃ Physiotherapy for muscle weakness and motor developmental delay.

 ⊃ Social and play therapy, speech therapy, occupational therapy, behavioral therapy, special education.

B. **Specific management of associated systemic complications:**

- Ophthalmological, cardiac, renal, liver, structural brain defects
- Hypothyroidism and some of the metabolic disorders.
- Surgical correction of heart defect.

C. **Follow-up**

- Growth and development assessment
- Progression and nature of the disease
- Suggest new diagnostic and therapeutic treatment to the family.

Q 7. **Explain the recurrence risk, genetic counseling and prenatal management for dysmorphism and congenital malformation in the sibling and other family members of an affected child.**

Ans. **Recurrence risk:**

- Recurrence risk in congenital malformation is low if the etiological factor in pregnancy does not recur.
- *De novo* **chromosomal mutations:** Recurrence risk is <1%.
- **Single gene disorder:** Based on mutated target gene risk, inheritance pattern risk is
  - 25% for autosomal recessive
  - 50% for autosomal dominant
  - 50% for X-linked disorders in male child.

Genetic counseling: Discussed in Chapter 8.

Prenatal management:

- In view of recurrence risk ranging from 1–50% in a couple with previous child with dysmorphism and congenital abnormality, prenatal testing for targeted mutation analysis is recommended in each conception.
- Prenatal testing can be done either at 11–13 weeks of gestation by chorionic villus sampling or through amniocentesis after 16 completed weeks of gestation.

Before prenatal testing for target mutation family should be informed regarding:

- Prenatal procedure and prenatal test details.

Q 8. **Describe the etiology, genetic basis of Noonan syndrome.**

Ans. **Etiology:** Noonan syndrome is a common disorder caused by pathogenic variants in genes involved in RAS-MAPK (Mitogen activated) pathway (RASopathies)—a signal transduction pathway responsible for transcription of various genes controlling multiple cellular processes (proliferation, differentiation and apoptosis) and thus responsible for normal development processes.

Genetic basis and inheritance pattern:

- It is a heterogeneous disorder. (Table 13.1)

TABLE 13.1: List of genes implicated in Noonan syndrome

Gene	% of Noonan syndrome
PTPN11	50
SOS1	13
RAF1	5
RIT1	5
KRAS	<5
NRAS	<1
BRAF	<1
MAP2K1	<1
LZTR1	NA

- Commonly has an autosomal dominant pattern of inheritance with variable expressivity.
- Rarely LZTRI pathogenic variants may show autosomal recessive pattern.
- Most variations are missense or gain of function mutations; deletion/duplication are rarely reported.
- PTPN11 mutation causes increased activity of phosphatase and RAS-MAPK pathway, due to dysregulation of auto-inhibitory mechanism between SH2 and phosphatase enzyme domain, which is responsible for binding of growth factor receptor to tyrosine kinase.

○ KRAS mutation causes increased active form of GTP-RAS (responsible for cell growth and proliferation) due to decreased activity of GTP-ase and decreased interaction of KRAS with guanosine.

Q 9. Write the characteristic features of Noonan syndrome.

Ans. Characteristic features (Table 13.2)

TABLE 13.2: Systemic findings are variably present and described

Characteristic systemic manifestations	
Growth	○ Normal at birth ○ Failure to thrive in infancy ○ Short stature—delayed bone age
Cardio-vascular (50–80%)	○ Pulmonary valve stenosis with dysplasia (20–50%) ○ Hypertrophic cardiomyopathy (20–30%)—usually detected before 1 year (~5 months). ○ Other defects—Atrial and ventricular septal defects, pulmonary artery stenosis, tetralogy of Fallot and coarctation of the aorta ○ Rhythmic disturbances
Genito-urinary	○ Renal abnormalities (11%)—pelvis dilatation, duplex collecting system, uretic stenosis, real hypoplasia, renal agenesis ○ Delayed puberty ○ Fertility in females is normal. In males, it can be normal, delayed or inadequate.
Bleeding diathesis	○ One or more coagulation defects
Lymphatic edema	○ Localized/widespread ○ Prenatal and/or postnatal
Ocular abnor-malities	○ Strabismus ○ Refractive errors ○ Amblyopia
Dermato-logic	○ Café au lait spots and lentigines ○ Follicular keratosis over extensor surfaces and face
Malignancies	○ Childhood leukemia and myeloproliferative disorders especially Juvenile myelomonocytic leukemia (JMML) ○ Solid tumors—rhabdo-myosarcoma and neuroblastoma
Psychomotor development	○ Delayed early milestones (mild-moderate) ○ Articulation defects (72%) ○ Learning disability (25%) ○ Intellectual delay (5–20%)

○ Key dysmorphic features classically seen in early childhood are (Figure 13.3):

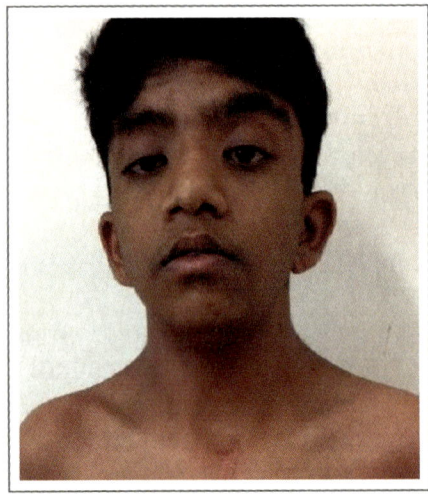

Figure 13.3: : Boy with Noonan syndrome with the typical facial dysmorphism (ptosis, downslanting eyes, hypertelorism, low-set ears), and webbed neck (*Courtesy:* Dr Prajnya Ranganathan, NIMS, Hyderabad)

- Low set posteriorly rotated ears with fleshy helices.
- Hypertelorism, downslanting eyes and epicanthal folds
- Ptosis
- Broad-webbed neck
- Deformed chest—superior pectus carinatum and inferior pectus excavatum
- Low set widely spaced nipples.
- It has a typical facial appearance known to change with age. (Figure 13.4)

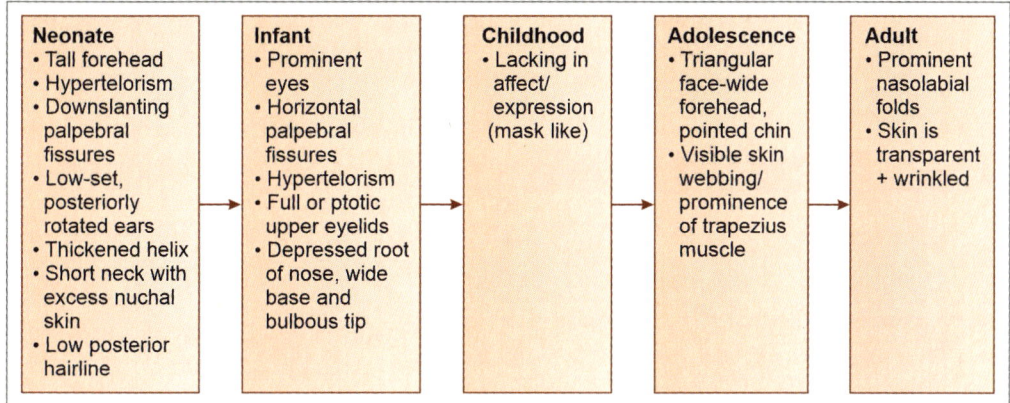

Figure 13.4: : Characteristics of facial features according to age

Q 10. How will you diagnose and do management for Noonan syndrome?

Ans. **Diagnosis** Table 13.3:

TABLE 13.3: Evaluation following initial diagnosis
○ Complete physical and neurological examination
○ Plotting of growth parameters on growth charts
○ Cardiac evaluation with echocardiography and electrocardiography
○ Hearing evaluation
○ Coagulation screen to include CBC with differential, differential PT/PTT
○ Ophthalmologic evaluation
○ Renal ultrasound examination; urinalysis if the urinary tract is anomalous
○ Clinical and radiographic assessment of spine and rib cage
○ Brain and cervical spine MRI, if neurologic symptoms are present
○ Multidisciplinary developmental evaluation
○ Consultation with a clinical geneticist and/or genetic counselor

When suggestive clinical findings are noted, further confirmation is by genetic testing. This may be achieved by a multigene panel (including all genes associated with the phenotype close differentials cardiofacial-cutaneous syndrome, Costello syndrome, LEOPARD syndrome, neurofibromatosis, Legius syndrome) or comprehensive genomic (exome/genome sequencing) testing.

MANAGEMENT
○ Following diagnosis, complete evaluation as described in Table 13.3, for possible systemic abnormalities is must.
○ Treatment of systemic manifestations detected. Example: Cardiovascular anomalies.
○ Developmental disabilities should be evaluated, and appropriate early intervention is initiated.
○ Growth hormone therapy: In view of a possible impairment of the GH-insulin like growth factor type 1 axis and documented response to growth hormone in past studies, it is now approved by FDA (2007) for short stature in Noonan syndrome. No specific dose has been established so far.

Q 11. Discuss recurrence risk, genetic counseling and prenatal management for Noonan syndrome.

Ans. **Recurrence risk:**

⊃ **Autosomal dominant:**

- In case of *de novo* pathogenic variants (most common), risk to proband's sibling is very low (<1%).
- The risk to siblings is 50% when one of the parents is affected (30–75%).
- The child of a proband has a 50% chance of inheriting the pathogenic variant.

Ↄ Autosomal recessive (LZTR1):
- Each sibling has a 25% chance of being affected and 50% chance of inheriting a single variant.

GENETIC COUNSELING
Considering all the general principles of genetic counseling and psychosocial aspects, the following is discussed with families:
○ Details of the disease like etiology, genetic basis, natural history, prognosis, management options, inheritance pattern, recurrence risk in future generation.
○ Details of prenatal procedure and testing for target mutation analysis if needed.
○ Likely benefits of early diagnosis and preparedness if the result returns positive

○ If the test comes positive, parents can take reproductive decision on their own.

Prenatal Management

Ↄ Common fetal characteristics detected on antenatal ultrasound:
- Polyhydramnios increased nuchal translucency, cystic hygroma (lymphatic dysplasia): 5–15% of chromosomally normal fetuses with increased nuchal translucency are likely to be Noonan syndrome.
- Relative macrocephaly.
- Cardiac and renal anomalies.

Ↄ Preimplantation genetic diagnosis and/or prenatal testing can be offered to families with identified pathogenic variants in the affected family member.

BIBLIOGRAPHY

1. GeneReviews® [Internet]. Seattle (WA): University of Washington, Seattle; 1993–2020. Available from: https://www.ncbi.nlm.nih.gov/books/NBK1124/
2. Narayanan DL, Pandey H, Moirangthem A, Mandal K, et al. Indian Pediatrics. 2017 Aug 15;54(8):638–43.
3. Rasmussen SA, Olney RS, Holmes LB, Lin AE, Keppler-Noreuil KM, Moore CA. Guidelines for case classification for the National Birth Defects Prevention Study. Birth Defects Res A Clin Mol Teratol. 2003; 67:193– 201.

Congenital Deafness

Inusha Panigrahi, Divya Kumari

Q 1. Describe the various parameters of classification of hereditary hearing loss.

Ans. Hearing loss is a sensory defect that affects 1–3 in every 1,000 children worldwide. Most of these cases are attributed to genetic factors, 35% to acquired/environmental or 30% to **idiopathic** causes. The classification of hearing loss is categorized based on different parameters.

a. **Age of onset:** Prelingual and postlingual
b. **Symptoms and severity:** Mild, moderate, severe, and profound
c. **Based on pure tone audiometry:** Conductive, sensorineural and mixed
d. **Genetic basis:** Syndromic and nonsyndromic
e. **Mode of inheritance:** Autosomal dominant, autosomal recessive, X-linked or mitochondrial.

Q 2. Explain the acquired etiological factors of hereditary hearing loss.

Ans. Acquired/environmental factors of hearing loss (35%)

⊃ **Prenatal infections** like cytomegalovirus (CMV), rubella virus, herpes virus infection and toxoplasmosis. The most common environmental cause is CMV infection. Around 18% of congenital CMV infected newborns will have some neurological sequelae, the major component of which is sensorineural hearing loss.

⊃ **Teratogens** like thalidomide, retinoic acid, and fetal alcohol syndrome.
⊃ **Postnatal infection,** mainly caused by *Neisseria meningitidis, Streptococcus pneumoniae, E. coli, Enterobacter cloacae* also cause hearing loss.
⊃ **Other postnatal factors:** Trauma, kernicterus, hypothyroidism, medicines like aminoglycosides, quinine, loop diuretics, etc.

Q 3. Explain the genetic nonsyndromic etiological factors of hereditary hearing loss.

Ans. Genetic factors (35%) are broadly divided into groups syndromic and non-syndromic.

Nonsyndromic hearing loss (NSHL)(60%)

i. It has no associated abnormalities of the external ear though it can be associated with abnormalities of the middle ear and/or inner ear.
ii. Nonsyndromic hearing loci are chosen as DFN and further classified on the basis mode of inheritance:
  ⊃ **DFNA:** Autosomal dominant (24 genes, common ones are *ACTG1, WFS1, GJB3, GJB6, KCNQ4*)
  ⊃ **DFNB:** Autosomal recessive (AR) (out of various AR genes, 5 genes *MYO3A, PJVK, LOXHD1, TMPRSS3* and *GJB2 are the common ones.*)
  ⊃ **DFNX:** X-linked (*PRPS, POU3F4, DMD*).

iii. Prelingual nonsyndromic hearing loss is 80% autosomal recessive, 20% autosomal dominant, 1–1.5% X-linked and <1% mitochondrial (most common *rRNA* gene and *UCNtRNA* gene).

iv. The most common cause of severe-to-profound autosomal recessive non-syndromic hearing loss in most populations is mutation in connexion 26 or *GJB2* gene (DFNB1). Mutation in GJB2 gene (connexion 26) is responsible for the failure of gap junction formation between the cells in the cochlea and causing failure of transduction of sound signals to electrical waves across these gaps leading to cochlear function impairment.

Q 4. Describe the genetic syndromic etiological factors of hereditary hearing loss.

Ans. Syndromic hearing loss (40%): Associated with malformations of the external ear or clinical problems associated with other organs or organ systems like renal anomalies or cardiac anomalies.

Few examples:

i. In Usher syndrome, there is additional eye involvement in the form of retinitis pigmentosa (RP).

ii. In Wolfram syndrome, presentation can also be with diabetes. In some cases, the problems run in families with multiple family members affected.

iii. In CHARGE syndrome, there can be additional ear anomalies, cardiac defect and ocular coloboma.

iv. In Pendred syndrome, there is additional hypothyroidism.

v. Waardenburg syndrome associated with hypopigmented, heterochromic iris and Hirschsprung disease.

vi. **Stickler syndrome:** Pierre Robin sequence, hypermobile joints, eye abnormalities.

Q 5. How will you approach a child with hereditary hearing loss?

Ans. The etiology of hearing loss is heterogenous. Algorithm approaches available

for the diagnostic evaluation depend on the clinical features associated with hearing loss, type of hearing loss, age of the patient, family history and other findings on the physical examination.

Aims of evaluation:

⮑ To know the etiology and associated co-morbidities.

⮑ To prevent further occurrence of hearing loss by doing genetic testing and genetic counseling.

Primary evaluation includes multidisciplinary team follow below mentioned steps:

1. **Physical examination:**

⮑ Measurement of growth parameters, i.e. height and weight

⮑ Assessment of the clinical features associated with various syndrome

⮑ Physical examination of outer ear, external auditory canal, middle ear abnormalities.

⮑ Tuning fork test for air or bone conduction, Romberg test to check vestibular system, and examination for nystagmus.

2. **Formal audiological assessment:** Following are the numerous different methods available.

⮑ *Pure tone audiometry (PTA):* It measures the ability to hear pure tone of different frequencies with both air and bone conduction as a function of intensity measurement.

⮑ Speech audiometry

⮑ *Behavioral audiometry:* This method is used to examine hearing function in infants below the age of 6–8 months.

⮑ *Visual reinforcement audiometry:* To evaluate the hearing of infants and young children from the age 6 months–2 years old.

⮑ Play audiometry

⮑ *Impedance testing:* It evaluates the function of the middle ear system, tympanic membrane mobility, eustachian tube function, etc.

- *Tympanometry:* It measures the change in the acoustic impedance of the middle ear in response to changes in air pressure.
- In younger children, a brainstem evoked response audiometry (BERA) is performed.

3. **If the etiology is uncertain on the basis of history and physical examination:**
- Prenatal infections (CMV/rubella infection) serology.
- Temporal bone imaging done by using magnetic resonance imaging (MRI) or computed tomography (CT) if there is progressive conductive hearing loss. If there is trauma to the temporal bone or persistent meningitis, preoperative evaluation earlier to cochlear implantation is to be done.
- Vestibular evoked potential

- Eye examination
- *Hormones:* Thyroid function test
- Renal function test
- *Genetic testing:* For infants and children with bilateral sensorineural hearing loss, the evaluation requires genetic testing of the patients and family members.

In case of nonsyndromic hearing loss selective testing for *GJB2* and *GJB6* variants by Sanger sequencing method.

Patients with bilateral sensorineural hearing loss without syndromic findings, genetic testing using NGS based whole exome sequencing or targeted multi-gene panel sequencing associated with hearing loss genes is preferred.

Approach to child with hearing loss is given in Figure 14.1.

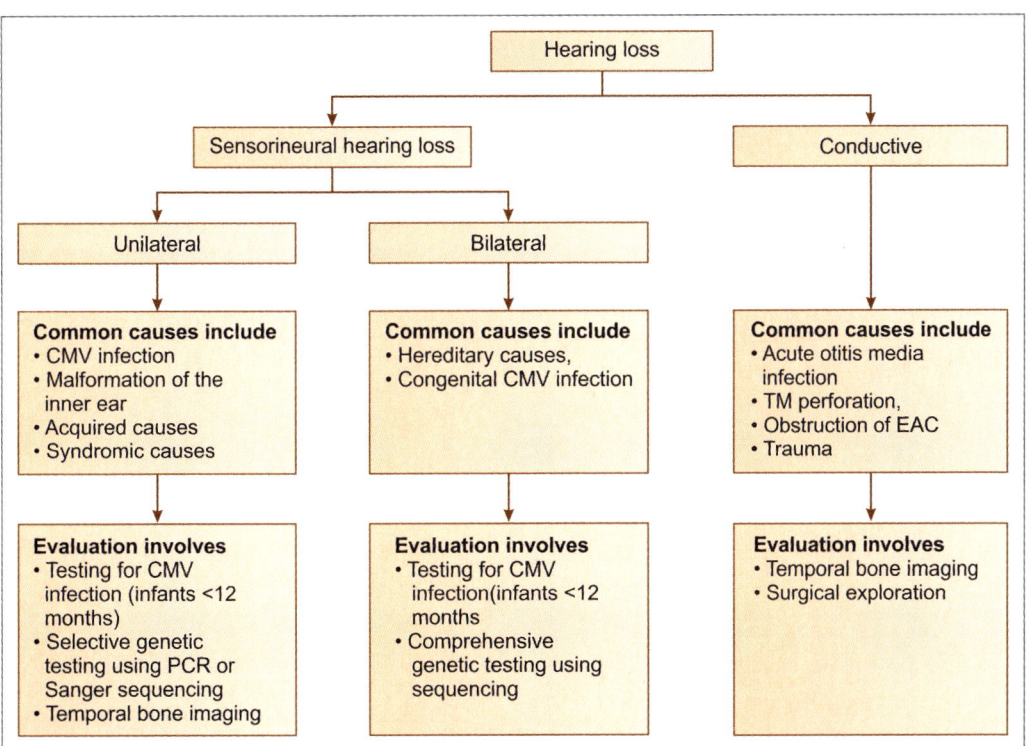

Figure 14.1: : Overview of the approach to identify the etiology of hearing loss. TM—Tympanic membrane; EAC—External auditory canal; CMV—Cytomegalovirus; NGS—Next generation sequencing

Q 6. How will you manage and do genetic counseling and prenatal management in congenital deafness?

Ans.

Management:

- **Multidisciplinary team** should intervene based on the associated symptoms.
- **Aim** of the treatment is to decrease the morbidity due to hearing loss, to reduce psychosocial effects and to improve learning in school.
- **Conductive deafness:** Surgical repair of pinna, auditory canal, tympanic membrane and ossicles.
- **Sensorineural hearing loss:** Hearing aids and cochlear implant.
- **Speech therapy and training** in understanding the sound signals.
- Vitamin A in Usher syndrome.
- **Surgery** for vestibular schwannomas in neurofibromatosis 2.
- **Hair cell regeneration** and **gene therapy** are under trials.

GENETIC COUNSELING AND PRENATAL MANAGEMENT

If genetic testing report reveals mutations, specific genetic counseling should be given followed by proper medical evaluations.

- Hearing risk assessment and routine hearing screening for children between 4–21 years of age, followed up with audiological tests.

- Communication with individuals regarding medical information, addressing the questions and concerns of the family or individual.

- It is preferable to offer genetic counseling about the probability of deafness in offspring to young couples and to inform about the availability of prenatal testing before pregnancy.

- In case of increased risk, prenatal diagnosis (PND) for a pregnancy can be offered. If mutations are identified earlier, PND can be done on chorionic villi samples in families with severe prelingual deafness.

Q 7. Write a note on the need of newborn screening for hereditary hearing loss.

Ans.

Hearing loss is one of the most common congenital disorders. One to three of all newborn babies, are born with some form of hearing loss, of which some may be identified later. Most of the neonatal hearing loss is sensorineural. Among children, about 60% have non-syndromic hearing loss and the remaining cause of neonatal sensorineural hearing loss includes various nongenetic factors.

- Symptoms of hearing loss are subtle because they often represent an erratic extent of environmental observation. Infants with hearing loss are basically identified with speech delay.
- The psychological and practical outcomes of hearing loss on the child or adult show impaired social and economic development, psychological stress, unemployment, etc. These can impact their social life clearly indicating the critical importance of newborn screening.
- Updated evidence from multiple studies show that early identification has improved language development, social behavior, and cognitive skills as compared to children with hearing impairment, undiagnosed or delayed diagnosed. Newborn screening significantly decreases the rate of morbidity due to deafness by early diagnosis and treatment of moderate to severe hearing loss in children. It can also help in genetic counseling of the family regarding the details of disease and recurrence risk.
- Those who do not undergo the initial hearing test due to either early hospital discharge, home delivery or non-availability of the test during newborn period, should be tested by BERA or otoacoustic emissions (OAE) by an audiologist later on. OAE is a simpler test and response is generally absent if the hearing loss is 30 dB or greater.
- Universal newborn hearing screening (UNHS) is being carried out across North America and Europe, so that early detection can be done, and effective interventions

can be provided to avoid speech problems and other psychosocial impacts because of difficulty in hearing.

Ɔ Use of dried blot testing for molecular testing of GJB2 and cytomegalovirus infection and population-based screening for hearing loss in high-risk communities are also in the pipeline.

BIBLIOGRAPHY

1. Emery & Rimoin's Principles & Practice of Medical Genetics, 7th edition.

2. Thompson & Thompson, Genetics in Medicine, 8th Edition.

Neurodevelopmental Disorders

Prajnya Ranganath

Q 1. Describe the etiology, genetic basis, risk factors for neurodevelopmental disorders and intellectual disability in children.

Ans. Neurodevelopmental disorders (NDDs) are a group of conditions with onset in the developmental period, i.e. from birth to 18 years of age are characterized by impairment of personal, social, academic, and/or occupational functioning. It can be associated with intellectual disability (ID) meaning person's intelligence will be below average as compared to a person with normal intelligence. The overall prevalence of ID across the world is 2–3%. ID is classified in to following categories based on intelligence quotient (IQ):

1. **Mild IQ:** 50–70
2. **Moderate IQ:** 35–50
3. **Severe IQ:** 20–35
4. **Profound IQ:** Less than 20

Etiology and genetic basis: Different genetic and non-genetic causes are identified for NDD. A cause is identifiable in only about 50 to 70% of children with intellectual disability (ID) and around 30–40% of children with autism spectrum disorders (ASDs). Down syndrome is the most commonly identified genetic cause of global developmental delay and ID. Fragile X syndrome is the most common monogenic disorder associated with intellectual disability.

1. **Genetic causes (see Appendix (Table 4) for ID syndromes):** The causes that account for around 25–50% of patients with ID, up to 60 to 70% of severe ID and 25–35% of ASDs include:
   a. **Gross chromosomal anomalies:** Down syndrome.
   b. **Chromosomal microdeletions and micro-duplications (submicroscopic chromosomal copy number variations):** Williams syndrome, DiGeorge syndrome.
   c. **Single gene disorders:** Fragile X syndrome, Rett syndrome, metabolic disorders, single gene syndromes which causes brain structural and functioning abnormalities.
   d. **Imprinting abnormalities:** Prader-Willi syndrome, Angelman syndrome.

2. **Nongenetic risk factors:** Risk factors during pregnancy and postnatal period that can lead to NDDs include:
   a. **Teratogenic exposures in the antenatal period especially in the first trimester of pregnancy:** Fetal phenytoin syndrome, fetal alcohol syndrome.
   b. **Intrauterine fetal infections:** Congenital toxoplasmosis, congenital cytomegalovirus infection.
   c. Perinatal and postnatal asphyxia
   d. Prematurity
   e. Postnatal intracranial infections
   f. Peri- and post-natal intracranial trauma and intracranial hemorrhage or infarction

3. **Idiopathic**

Q 2. Describe the clinical features and complications for neurodevelopmental disorders and intellectual disability in children.

Ans. Clinical features and complications: Children with NDDs can have the following:

1. Delayed attainment of developmental milestones, intellectual disability, autism, behavioral anomalies (such as attention-deficit, hyperactivity, aggression, self-injurious behavior, etc.), speech delay and/or learning disability.

2. Additional neurological features, such as seizures, muscle weakness, tone abnormalities (spasticity or hypotonia), abnormal movements, etc. also may be present.

3. Syndromic NDDs have associated dysmorphic features, malformations and other systemic manifestations.

Therefore, detailed dysmorphology evaluation, systemic examination, ophthalmological and hearing evaluation, abdominal ultrasound and cardiac imaging (2D echocardiography) have to be done in every child with an NDD, to look for these additional findings, to identify these diagnoses clinically and also to appropriately manage the associated systemic complications.

Q 3. How will you diagnosis and manage neurodevelopmental disorders and intellectual disability in children?

Ans. Diagnosis and management: Take the detailed medical history of patient, perinatal and postnatal history, family history with pedigree up to third generation, and do detailed general and systemic examination especially neurological examination.

Investigations:

BASELINE LABORATORY

- **Complete hemogram:** To see the type of anemia (Example: Vit B$_{12}$ deficiency).
- **Serum creatinine and electrolytes:** To assess renal function.
- **Thyroid function tests (serum TSH and free T4):** As hypothyroidism is one of the few treatable causes of ID.
- Serum creatine phosphokinase must be checked in unexplained non-syndromic developmental delay (as Duchenne muscular dystrophy) may present in early childhood with developmental delay.
- **Neuroimaging:** If microcephaly/macrocephaly, seizures, focal motor deficits or specific findings on neurological examination, and if other external malformations are noted.
- **Evaluation for inborn errors of metabolism:** In case of failure to thrive, seizures, hepatosplenomegaly, etc.
- EEG, TORCH serology.
- Ultrasonography of abdomen to see any organ malformation
- 2-D-Echo to see any cardiac abnormality.

SPECIFIC INVESTIGATIONS

Genetic evaluation should be done in all cases of intellectual disability without a proven environmental cause. The label of 'cerebral palsy due to adverse perinatal events' should not be given until there is definite history and evidence in neuroimaging. It depends on the clinical diagnosis:

- **Karyotyping:** Chromosomal disorders such as Down syndrome
- **Fluorescence *in situ* hybridization (FISH) and multiplex ligation-dependent probe amplification (MLPA):** Clinically suspected specific chromosomal microdeletion syndromes
- **Targeted gene sequencing:** Clinically suspected monogenic disorders
- **Methylation studies:** Imprinting-related disorders.
- **Testing for trinucleotide repeat expansion:** Fragile X syndrome.
- **Chromosomal microarray:** If the clinical features are not suggestive of any specific diagnosis, this is recommended as the first line genetic investigation.
- **Whole exome sequencing:** Detects gene variants in the exons, i.e. coding portions of all the genes.
- **Whole genome sequencing:** Detects both sequence variants and copy number variants in the entire genome; is gradually emerging as a second line diagnostic modality for undiagnosed cases.

> **Management**
> A multidisciplinary approach for symptomatic and supportive treatment is essential for appropriate management. The goal of the treatment is to lessen the morbidity due to disabilities and to improve the quality of life of the individual suffering from disorder.

> **Supportive care and different modalities of symptomatic treatment**
> (depending upon the age of the patient symptoms)
> • Control of seizures, feeding problems, etc.
> • Physiotherapy for muscle weakness and motor developmental delay
> • Social and play therapy, speech therapy, occupational therapy, behavioral therapy, special education.

> **Specific management of associated systemic complication**
> • Ophthalmological, cardiac, renal, liver, structural brain defects.
> • Hypothyroidism and some metabolic disorders: At present expect for a few causes such as hypothyroidism and certain metabolic causes such as phenylketonuria, for most causes there are no disease-specific treatment available.

Q 4. Describe genetic counseling, prenatal management and recurrence risk in subsequent pregnancy for neurodevelopmental disorders and intellectual disability in children.

Ans.

Genetic counseling: After complete evaluation and identification of the underlying cause, accurate genetic counseling must be provided to the family regarding the

- genetic basis of the condition
- course of the disorder   o prognosis
- anticipated complications
- appropriate management
- follow-up
- risk of recurrence in subsequent offspring
- reproductive options
- details of prenatal procedure

PRENATAL MANAGEMENT FOR SUBSEQUENT PREGNANCIES

- For all pregnancies, periconceptional folic acid (0.5 mg per day) starting from 1 month before conception till 12 weeks of gestation to prevent neural tube defects, and prenatal biochemical screening, fetal ultrasound and prevention of teratogenic exposures especially in the first trimester of pregnancy should be recommended.
- Specific prenatal diagnostic test can be offered for future pregnancies in the family only if the exact etiology is established in the proband or index patient.
- Details of prenatal testing done in the fetal sample (chorionic villus sample or cultured amniocentesis) with diagnosis time limit should be explained.

Recurrence risk: The risk of recurrence depends on the etiology identified:

1. For **chromosomal disorders** (like free trisomy 21) where neither parent is a carrier, the risk of recurrence is low (usually <1%).
   The risk of recurrence can be much higher for Down syndrome caused by chromosome 21 translocation. The risk is 2–5% if the father is a carrier, 10–15% if the mother is a carrier, and 100% if either parent is a carrier.

2. **For monogenic disorders like:**
   - *Autosomal recessive disorders:* The risk of recurrence in each offspring is 25%.
   - *Autosomal dominant disorders:* The risk of recurrence for each offspring is 50% if one of the parents is affected.
   - *X-linked recessive disorders:* The risk of recurrence for each male offspring is 50% if the mother is a carrier.

Recurrence is unlikely for non-genetic causes, but can occur if the causative agent persists antenatally or postnatally in the environment of the next child also.

When no etiology is identified, empiric risks of recurrence can be predicted, but a specific prenatal diagnostic test cannot be offered for the next pregnancy.

BIBLIOGRAPHY

1. Bélanger SA, Caron J. Evaluation of the child with global developmental delay and intellectual disability. Paediatr Child Health. 2018; 23:403–19.

2. Han JY, Jang W, Park J, Kim M, Kim Y, Lee IG. Diagnostic approach with genetic tests for global developmental delay and/or intellectual disability: Single tertiary center experience. AnnHum Genet. 2019; 83:115–23.

Triplet Repeat Disorders

Divya Agarwal

Q 1. What do you mean by triplet repeat mutations (unstable/dynamic mutations)? Enumerate some triplet repeat disorders.

Ans.

- ⊃ Triplet repeat mutations are unique unstable or dynamic mutations, which get expanded (CAGCAGCAG) as they are passed on from one generation to another.
- ⊃ They arise from normal polymorphic repeat sequences, usually of three nucleotides (and

hence, trinucleotide repeats), present in tandem, scattered in some genes.

- ⊃ The repeats may be present in 5′ untranslated (5′UTR) region of the gene or in the exon, intron or the 3′ UTR region of the gene (Figure 16.1).
- ⊃ The number of repeats vary from person to person and tissue to tissue in a person.
- ⊃ During mitosis/meiosis, these repeats may increase (expand) in copy number beyond a threshold.

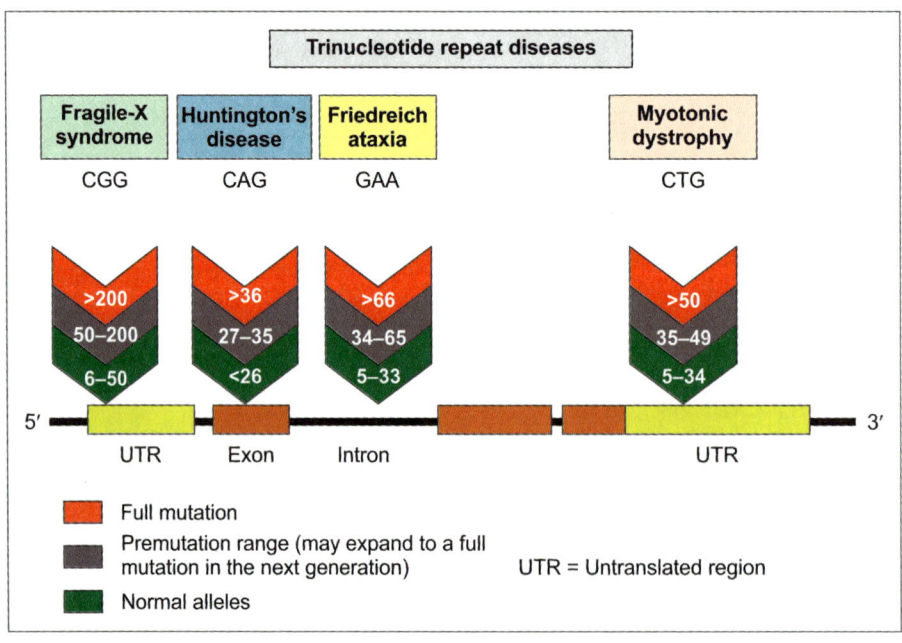

Figure 16.1: Common trinucleotide repeat disorders with the repeat size and location within specific genes

○ The chance of expansion is more in a person with a greater number of repeats.

○ The repeated expansion in a particular gene leads to instability of RNA or protein coded by that gene leading to more than 40 diseases especially neurologic.

Repeat expansion disorders have some unique characteristics.

a. They show marked inter and intrafamilial clinical variability.

b. They exhibit the phenomenon of anticipation.

Most common triplet repeat disorders include (Figure 16.1):

1. Huntington disease
2. Friedreich ataxia
3. Fragile X syndrome
4. Myotonic dystrophy

Q 2. Write the common triplet repeat disorders with their genetic basis and clinical features.

Ans. Common triplet disorders are shown in Table 16.1.

TABLE 16.1: Common triplet disorders

Disease	Trinucleotide repeat (region of gene, gene)	Repeat number		Change in gene function	Inheritance	Parent in whom expansion occurs usually	Clinical description
		Normal	Affected				
Fragile X syndrome	CGG (5'UTR of gene *FMR1*)	6–52	>200	Loss	XR	Mother	ID, ADHD, hyperactivity, autism, normal growth, macrocephaly, long face
Myotonic dystrophy	CGG (3'UTR of gene *DMPK*)	5–34	>50 to even >1000	mRNA stability	AD	Mother	Hypotonia, weakness, development delay, myotonia, cardiac conduction defects, cataract
Friedreich ataxia	GAA (Intron part of gene *FXN*)	5–33	>66	Loss	AR	Alleles from both parents	Tremors, ataxia, neuropathy, cardiomyopathy, diabetes, scoliosis
Huntington's disease	CAG (coding part of gene *HTT*)	<26	>36	Gain	AD	Father	Progressive motor, cognitive, psychiatric decline, chorea, gait problems
Spinocerebell of Ataxia type 1	CAG (coding part of gene A)	6–39	41–81	Gain	AD	Father	Progressive ataxia, dysarthria, dysmetria

Contd.

TABLE 16.1: Common triplet disorders *(Contd.)*

Disease	Trinucleo-tide repeat (region of gene, gene)	Repeat number		Change in gene function	Inheri-tance	Parent in whom expansion occurs usually	Clinical description
		Normal	Affected				
Spinal and bulbar muscular atrophy	CAG (Coding part of gene AR)	11–34	40–62	Gain	XR	Father	Adult onset motor neuron disease, androgen insensitivity
Dentatorubral pallidoluysian atrophy	CAG (coding part of gene ATN1)	7–25	49–88	Gain	AD	Father	Cerebellar atrophy, ataxia, myoclonic, epilepsy, choreoathetosis, dementia

(ID: Intellectual disability, ADHD: Attention deficit hyperactivity disorder, XR: X-linked recessive, AD: Autosomal dominant, AR: Autosomal recessive)
(Spinocerebellar ataxias are a group of triplet repeat disorders with overlapping clinical features and genetic mechanisms. Type 1 has been used as an example here.)

Q 3. Describe the etiology and genetic basis for Friedreich's ataxia.

Ans. Friedreich's ataxia (FRDA) is an autosomal recessive disorder due to mutations in the gene, *FXN*, leading to slowly progressive neurodegeneration and ataxia.

Etiology: *FXN* gene codes for a protein, Frataxin, predominantly located in the mitochondria. Frataxin binds iron and is important for synthesis of respiratory enzymes.

Mutations in the gene lead to deficiency of protein Frataxin which results in secondary deficiency of iron containing enzymes and mislocalization of iron in the mitochondria. This results in impaired mitochondrial respiratory function and increased oxidative stress especially in neurons and nerve cells which have high energy demands.

Genetic basis:

Various types of mutations in FXN gene could be:

I. GAA repeat expansions in intron 1 of the gene constitutes to 96%.

⊃ Normal alleles of the gene have 5–33 GAA repeats in intron 1.
⊃ Mutable normal (premutation) alleles have 34–65 GAA repeats. These alleles are unstable and can get expanded in next generation. Individuals with these alleles are normal themselves but can have offspring with the expanded allele and hence, with the disease.
⊃ Expanded (mutated) disease causing alleles have 66–1300 GAA repeats. The expanded repeats in the intron 1 of gene disrupt the DNA structure and interfere with the transcription of *FXN* gene.

II. Frameshift/nonsense mutations constitute for 4%.

Q 4. Describe the various clinical features and complications of Friedreich's ataxia.

Ans. Friedreich's ataxia is an autosomal recessive triplet repeat disorder, which shows various types of clinical features (Figure 16.2), with onset typically at 10–15 years but may vary between 5 and 25 years of age.

- **Neurologic:**
  - Progressive ataxia, dysarthria due to progressive cerebellar degeneration.
  - Loss of position and vibration sense due to degeneration of dorsal root ganglia and posterior columns.
  - Lower extremity weakness and extensor plantar related to corticospinal tract affection.
  - Mixed axonal peripheral neuropathy results in wasting, pes cavus and loss of deep tendon reflexes in the limbs.
  - Motor and mental reaction progressively slows down.
- Hypertrophic non-obstructive cardio-myopathy.
- **Endocrinologic:** Diabetes mellitus.
- Optic atrophy and/or deafness.
- Scoliosis.

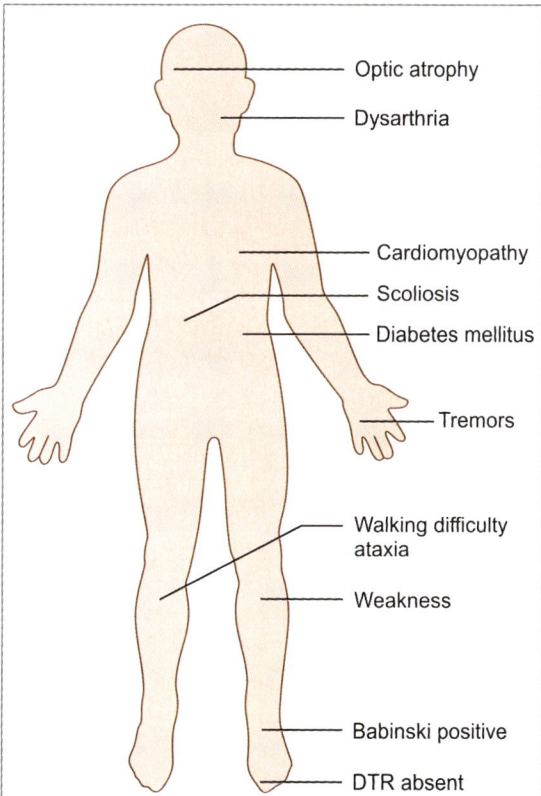

- Optic atrophy
- Dysarthria
- Cardiomyopathy
- Scoliosis
- Diabetes mellitus
- Tremors
- Walking difficulty ataxia
- Weakness
- Babinski positive
- DTR absent

Figure 16.2: Clinical features of Friedreich's ataxia (*Source of human body outline*: DLPNG.com)

- Some individuals show atypical signs and symptoms after the age of 25 years.

Q 5. Describe the recurrence risk, diagnosis and management of Friedreich's ataxia.

Ans.

RECURRENCE RISK AND GENETIC COUNSELING

- Friedreich ataxia is an autosomal recessive disorder.
- Recurrence risk in each sibling is 25%.
- Molecular gene testing for the mutations identified in *FXN* gene can be done in prenatal diagnosis or preimplantation genetic diagnosis and the family members.

DIAGNOSIS

- Take medical history, family history and do complete physical and neurological examination.
- Diagnosis is confirmed by specialized molecular gene test:
  1. Triplet primed PCR test is used to detect triplet repeat mutation GAA repeats in *FXN* gene.
  2. If the triplet repeat mutation is present on one of the alleles, then sequencing of the gene should be done for point mutations (frameshift/ nonsense) on the other allele.
  3. If no mutations are found on either allele of the *FXN* gene, then consider alternative diagnosis and rule out other causes of childhood onset ataxia and neurodegeneration.

MANAGEMENT

- No definitive gene therapy for correction of the gene defect is available.
- **Treatment of manifestations:** A multidisciplinary approach is required as Friedreich's ataxia affects multiple organ systems (Figure 16.3).
- **Iron chelation:** Deferiprone to remove abnormal accumulation of intramitochondrial iron due to deficiency of frataxin.
- **Antioxidant therapy:** Antioxidant therapy like Idebenone, coenzyme Q10 and vitamin E decrease the progression of neurodegeneration and cardiomyopathy due to free radicals' damage.

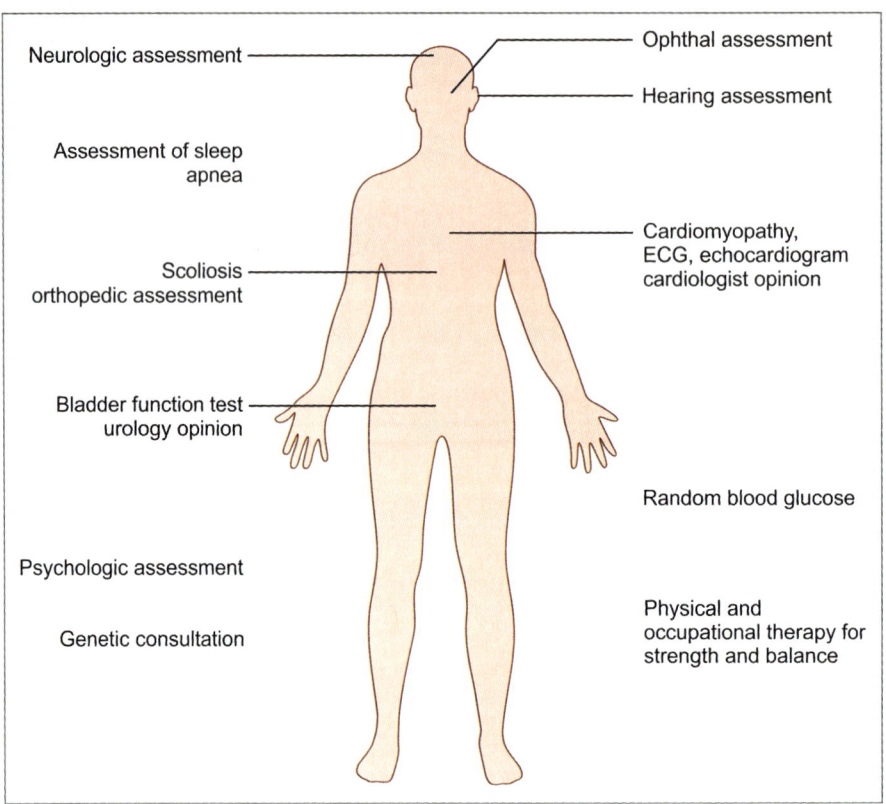

Figure 16.3: : Multidisciplinary management of widespread systemic involvement in Friedreich's ataxia

Q 6. Write a note on genetic basis, clinical features, diagnosis and management of Huntington disease.

Ans. Genetic Basis:
Huntington disease (HD) (Figure 16.1, Table 16.1) is a classic example of a triplet repeat disorder and shows anticipation.

- In HD, CAG triplet repeats in the exon of *HTT* gene, expand as they are passed down in the offspring particularly from the father.
- Normal individuals have CAG repeats less than 26. Individuals who have 27 to 35 CAG repeats in the *HTT* gene do not develop Huntington disease, but they are at a risk of having children who will develop the disorder due to expansion of the CAG trinucleotide repeats into the range associated with HD (36 repeats or more).
- The larger the number of repeats, the earlier the onset of disease and more severe are the symptoms. This phenomenon is called

anticipation. People with 40 to 50 CAG repeats in the *HTT* gene will have the adult onset form of Huntington disease, while people with more than 60 CAG repeats tend to have juvenile onset and severe neurodegeneration.

Clinical features: These could be progressive motor disability, involuntary movements like chorea, dystonia, bradykinesia, mental disturbances including cognitive decline, changes in personality, and/or depression.

DIAGNOSIS

- By clinical findings and similar positive family history.
- Neuroimaging by MRI reveals progressive grey and white matter atrophy.
- The confirmatory genetic test: Triplet repeat PCR test for detection of number of triplet repeats in the *HTT* gene.

MANAGEMENT OF HD

1. Pharmacologic treatment of motor manifestations like chorea, bradykinesia, rigidity or psychiatric disturbances like depression, aggression.

2. Supportive care like good nursing, diet advice, emotional support and psychologic counseling.

   o **Inheritance** of Huntington disease is autosomal dominant.

   o **Recurrence risk:** An affected person has 50% chance of transmitting the pathogenic mutation to his offspring. But during risk assessment, reduced penetrance or possibility of expansion from asymptomatic carrier of intermediate repeat allele (27–35 repeats) should be kept in mind.

   o **Prenatal diagnosis:** If HTT allele has been confirmed in the affected parent, prenatal testing for a pregnancy at increased risk is possible.

   o **Presymptomatic diagnosis** involves testing of asymptomatic adults (>18 years of age) at risk for HD who are children of confirmed patients.

3. **Recent clinical trial:** Various clinical trials at the level of gene, transcript and protein are going onto reduce Huntington levels. IONIS-HTTRx/RG6042 a synthetic allele unspecific oligomer acting at mRNA level, showing reduced level of Huntington in cerebrospinal fluid is under phase III clinical trial.

FRAGILE X SYNDROME

Q 7. Describe the genetic mechanism of fragile X syndrome.

Ans. Fragile X syndrome (FXS), a triplet repeat expansion disorder, is the most frequent (1:5000) cause of inherited intellectual disability in males, also called Martin-Bell syndrome.

Genetic mechanism (Table 16.1):

⮑ Fragile X is an X-linked dominant inherited disease with reduced penetrance caused by dynamic mutations triplet repeat expansion in the promoter region (5′ untranslated region) of the *FMR1*(Fragile X mental retardation) gene located at Xq27.3 (Figure 16.1).

⮑ The gene codes for FMRP protein found in many cell types including the neurons to maintain neurotransmission across synapses.

⮑ In normal individuals, 6–52 CGG repeats are stably transmitted from generation to generation (Table 16.2).

⮑ The CGG DNA segment repeats more than 200 times cause hypermethylation (addition of methyl group) to the nearby promoter region and inactivates or switches off the gene resulting in absent FMRP.

⮑ CGG repeats between ~55 and 200 in premutation carrier mothers can expand, causing clinical variation in their sons. The carriers of premutation do not have hypermethylated promoter region and hence are unaffected.

TABLE 16.2: Types of FMR1 repeat expansion pathogenic variants				
Variant type	*No. of CGG trinucleotide repeats*	*Methylation status of FMR1*	*Clinical status*	
			Male	*Female*
Normal	6-52	Unmethylated	Normal	Normal
Premutation	~55–200	Unmethylated	At risk for FXTAS	At risk of FXPOI & FXTAS
Full mutation	>200	Completely methylated	100% have ID	~50% with mild ID, ~50% normal intellect

FXTAS—Fragile X tremor ataxia syndrome, FXPOI—Fragile X premature ovarian insufficiency, ID—Intellectual disability

Q 8. Describe the clinical features and complications of fragile X syndrome.

Ans. Clinical features (full mutation):

- **Intellectual disability:** FXS primarily affects males causing mild to profound intellectual disability. About one-third of the carrier females are also found to be affected with less severity.
- **Behavioral problems:** FXS includes hyperactivity, short attention span and problems with impulse control (in up to 80% of affected) and autistic features (in 50–70%) during childhood.
- **Growth and development:** Normal or on the higher side. The head circumference is usually >50th centile for age.
- **Dysmorphism:** Fragile X males have long face with prominent mandible, large and mildly dysmorphic ears and macroorchidism which become prominent during puberty (Figure 16.4).

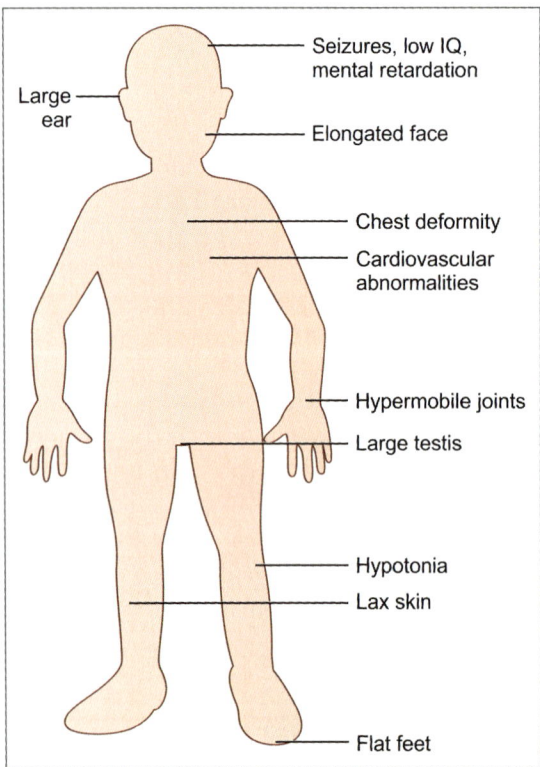

Figure 16.4: Clinical features of fragile X syndrome

Seizures, low IQ, mental retardation

Large ear

Elongated face

Chest deformity

Cardiovascular abnormalities

Hypermobile joints

Large testis

Hypotonia

Lax skin

Flat feet

Fragile X premutation carriers are usually asymptomatic:

- **Fragile X tremor ataxia syndrome (FXTAS):** About 40% of males above 50 years of age carrying a premutation allele have a late onset progressive cerebellar ataxia and tremor syndrome.
- **Premature ovarian failure:** Female premutation carriers are at an increased risk (20%) of hypogonadotropic hypogonadism before the age of 40 years.

Q 9. How will you diagnose a case of fragile X syndrome?

Ans. Diagnosis: History of any male with intellectual disability and/or autistic features unless clear evidence of a different etiology and in any female with unexplained intellectual disability or with a suggestive family history. Diagnosis cannot be established by routine genomic sequencing tests. It can be established by following tests:

- **Cytogenetic diagnosis of fragile X:** One of the first tests developed, but now obsolete with high false positives and negatives. Cells from fragile X patients grown in folic acid deficient cell culture medium induces a chromosomal fragile site at Xq27.3, which could be seen under a microscope.
- **Southern blot analysis:** It is considered as the golden standard for fragile X diagnosis. It can distinguish between mutation and premutation alleles and can also provide information regarding methylation status of the gene. It is a cumbersome and time-consuming technique, hence no longer used widely.
- **PCR:** Polymerase chain reaction.
  a. An easy, rapid test followed by a specific test to know the exact size of repeats and for methylation of the gene.
  b. Cannot be used in heterozygous females reliably.
- **Methylation specific PCR:** It can detect the methylation status of *FMR1* gene promoter region.
- **Triplet primed PCR:** It can diagnose both affected males and carrier females. Reliably

detects the exact repeat allele size and hence differentiates between affected, premutation carriers and normal individual.

Q 10. Describe the treatment, mode of inheritance, recurrence risk, genetic counseling and prenatal management for subsequent pregnancy in fragile X syndrome.

Ans.

1. **Treatment:** No definitive treatment is available.
   - *Supportive treatment:*
     a. Multidisciplinary supportive treatment of manifestations.
     b. Regular development assessment and early intervention programs are suggested.
   - *Therapeutic services:*
     a. Behavioral intervention, speech and language therapy, occupational therapy, and individualized educational support.
     b. Psychopharmacologic treatment of symptoms in behavior problems.
     c. Vision and hearing assessments.
   - *Surveillance and treatment:* For fragile X tremor ataxia syndrome and premature ovarian failure in premutation carriers in the family should be advised.

Recent advances: There are multiple ongoing trials like:
- *Metformin* in children and adults for behavioral defects, intellectual disability and language deficits in fragile X.
- *Negative regulators of mGluR5* signaling in neurons are being tested for improved language outcomes.

Mode of inheritance and genetic counseling:
- Fragile X is inherited in X-linked dominant with reduced penetrance. So, there is a big challenge to counseling process.
- All males with mutation will be affected and all females with heterozygous mutations will be unaffected. But in females with full mutation, severity cannot be predicted.
- Carrier females with heterozygous mutation or premutation range can transmit the disease to their offspring up to 50% in each pregnancy. Expansion depends upon the number of repeats.
- Males with the permutation will not transmit the X-linked mutation to their sons. They will transmit only to daughters who will be carriers.
- **Screening testing:** Premutated female and male carrier should be advised to get screening test after explaining about symptoms, to intervene early.

Prenatal test or preimplantation genetic test can be done to ascertain the fetal affection in high-risk families with molecularly confirmed fragile X patient previously or confirmed carrier status in the mother. But the severity in a full mutated male can be predicted and for a female with full mutation cannot be predicted should be explained to the family.

BIBLIOGRAPHY

1. Emery & Rimoin's Principles & Practice of Medical Genetics, 7th edition.
2. Genetic Clinics, IAMG.
3. Nelson's Textbook of Pediatrics, 21st edition.
4. Thompson & Thompson, Genetics in Medicine, 8th Edition.

Disorders of Sexual Development

Chapter

17

Divya Agarwal

Q 1. Describe normal sex determination, gonadal differentiation and sexual developmental process during embryonic life.

Ans. The normal process of sexual development between 6 and 14 weeks of embryonic life involves the following three stages:

The normal process of male sexual development:
1. Presence of intact Y chromosome with *SRY* gene region leads to male sex XY.
2. WT1 and SF-1 helps in development of primordial germ cells to urogenital ridge.
3. *SRY gene* activates *SOX9 gene* to develop the testes.

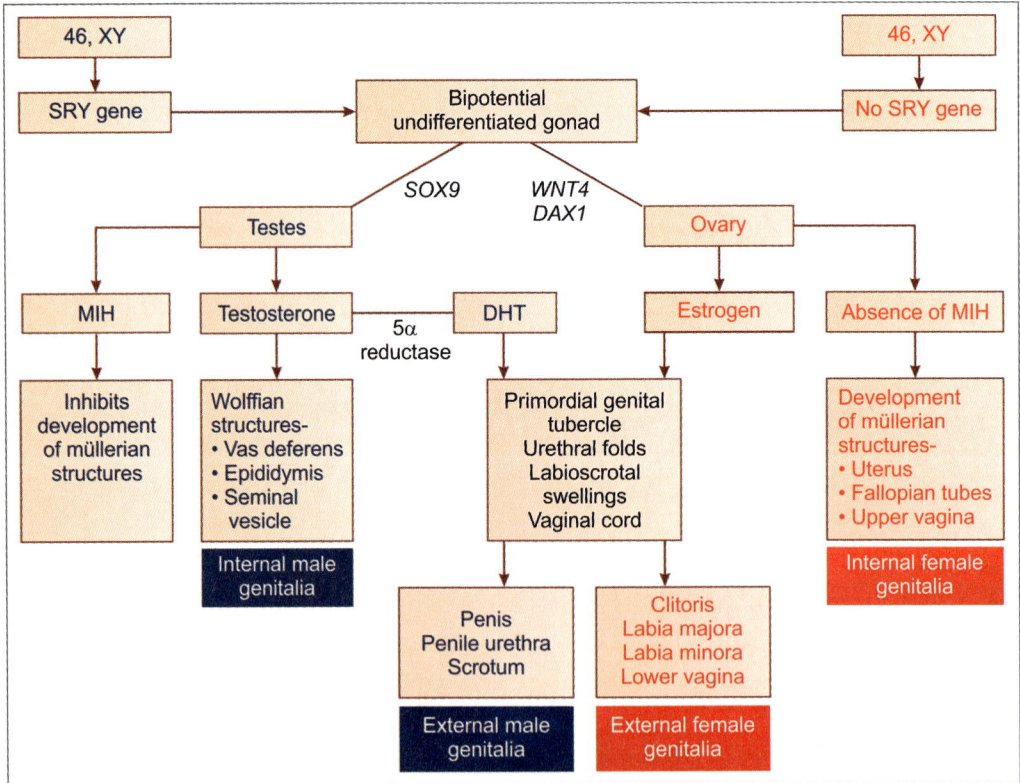

Figure 17.1: The normal process of sexual development (MIH: Mullerian inhibiting hormone, DHT-Dihydrotestosterone)

4. Testosterone secreted by Sertoli cells develop the male internal genitalia or wolffian structures and changes to dihydrotestosterone by 5-alpha reductase enzyme which develops the male external genitalia.
5. MIH secreted by Leydig cells regresses müllerian structures.

The normal process of female sexual development:

1. Ovarian differentiation occurs due to absence of *SRY* gene and suppression of *SOX9* through the activities of *DAX1* and *Wnt4* genes.
2. **Ovary** secretes estrogen which develops normal female external genitalia and müllerian structures.

Q 2. Write the classification of different disorders of sex development (DSD).

Ans. Disorders of the sex development (DSD) are congenital conditions where chromosomal, anatomical or gonadal sex development is abnormal or discordant with each other.

The term **DSD** replaces previous terms like intersex, pseudohermaphroditism, true hermaphroditism and sex reversal. The affected person can present with ambiguous genitalia, delayed puberty, sexual precocity or infertility.

DSD is classified into three major groups:

Sex chromosomal disorders	46, XY DSD	46, XX DSD
○ Chromosomal constitution is abnormal, i.e. other than the normal XX or XY. ○ Results in abnormal gonads, external and internal genitalia development.	○ Chromosomal constitution is XY. ○ Maldevelopment of external/internal genitalia either due to abnormal gonadal formation or testosterone synthesis or action.	○ Chromosomal constitution is XX. ○ Ambiguity occurs due to abnormal gonad or excessive androgens or isolated defects in müllerian structures.

TABLE 17.1: Classification of disorders of sexual development (DSD)

Sex chromosome DSD	46, XY DSD	46, XX DSD
45,X (Turner) **47,XXY** (Klinefelter)	**Testicular hormone synthesis defects** a. LHR—Luteinizing hormone receptor defect b. Enzymatic defects in testosterone synthesis	**Excess androgens** a. *Fetal:* Congenital adrenal hyperplasia (CAH) b. *Maternal:* Androgen intake during pregnancy, virilising disorders/virilising tumors in mother c. *Placental:* Aromatase deficiency
46,XX/46,XY (Ovotesticular) **45,X/46,XY** (MGD:Mixed gonadal dysgenesis)	**Testicular formation defects** a. CGD: Complete gonadal dysgenesis b. PGD: Partial gonadal dysgenesis c. Testicular regression d. Ovotesticular DSD	**Ovarian formation** defects a. CGD b. Ovotesticular c. Testicular
	Testosterone action defects a. CAIS/PAIS: Complete/partial androgen insensitivity b. 5-alpha reductase defect	**MURCS:** Müllerian duct anomaly-renal agenesis-cervical somite anomaly **Cloacal exstrophy**

Q 3. Write the clinical features and causes of 46,XY DSD.

Ans. 46,XY DSD can present with:

a. Complete female external genitalia and primary amenorrhea/delayed puberty/infertility.

b. Apparent male DSD child can present as:
- Perineal hypospadias
- Unilateral undescended testes with hypospadias
- Bilateral undescended testes
- Micropenis < 2.5 cm

c. Apparent female DSD child can present as:
- Clitoromegaly > 1 cm
- Labial fusion
- Inguinal hernia
- Foreshortening vulva with single opening.

d. Associated systemic features in syndromic cases.

The causes of 46,XY DSD:

1. **Syndromic:** Many genetic syndromes like Denys-Drash, WAGR, Frasier, Campomelic, etc.

2. **Non-syndromic or isolated defects:**

   a. *Disorders of testes formation:*
   - Mutations in genes *SF1, SRY, SOX9* or duplication of genes for ovarian development like *DAX1, WNT4*.
   - *Ovotesticular DSD:* Ovary on one side and testes on the other side or ovotesticular tissue on both the sides.
   - *Testicular regression:* Testes was present in embryonic life undergoes vascular disruption with low testosterone. Müllerian structures are usually absent as MIS was secreted by previously functioning testes in embryo.

   b. *Disorders of testosterone biosynthesis:*
   - Due to deficiency of enzymes like 17β-hydroxysteroid dehydrogenase, 17–20 lyase, 3β-hydroxysteroid dehydrogenase, P 450 oxidoreductase, etc.
   - It leads to defective development of internal and external genitalia.

- Gonads would be palpable.
- Testosterone levels will be low and steroid precursors rise in plasma and urine depending upon where the biosynthetic enzymatic defect is.

   c. *Disorders of testosterone action:*
   - *Androgen receptor defect or androgen insensitivity:* Most common 46, XY DSD. Occurs due to mutation of X-linked gene *AR*.
   - *5-alfpha reductase defect:* Autosomal recessive disorder due to mutation in *SRD5A2* gene and testosterone: DHT ratio in blood is >20.

Q 4. How will you diagnose and do management of 46,XY DSD?

Ans. An approach to the diagnosis and evaluation of 46,XY DSD is (Figure 17.2):

- Clinical history and examination.
- **Chromosomal karyotype:** For establishment of genetic sex.
- **USG of abdomen and pelvis** to see the male/female gonads and internal genitalia (wolffian structures/müllerian structures).
- **Genetic test** should be done for the definitive diagnosis and for characterization of mutation for further counseling and prenatal diagnosis.

Management of 46,XY DSD:

It is a multispeciality team approach and includes:

a. **Assignment of gender:** After proper diagnosis, assessing psychosocial issues and counseling of the family.

b. **Surgical intervention:** Assignment of gender includes hypospadias repair, orchidopexy, vaginoplasty, clitoroplasty. Gonadectomy is recommended in almost all 46, XY DSDs as soon as possible because of risk of carcinoma in dysgenetic gonads.

c. **Hormone replacement:** Testosterone in Klinefelter and biosynthetic defects to develop secondary sexual characters.

d. **Genetic counseling:**
- The risk of recurrence depending upon the diagnosis and exact etiology of 46, XY

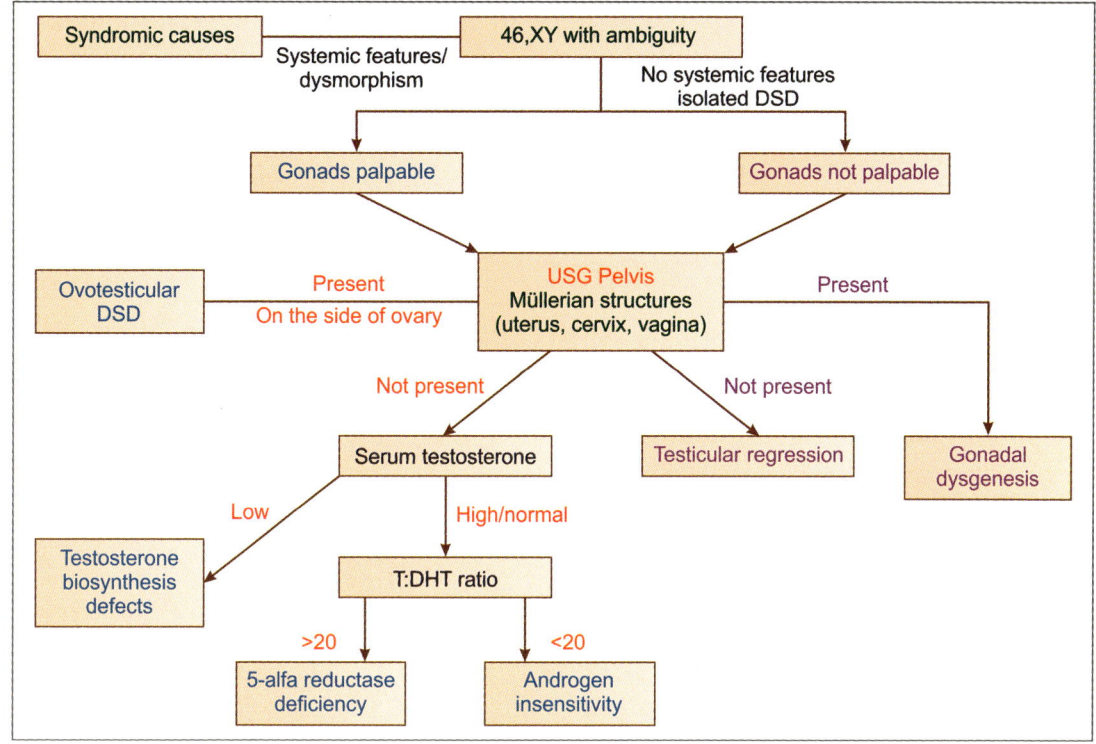

Figure 17.2: Approach to evaluation of child with 46,XY DSD (T—Testosterone, DHT—Dihydrotestosterone)

DSDs should be explained. Most of these disorders are sporadic and have low-risk of recurrence.

○ Prenatal diagnosis for target mutation in the next pregnancy can be provided.

Q 5. Write the causes of 46,XX DSD.

Ans. 46,XX DSD are disorders where complete or partial failure of development of female internal and/or external organs and masculinization of the same occurs.

The patients may present with:

a. Complete sex reversal/male external genitalia.

b. Ambiguous external genitalia.

c. Primary amenorrhea or delayed puberty or infertility.

The causes of 46,XX DSD could be:

1. **Abnormal gonadal development:** It includes conditions with 46,XX but absence of normal ovarian tissue with the presence of palpable gonads. Any gonad which

is palpable below the level of inguinal ligament is testes unless proved otherwise. It could be either:

a. *Testicular DSD* with partial/complete dysgenetic testicular tissue.

○ *46, XX, SRY (+):* SRY gene is present along with XX chromosomal constitution. Individual presents with complete sex reversal/hypospadias/ambiguous genitalia.

○ *46, XX, SRY (−):* In conditions like *SOX 9* gene duplication or *ROSP 1* gene mutations (required for normal ovarian development).

b. *Ovotesticular DSD*

2. **Excess androgens**

○ Various types of congenital adrenal hyperplasia (most common cause of DSD).

○ Aromatase deficiency.

○ P450 oxidoreductase deficiency.

○ Maternal tumors and intake of androgenic medicines.

Other causes: Müllerian structure abnormalities (Table 17.1).

Q 6. How will you diagnose and do management of 46,XX DSD?

Ans. An approach to the diagnosis and evaluation of 46,XX DSD is shown below:

- **Karyotype or FISH (fluorescence *in situ* hybridization):** Establishment of chromosomal sex.
- **Clinical examination** for palpable gonad (testes).
- An **USG** of pelvis to characterize the presence or absence of müllerian structures.

Based on presence or absence of testes and müllerian structures, specific conditions are suspected (Figure 17.3) and specific tests are done:

- **Serum 17-OHP** (17-hydroxy progesterone) for congenital adrenal hyperplasia.
- **Molecular genetic test.**

Q 7. Write about different types of congenital hyperplasia and their clinical features.

Ans. Congenital adrenal hyperplasia (CAH) occurs due to defect in the genes coding for enzymes required for synthesis of steroid hormones (including mineralocorticoids, glucocorticoids, and sex hormones) in the adrenal gland.

Various forms are recognized depending upon the defective enzyme (Figure 17.4). The most common form which accounts for 90% of all defects, is 21 hydroxylase enzyme deficiency due to mutations in CYP21A2 gene. Other less common enzyme deficiencies are 11 β-hydroxylase, 3 β-dehydrogenase and 17 α-hydroxylase.

They present with some overlapping and some unique clinical features, depending upon the deficiency or accumulation of either mineralocorticoids, glucocorticoids or sex hormones, particularly androgens.

The newborns could present with:

a. **Classical form (salt wasting type):** It occurs due to severe defects in the gene *CYP21A2*, leading to absent 21 hydroxylase enzyme, causing decreased glucocorticoid and mineralocorticoid and excessive androgens production (Figure 17.4).

The newborns present with life-threatening salt wasting crisis due to inadequate aldosterone production, hyperpigmentation, poor feeding, weight loss, failure to thrive, vomiting, dehydration, hypotension, hyponatremia, and hyperkalemic metabolic acidosis, prenatal virilization and masculinization of the female genitalia in a 46,XX female fetus.

b. **Classic form (simple virilizing type):** Less severe gene defects lead to some residual activity of 21 hydroxylase enzyme enough for normal production of glucocorticoids and mineralocorticoids and excessive androgen production.

The newborns present with prenatal virilization but no adrenal crisis or salt wasting.

c. **Nonclassic form:** Mild deficiency of the enzyme presents in childhood or later with hyperandrogenism like acnes, hirsutism, baldness and menstrual irregularities in females or precocious puberty in males.

Q 8. How will you manage a newborn baby with congenital hyperplasia?

Ans. Management of a newborn baby with congenital hyperplasia is as follows:

A. ESTABLISHING THE DIAGNOSIS
o Karyotype or FISH to identify gender.
o Ultrasound abdomen to see müllerian structures.
o Serum electrolytes.
o Serum 17-OHP which is the substrate of 21-hydroxylase enzyme (**Figure 17.4**) is marked elevated.
o Elevated 11 deoxycortisol in 11-beta-hydroxylase and decreased deoxycorticosterone in 21-hydroxylase deficiency.
o Adrenal androgens are elevated: Δ^4-androstenedione, 21-deoxycortisol and progesterone.
o Plasma renin activity is markedly elevated.
o Increased pregnanetriol in urine.
o Gene analysis shows deletions or sequence variations in gene *CYP21A2*.

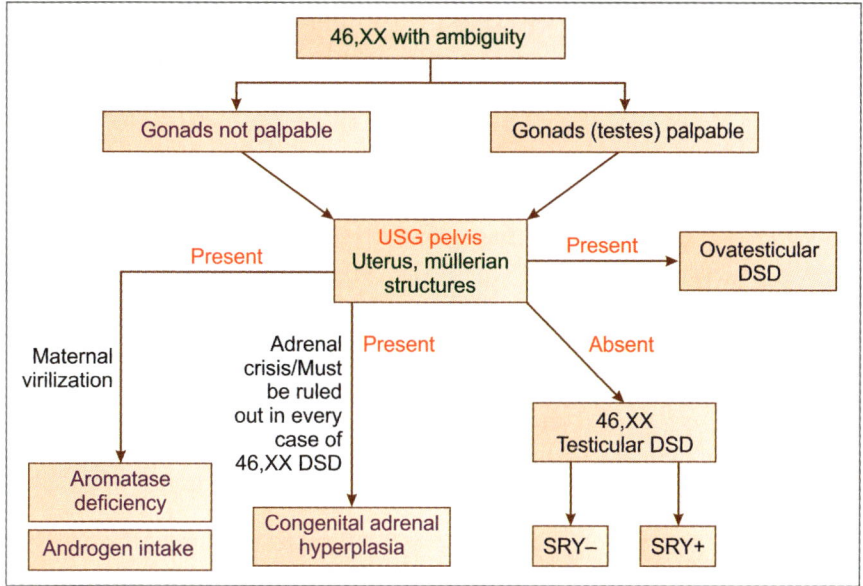

Figure 17.3: Approach to evaluation of a child with 46,XX DSD (USG: Ultrasonography)

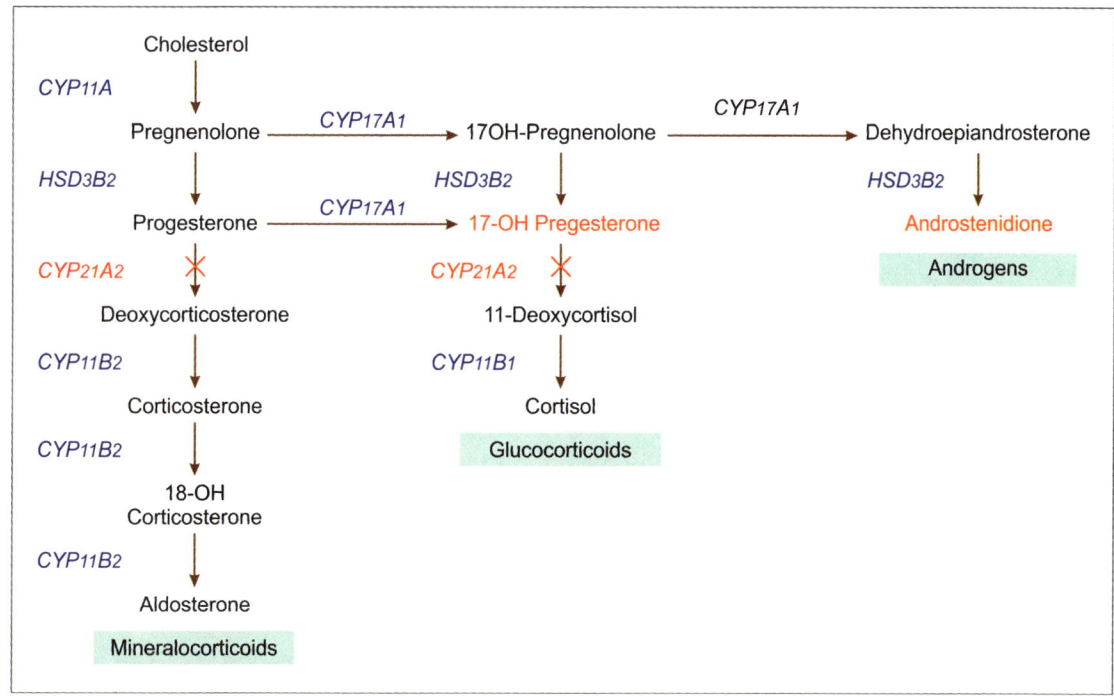

Figure 17.4: Normal steroid hormone synthesis in adrenal gland
(*HSD3B2*: Gene for enzyme 3β-hydroxysteroid dehydrogenase, *CYP11A*: Gene encoding cytochrome group of enzyme 11α-hydroxylase, *CYP21A2*: Gene for 21α-hydroxylase, *CYP17A1*: Gene for 17α-hydroxylase, *CYP11B2*: Gene for 11β-hydroxylase)

B. TREATMENT OF MANIFESTATIONS

o **Glucocorticoid replacement therapy:** It needs to be increased during periods of stress.

o Blood pressure monitoring needs to be done.

o **Salt-wasting form:** It needs mineralocorticoid 9α-fluorohydrocortisone therapy and often sodium chloride.

o **Newborn babies:** By screening newborns, we can intervene early and decrease the disease manifestations.

o **Virilization in female fetuses:** If detected during pregnancy, CAH should be treated by administering dexamethasone to the pregnant female to prevent virilization in the female fetus. In newborns, family counseling and gender assignment should proceed definitive genitoplasty for ambiguous genitalia.

Genetic counseling:

⊃ *CYP21A2* gene-related CAH is an autosomal recessive disorder with a risk of recurrence of 25% in families.

⊃ Prenatal testing or fetal testing in pregnancy has been recommended so that female fetus virilization can be prevented by administering dexamethasone.

Q 9. Write the prenatal management approach for a pregnant mother who is at a risk of CAH.

Ans. Prenatal test:

a. **High-risk pregnancies:** When there is an identified CYP21A2 mutation in a family member, start dexamethasone 20 µg/kg of maternal pre-pregnancy weight 3 times a day at 9 weeks. If at 11–12 weeks, prenatal mutation analysis is positive and fetus is female, dexamethasone is to be continued but for male fetus we can stop it. (In India, fetal sex cannot be determined in accordance with PCPNDT Act.)

b. **Low-risk pregnancies:** When there is no previously affected child in the family, CAH might be suspected, if ambiguous genitalia are seen on routine prenatal ultrasonography. In such cases, if fetal sampling and chromosomal test establishes 46,XX karyotype, then *CYP21A2* gene test should be done.

Q 10. Write a note on androgen insensitivity syndrome.

Ans. Androgen insensitivity syndrome (AIS) is a 46,XY DSD typically characterized by feminization (i.e. under-masculinization) of the external genitalia at birth.

AIS occurs due to defects in androgen action as a result of mutation in gene *AR*, which codes for the androgen receptor.

It can be subdivided into three broad phenotypes:

⊃ **Complete androgen insensitivity syndrome (CAIS)** leads to complete sex reversal with typical female external genitalia. These patients are usually raised as females, affected with primary amenorrhea or infertility.

⊃ **Partial androgen insensitivity syndrome (PAIS)** with ambiguous external genitalia.

⊃ **Mild androgen insensitivity syndrome (MAIS)** with typical male external genitalia, affected with delayed puberty, gynecomastia or infertility.

The clinical suspicion of androgen insensitivity in an individual can be made who presents with:

⊃ Under-masculinization of the external genitalia.

⊃ Impaired spermatogenesis with otherwise normal testes, absent or rudimentary mullerian structures.

⊃ Evidence of normal or increased synthesis of testosterone and its normal conversion to dihydrotestosterone.

The diagnosis of AIS:

⊃ **Hormone analysis:** Normal testosterone, dihydrotestosterone and ratio of testosterone and dihydrotestosterone.

⊃ A hemizygous pathogenic variation *AR* gene identified by molecular genetic testing.

Treatment of AIS:

a. **CAIS:**
- These patients are raised as females.
- Gonadectomy/removal of testes after puberty when feminization is complete.
- Prepuberty: Estrogen supplementation.

b. **PAIS:**
- Gender assignment should be done after complete assessment of genitalia and counseling.
- Surgical intervention might be needed according to the assignment of gender like vaginal dilatation, clitoroplasty, hypospadias repair or orchidopexy.
- Gonadectomy with hormone replacement.

c. **MAIS:**
- Mammoplasty for gynecomastia.
- Androgen/testosterone therapy may be required for virilization.

BIBLIOGRAPHY

1. Emery & Rimoin's Principles & Practice of Medical Genetics, 6th edition.
2. Nelson's Textbook of Pediatrics, 21st edition.
3. Thompson & Thompson, Genetics in Medicine, 8th Edition.

Metabolic Disorders

Chaitanya A Datar, Snehal Patil, Sarah Bailur, Siyaram Didel, Varuna Vyas, Kuldeep Singh

INBORN ERROR OF METABOLISM (IEM)
Chaitanya A Datar

Q 1. Describe the etiopathogenesis, genetic basis of inborn error of metabolism (IEM).

 Ans. Etiology: Inborn errors of metabolism (IEMs) are inherited disorders of the metabolic pathways. These disorders can also be classified into three major groups as per their pathophysiology. (Figure 18.1).

➲ First group includes the disorders characterized by toxic accumulation of various metabolites of protein metabolism (like amino acid disorders, organic acidemia and urea cycle defects), carbohydrate metabolism, copper metabolism and porphyria.

➲ Second group includes disorders that occur due to energy failure of various pathways like carbohydrate utilization and production disorders (glycogen storage disorders, disorders of gluconeogenesis and glycogenolysis pathway), mitochondrial disorders, and fatty acid oxidation disorders due to deficiency of end product or intermediate metabolite.

➲ Third group includes complex molecule metabolism defects like lysosomal storage disorders, congenital disorder of glycosylation, peroxisomal disorders and α_1-antitrypsin deficiency.

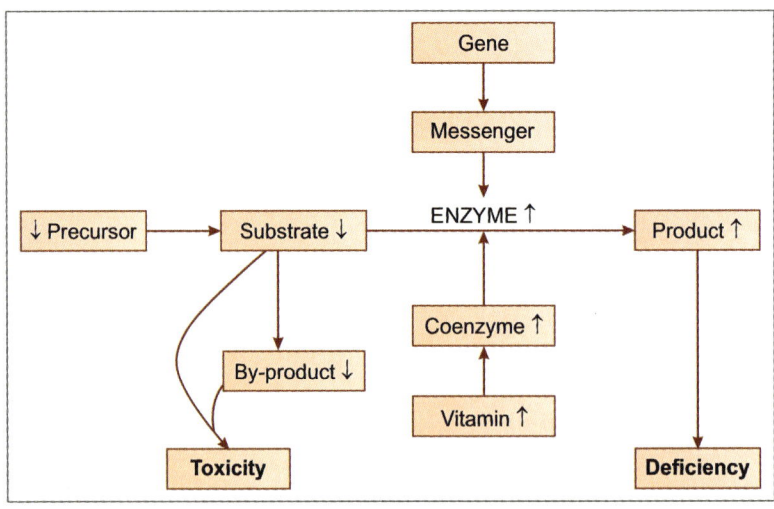

Figure 18.1: Genesis of IEM

Q 2. Describe the clinical features and complications of IEM.

Ans. Clinical features: Accumulation of toxic metabolites and energy deficiency together lead to symptoms that characterize IEMs.

Acute presentation:

- Irritability, peculiar odor (maple syrup in maple syrup urine disease), excessive cry, hypotonia, drowsiness, coma, vomiting, diarrhea, seizures, etc.
- Organomegaly in storage disorders.

Chronic manifestations:

- **Irreversible brain damage** leads to abnormal tone, seizure disorders, developmental delay, psychomotor retardation, neuroregression, hearing loss, dystonias, myopathy (Pompe's disease), etc.
- **Specific organ involvement:** Eye (homocystinuria), liver/kidneys (tyrosinemia), heart (fatty acid oxidation defects), skin and renal (Fabry's disease), teeth, hair (biotinidase deficiency), endocrine system (adrenal in adrenoleucodystrophy), hematological (organic acidemia and Gaucher disease) and immunological system (Gaucher disease), etc.
- **Dysmorphism:** Zellweger, glutaric acidemia, etc.
- **Skeletal abnormality:** Mucopolysaccharidosis.

Q 3. How will you make diagnosis of IEM?

Ans. Diagnosis of IEMs is generally carried out on blood, urine and cerebrospinal fluid (CSF) samples.

Basic investigations	o Complete blood counts (anemia, thrombocytopenia, leucopenia) o GALEK—Glucose (hypoglycemia) o Acid–base gases (acidosis) o Ammonia o Lactate o Electrolytes o Ketones o Urine for reducing substances o Liver and renal function test o Lactate and pyruvate ratio.
Advanced investigations	o Tandem mass spectrometry (blood)—amino acids, organic acids and fatty acid oxidation disorders o Gas chromatography/mass spectrometry (urine)—organic acid disorders o VLCFA analysis—peroxisomal disorders, plasma carnitine and acyl-carnitine o Creatine phosphokinase in myopathies o Lipid profile
Enzyme studies (fibroblast or leucocytes)	o Lysosomal storage disorders: MPS, etc.
Genetic studies	o Single gene analysis or panel-based testing to determine the exact genetic cause.

VLCFA—Very long chain fatty acid, MPS—Mucopolysaccharides

Other auxiliary investigations:

- **Abdominal scan** to see organomegaly
- Magnetic resonance imaging of brain, 2D Echo, electroencephalography, bone density scan, ophthalmology and hearing assessment.

Q 4. How will you do management of IEM?

Ans. Management of IEMs: Despite treatment, a normal outcome may not always be guaranteed in case of some severe IEMs such as—phenylketonuria (PKU), tyrosinemia, propionic acidemia, maple syrup urine disease (MSUD), etc. but by early newborn screening and by intervening early, the morbidity and mortality can be decreased. The basic principles to manage IEMs are:

a. Reduce the substrate/toxic substances
b. Provide the product/energy.

Acute management:

- **Stop all exogenous feeds** causing accumulation of the offending substrate, e.g. proteins have to be stopped for urea cycle disorders or organic acid disorders; milk/milk products are eliminated in galactosemia.

- **To reduce the already generated toxic products:**
  i. Administer glucose or normal saline.
  ii. Correct acid–base imbalance: Bicarbonate infusion.
  iii. Give medications which hasten removal of the toxic chemical, e.g. sodium benzoate in urea cycle defect.
  iv. Provide the deficient product, e.g. biotin in biotinidase deficiency
  v. Provide the coenzymes for the defective enzymatic pathways, e.g. thiamine in MSUD, pyridoxine in homocystinuria.
  vi. Improve energy generation to reduce catabolism—by giving glucose, intralipids, etc.
  vii. Hemodialysis: in urea cycle defect.

Chronic management (Figure 18.2):

- The principles of long-term management include prevention of major acute episodes, provide adequate nutrition to ensure proper growth and development.
- Oral supplementation to reduce toxic products (penicillamine in Wilson disease), to provide the product/energy, enhancing the enzyme by providing cofactors, Chaperone therapy (Miglustat for Gaucher disease), etc. has to be continued.
- **Restriction of diet:** In phenylketonuria.
- Special medical foods (diet) customized as per the metabolic defect has to be provided in many IEMs.
- **Enzyme replacement:** Gaucher disease.
- **Liver and renal transplantation:** Methyl malonic aciduria.
- **Bone marrow transplantation:** Krabbe disease.
- **Gene therapy:** Adenosine deaminase deficiency.

Q 5. What is the inheritance pattern and recurrence risk of IEM?

Ans. Inborn errors of metabolism (IEMs) are inherited disorders of the metabolic pathways. IEMs follow variable patterns of inheritance as follows.

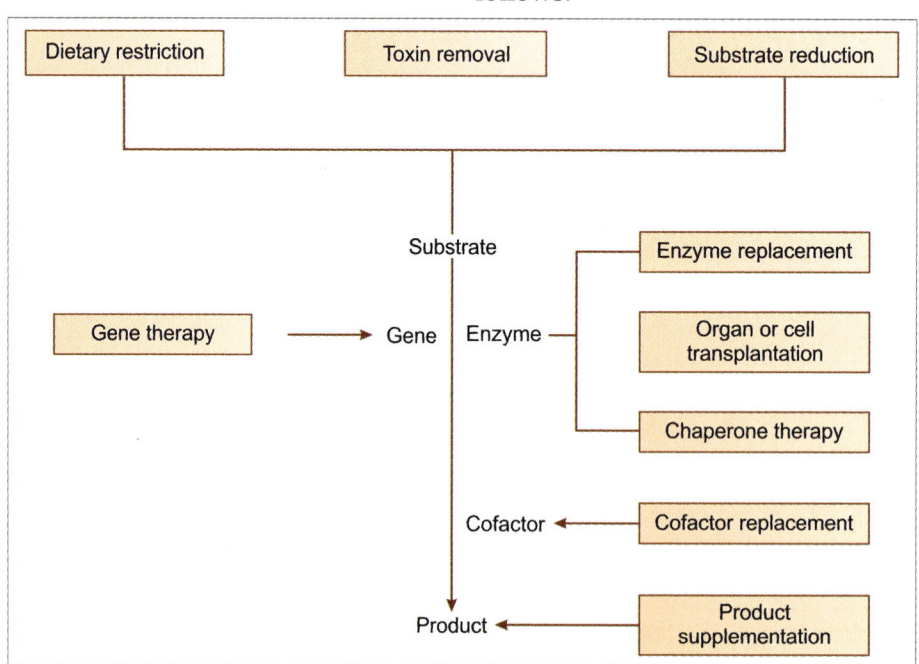

Figure 18.2: Management approach of inborn error of metabolism

Inheritance patterns	Examples	Risk of recurrence in subsequent siblings
○ Autosomal recessive	○ Majority IEMs ○ Phenylketonuria ○ Galactosemia ○ Mucopolysaccharidosis (MPS) ○ Gaucher disease	○ 25%
○ X-linked	○ OTC deficiency ○ Hunter syndrome	○ Male sibs—50% affected, 50% normal ○ Female sibs—50% carriers, 50% normal
○ Autosomal dominant	○ Familial hypercholesterolemia	○ If the parent of the child is affected, risk of recurrence will be 50%. ○ Risk is only ~1–3% in case the mutation is *de novo*.
○ Mitochondrial	○ Leigh syndrome ○ MELAS ○ Mitochondrial complex deficiencies	○ ~90% disorders occur due to mutations in nuclear genes (autosomal recessive inheritance) ○ Risk of recurrence in sibs is 25% ○ 10% mitochondrial disorders follow matrilineal inheritance pattern. ○ Risk and degree of affection depends on status in mother (homoplasmy/heteroplasmy) and quantity of mutated mitochondria received per cell/organ

Hence, the exact disorder must be identified in the index child to be able to offer prenatal counseling for the future pregnancies of the parents.

Q 6. How will you do genetic counseling for inherited metabolic disorders? Write the prenatal management for a couple who is planning for subsequent pregnancy with the previous child affected with IEM.

Ans. **Genetic counseling:** Following all the general principles of counseling and respecting the psychosocial aspects of family, discuss the following with families during counseling:
a. Need of genetic testing in the proband and parents, details of the disease like etiology, natural history, prognosis, management options, inheritance pattern, recurrence risk in future generation and prenatal testing.
b. Before prenatal testing family should be informed regarding:
    ⊃ Prenatal procedure and prenatal test details.
    ⊃ Likely benefits of early diagnosis
    ⊃ Appropriate support and preparedness if the result returns positive.

Prenatal diagnosis for IEMs is offered for prevention of recurrence of the condition in the family as IEMs can lead to significant mortality or morbidity including major neurological impairments in the child. However, it may also be considered for some of the treatable IEMs to be able to offer better quality of life for the child and family. Prenatal biochemical diagnosis is not preferred as it is not reliable in amniotic fluid.

Gene-based prenatal testing can be offered for the couple's pregnancy either on the chorionic villus sample collected at 11–12 weeks or amniotic fluid sample collected at 16 weeks of gestation after identifying the mutation in the proband and after doing parental carrier testing for the same mutation. If the result returns positive, decision regarding continuation of pregnancy is left on the parents.

AMINOACIDOPATHIES
SNEHAL PATIL

Q 7. Write the incidence and classification of aminoacidopathies.

Ans. Aminoacidopathies are inherited metabolic disorders that occur either due to decreased or increased levels of amino acids in the blood or urine due to various enzyme deficiencies. Signs and symptoms can vary from asymptomatic to fatal disease due to accumulation of toxic metabolite affecting various major systems of the body especially brain. Severity of the disease depends upon:

- Type of deficient enzyme
- Amount of protein in the diet and its metabolism.

These disorders generally manifest acutely (vomiting, diarrhea, seizures, acidosis, hyperammonia, encephalopathy) during early neonatal period but can also present as a chronic disorder during later period of life. These can be detected by tandem mass spectrometry and plasma high-performance liquid chromatography. The cumulative incidence of these disorders is approximately 1:1000 worldwide. Aminoacidopathies can be classified based on the following groups:

1. **Abnormal catabolism of amino acids:** Maple syrup urine disease, phenylketonuria.

2. **Anabolic defects:** Proline and serine synthesis defects.

3. **Defective transport of amino acids:** Cystinuria, Hartnup disease.

Q 8. Write the etiology, inheritance pattern, clinical features and complications of phenylketonuria.

Ans.

Disorder	Phenylketonuria (PKU) i. Classic PKU (>98%) ii. Mild/moderate PKU
Etiology enzyme & candidate gene	Phenylalanine hydroxylase (PAH) enzyme deficiency due to mutation in PAH gene
Inheritance pattern	Autosomal recessive
Enzyme deficiency & mechanism	PAH deficiency causes increased phenylalanine (Phe) in blood, tissues, and urine. And there is increased excretion of its metabolites phenylacetate and phenyl pyruvic acid (Figure 18.3)
Specific clinical features	All are normal at birth. If untreated, patient can present as : o Moderate to profound intellectual disability – IQ <= 50 o Musty or mousy odor due to phenylacetic acid o Eczema (20–40%) o Depigmented/light colored hair, skin and iris due to decreased melanin synthesis o Microcephaly, prominent maxillae o Neurologic impairment, seizures 25%, tremors 30%, spasticity 5%, athetosis, hyperreflexia o Behavioral problems
Complications	o Intellectual disability persists. o **Maternal PKU:** If pregnant women with PKU are not on Phe restricted diet, the offspring may be born with intellectual disability, microcephaly, growth retardation, congenital malformations, and congenital heart disease.

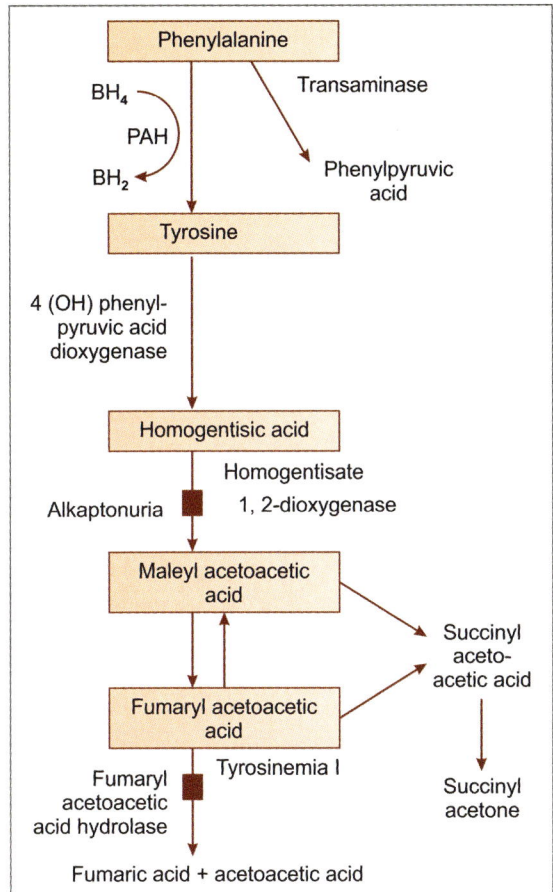

Figure 18.3: Phenylalanine and tyrosine metabolism pathway (PAH: Phenylalanine hydroxylase)

Q 9. How will you diagnose phenylketonuria?
Ans.

DIAGNOSTIC LABORATORY INVESTIGATIONS AND LABORATORY FINDINGS OF PHENYLKETONURIA		
Disorder	*Diagnostic investigations*	*Laboratory findings*
Phenylketonuria: 1. Classic PKU (>98%) 2. Mild/moderate PKU	○ MS/MS in all newborns (between day 1–5) ○ Plasma amino acid levels (PAA) ○ BH4 (tetrahydro-biopterine) cofactor analysis/challenge	○ Hyperphenylalaninemia (plasma phenylalaninemia levels persistently higher than 120 micromoles/L). ○ Classic PKU has Phe levels of >1200 micromoles/lit ○ Altered plasma phenylalaninemia: Tyrosine ratio in untreated patient (normal >1, ratio >3) considered significant. ○ Normal urine/dried blood spot pterines (neopterin, biopterin) studies ○ Normal dihydropterin reductase measurement in red blood cells from dried blood spot. ○ Mutational testing of PAH gene.

Q 10. How will you treat phenylketonuria?
Ans.

Disorder	Specific management	Recent advances
Phenylketonuria: 1. Classic PKU (> 98%) 2. Mild/moderate PKU	**Principles of management** *Dietary treatment:* o *Principle:* To reduce plasma phenylalanine concentration sufficiently to prevent neuropathological effects and also fulfil age dependent requirement for protein synthesis. o Low phenylalanine diet. o Diet treatment started in patients with phenylalanine levels >10 mg/dl. o Maintain blood Phe levels between 2–6 mg/dl throughout the life. o Tyrosine and tryptophan levels also need to be maintained. o Maintain other nutrients and micro-nutrients at RDA levels, including calcium, vitamin D, iron, folic acid and B vitamins. o Glycomacropeptide is special formula with low Phe and optimal protein. o Milder versions of PKU do not need dietary restriction though regular monitoring of Phe levels and neuropsychiatric symptoms need to be monitored. o Also, women of childbearing age with mild to moderate PKU need to be counseled about teratogenic effects of high maternal phenylalanine levels. o To prevent this, women with PKU should be on strict Phe restricted diet before and during pregnancy (Phe level should be in between 2–6 mg/dl)	**Large neutral amino acids (LNAAs):** o LNAAs (Lanaflex, PreKUnil) in the diet, adjunct therapy for those who have a poorly controlled diet decreases the brain Phe levels. **Tetrahydrobiopterin (BH4; sapropterin dihydrochloride, Kuvan®):** o Kuvan was the first drug for PKU approved in 2007 by FDA as standard therapy for children with phenylalanine hydroxylase deficiency that showed a decrease of Phe levels after BH4 loading **Pegvaliase is an enzyme** replacement therapy approved for adults with PKU in 2018 by FDA. o Studies are also going on for gene therapy for PKU

Q 11. Write the etiology, inheritance pattern, clinical features and complications of tyrosinemia.
Ans.

Disorder	Etiology enzyme & candidate gene	Inheritance pattern	Enzyme deficiency & mechanism	Specific clinical features	Complications
Tyrosinemia Type I (hepatorenal tyrosinemia)	FAH deficiency; *FAH* Gene: Expressed in liver and kidney	Autosomal recessive (AR)	Deficiency of FAH leads to accumulation of fumarylacetoacetate and succinylacetone which cause liver, kidney, and nerve damage (Figure 18.3)	Earlier the presentation, poorer the prognosis. 1. **Liver:** ○ Acute liver failure, cirrhosis, or hepatocellular carcinoma ○ **Severe presentation in infants:** Septicemia, vomiting, diarrhea, bleeding diathesis, direct jaundice, hepato-megaly, and other signs of acute hepatic failure ○ Chronic liver disease 2. **Renal:** Variable from mild tubular dysfunction to renal failure: ♦ Fanconi-like syndrome ♦ Proximal tubular disease ♦ Hypophosphatemic rickets 3. **CNS:** Acute neurologic crises in 2 phases: ♦ *Active phase* lasting 1–7 days painful pares-thesias and autonomic signs ♦ *Recovery phase* of many days to months	Seizures, self-mutilation, respiratory paralysis, hypertrophic cardiomyopathy.
Tyrosinemia Type II (oculo-cutaneous tyrosinemia) (Richner-Hanhart syndrome)	Hepatic cytosolic tyrosine aminotrans-ferase deficiency; *TAT* gene	AR	Deficiency of the enzyme causes accumulation of tyrosine in blood and tissues including *corneal epithelial cells* and *skin* (it affects the tonofilament structure and number and stability of microtubules.)	Usual presentation at infancy but can manifest at any age. Combination of eye, skin and neurologic manifestations are seen. 1. **Ocular lesions (75%):** • First months of life with photophobia, lacrimation, and intense burning pain • Conjunctivitis • Bilateral corneal ulcerations on slit lamp examination (herpetiform lesions) ♦ Neovascularization	Corneal scar-ring, visual impairment, glaucoma.

Contd.

Disorder	Etiology enzyme & candidate gene	Inheritance pattern	Enzyme deficiency & mechanism	Specific clinical features	Complications
				2. **Skin lesions (80%):** Specifically affect pressure areas. ♦ *Most common site:* Palms and soles ♦ Blisters or erosions with crusts ♦ Progress to painful, nonpruritic hyperkeratotic plaques	
				3. **CNS:** ♦ Normal to variable developmental retardation ♦ Microcephaly, seizures, self-mutilation, and behavioral abnormalities	
Tyrosinemia Type III	Deficiency of HPD; HPD gene	AR	Enzyme block causes hypertyrosinemia and increased excretion of HPD and its derivatives.	○ Developmental delay ○ Seizures ○ Intermittent ataxia ○ Self-mutilation ○ No hepatic or renal manifestations	Intellectual impairment in 75% cases
Hawkinsi- nuria	Thought to be allelic to tyrosi- nemia type III. *HPD* gene.	Autosomal dominant (AD)	Abnormal HPD leads to formation of abnormal metabolite 'hawkinsin' which causes secondary glutathione deficiency.	Manifests in first few months of life after weaning from breastfeeding and introduction of high protein diet. ○ Severe metabolic acidosis ○ Ketosis ○ Failure to thrive ○ Mild hepatomegaly ○ Renal tubular acidosis ○ Anemia ○ Unusual odor	-
Transient tyrosinemia of the newborn	Delayed fetal matu- ration of HPD	-	Hypertyrosinemia resolves spontaneously by 4–6 weeks	Generally asymptomatic but may present with lethargy, poor feeding and decreased motor activity	

FAH: Fumarylacetoacetate hydrolase; HPD: 4-hydroxyphenylpyruvate dioxygenase

Q 12. How will you diagnose tyrosinemia?
Ans.

Disorder	Diagnostic investigations	
Tyrosinemia type I (hepatorenal tyrosinemia)	o Severely deranged synthetic liver function o Grossly elevated alpha fetoprotein levels o MS/MS o Increased succinylacetone in urine and dried blood spot.	o Elevated plasma levels of tyrosine, phenylalanine and methionine, reduced erythrocyte 5-ALA dehydratase activity and increased urinary 5-ALA excretion. o Decreases FAH enzyme activity o Homozygous or compound heterozygous mutation in *FAH* gene.
Tyrosinemia type II (Oculocutaneous tyrosinemia) (Richner-Hanhart syndrome)	o MS/MS o Plasma tyrosine concentrations are usually above 1200 µmol/l o Urinary excretion of the phenolic acids 4-hydroxyphenylpyruvate,4-hydroxyphenyl lactate and 4-hydroxyphenylacetate is highly elevated.	o N-acetyltyrosine and 4-tyramine are also increased. o Homozygous or compound heterozygous mutation in *TAT* gene
Tyrosinemia type III	o Elevated plasma tyrosine levels of 300–1300 µmol/l have been found at diagnosis. o Elevated urinary excretion of 4-hydroxyphenylpyruvate,4- hydroxyphenyl lactate and 4-hydroxyphenylacetate associated with increase in plasma tyrosine	Diagnosis can be confirmed by 1. Enzyme assay in liver. 2. Kidney biopsy. 3. Mutation analysis.
Hawkinsinuria	Identification of urinary hawkinsin or 4-hydroxycyclohexylacetate by GCMS is diagnostic	
Transient tyrosinemia of the newborn	MS/MS (newborn screening)	o Elevated plasma tyrosine levels to >2000 micromol/L which decreases by 4–6 weeks of age

Q 13. How will you treat tyrosinemia?
Ans.

Disorder	Specific Management
Tyrosinemia type I (hepatorenal tyrosinemia)	**Nitisinone (NTBC):** o Treatment of choice o It inhibits 4-hydroxyphenylpyruvate dioxygenase and reduces the flux of tyrosine metabolites to FAH, decreasing the production of fumarylacetoacetate and succinylacetone.

Contd.

Disorder	Specific Management
	o Dose is titrated to lowest effective dose (start at 1 mg/kg/day) to plasma levels of 20–40 micromol/L to suppress production of succinylacetone and maintain plasma tyrosine levels to <400 micromol/L. o This prevents acute neurologic and hepatic crises. o Liver function test monitoring. o Patients not responding to nitisinone require liver transplant. o Nitisinone increases plasma tyrosine levels hence low tyrosine low phenylalanine diet is recommended.
Tyrosinemia Type II (oculocutaneous tyrosinemia) (Richner-Hanhart syndrome)	o Diet low in tyrosine and phenylalanine aiming to achieve plasma tyrosine levels <500 µmol/L improves skin and eye manifestations and reduces intellectual disability.
Tyrosinemia Type III	o Dietary restriction of tyrosine and phenylalanine o Trial of vitamin C.
Hawkinsinuria	o Low-protein diet during infancy. o Breastfeeding is encouraged. o Avoid protein over-restriction as it can lead to failure to thrive. o Successful long-term use of N-acetyl-L-cysteine to treat secondary glutathione deficiency has been reported. o A trial with vitamin C.
Transient tyrosinemia of the newborn	o Hypertyrosinemia resolves by first 2 months of life. o Reducing dietary protein to below 2 g/kg/24 hr and with vitamin C supplementation.

Q 14. Write the etiology, inheritance pattern, clinical features and complications of alkaptonuria.

Ans.

Disorder	Alkaptonuria
Etiology enzyme & candidate gene	Deficiency of homogentisate dioxygenase; HGD gene
Inheritance pattern	Autosomal recessive
Enzyme deficiency & mechanism	Defect of enzyme homogentisate dioxygenase (mainly in liver and kidney) leads to accumulation of homogentisate and its oxidized derivative benzoquinone acetic acid precursor to the dark pigment, which is deposited in various tissues.
Specific clinical features	**Adults:** o **Ochronosis:** Dark spots on sclera and ear cartilage o **Arthritis:** Involves spine and large joints (shoulders, hips, and knees) • More severe and acute in males • Radiologic findings are typical of osteoarthritis characteristic narrowing of the joint spaces and calcification of the intervertebral disks. • Cardiac valvular defects, myocardial infarction. Only sign in children is blackening of the urine on standing, caused by oxidation and polymerization of homogentisic acid.

Q 15. How will you diagnose and treat alkaptonuria?
Ans.

Disorder	Laboratory findings
Alkapto-nuria	○ Gross elevated urinary homogentisic acid levels ○ Normal tyrosine levels ○ Mutation analysis.

Disorder	Specific management
Alkapto-nuria	○ Treatment of the arthritis is symptomatic. ○ Mild protein restriction is recommended in childhood to limit pigment deposition ○ Dietary restrictions and nitisinone are then introduced in adulthood. ○ Nitisinone efficiently reduces homogentisic acid production in alkaptonuria. ○ Vitamin C: 1g/day decreases benzoquinone acetic acid excretion.

Q 16. Write the metabolic pathway, etiology, inheritance pattern, clinical features and complications of homocystinuria.

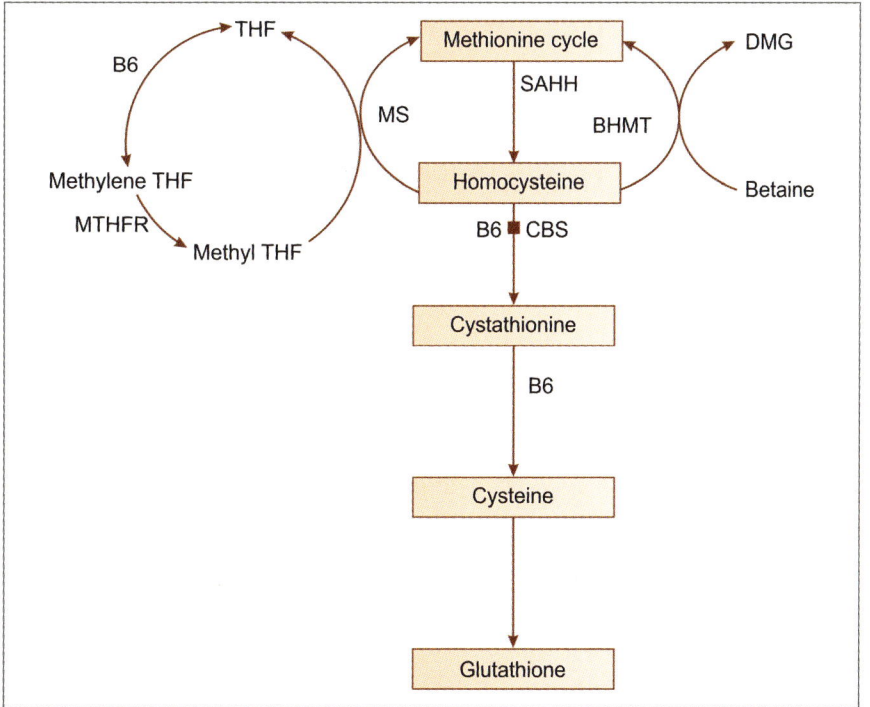

Fig. 18.4: Metabolic pathway of homocystinuria

SAHH—S-Adenosylhomocysteine hydrolase; MS—Methionine synthetase DMG: Dimethylglycine; MTHFR—Methyl-tetrahydrofolate reductase; CBS—Cystathionine-β-synthetase; BHMT—Betaine homocysteine S-methyltransferase

Disorder	Etiology enzyme & candidate gene	Inheritance pattern	Enzyme deficiency and mechanism	Specific clinical features	Complications
Homocysti-nuria: Classic homocystinuria	Cystathionine β-synthase (CBS) deficiency; *CBS* gene	AR	CBS enzyme mainly expressed in liver, pancreas, kidneys and brain. Deficiency leads to accumulation of homocysteine, causes increased thrombo-embolism and vascular disease. Also leads to connective tissue abnormalities.	**Two phenotypic variants are known:** ○ B_6 responsive homocystinuria (mild) ○ B_6 non-responsive homocystinuria (severe) **Eye:** ○ Progressive lenticular myopia ○ Ectopialentis ○ Iridodonesis ○ Astigmatism, glaucoma, staphyloma, cataracts, retinal detachment, and optic atrophy **Nervous system:** ○ Developmental delay. ○ Intellectual disability with IQ (10–135), better in B_6 responsive homocystinuria ○ Behavioral and psychiatric problems (50%). ○ Seizures 20% **Marfanoid habitus** ○ **Thromboembolism:** Involving both large and small vessels especially in brain, occur at any age.	○ Paralysis ○ Cor pulmonale ○ Severe hypertension (from renal infarcts) ○ Spontaneous pneumothorax ○ Acute pancreatitis

Contd.

Disorder	Etiology enzyme & candidate gene	Inheritance pattern	Enzyme deficiency and mechanism	Specific clinical features	Complications
Homocystinuria due to defects in methyl-cobalamin formation	Cbl E (methionine synthase reductase) (*MTRR* gene)	AR	o Methylcobalamin is a cofactor for methionine synthase which causes remethylation of homocysteine to methionine. o Defects in cobalamin metabolism interfere with methylcobalamin formation which leads to homocystinemia and homocystinuria (Figure 18.4)	**In 1st few months of life:** o Vomiting o Poor feeding o Failure to thrive o Lethargy o Hypotonia o Seizures o Developmental delay **Late onset forms have:** o Neurocognitive defects o Psychosis o Peripheral neuropathy.	**Rarer serious presentations:** o Renal artery thrombosis o Hemolytic uremic syndrome o Pulmonary hypertension o Optic nerve atrophy.
	Cbl G (methionine synthase reductase) (*MTRR* gene)	AR			
	Cbl D variant 1	AR			
Homocystinuria: Methylmalonic acidemia due to defects in methyl-cobalamin formation	Cbl C (most common)	AR	Methylmalonic acidemia in addition to homocystinuria because the formation of both adenosylcobalamin and methylcobalamin is impaired.	*Cbl C* may also have: o **Early onset symptoms:** Microcephaly, hydrocephalus, cortical atrophy. o **Late onset symptoms:** ♦ Acute neurologic decompensation, extrapyramidal symptoms ♦ Pigmentary retinopathy, visual problem.	—
	Cbl D	AR			
	Cbl F	AR			
	Cbl J	AR			
	Cbl X defects	X-linked			
Homocystinuria due to MTHFR deficiency	Methylene tetrahydrofolate reductase (*MTHFR* gene) deficiency (severe)	AR	o Methyl-tetrahydrofolate is the methyl donor for the conversion of homocysteine to methionine. o In MTHFR deficiency absence of Methyl THF causes elevation of total plasma homocysteine levels and decreased levels of methionine.	**In infancy:** o Progressive encephalopathy o Apnea o Seizures o Microcephaly. **In older patients:** o Ataxic gait o Psychiatric problems o Thromboembolism	

AR—Autosomal recessive

Q 17. How will you diagnose homocystinuria?
Ans.

Disorder	Laboratory findings
Classic homocystinuria	o Elevated plasma homocysteine and methionine o Low or absent plasma cysteine level o Homocystinuria in freshly voided urine o CBS enzyme analysis o Homozygous or compound heterozygous mutation in CBS gene
Homocystinuria due to defects in methyl-cobalamin formation	o Megaloblastic anemia o Hyperhomocysteinemia o Homocystinuria o Hypomethioninemia o Mutation analysis
Homocystinuria: Methylmalonic acidemia due to defects in methyl-cobalamin formation	o Mild to moderate increase in methylmalonic acid significant elevations in total plasma homocysteine. o Unlike classic homocystinuria, in untreated Cbl C patients plasma methionine is low to normal o Megaloblastic anemia o Rarely hyperammonemia o Mutation analysis
Homocystinuria due to MTHFR deficiency	o Moderate homocystinemia o Moderate homocystinuria o Low or low-normal methionine concentration: This finding helps differentiate this condition from classic homocystinuria caused by cystathionine β-synthase deficiency. o Enzyme assay in cultured fibroblasts or leukocytes o Homozygous/heterozygous mutation in MTHFR gene

Q 18. How will you treat homocystinuria?
Ans.

Disorder	Specific management
Classic homocystinuria	o Response to vitamin B_6 is variable. o High doses of vitamin B_6 (100–500 mg/24 hr) causes dramatic improvement in patients who are responsive to this therapy. o Patient should not be considered unresponsive to vitamin B_6 until folic acid (1–5 mg/24 hr) has been added to the treatment regimen. o Patients unresponsive to Vit B_6 may respond to methionine intake restriction and cysteine supplementation. o Betaine (trimethylglycine, 6 g/24 hr for adults or 200–250 mg/kg/day for children) lowers homocysteine levels in body fluids by remethylating homocysteine to methionine. o It has been found to be effective in preventing vascular events in B_6 unresponsive patients.

Contd.

Disorder	Specific management
Homocystinuria due to defects in methyl-cobalamin formation	o High dose hydroxycobalamin (Vit B$_{12}$–1 mg/day)
Homocystinuria: Methyl-malonic acidemia due to defects in methyl-cobalamin formation	o Patients with Cbl C, Cbl D, Cbl F, Cbl J, and Cbl X defects—large doses of hydroxocobalamin (up to 0.3 mg/kg/day) with betaine (up to 250 mg/kg/day) o Folic or Folinic acid supplementation o Avoid dietary methionine deficiency
Homocystinuria due to MTHFR deficiency	o Folinic acid orally 15 mg/day o Betaine orally 100–250 mg/kg/day in neonates and infants o In children and adults, 6–9 g/day in three divided doses with a maximum daily dose of up to 20 g/day o Hydroxycobalamin 0.5–1 mg orally or 1 mg IM monthly o Methionine orally 40–50 mg/kg/day o Vitamin B$_6$ orally 100–250 mg/day o Early treatment with betaine has been found to be useful.

Q 19. Write the etiology, inheritance pattern, clinical features and complications of Maple syrup urine disease.

Ans.

Disorder	Etiology enzyme & candidate gene	Inheritance pattern	Enzyme deficiency & mechanism	Specific clinical features
Maple syrup urine disease (MSUD)	Branched-chain ketoacid dehydroge-nase (BCKDH) complex deficiency (Figure 18.7) *BCKDHA, BCKDHB, DBT*	Autosomal Recessive	Decreased activity of BCKD leads to increased branched chain amino acids in plasma, alpha ketoacids in urine and production of pathognomonic disease marker alloisoleucine	Based on clinical findings and response to thiamine administration, MSUD is classified into o Classic maple syrup urine disease o Intermediate maple syrup urine disease o Intermittent maple syrup urine disease o Thiamine-responsive maple syrup urine disease o Maple syrup urine disease caused by deficiency of E3 subunit (MSUD type 3)
Classic maple syrup urine disease				**Most severe clinical manifestations** o Affected infants appear healthy at birth

Contd.

Disorder	Etiology enzyme & candidate gene	Inheritance pattern	Enzyme deficiency & mechanism	Specific clinical features
				○ Maple syrup odor in cerumen and urine ○ Poor feeding and vomiting ○ Lethargy and coma. **Physical examination** ○ Hypertonicity and muscular rigidity with severe opisthotonos ○ Periods of hypertonicity may alternate with bouts of flaccidity ○ Repetitive movements of the extremities ("boxing" and "bicycling") ○ Often mistakenly thought to be generalized sepsis and meningitis ○ Cerebral edema ○ Seizures ○ Hypoglycemia ○ Acute cerebral edema ○ Encephalopathy
Intermediate MSUD				○ Milder disease after the neonatal period ○ Mild to moderate intellectual disability with or without seizures ○ Odor of maple syrup present
Intermittent MSUD				○ Asymptomatic ○ In stress situations, may present similar to classic MSUD
Thiamine-responsive MSUD				○ Similar to the intermediate form but respond dramatically to high doses of thiamine
MSUD type 3 caused by deficiency of E3 subunit				○ Clinical spectrum from early-onset neurologic manifestations to adult-onset isolated liver disease.

Q 20. How will you diagnose Maple syrup urine disease?
Ans.

Disorder	Laboratory findings
Classic maple syrup urine disease	o Hypoglycemia o Ketoacidosis o Marked elevations in plasma levels of leucine, isoleucine, valine, and alloisoleucine o Leucine higher than rest 3 amino acids o Decreased level of alanine o Urine contains high levels of leucine, isoleucine, and valine and their respective ketoacids. o BCKDH complex activity varies between 0% and 2% of controls. o Neuroimaging during the acute state may show cerebral edema most prominent in the cerebellum, dorsal brainstem, cerebral peduncle, and internal capsule. o Molecular analysis.
Intermediate maple syrup urine disease	o Plasma lactate and pyruvate normal o Rest similar to classic MSUD.
Intermittent maple syrup urine disease	Similar to classic MSUD.
Maple syrup urine disease caused by deficiency of E3 subunit (MSUD Type 3)	o Persistent lactic acidosis o Rest similar to classic MSUD o Patients excrete large amounts of lactate, pyruvate, α-ketoglutarate and the 3 branched-chain ketoacids in their urine.

Q 21. How will you treat maple syrup urine disease?
Ans.

Disorder	Specific management
Maple syrup urine disease (MSUD)	

Classic maple syrup urine disease	**Acute Decompensation:**
	o Aim:
	  ♦ To maintain hydration
	  ♦ To remove excess branched chain amino acids and their metabolites from tissues and body fluids at the earliest.
	o Toxin removal by peritoneal dialysis or hemodialysis

Contd.

Disorder	Specific management
	o High energy dietary treatment o Restart enteral feeds early: Nasogastric feeds with BCAA free formula o Adjust BCAA intake as per plasma levels taken daily till optimum levels of BCAA are reached. o Supplementation of isoleucine and valine as their fall becomes rate limiting for protein synthesis o Isoleucine and valine also compete with leucine for LNAA transporters and decrease leucine's entry into central nervous system, decreasing chances of leucine encephalopathy. **Maintenance phase:** o BCAA restricted diet to be followed for life with age appropriate BCAA provided through diet and frequent titration based on plasma amino acid levels o Liver transplant.
Intermediate maple syrup urine disease	o **Thiamine trial:** 4-week trial of enteral thiamine (50–100 mg/day, divided in two doses) o Diet therapy like that of classic MSUD.
Intermittent maple syrup urine disease	o **Acute attack:** Treatment similar to that in classic MSUD o **After recovery:** Although a normal diet can be tolerated, a low-BCAA diet is recommended.
Thiamine-responsive maple syrup urine disease	o Tab Thiamine 10 mg/24 hours in two divided doses to 100 mg/24 hours BD for at least 3 weeks can be required to get a response. o BCAA-restricted diet.
Maple syrup urine disease caused by deficiency of E3 subunit (MSUD type 3)	o No effective treatment is available.

Q 22. Write the etiology, inheritance pattern, clinical features and complications of non-ketotic hyperglycinemia.
Ans.

Disorder	Etiology enzyme & candidate gene	Inheritance pattern	Enzyme deficiency & mechanism	Specific clinical features	Complications
Non-ketotic hyper-glycinemia (NKH) Two types based on ultimate outcome o **Severe NKH**	o Deficient activity of glycine cleavage enzyme system (GCS) made of 4 proteins. o GLDC gene (80% NKH) encodes P protein and AMT gene (20% NKH) encodes T protein	AR	GCS deficiency results in accumulation of glycine in blood and cerebrospinal fluid causing symptoms of NKH	Present in mostly neonatal and sometimes in early infancy. Patient presents with o hypotonia o lethargy o coma o apnea o myoclonic jerks o seizures o pin-point pupils o may require ventilator for first 10–20 days o congenital brain malformations o developmental delay.	**1st year of life** o Spastic quadriparesis and truncal hypotonia. o Cortical blindness o Microcephaly **Further long-term problems:** o No developmental progress o Feeding difficulties requiring tube feeding o Gastroesophageal reflux o Hip dislocation and scoliosis o Sudden life-threatening electrolyte imbalances of hypokalemia or hyper-natremia
o Attenuated NKH	Deficient activity of GCS	AR		o Variable developmental progress o Treatable o No epilepsy o Behavioral problems o Intermittent episodes of lethargy and ataxia o Patients often achieve various motor skills o Expressive speech much more delayed than receptive speech o Three types based on developmental quotient: <20 – >50.	o Sudden life-threatening electrolyte imbalances of hypokalemia or hypernatremia

Q 23. How will you diagnose non-ketotic hyperglycinemia?
Ans.

Disorder	Laboratory findings
Non-ketotic hyper-glycinemia—two types based on ulti-mate outcome: Severe and attenuated NKH	o Grossly elevated plasma glycine levels (about 8× more than normal) o Grossly elevated CSF glycine (15–30× normal) o Abnormal CSF: Plasma glycine levels (normal <0.02, in NKH >0.08) o Enzyme analysis in liver o Molecular analysis.

Q 24. How will you treat non-ketotic hyperglycinemia?
Ans.

Disorder	Treatment

Non-ketotic hypergly-cinemia
o **Severe NKH**
o **Attenuated NKH**
	First principle of medical treatment: Reduction of glycine plasma levels by
	1. **Sodium benzoate** with 250–750 mg/kg/day in 3–6 daily doses, in severely affected patients (500–750 mg/kg/day) compared to attenuated patients (250–500 mg/kg/day)
	   ◆ Watch for overdosage and noncompliance due to unpalatable taste of benzoate.
	2. Those with severe NKH requiring high doses of benzoate consider:
	   ◆ Glycine and serine restricted diet with glycine free amino acid formula.
	   ◆ Avoid gelatine and protein rich diet.

	Second principle of treatment: NMDA receptor site antagonists: N-methyl-D-aspartate receptors are allosterically stimulated by glycine. Hence it is thought that hyperglycinemia causes seizures and developmental delay. Clinically used NMDA receptor antagonists include: o **Dextromethorphan:** 3–15 mg/kg/day with highest dose used in neonates and lowest in adults with sodium benzoate has shown improved neurocognitive outcomes and decreased frequency of seizures. Results have been poor in severe NKH. o **Oral ketamine** is effective in attenuated NKH.
	Third principle: Symptomatic treatment: **Seizure control** is very difficult especially in severe NKH. o Clobazam is drug of choice for neonatal seizures in NKH. o Valparin, vigabatrin are contraindicated. o Other antiepileptic drugs have been used with variable results o Ketogenic diet has been used with variable success too
	Others: Gastrostomy tubes, management of scoliosis, physical therapy.

UREA CYCLE DEFECTS
SNEHAL PATIL

Q 25. Draw the metabolic pathway of urea cycle defects.

Ans. Urea cycle disorders (UCDs) are inborn errors of metabolism (IEMs) resulting from defects in any 1 of the six enzymes or 2 transporters involved in the hepatic removal of ammonia from the bloodstream by conversion to urea which is excreted by the kidneys (Figure 18.5). Deficiencies in specific enzymes needed to breakdown amino acids or other metabolites lead to accumulation of ammonia which in turn causes toxicity primarily to central nervous system causing catastrophic manifestations seen in UCDs.

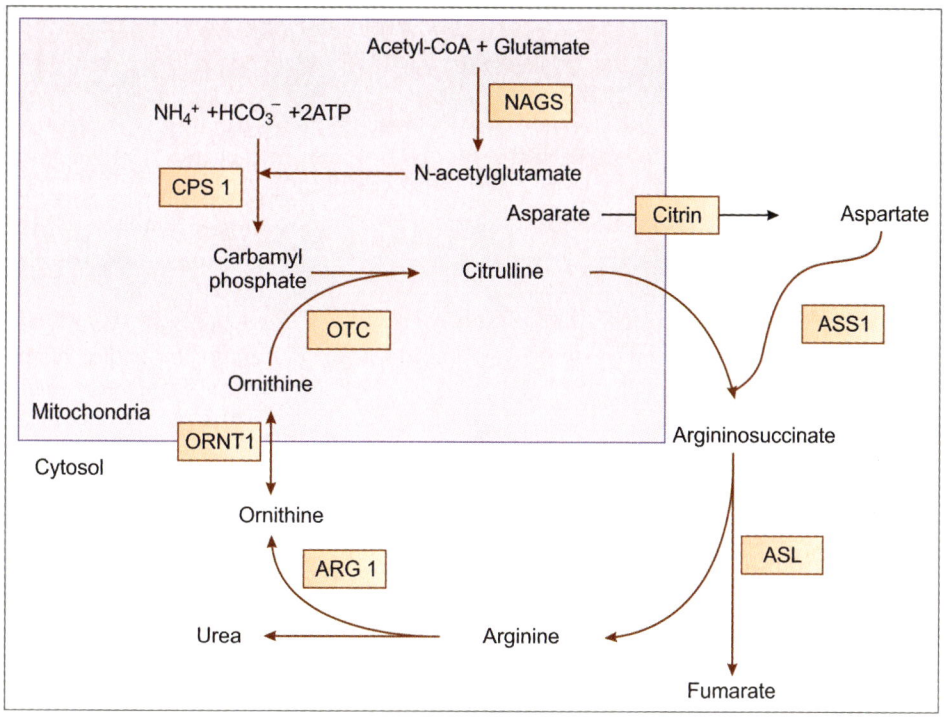

Figure 18.5: : Metabolic pathway of urea cycle defects

NAGS—N-acetyl glutamate synthetase, CPS1—Carbamoyl phosphate synthetase, ASS1—Argininosuccinate synthetase; ASL—Argininosuccinate lyase, ARG1—Arginase 1, ORNT1—Orinthine transporter 1, OTC—Ornithine transcarbamylase

Q 26. Write the etiology, inheritance pattern and clinical features of urea cycle defects.
Ans.

Disorder	Etiology	Inheritance pattern	Enzyme deficiency and mechanism	Specific clinical features
Mitochondrial urea cycle disorders:				
Carbamoyl phosphate synthetase 1 (CPS1) deficiency	CPS 1 deficiency CPS1 gene	AR	CPS 1 is required to incorporate ammonia into carbamoyl phosphate (*see* Figure 18.5). Its deficiency leads to hyperammonemia and low or absent levels of citrulline in plasma.	Marked hyperammonemia. **Newborn:** ○ Normal at birth. ○ Rapidly progressing encephalopathy by day 2 ○ Vomiting, refusal to feed, ○ Coma ○ Hypotonia, seizures, hyper or hypoventilation ○ Hypo or hyperthermia ○ Respiratory alkalosis.

Contd.

Disorder	Etiology	Inheritance pattern	Enzyme deficiency and mechanism	Specific clinical features
				Children, adolescents and adults: ○ Variable presentation ○ Present during or after an inter-current illness or catabolic state ○ Unexplained change in consciousness ○ Novel neurological signs (e.g. tremor, irritability, seizures) often mistaken for encephalitis, drug intoxication or brain tumor.
N-acetyl-glutamate synthase (NAGS) deficiency	NAGS deficiency -NAGS gene	AR	NAGS is a CPS1 activating enzyme and its deficiency leads to *hyper-ammonemia* and low to absent plasma citrulline.	Clinical features similar to CPS 1 deficiency.
Ornithine trans-carbamylase (OTC) deficiency: Most common of all UCDs	OTC deficiency OTC gene	X-linked recessive	OTC is required for formation of citrulline from carbamoyl-phosphate (CP) and ornithine. ○ Its deficiency leads to accumulation of CP which inhibits CPS1 causing **hyperammonemia** ○ CP leaks from mitochondria causing increased pyrimidine biosynthesis and **increased production of orotic acid** and uracil.	○ Hemizygous males more severely affected than heterozygous females ○ Heterozygous females: Some have mild disease but most (75%) are asymptomatic with subtle neurologic defects even without frank hyperammonemia **Male newborn:** ○ Marked hyperammonemia leading to refusal to feed, vomiting, lethargy, convulsion, coma. **Late presentation (>4th decade of life):** ○ Acute bout of hyperammonemia (lethargy, headache, seizures, psychosis) ○ Coma and death may occur.
Cytosolic urea cycle disorders				
Citrullinemia Type I/arginino-succinate synthetase deficiency/ classic citrullinemia	ASS deficiency ASS1 gene	AR	ASS1 is required for conversion of citrulline to argininosuccinate. ○ Due to its deficiency, there is marked increase in citrulline in plasma and formation of orotic acid leads to poor	Depending on degree of enzyme deficiency **Two forms:** 1. *Severe/Neonatal form:* ◆ most common ◆ hyperammonemia in first few day of life

Contd.

Disorder	Etiology	Inheritance pattern	Enzyme deficiency and mechanism	Specific clinical features
			availability of ornithine and secondary impairment of OTC thus causing **hyperammonemia**.	2. *Subacute or mild form:* ♦ Failure to thrive ♦ Frequent vomiting ♦ Developmental delay ♦ Dry and brittle hair appear gradually after 1-year age.
Citrullinemia type II/citrin deficiency/ AGC2 deficiency	Citrin, aspartate/ glutamate antiporter deficiency gene SLC25A13	AR	Citrin transports aspartate from mitochondria into cytoplasm and replenish the cytosolic aspartate pool required for converting citrulline to argininosuccinic acid (*see* Figure 18.5). Citrin deficiency causes decreased aspartate to the cytoplasmic component of the urea cycle, so urea will not be formed at a normal rate, and citrulline will accumulate.	Two main age dependent clinical presentations: 1. **Neonatal form (neonatal intrahepatic cholestasis):** Condition is usually self-limiting with recovery by 1 year of age. 2. **Adult form:** Age at onset is usually between 20 and 40 years (range: 11 to >100 years) ♦ Starts acutely in a previously apparently normal individual. ♦ Manifests with neuropsychiatric symptoms such as disorientation, delirium, delusion, aberrant behavior, tremors, and frank psychosis. ♦ Moderate degrees of hyperammonemia. ♦ Patients who recover from the 1st episode may have recurrent attacks. ♦ Pancreatitis, hyperlipidemia and hepatoma.
Argininosuccinate lyase deficiency (argininosuccinic aciduria)	Argininosuccinate lyase deficiency (ASL) ASL gene	AR	○ ASL is required for conversion of argininosuccinate to arginine. ○ Thus, its deficiency leads to increased argininosuccinate in plasma and urine. ○ Increased excretion of orotic acid leading to poor availability	Variable severity: **In severe form:** ○ Signs and symptoms develop in the 1st few days of life. ○ Acute attacks of severe hyperammonemia seen during intercurrent catabolic state. ○ Intellectual disability, failure to thrive, hypertension, gallstones, liver fibrosis and hepatomegaly.

Contd.

Disorder	Etiology	Inheritance pattern	Enzyme deficiency and mechanism	Specific clinical features
			of ornithine and secondary impairment of OTC causes **hyperammonemia.**	○ **Trichorrhexis nodosa** (dry and brittle hair)
Arginase deficiency/ hyper-argininemia	Arginase 1 (ARG1) deficiency ARG1 gene	AR	Arginase 1 is required to convert arginine to ornithine and to urea. Inhibition of arginase 1 leads to increased citrulline levels (*see* Figure 18.5) (although not as high as in ASS deficiency). ARG1 deficiency induces second arginase (ARG2) in extrahepatic tissues because of which arginine levels do not go very high and also plasma ornithine becomes near normal and urea is present (but still it is generally decreased).	Clinical features different than other UCDS. ○ **Acute neonatal form** with intractable seizures, cerebral edema, and death. ○ **Infant** can remain asymptomatic in the 1st few months or years of life. ○ Onset is insidious. ○ Cerebral palsy mimic. **In a previously normal infant:** ○ Progressive spastic diplegia with scissoring of the lower extremities, choreoathetotic movements, loss of developmental milestones, and failure to thrive. ○ Intellectual disability. ○ Seizures. ○ Hepatomegaly.
Hyper-ammonemia hyper-ornithinemia	ORNT1 transporter defect *SLC25A15* gene	AR	The defect is in the transport system of ornithine from the cytosol into mitochondria.	**Variable clinical manifestations** ○ Patient may present shortly after birth or may be delayed until adulthood.
Homo-citrullinemia syndrome (HHH syndrome)			This causes accumulation of ornithine in the cytosol (causing **hyperornithinemia**) and its depletion in mito-chondria (disrupting urea cycle) and results in **hyperammonemia.** **Homocitrulline** is formed from the reaction of mitochondrial carbamoyl phosphate with lysine, which can become a substrate for the OTC reaction when ornithine is deficient.	○ Presents with acute episodes of hyperammonemia. ○ Psychomotor retardation.

Contd.

Disorder	Etiology	Inheritance pattern	Enzyme deficiency and mechanism	Specific clinical features
Transient hyperammonemia of the newborn (THAN)	--	—	—	o Seen in some newborn preterm babies with mild respiratory distress syndrome. o **Present with severe transient hyperammonemia:** Hyperammonemic coma may develop within 2–3 days of life, and the infant may succumb to the disease if treatment is not started immediately

AR—Autosomal recessive

Q 27. How will you diagnose urea cycle defects?

Ans.

DIAGNOSTIC LABORATORY TESTS AND LABORATORY FINDINGS—UREA CYCLE DEFECTS	
Disorder	Laboratory findings
Carbamoyl phosphate synthetase 1 (CPS1) deficiency	o Hyperammonemia o Marked increase of plasma glutamine and alanine with relatively low levels of citrulline and arginine. o Low or absent urinary orotic acid. o Enzyme analysis in liver. o Mutation analysis in CPS1 gene.
N-acetylglutamate synthase (NAGS) deficiency	o Hyperammonemia o Marked increase of plasma glutamine and alanine with relatively low levels of citrulline and arginine. o Low or absent urinary orotic acid. o Enzyme analysis in liver. o Mutation analysis in NAGS gene.
Ornithine transcarbamylase deficiency	o Hyperammonemia o Marked elevations of plasma concentrations of glutamine and alanine with low levels of citrulline and arginine. o Low serum urea. o Marked increase in the urinary excretion of orotic acid. o Enzyme analysis in liver. o Mutation analysis in OTC gene.
Citrullinemia type I/argininosuccinate synthetase deficiency/ classic citrullinemia	o Hyperammonemia o Plasma citrulline concentration is greatly elevated (50–100 times normal). o Moderately increased urinary excretion of orotic acid. o Crystalluria as a result of precipitation of orotates. o Enzyme analysis in liver. o Mutation analysis
Citrullinemia type II/citrin deficiency/ AGC2 deficiency	**Neonatal form:** o Mild to moderate direct hyperbilirubinemia, marked hypoproteinemia. o Increased prothrombin time and partial thromboplastin time. o Increased serum γ-glutamyl transferase and alkaline phosphatase activities. o Elevated levels of serum galactose. o Marked elevation in the serum α-fetoprotein. o Plasma ammonia and citrulline normal or moderate elevations. o Increases in plasma concentrations of methionine, tyrosine, alanine and threonine. o Mutation analysis.

Contd.

	Adult form: ○ Moderate degrees of hyper-ammonemia ○ Hypercitrullinemia ○ Mutation analysis.
Arginino-succinate lyase deficiency (ASL) (arginino-succinic aciduria)	○ Hyperammonemia ○ Moderate elevations in liver enzymes. ○ Nonspecific increases in plasma glutamine and alanine. ○ Moderate increase in plasma citrulline (less than in citrulli-nemia). ○ Marked increase arginino-succinic acid in plasma, urine and cerebrospinal fluid (CSF). CSF levels are usually higher than plasma ○ ASL assay ○ Mutation analysis.
Arginase deficiency/ hyperargini-nemia	○ Hyperammonemia ○ Marked elevations of arginine in plasma and CSF. ○ Increased urinary orotic acid. ○ Markedly increased guanidino compounds (α-keto-guanidinovaleric acid and α-keto-argininic acid) in urine. ○ Decreased arginase activity in erythrocytes. ○ Mutation analysis.
Transient hyper-ammonemia of the newborn (THAN)	○ Hyperammonemia ○ Citrulline, glutamine and alanine levels are moderately elevated. ○ Rest plasma amino acids are normal.

Q 28. How will you treat urea cycle disorders?
Ans. Urea cycle disorders: Emergency immediate treatment in acute decompensation and hyperammonemia:

AIM

1. Minimize ammonia production by preventing protein breakdown.

2. Simultaneously increase ammonia removal.

MANAGEMENT

○ **Withhold dietary proteins** immediately for maximum 48 hours following which at least essential amino acids should be supplemented.

○ **Ensure high energy supply** through high dose intravenous glucose (with or without insulin). This is to prevent endogenous protein breakdown which will cause catabolism and further increase in ammonia levels.

○ **Medications to reduce hyperammonemia:**
  • Nitrogen scavenges sodium benzoate and sodium phenylacetate/phenylbutyrate increase urinary nitrogen excretion bypassing the urea cycle and are excreted as conjugates of glycine and glutamine, respectively.
  • L-arginine (oral or intravenous) or L-citrulline (oral) enhances residual urea cycle function and urinary excretion of urea cycle intermediates.
  • Carbamylglutamate administration (oral) restores CPS1 function in NAGS deficiency.

○ **Nitrogen scavenger drugs and L-arginine are given at the beginning of treatment** of acute hyperammonemia as boluses followed by continuous infusions.

○ **If plasma ammonia exceeds 500 µmol/L,** extracorporeal detoxification is needed, either through peritoneal dialysis in infants and young children and hemodialysis in older children and adults.

○ **Maintenance** of fluid and electrolytes and acid–base balance and removal of provoking factors can make recovery fast.

DOSES OF VARIOUS MEDICATION IN UCD

Disorder	IV Sodium benzoate in D10%	IV L-Arginine in D10%	N-Carbamyl-glutamate (oral)	IV Sodium phenyl-acetate in D10%
Carbamoyl phosphate synthetase 1 (CPS1) deficiency	250 mg/kg bolus over 90–120 min, then 250–500 mg/kg/day maintenance 8 hourly	250 mg/kg bolus over 90–120 min, then 250 mg/kg/day maintenance 8 hourly	—	250 mg/kg bolus over 90–120 min, then 250–500 mg/kg/day maintenance 8 hourly
N-acetylglutamate synthase (NAGS) deficiency	Same	Same	100 mg/kg bolus through nasogastric tube then 25–62.5 mg/kg 6 hourly	—
Ornithine transcarbamylase deficiency	Same	Same	—	Same
Citrullinemia type I/argininosuccinate synthetase deficiency/classic citrullinemia	Same	Same	—	Same
Citrullinemia type II/citrin deficiency /AGC2 deficiency	—	10–15 gm/day	—	—
Argininosuccinate lyase deficiency (argininosuccinic aciduria)	Same	200–400 mg/kg bolus over 90–120 min, then 200–400 mg/kg/day maintenance 8 hourly	—	Same
Arginase deficiency/hyper-argininemia	Same	Avoid	—	—
Hyperammonemia-hyperornithinemia-homocitrullinemia syndrome (HHH syndrome)	Same	—	—	Same
Transient hyper-ammonemia of the newborn (THAN)	Same	250–400 mg/kg bolus over 90–120 min, then 250 mg/kg/day maintenance 8 hourly		

If injectable sodium benzoate and L-arginine are not available, powder forms/granules of the same are easily available in grocery stores and pharmacies, respectively. They can be given through nasogastric/orogastric tubes after adequate dilution in following doses:

1. Sodium benzoate 250–500 mg/kg/day in 3 divided doses.
2. L-Arginine granules as 250 mg/kg/day in 3 divided doses.

STANDARD MAINTENANCE THERAPY IN UREA CYCLE DEFECTS					
Disorder	Diet	Sodium benzoate (mg/kg/day)	L-arginine (mg/kg/day)	L-citrulline (mg/kg/day)	Specific treatment
Carbamoyl phosphate synthetase 1 (CPS1) deficiency	Protein restricted	250	<20 kg:100–200 > 20 kg:2.5–6 g/m²/day	100–200	
N-acetylglutamate synthase (NAGS) deficiency	Normal but avoid excess proteins	–	–	–	○ N-carbamyl L-glutamate (carglumic acid, licensed drug carbaglu) a synthetic analogue of the physiological activator of CPS1, NAG, given orally activates ○ CPS1 and thereby urea cycle function. The recommended maintenance treatment is 100 mg/kg/d in 3 dosages prior to meals, but it may be possible to reduce the dose to as low as 10 mg/kg/d.
Ornithine transcarbamylase deficiency	Protein restricted	250	<20 kg: 100–200 >20 kg:2.5–6 g/m²/day	100–200	–
Citrullinemia type I/arginino-succinate synthetase deficiency/classic citrullinemia	Protein restricted	250	<20 kg: 100–300 >20 kg:2.5–6 g/m²/day	–	–

Contd.

STANDARD MAINTENANCE THERAPY IN UREA CYCLE DEFECTS *(Contd.)*

Disorder	*Diet*	*Sodium benzoate (mg/kg/day)*	*L-arginine (mg/kg/day)*	*L-citrulline (mg/kg/day)*	*Specific treatment*
Citrullinemia type II/citrin deficiency/AGC2 deficiency	Low carbohydrate, protein rich	Children: Fat soluble vitamins and lactose free formula Adults: L-arginine, pyruvate, liver transplant			
Argininosuccinate lyase deficiency (argininosuccinic aciduria)	Protein restricted	250	<20 kg:100–300 >20 kg:2.5–6 g/m²/day	–	–
Arginase deficiency/ hyperargininemia	Protein restricted	250	–	–	–
Hyper-ammonemia-hyper-ornithinemia-homocitrullinemia syndrome (HHH syndrome)	Protein restricted	250	<20 kg:100–200 >20 kg:2.5–6 g/m²/day	100–250	–
Transient hyper-ammonemia of the newborn (THAN)	Not applicable				

Recent advances: In severe urea cycle defects, liver cell transplant and stem cell transplant are being studied at present.

- ➲ **Anticonvulsants** for seizures. Avoid valproic acid.
- ➲ **Monitoring:**
  - ▪ Growth, development, neurodevelopment assessment.
  - ▪ Protein levels, ammonia, hemoglobin, vitamins and amino acid levels.
- ➲ **Prognosis:** Even after treatment, prognosis is poor. So, to prevent UCD in next child, prenatal target mutation analysis should be suggested to the family.

Approach to urea cycle diagnosis: Figure 18.6 depicts approach to urea cycle diagnosis.

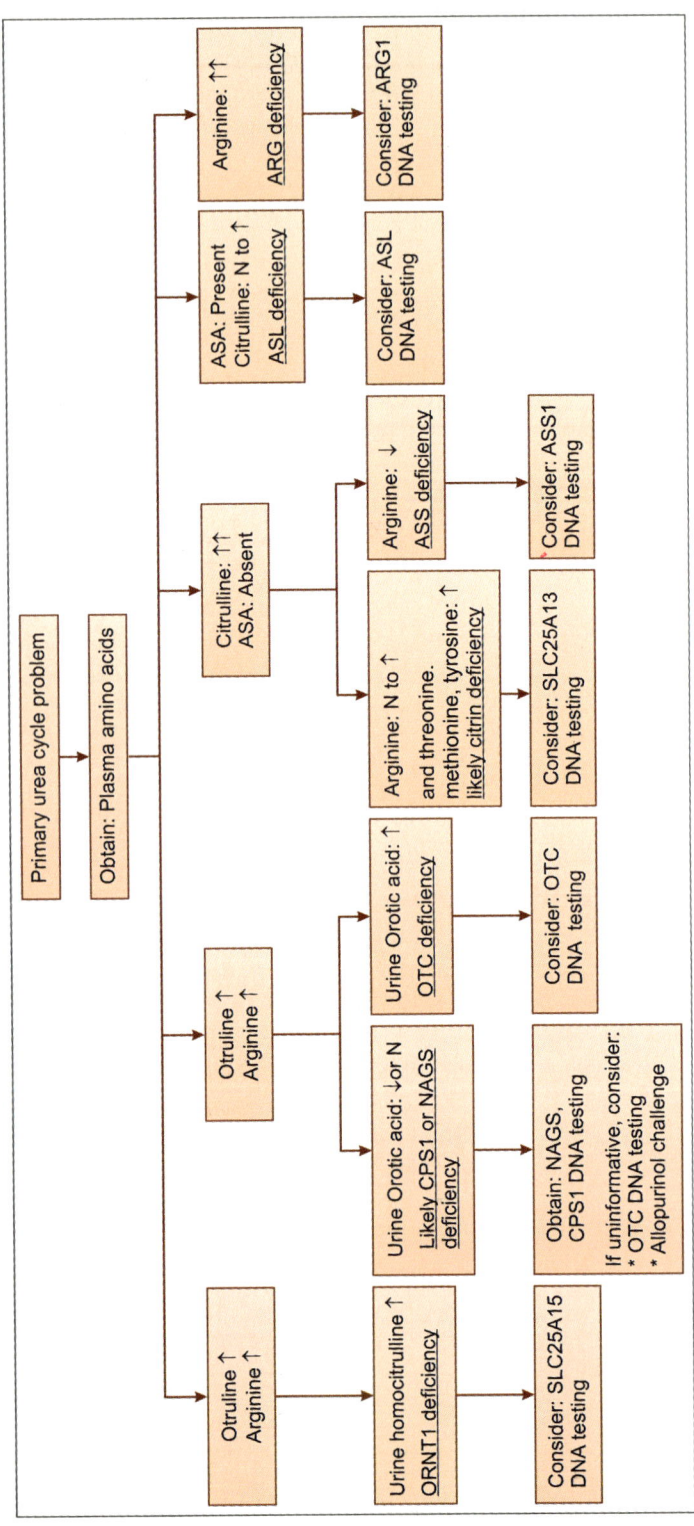

Figure 18.6: Approach to urea cycle diagnosis

ASA: Argininosuccinic aciduria; ASL: Argininosuccinate lyase; ARG: Arginase deficiency; OTC: Ornithine transcarbamylase deficiency; CPS1: Carbamoyl phosphate synthetase 1; ASS: Argininosuccinate synthetase; NAGS: N-acetylglutamate synthase

ORGANIC ACIDEMIAS
SARAH BAILUR

Q 29. Write the metabolic pathway of common organic acidemias.

Ans. Organic acids are the intermediate metabolites of all branched-chain amino acid (valine, leucine and isoleucine). Organic acidemia is caused by a deficiency of any of the degradative enzymes which leads to accumulation of organic acids in body fluids and are excreted in the urine. These disorders commonly occur during infections either as acute intermittent form during neonatal period or during infancy or as late onset form in adolescence-adulthood and causes metabolic acidosis and life-threatening condition. Common organic acidemias metabolic pathway is shown in Figure 18.7.

1. Isovaleric acidemia (IVA)
2. Maple syrup urine disease (MSUD)
3. Glutaric acidemia: 2nd most common.
4. Propionic aciduria (PPA)
5. Methylmalonic aciduria (MMA): Most common.
6. Other rare ones are multiple carboxylase deficiency and 3-methylglutaconic acidurias.

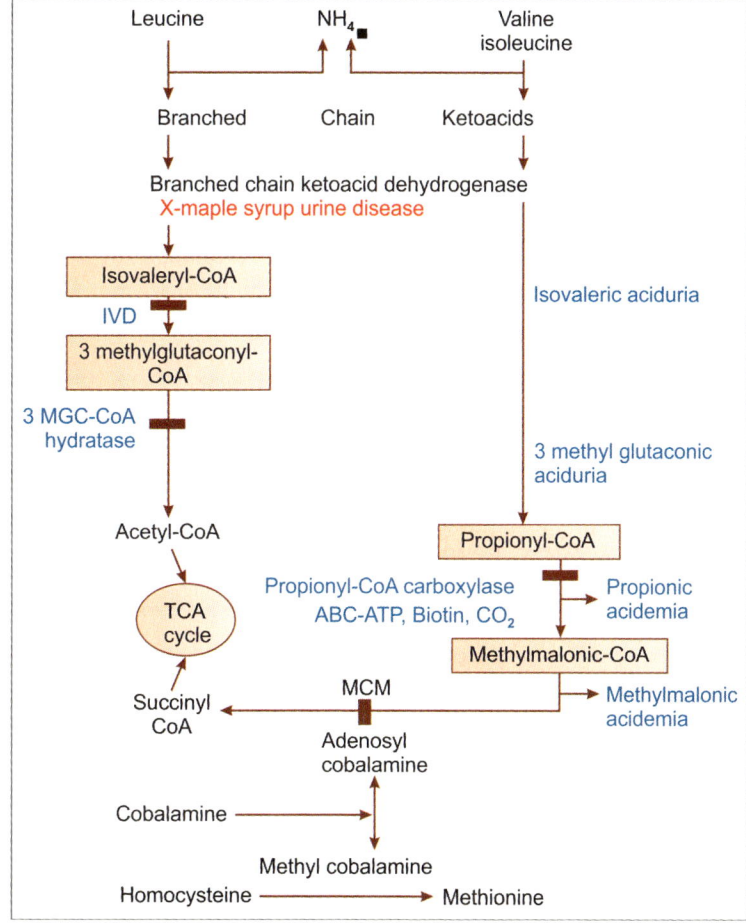

Figure 18.7: Metabolic pathway of branched chain amino acids leading to formation of different organic acids. IVD—Isovaleric acid CoA dehydrogenase; 3 MGC—3-methylglutaconyl; MCM—Methylmalonyl-CoA mutase; TCA—Tricarboxylic acid cycle

Q 30. Write the inheritance, etiology, genetic basis and clinical features of organic acidemia.
Ans.

ORGANIC ACIDEMIAS				
	Glutaric acidemia Type 1	*Isovaleric acidemia (IVA)*	*Propionic aciduria (PPA)*	*Methylmalonic aciduria (MMA)*
Enzyme deficiency	Glutaryl-CoA dehydrogenase: catabolism of lysine, hydroxylysine, tryptophan.	Isovaleryl-CoA dehydrogenase	Propionyl-CoA carboxylase	Methylmalonyl-CoA mutase
Coenzyme deficiency	–		Biotin	Adenosylcobalamin
Gene	*GCDH* gene	*IVD*	*PCCA/PCCB*	*MUT* coding *MCM, MMAA, MMBB, MMAI.*
Mode of inheritance	AR	AR	AR	AR
Pathology	Increased plasma glutaryl carnitine C5. Elevated urine glutaric acid, 3-hydroxyglutaric acid, glutaconic acid	Accumulation of derivatives of Isovaleryl-CoA	Accumulation of propionic acid and its derivatives	Accumulation of methylmalonyl-CoA, propionic acid
Clinical features	Symptoms in 2–36 months of age aggravated due to stress: hypotonia, feeding difficulty, dystonia, large head, developmental regression, irritability	Vomiting, lethargy, hypotonia, seizures, coma, sweat feet odor	Vomiting, lethargy, hypotonia, seizures, dystonia **Chronic symptoms:** Growth failure, seizures, development delay, ataxia, cardiomyopathy, facial dysmorphism	Vomiting, lethargy, hypotonia, seizures, dystonia, **Chronic symptoms:** Growth failure, seizures, development delay, ataxia. cardiomyopathy, facial dysmorphism. Stroke-like episodes

Q 31. How will you diagnose organic acidemia?

Ans. Diagnostic tests:

COMMON BASIC INVESTIGATIONS
o **Blood sugar:** N/decreased
o **Metabolic acidosis:** No/+ (Anion gap > 20 m mol/L)
o **Serum ammonia :** ++/+++(>200 micromol/L in metabolic disorders in neonates and >100 micromol/L after neonatal period)
o **Serum lactate:** N/++ (Normal: 0.5–1 mmol/L)
o **Blood cell count:** N/neutropenia or thrombocytopenia.

o **Urine ketone bodies:** ++

o **Liver and renal function test:** N/Abnormal.

o Calcium low in **isovaleric acidemia, PPA, MMA**

o **Uric acid:** ++

SPECIFIC TESTS
o **Tandem mass spectroscopy:** Abnormal acylcarnitines (increased C3, low free carnitine in PPA, MMA) and increased glutaryl carnitine in glutaric acidemia.
o **Gas chromatography mass spectroscopy:** Increased unmeasured urine organic acids.

o **Neuroimaging:** In glutaric acidemia shows hyperintense lesions in basal ganglia, Wide Sylvian fissure, frontotemporal atrophy.

o **Gene testing of specific gene:** Next generation sequencing.

o **Prenatal testing of target mutation:** By amniocentesis, chorionic villi sampling.

Q 32. How will you do treatment of organic acidemia?

Ans. Even after doing treatment the outcome in organic acidemia is poor. Methylmalonic acidemia (MMA) which responds to vitamin B_{12} shows good response.

TREATMENT OF ACUTE ATTACK

o Hydration	o Reversal of catabolic state
o Low protein diet (1gm/kg/day)	
o Correct metabolic acidosis	
o Treat hyperammonemia: Sodium benzoate	
o Remove excess isovaleric acid by giving glycine and L-carnitine.	
o Hemodialysis	

PRINCIPLES OF LONG-TERM DIETARY MANAGEMENT BASED ON AGE

A. **General**

- Decreased toxic metabolites
- Nutritional status normal
- Prevent catabolism

- Limit one/more amino acids
- Protein (1–1.5 g/kg/day)
- Give essential amino acids.
- Lysine and tryptophan restricted diet in glutaric acidemia.

B. **Drugs in MMA, propionic acidemia (PPA), glutaric acidemia:**

- Carnitine supplementation oral (100–200 mg/kg/day) two divided doses.
- Vit B_{12} in vit B_{12} MMA (1000–2000 μg/day) for 5–10 days
- *Metronidazole:* Reduces intestinal production of propionyl-CoA due to fermentation of carbohydrate in the gut by anaerobic bacteria (10–20 mg/kg/day two divided doses for 10 days).
- *Betaine:* If homocystinuria (100 mg/kg/day) two divided doses.
- *Glutaric acidemia:* Riboflavin (100–300 mg/day), drugs for movement disorders like baclofen or trihexyphenidyl.

C. **Liver transplantation:** Limited studies done in MMA and PPA.

CARBOHYDRATE METABOLIC DISORDERS
SNEHAL PATIL

Q 33. Draw the carbohydrate metabolism pathway.

Ans.

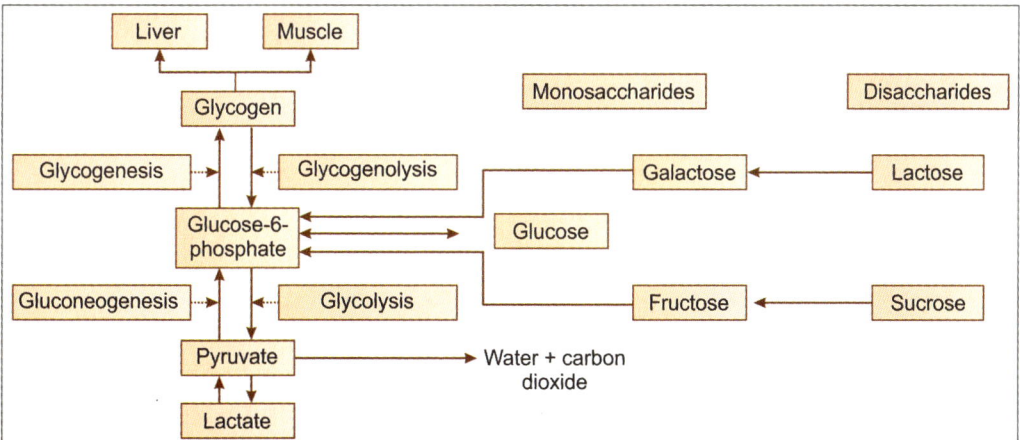

Figure 18.8: : Carbohydrate metabolic pathway

Q 34. Write the etiology, inheritance pattern, clinical features and complications of glucose monosaccharides metabolic disorders.

Ans.

Monosaccharides:
Glucose metabolism: Glucose transport defects

Disorder	Etiology	Inheritance pattern	Enzyme deficiency & mechanism	Specific clinical features	Complications
Congenital glucose/galactose malabsorption	Mutations in the *SLC5A1* gene.	Autosomal recessive (AR)	*SLC5A1* gene mutations cause decrease or loss of ability of SGLT1 protein to transport glucose and galactose across cell membrane, coma leading to the malabsorption of monosaccharides glucose and galactose.	Present within days of birth and feeding with o profuse watery diarrhea o bloating o severe dehydration o chronic dehydration can cause renal stones.	Can be fatal.
Glucose transporter 1 deficiency (GLUT 1 deficiency)	Mostly heterozygous *de novo* mutations and rarely homozygous mutations in SLC2A1 gene encoding GLUT1 transporter protein.	Autosomal dominant AD/AR	o More than 150 mutations in SLC2A1 gene are associated with GLUT1 deficiency. o GLUT1 defect affects glucose transport across blood–brain barrier, leads to hypoglycorrhachia	o **Classic form:** Normal antenatal and neonatal period followed by early onset epileptic encephalopathy. **3 cardinal features:** o Severe epilepsy mimic cyanotic spells, or abnormal eye movements. o Complex movement disorder. o Developmental delay. **Adolescents present with:** o Variable seizures refractory to anticonvulsants. o Abnormal movements like ataxia, dystonia, chorea. o Spasticity may develop parkinsonism, alternating hemiplegia, etc. triggered by poor oral intake.	o Secondary microcephaly

Contd.

Disorder	Etiology	Inheritance pattern	Enzyme deficiency & mechanism	Specific clinical features	Complications
Fanconi-Bickel syndrome (GLUT2 deficiency)	Mutations in the *SLC2A2* gene (3q26.2-q27), encoding GLUT2 transporter protein.	AR	Absence or decreased expression of GLUT2 transporter protein leads to impaired glucose transport through liver and kidneys and therefore accumulation of glucose as glycogen, leading to hepatorenal manifestations.	Typical presentation at 3–10 months of age with combination of: o Hepatomegaly o Fanconi-type nephropathy with severe glycosuria o Hypoglycemia when fasting o Glucose-galactose malabsorption when in fed state. **Kidneys:** o Proximal renal tubular dysfunction: Hypophosphatemic rickets. o Normal mental development.	
Arterial tortuosity syndrome (GLUT10 deficiency)	Mutations in the *SLC2A10* gene encoding GLUT10 transporter protein.	AR	Deficiency of GLUT 10 causes upregulation of transforming growth factors beta-pathway in arterial wall leading to clinical manifestations.	Generalized tortuosity, elongation, stenosis and aneurysm formation of major arteries including aorta. o Acute infarction due to ischemic stroke o Aortic regurgitation o Multiple pulmonary artery stenoses o Telengiectasias o Excessively stretchable skin o Diaphragmatic abnormalities.	o Life-threatening stroke o Aortic regurgitation

Q 35. How will you diagnose glucose monosaccharides metabolic disorders?
Ans.

Disorder	Laboratory findings
Monosaccharides: Glucose metabolism: Glucose transport defects	
Congenital glucose/galactose malabsorption	○ Breath hydrogen test suggestive of glucose-galactose malabsorption ○ Stool shows large amount of reducing sugars (>2 gm%)
Glucose transporter 1 deficiency (GLUT 1 deficiency)	○ Low CSF glucose of <2.5 mmol/L (>3.3 mmol/L). ○ CSF blood glucose level <0.5 with no CSF infection, or hypoglycemia is strongly suggestive of GLUT1 deficiency. ○ CSF lactate is normal.
Fanconi-Bickel syndrome (GLUT2 deficiency)	○ Hypoglycemia ○ Metabolic acidosis (+/-) ○ Mildly elevated transaminases ○ Increased plasma. lactate, uric acid and plasma lipids ○ Hypercalciuria, phosphaturia, bicarbonaturia ○ Severe glycosuria, proteinuria. ○ Hyperaminoaciduria ○ Decreased gamma globulins, hyperlipidemia. ○ Urine routine and microscopy ○ Mutation analysis.

Q 36. How will you treat glucose metabolic disorders?
Ans.

Disorder	Specific management	Recent advances
Monosaccharides: Glucose metabolism: Glucose transport defects		
Congenital glucose/galactose malabsorption	**Hypertonic dehydration:** Intravenous fluid therapy with dextrose and electrolytes. **Long-term:** ○ Avoid both glucose and galactose as monomers, as well as disaccharides and polymers of these sugars. ○ Specialized commercial infant formulas containing fat and protein but free of a carbohydrate component can be used. ○ Fructose added as per the dietary allowances for carbohydrates to meet caloric needs. ○ High fluid intake is recommended to prevent renal stone formation.	

Contd.

Disorder	Specific management	Recent advances
Glucose transporter 1 deficiency (GLUT 1 deficiency)	**Aim:** ○ To prevent low cerebrospinal fluid (CSF) glucose concentration (hypoglycorrhachia) ○ Provide other substrates for brain metabolism. **Treatment:** Modified Atkins diet or ketogenic diet: Both provide ketones as an alternative fuel for the brain. Ketones enter the brain via the facilitative MCT1 transporter. ○ 3 : 1 ratio (fat vs. non-fat intake in grams) using long-chain triglycerides usually sufficient for seizure control in infantile cases. ○ Fluids and calories are not restricted. ○ Supplements (multivitamins, calcium and often carnitine). ○ Anticonvulsive drugs (phenobarbital, chloral hydrate, valproate, topiramate) should not be given.	**Clinical trial:** ○ Oral triheptanoic acid, an artificial C7-ketone body is under trial as additional source for brain energy metabolism. ○ In individual patients, acetazolamide has shown good responses in movement disorders caused by GLUT1-deficiency. ○ α-lipoic acid, an antioxidant, has been shown to increase glucose transport in cultured muscle cells but *in vivo* data is not yet available.
Fanconi-Bickel syndrome (GLUT2 deficiency)	Clinically present with hepatic glycogen storage disorder type1(GSD), hence treatment is similar to GSD type1. It includes: ○ Frequent feeds and use of slowly absorbed carbohydrates. ○ Maintaining blood glucose levels. ○ Frequent feeds, cornstarch, nasogastric oligosaccharide drip feeding. **For tubulopathy:** ○ Water and electrolytes must be replaced. ○ Administration of alkali for renal tubular acidosis. ○ Hypophosphatemic rickets require supplementation with phosphate and vitamin D. With these measures, prognosis is fairly good.	
Arterial tortuosity syndrome (GLUT10 deficiency)	○ No curative treatment is available. ○ Surgical correction of single blood vessels, e.g. pulmonary stenosis needed.	

Q 37. Write the etiology, inheritance pattern, clinical features and complications of galactose metabolic disorders.

Ans. Disorders of galactose metabolism: Galactose is derived from lactose metabolism, primarily found in milk and other dairy products. Galactose metabolism produces fuel for cellular metabolism. It is also necessary for formation of galactosides including glycoproteins, glycolipids and glycosaminoglycans. Primarily 3 enzyme deficiencies in galactose metabolism pathway (Leloir pathway) are significant and all lead to accumulation of excess galactose in the blood and clinical manifestations due to the same.

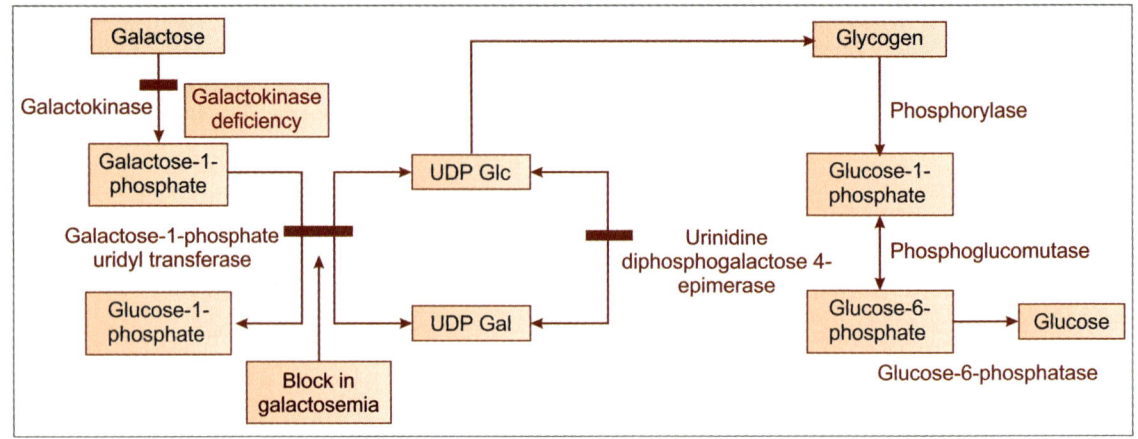

Figure 18.9: Galactose metabolic pathway

Disorder	Etiology	Inheritance pattern	Enzyme deficiency and mechanism	Specific clinical features	Complications
Galactose-1-phosphate uridyl transferase (GALT) deficiency (galactosemia)	Mutation in *GALT* gene coding for *GALT* enzyme	AR	Mutation in GALT gene causes decreased or absent activity of transferase enzyme leading to accumulation of galactose, Gal-1P, galactitol and galactonate in blood and tissues, especially after a diet with high levels of lactose or galactose. ○ Galactitol accumulation is responsible for recurrent cataract. ○ Gal-1-p is responsible for hepatic, renal and cerebral	Depending on the residual erythrocyte enzyme activity, GALT deficiency is classified into: 1. **Classic galactosemia:** Baby develops life-threatening illness with ♦ feeding problems ♦ failure to thrive ♦ hypoglycemia ♦ hepatomegaly ♦ bleeding diathesis ♦ jaundice ♦ nuclear cataracts ♦ sepsis most commonly with *E.coli* ♦ pseudotumor cerebri	**Classic galactosemia:** May develop severe brain damage. **Long-term outcome even with proper treatment:** ○ Speech defects ○ Poor intellectual function ○ Neurologic deficits.

Contd.

Disorder	Etiology	Inheritance pattern	Enzyme deficiency and mechanism	Specific clinical features	Complications
				2. **Partial transferase deficiency:** ◆ More common than classic galactosemia ◆ Generally asymptomatic ◆ Diagnosed on newborn screening ◆ May show some changes on liver biopsy. 3. **Primary or secondary amenorrhea**	
Galacto-kinase (GALK) deficiency		AR	○ Galactokinase enzyme catalyses phosphory-lation of galactose. ○ Its deficiency leads to accumulation of galactose and galactitol.	○ Primarily associated with diet dependent cataracts. ○ Rarely pseudotumor-cerebri. **Long-term complications in 30% of affected individuals with poor diet control:** ○ Hypoglycemia ○ Failure to thrive ○ Microcephaly ○ Intellectual disability ○ Hypercholes-terolemia.	
Uridine diphosphate galactose-4-epimerase (GALE) deficiency	Mutation in *GALE* gene encoding galactose-4-Epimerase enzyme.	AR	Deficiency or absence of epimerase leads to accumulation of galactitol, galactose 1-phosphate and other metabolites in different cells.	Continuum of 3 forms: 1. **Generalized/severe:** Similar to classic galacto-semia 2. **Peripheral/benign:** Asymptomatic 3. **Intermediate form:** Developmental delay if dietary restriction of galactose/lactose is not followed.	○ Sensorineural hearing impairment ○ Physical and cognitive developmental delay ○ Learning difficulties.

Q 38. How will you diagnose disorders of galactose metabolism?

Ans.

Diagnostic lab investigations	Laboratory findings
Galactose-1-phosphate uridyl transferase (GALT) deficiency (galactosemia)	o Hypoglycemia o Hyperbilirubinemia o Elevated transaminases o Deranged PT/aPTT o Mild acidosis o Glycosuria o Generalized aminoaciduria o Reducing substances in urine o Reduced GALT activity o Homozygous/double heterozygous mutation in *GALT* gene.
Galactokinase (GALK) deficiency Pseudotumor cerebri	o Decreased galactokinase activity o Homozygous/double heterozygous mutation in *GALK* gene.
Uridine diphosphate galactose-4-epimerase (GALE) deficiency	o Decreased epimerase activity o Homozygous/double heterozygous mutation in *GALE* gene.

Q 39. How will you treat disorders of galactose metabolism?

Ans.

Disorder	Specific management
Galactose-1-phosphate uridyl transferase (GALT) deficiency (galactosemia)	o **Suspected newborns:** Immediate exclusion of all lactose from the diet, including both breast milk and milk-based formula and switch to a soya-based formula.
	o **In significant liver disease:** Medium-chain triglyceride containing case in hydrolysate. o In seriously ill infants, consider supportive care. o Adequate calcium supplementation can reverse growth failure. o Hormones for ovarian failure with primary or secondary amenorrhea. o Neurological and development assessment.
Galactokinase (GALK) deficiency	Galactose restriction in diet
Uridine diphosphate galactose-4-epimerase (GALE) deficiency	o **Peripheral/benign form:** Does not require dietary restriction of galactose/lactose o **Severe form:** Galactose restricted diet instead of galactose-free diet is given.

Q 40. Write the etiology, inheritance pattern, clinical features and complications of fructose metabolic disorders.

Ans. Disorders of fructose metabolism: Fructose metabolism primarily occurs in liver and to a lesser extent in other tissues of the body like kidney and in intestinal mucosa. In the liver, fructose is phosphorylated to fructose-1-phosphate (F-1-P), by fructokinase. In the liver, F-1-P is further metabolized to d-glyceraldehyde and dihydroxyacetone phosphate by F-1-P aldolase. There are two common errors of fructose metabolism pathway (Figure 18.10).

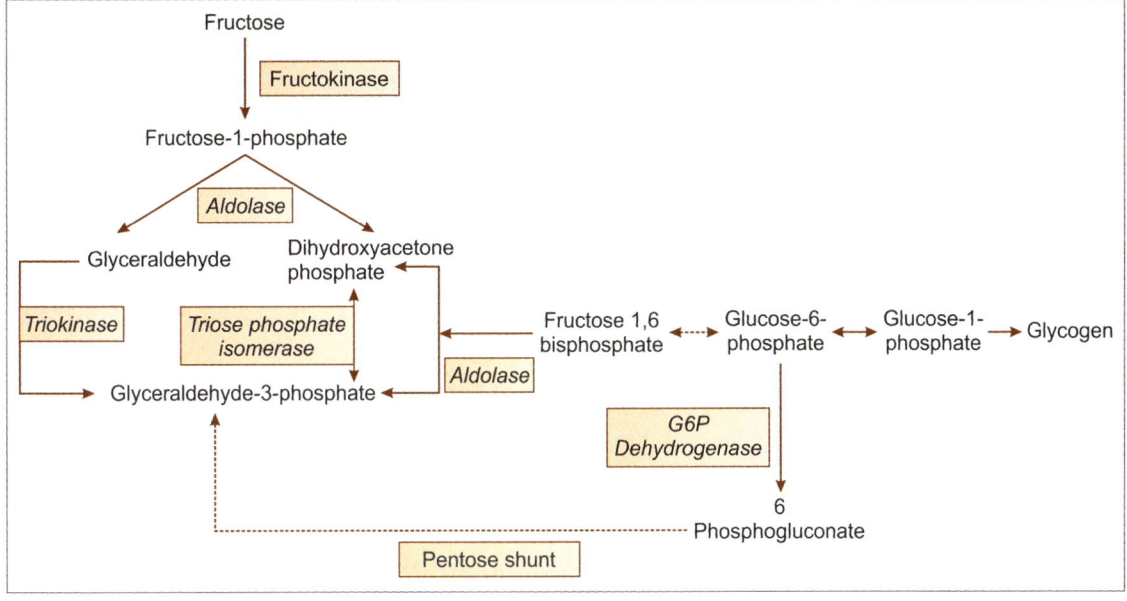

Figure 18.10: Fructose metabolic pathway

Disorder	Etiology	Inheritance pattern	Enzyme deficiency & mechanism	Specific clinical features
Essential fructosuria	Mutation in KHK gene leading to absence or deficiency of hepatic fructokinase enzyme.	AR	○ Deficiency of hepatic fructokinase or ketohexokinase leads to accumulation of fructose of which 10–20% is excreted through urine while remaining is metabolized through alternative pathway in adipose tissue and muscles by hexokinase.	○ Asymptomatic. ○ Fructosuria is incidentally diagnosed on finding reducing substances in urine of a patient.
Hereditary fructose intolerance (HFI)	Mutation in ALDOB gene leading to absence or deficiency of fructose-1,6-bisphosphate aldolase (aldolase-B).	AR	○ Aldolase-B enzyme catalyses the hydrolysis of fructose-1,6-bisphosphate into triose phosphate and glyceraldehyde phosphate. It also hydrolyses fructose-1-phosphate. ○ In the absence of enzyme activity, there is a rapid accumulation of fructose-1-phosphate which leads to clinical manifestations.	○ Affected individuals often present when weaning are introduced with fruits, fruit juice (fructose) or cereals sweetened with sugar (sucrose). **Early clinical features resemble galactosemia and include:** ○ Jaundice ○ Hepatomegaly ○ Lethargy ○ Vomiting ○ Irritability

Contd.

Disorder	Etiology	Inheritance pattern	Enzyme deficiency & mechanism	Specific clinical features
				○ Convulsions ○ Symptomatic Hypoglycemia ○ Celiac disease (10%) **If dietary intake persists:** ○ Failure to thrive ○ Recurrent hypoglycemia ○ Progressive renal and hepatic failure ○ Death.

AR: Autosomal recessive

Q 41. How will you diagnose disorders of fructose metabolism?
Ans.

Disorder	Laboratory findings
Essential fructosuria	○ Fructosuria (reducing substances positive in sugar, on chromatography identified as fructose)
Hereditary fructose intolerance	○ Positive for urinary reducing substances (fructose). ○ Increased uric acid and lactic acid. ○ Deficient aldolase B activity. ○ Homozygous/double heterozygous mutation in *ALDOB* gene.

Q 42. How will you treat disorders of fructose metabolism?
Ans.

Disorder	Specific management
Essential fructosuria	No treatment needed. Excellent prognosis
Hereditary fructose intolerance	**Acute episodes:** ○ Correct hypoglycemia with IV dextrose administration. ○ Supportive treatment of hepatic insufficiency. ○ Correcting metabolic acidosis. ○ Complete elimination of fructose usually rapidly reverses symptoms.

Long-term treatment: Complete restriction of all sources of sucrose, fructose, and sorbitol from the diet.

With treatment there would be:
○ Improvement in hepatic and renal function
○ Good catch-up in growth
○ Unimpaired intellectual development, usually
○ Few dental caries
○ Milder symptoms even after fructose ingestion as the patient matures
○ The long-term prognosis is good.

Q 43. Write the etiology, inheritance pattern, clinical features and complications of disorders of gluconeogenesis.
Ans. Disorders of gluconeogenesis: Gluconeogenesis primarily involves formation of glucose in fasting conditions from lactic acid and certain amino acids in liver and kidneys.

During prolonged fasting, levels of glucocorticoids increase leading to increased synthesis of pyruvate carboxylase, aminotransferases and glucose-6-phosphatase which then participates in gluconeogenesis.

Alanine, aspartic acid and glutamic acid are converted to pyruvate, oxaloacetate and alpha-ketoglutarate which by gluconeogenesis form glucose.

Three key enzymes regulate gluconeogenesis, whose deficiencies lead to significant clinical manifestations with severe lactic acidosis. (Figure 18.11)

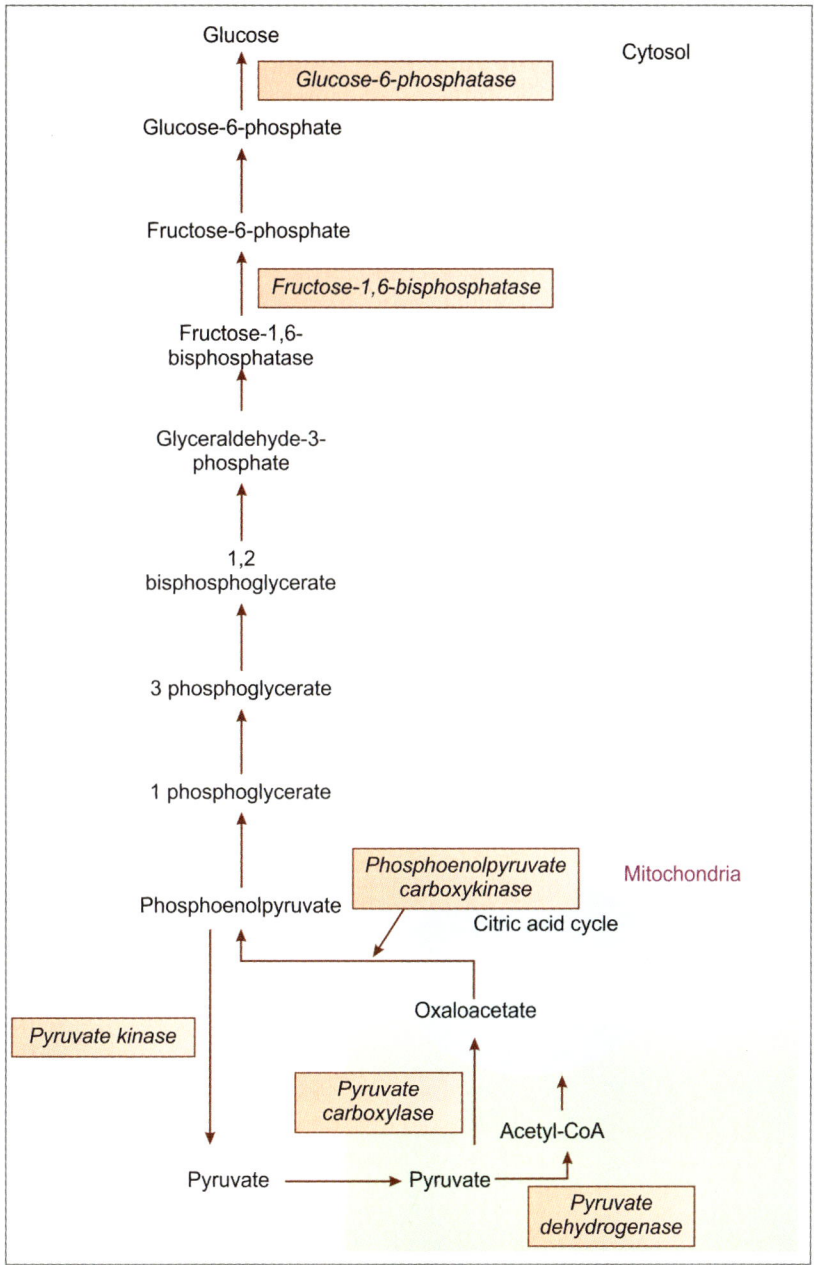

Figure 18.11: Gluconeogenesis pathway

Disorder	Etiology	Inheri- tance pattern	Enzyme deficiency & mechanism	Specific clinical features
Fructose-1,6-diphosphatase deficiency	Mutations in FBP1 gene causing deficiency of Fructose-1,6-bisphosphatase enzyme.	AR	○ Fructose-1,6-diphos-phatase deficiency impairs the formation of glucose from all gluco-neogenic precursors, including dietary fructose. ○ It also causes accumu-lation of pyruvate, lactate, alanine and glycerol	Characterized by life-threatening episodes of: ○ Lactic acidosis ○ Hyperventilation ○ Hypoglycemia ○ Convulsions ○ Coma ♦ Half of cases present in first week of life. ♦ Decreased oral intake seen with febrile illnesses lead to acute decompensation. ♦ Frequency of attacks decrease with advancing age
Pyruvate carboxylase deficiency	Mutations in *PC* gene causing deficiency of pyruvate carboxylase enzyme	AR	Pyruvate carboxylase is a mitochondrial, biotin-containing enzyme. ○ It catalyses the conver-sion of pyruvate to oxaloacetate for Krebs cycle and for the glutamine-glutamate cycle in astrocytes. ○ It is involved in lipo-genesis and formation of nonessential amino acids.	Three forms based on severity are: 1. Type A (infantile onset) 2. Type B (neonatal onset) 3. Type C (benign form) **Most patients present with** ○ failure to thrive ○ developmental delay ○ recurrent seizures ○ lactic acidosis ○ hypotonia ○ pyramidal tract signs ○ convulsions ○ hypoglycemia ○ hyperammonemia ○ hypernatremia ○ hepatomegaly ○ stupor ○ abnormal movements: Tremor and dyskinesia ○ abnormal ocular behavior

Contd.

Disorder	Etiology	Inheritance pattern	Enzyme deficiency & mechanism	Specific clinical features
				○ acute decompensation seen with stress ○ death common in infancy or early childhood ○ on survival, intellectual disability requiring special care and schooling
Pyruvate Dehydrogenase Complex Deficiency (PDHC): Pyruvate in the mitochondria is converted into acetyl-CoA by PHDC, which enters the TCA cycle for ATP production. The complex consists of 5 components: 1. E1: α-ketoacid decarboxylase (E1-alpha subunit and E1-beta subunit) 2. E2: Dihydrolipoyltransacylase 3. E3: Dihydrolipoyl dehydrogenase 4. Protein X: An extra lipoate-containing protein 5. Pyruvate dehydrogenase phosphatase Deficiency of any of these components leads to manifestations of PDHC deficiency.				
Pyruvate dehydrogenase E1-alpha deficiency	Most mutations in *PDHA1* gene are *de novo* mutations: Males mostly have missense mutations, females have deletions and insertions.	X-linked dominant	Absence or deficiency of PDHC leads to accumulation of pyruvate, lactate and alanine, leading to deficient energy production through alternative pathways in brain and leads to severe neurological manifestations.	Wide spectrum of presentation seen with E1-alpha deficiency: **Neonatal form:** Most severe and often fatal, presents in first days or weeks of life and death before 6 months of age. **Characterized by:** ○ Lethargy ○ Hypotonia ○ Seizures ○ Episodic apnea ○ Failure to thrive ○ Severe lactic acidosis ○ Frequent agenesis of corpus callosum

Contd.

Disorder	Etiology	Inheritance pattern	Enzyme deficiency & mechanism	Specific clinical features
				Infantile form: Onset before 6 months age, characterized by ○ Neonatal form manifestations. ○ Psychomotor delay ○ Optic atrophy ○ Ophthalmoplegia ○ Death before 3 years age ○ Neuropathologically similar to Leigh's syndrome **Benign form:** Seen only in males ○ Mild developmental delay ○ Intermittent ataxia ○ Exercise intolerance
Pyruvate dehydrogenase E1-beta deficiency	*PDHB* gene	–	–	
Pyruvate dehydrogenase E2 deficiency	*DLAT* gene	AR	–	Moderate clinical course with slowly progressive neurological features reflecting basal ganglia and brainstem involvement with typical findings of Leigh syndrome.
Protein X lipoate deficiency	–	AR	–	
Pyruvate dehydrogenase E3-deficiency (lactic acidemia due to PDX1 deficiency)	*PDHX* gene	AR	–	
Pyruvate dehydrogenase phosphatase deficiency	*PDP1* gene	AR	–	

AR: Autosomal recessive

Q 44. How will you diagnose disorders of gluconeogenesis?

Ans.

Disorder		Laboratory findings
Fructose-1,6-diphosphatase deficiency		○ Hypoglycemia ○ Metabolic acidosis ○ Increased lactate ○ Elevated uric acid levels ○ Fructose-1,6-diphosphatase deficiency in liver or intestinal biopsy ○ Homozygous/double heterozygous mutation in *FBP1* gene.
Pyruvate carboxylase deficiency	**Type A**	○ Elevated alanine ○ Elevated lactate ○ Increased pyruvate ○ Ketonuria ○ Mild to moderate lactic acidosis ○ *PC* gene sequencing
	Type B	○ Hyperlysinemia ○ Citrullinemia ○ Decreased aspartate ○ Severe lactic acidosis ○ Hyperammonemia ○ *PC* gene sequencing
	Type C	○ Recurrent lactic acidosis
Pyruvate dehydrogenase complex deficiency		○ Elevated cerebrospinal fluid lactate compared to blood lactate levels ○ Plasma lactate: Pyruvate ratio is generally normal/low. ○ Blood lactate, pyruvate, alanine might be normal but increase after carbohydrate load. ○ Plasma amino acid levels ○ Enzyme assay through skin fibroblasts or leukocytes ○ Gene sequencing.

Q 45. How will you treat disorders of gluconeogenesis?

Ans.

Disorder	Specific management
Fructose-1,6-diphosphatase deficiency	**Acute decompensation:** Correction of hypoglycemia and acidosis by IV dextrose infusion; the response is usually rapid. **To prevent further episodes:** ○ Avoid fasting ○ Management of infections ○ Restriction of fructose and sucrose from the diet ○ Long-term prevention of hypoglycemia with cornstarch. ○ Patients who survive childhood develop normally.
Pyruvate carboxylase deficiency	**Acute episodes:** ○ IV Dextrose ○ Peritoneal dialysis. **Long-term management:** ○ Avoid fasting, advise eating a carbohydrate meal before bedtime. ○ Aspartate and citrate supplements to restore the metabolic abnormalities. ○ No ketogenic diet. ○ Biotin and thiamine supplements. ○ Liver transplantation has been attempted though its benefit remains unknown.
Pyruvate dehydrogenase complex deficiency	○ General prognosis poor. ○ In rare patients associated with altered affinity for thiamine pyrophosphate, they may respond to **thiamine supplementation.** ○ **Ketogenic diet.** ○ A potential treatment strategy to maintain any residual PDHC in its active form is by oral administration of **dichloroacetate**, an inhibitor of E1kinase.

Q 46. Write the etiology, inheritance pattern, genetic basis, specific clinical features and complications of disaccharide carbohydrate metabolic defects.

Ans.

DISACCHARIDASE DEFICIENCY				
Disorder	*Etiology*	*Inheritance pattern*	*Enzyme deficiency & mechanism*	*Specific clinical features*
1. **Lactase deficiency:** Most common type of carbohydrate malabsorption				
i. **Congenital lactase deficiency (alactasia)**	Mutations in *LCT* gene leading to lactase enzyme deficiency.	AR	Lactase enzyme deficiency leads to severely impaired ability to digest lactose in breast milk or formula feeds.	Symptoms appear several days (1–10 days) after birth with initiation of breastfeeding or lactose containing formula. **Symptoms include:** ○ Acidic watery diarrhea ○ Abdominal distension ○ Dehydration ○ Acidosis ○ Severe malnutrition ○ Infant appears hungry ○ Rarely vomiting.
ii. **Primary lactase deficiency (adult onset hypolactasia)**	*MCM6* gene, *LCT* gene	AD	Genetic polymorphism C/T 13910 and G/A 22018 in *MCM6* gene are associated with persistence of lactase activity. If either of these are absent the person has primary adult onset lactose intolerance.	○ Symptoms can occur any time after age 2–3 years but mostly in adulthood. ○ Abdominal discomfort begins soon after consuming milk or milk products. ○ Symptoms include pain, diarrhea, and flatulence. ○ Osteoporosis in older age.
2. **Congenital sucrase-isomaltase deficiency**	*SI* gene on Chr3q26.1	AR	Deficiency of enzymes sucrase and isomaltase hampers breakdown of sucrose and maltose to glucose and fructose leading to symptoms.	Patient presents at the time of weaning when the baby starts consuming fruits, juices and grains similar to lactase deficiency.
AR: Autosomal recessive; AD: Autosomal dominant				

Q 47. How will you diagnose disorders of disaccharide metabolism?

Ans.

DISORDERS OF DISACCHARIDASE DEFICIENCY	
Disorder	*Laboratory findings*
Lactase deficiency	○ Breath hydrogen concentration increased ○ Acidic stool pH ○ Deficient activity of lactase enzyme ○ Intestinal biopsy for lactase activity
Congenital sucrase-isomaltase deficiency	○ Carbon-13 breath test/hydrogen-methane breath test ○ Acidic stool. ○ Disaccharide tolerance test ○ Decreased sucrase activity ○ Homozygous/double heterozygous mutation in *SI* gene

Q 48. How will you treat disorders of disaccharide metabolism?

Ans.

DISACCHARIDASE DEFICIENCY	
Disorder	*Specific management*
Lactase deficiency	o **Congenital lactase deficiency:** Strict lactose free diet. o **Primary adult onset hypolactasia:** Lactose avoidance/limitation as well as supplemental lactase ingestion.
Congenital sucrase-isomaltase deficiency	**Sucraid (sacrosidase)** enzyme replacement therapy: o Available as oral solution. o Dose: <15 kg–1 ml (8,500 IU) per meal/snack >15 kg–2 ml (17,000 IU) per meal/snack Diet with severely limited sucrose intake

CONGENITAL DISORDERS OF GLYCOSYLATION
SNEHAL PATIL

Q 49. Write the classification of congenital disorders of glycosylation (CDG).

Ans. Glycosylation is a multistep complex metabolic process where sugar (oligo-saccharides) 'trees' are formed and then attached to either proteins or lipids to form glycoproteins and glycolipids, respectively. Congenital disorders of glycosylation are extremely rare and require a strong suspicion to diagnose.

CDG are further divided based on biochemical structures into:
1. Defects in protein N-linked glycosylation
2. Defects in protein O-linked glycosylation
3. Defects in glycosphingolipid and in glycosylphosphatidylinositol anchor glycosylation
4. Defects in multiple glycosylation pathways and in other pathways.

Congenital disorders of glycosylation (CDG) are predominantly multisystem disorders, caused by >140 different genetic defects in glycoprotein and glycolipid glycan synthesis.

The commonest to rarest amongst the CDG are N-glycosylation defects, followed by CDG involving multiple glycosylation pathways and dolichol phosphate synthesis and then O-glycosylation disorders and disorders of glycosylphosphatidylinositol, respectively.

Q 50. What are the different N-linked glycosylation defects?

Ans. N-linked glycosylation pathway (Figure 18.12).

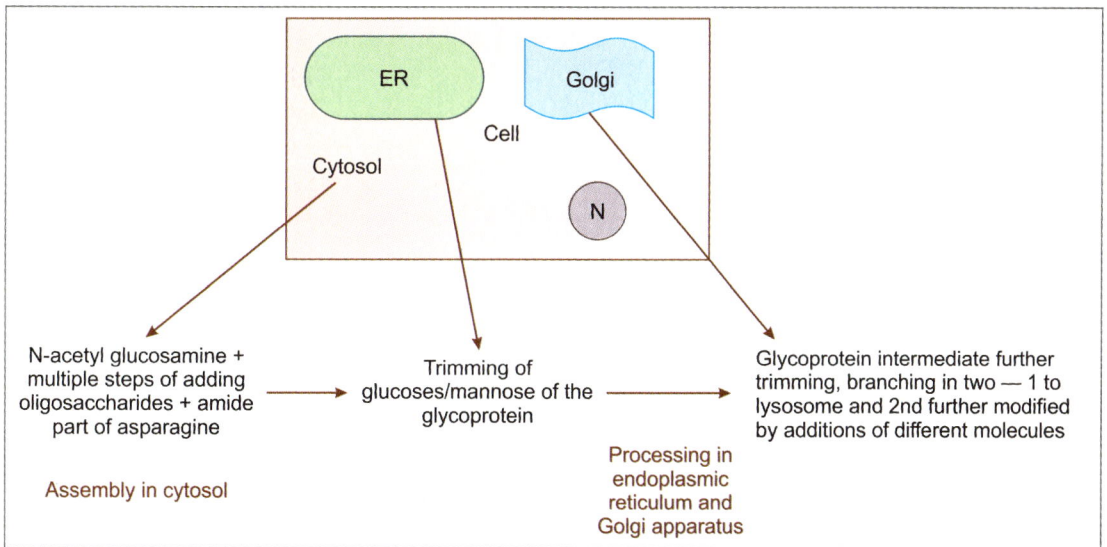

Figure 18.12: : N-linked glycosylation pathway. (ER: Endoplasmic reticulum)

DEFECTS IN PROTEIN N-GLYCOSYLATION

Disorder	Etiology	Inheritance pattern	Enzyme deficiency & mechanism	Specific clinical features	Complications
PMM2-CDG: Most common	Mutation in *PMM2* gene leading to deficiency of phosphomannomutase 2 (PMM2) enzyme	AR	o Phosphomannomutase 2 catalyses the conversion of mannose-6-phosphate to mannose-1-phosphate, used in glycosylation. o Deficiency of PMM2 causes hypoglycosylation which impairs functioning of important glycoproteins which affects coagulation and anticoagulation factors, endocrine regulation, transport proteins and liver function, etc.	o Characteristic facies (smooth philtrum, large ears) o Nystagmus o Alternating strabismus o Inverted nipples and/or abnormal fat pads o Failure to thrive o Axial hypotonia o Ataxia o Psychomotor disability o Stroke-like episodes Not progressive disorder but different features appear at different age: o **Neonate:** Cardiomyopathy, pericardial effusion o **7 years:** Retinitis pigmentosa, cataract o **After puberty:** Scoliosis, neuropathy, thrombotic events.	o Hypergonadotropic hypogonadism o Mild to severe intellectual disability o Delayed to absent speech o Autistic behavior.
MPI-CDG	Mutation in MPI gene leading to deficiency of mannose-phospho-isomerase (MPI) enzyme	AR	o Mannose-phospho-isomerase catalyses the conversion of fructose-6-phosphate to mannose-6-phosphate, 1 step before PMM2. o Hypoglycosylation causes abnormal glycoprotein function similar to PMM2-CDG.	o Early hepatic cholestasis o Hypoglycemia.	o Recurrent thrombosis o Severe gastro-intestinal bleeding.

Contd.

DEFECTS IN PROTEIN N-GLYCOSYLATION (CONTD.)

Disorder	Etiology	Inheritance pattern	Enzyme deficiency & mechanism	Specific clinical features	Complications
ALG6-CDG	Mutation in ALG6 gene leading to deficiency of glucosyltransferase-1	AR	Glucosyltransferase-1 deficiency leads to hypoglycosylation similar to PMM6CDG.	2nd most common CDG. Similar to PMM2.	Autistic behavior
DPAGT 1-CDG	Mutation in DPAGT1 gene leading to deficiency of DPAGT1 enzyme.	AR	UDP-GlcNAc:Dol-P-GlcNAc-P transferase deficiency leads to arrest of glycan synthesis outside the ER. ○ This leads to abnormal receptor glycosylation causing myasthenia like symptoms. ○ Hypoglycosylation causes features similar to PMM2-CDG.	○ Relatively good prognosis ○ Congenital myasthenia Phenotype ○ Some patients also show: ◆ Microcephaly ◆ Brain malformations, hypotonia ◆ Severe psychomotor disability ◆ Seizures ◆ Spasticity ◆ Failure to thrive ◆ Joint contractures ◆ Cataracts.	

CDG: Congenital disorders of glycosylation; ER: Endoplasmic reticulum; AR: Autosomal recessive; DPAGT: UDP-N-acetylglucosamine-dolichyl-phosphate N-acetylglucosaminephosphotransferase

Q 51. What are the different O-linked glycosylation defects?

Ans. Pathway of protein O glycosylation (Figure 18.13).

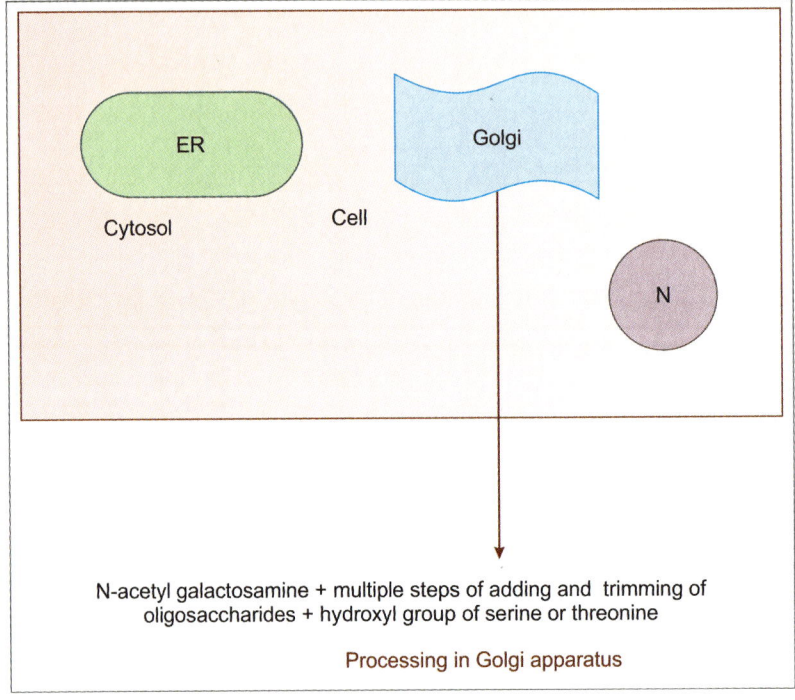

Figure 18.13: : Pathway of protein O glycosylation

Disorder	Etiology	Inheritance pattern	Enzyme deficiency & mechanism	Specific clinical features	Complications
Cerebro-ocular dysplasia– Muscular dystrophy and muscle-eye- brain disease spectrum (POMT1- CDG, POMT2- CDG, POMGNT1- CDG)	Mutations in POMT1, POMT2, and POMGNT1 genes lead to abnormal synthesis of the O- mannosyl glycan core.	AR	Defective mannosylation of α-dystro- glycan causes neuronal migration defects and muscle degeneration.	○ **Eye abnormalities:** • Anophthalmia • Microphthalmia • Congenital cataract • Colobomas ○ **Congenital muscular dystrophy** ○ **Brain abnormalities:** • Pachygyria • Hydrocephalus • Polymicrogyria • Heterotopias • Corpus callosum agenesis	○ Severe psycho- motor disability.

DEFECTS IN LIPID GLYCOSYLATION AND IN GLYCOSYLPHOSPHATIDYLINOSITOL ANCHORBIOSYNTHESIS

Disorder	Etiology	Inheritance pattern	Enzyme deficiency & mechanism	Specific clinical features	Complications
PIGA-CDG	PIGA gene	X-linked	○ Glycophosphatidyl-inositol synthesis is hampered. ○ Abnormal anchoring of alkaline phosphatase causes hyperphospha-tasemia in blood and loss of specific surface antigens on blood cells.	Clinically recognizable epilepsy syndrome with: ○ Dysmorphic facial features ○ Congenital brain malformations ○ Intellectual disability ○ Hypotonia ○ Behavioral abnormalities autism ○ Cardiac and renal defects. ○ Skin anomalies	—

Q 52. How will you diagnose congenital disorders of glycosylation (CDG)?

Ans.

DEFECTS IN PROTEIN N-GLYCOSYLATION

Disorder	Laboratory findings
PMM2-CDG	○ Serum transferrin glycoform analysis by transferrin isoelectric focusing (TIEF) or mass spectrometry (MS). ○ TIEF s/o type 1 pattern ○ Hypoalbuminemia ○ Elevated transaminases ○ Decreased factors IX, XI and antithrombin activity ○ Low serum ceruloplasmin and serum thyroxine binding globulin TBG levels ○ Decreased activity of PMM enzyme ○ Homozygous or double heterozygous mutation in *PMM2-CDG* gene.
MPI-CDG	○ TIEF s/o type 1 pattern ○ Hypoalbuminemia ○ Elevated transaminases ○ Decreased factors IX, XI and antithrombin activity ○ Nonketotic hypoglycemia ○ Hyperinsulinism ○ Decreased activity of Manno-sephosphoisomerase (MPI) enzyme ○ Homozygous or double hetero-zygous mutation in *MPI-CDG* gene.
ALG6-CDG	○ Type 1 pattern on TIEF or MS ○ *ALG6-CDG* gene homozygous or double heterozygous mutation.

DPAGT1-CDG	○ Type 1 pattern on TIEF or MS ○ Creatine phosphokinase CPK levels are normal. ○ DPAGT1-CDG gene homozygous or double heterozygous mutation

DEFECTS IN PROTEIN O-GLYCOSYLATION

Disorder	Laboratory findings
Cerebro-ocular dysplasia–Muscular dystrophy and muscle-eye-brain disease spectrum (POMT1-CDG, POMT2- CDG, POMGNT1-CDG)	○ CPK levels are very high if clinically present as congenital muscular dystrophy. ○ Muscle biopsy shows abnormal alpha-dystroglycan staining on immunohistochemistry. ○ 6 genes are involved— *POMK, FKTN, FKRP, LARGE, B4GAT1, TMEM5,* and *ISPD.* Homozygous or double heterozygous mutation will give the diagnosis.

DEFECTS IN LIPID GLYCOSYLATION AND IN GLYCOSYLPHOSPHATIDYLINOSITOL ANCHOR BIOSYNTHESIS

Disorder	Laboratory findings
PIGA-CDG	○ Fluorescence-activated cell sorting FACS analysis of the membrane-anchored markers CD16 and CD24 in leukocytes is highly suggestive for a GPI-anchor abnormality. ○ Elevated serum alkaline phosphatase. ○ TIEF is normal.

Q 53. How will you treat congenital disorders of glycosylation?
Ans.

Disorder	Specific management	Recent advances
PMM2-CDG	**Supportive management:** ○ Adequate nutrition ○ Diet or tube feeding if needed ○ Cardiac support ○ Hormone supplements ○ Physical and occupational therapy ○ Speech therapy ○ Seizure management ○ Strabismus surgery.	**Preclinical trial phases** ○ Targeted mannose-phosphate treatment ○ Chaperone therapy

MPI-CDG	First CDG type treatable by dietary therapy:
	1. **Mannose therapy:** Clinically effective by both IV and oral supplementation.
	   ◆ *Dose:* 1 g/kg/day divided into 3–4 doses. Side effect is hemolysis.
	   ◆ *Mechanism of action:* Use of alternative pathway: Mannose phosphorylated by hexokinases to mannose 6-phosphate, bypassing the MPI defect.
	   ◆ *Result:* Rapid improvement in clinical symptoms but liver function might further deteriorate
	2. **Liver transplantation.**
		—

ALG6-CDG	○ Supportive treatment	
DPAGT1-CDG	1. Congenital myasthenia phenotype: High dose pyridostigmine and salbutamol. 2. *Multisystem phenotype:* Supportive treatment	

DEFECTS IN PROTEIN O-GLYCOSYLATION	
Disorder	Specific management
Cerebro-ocular dysplasia—muscular dystrophy and muscle-eye-brain disease spectrum (POMT1-CDG, POMT2-CDG, POMGNT1-CDG)	Supportive symptomatic management

DEFECTS IN LIPID GLYCOSYLATION AND IN GLYCOSYLPHOSPHATIDYLINOSITOL ANCHOR BIOSYNTHESIS	
Disorder	Specific management
PIGA-CDG	Supportive symptomatic management

GLYCOGEN STORAGE DISORDER (GSD)
Sarah Bailur

Q 54. Write the glycogen storage pathway mechanism.

Ans. **Glycogen storage disorder (GSD) pathway** (Figure 18.14).

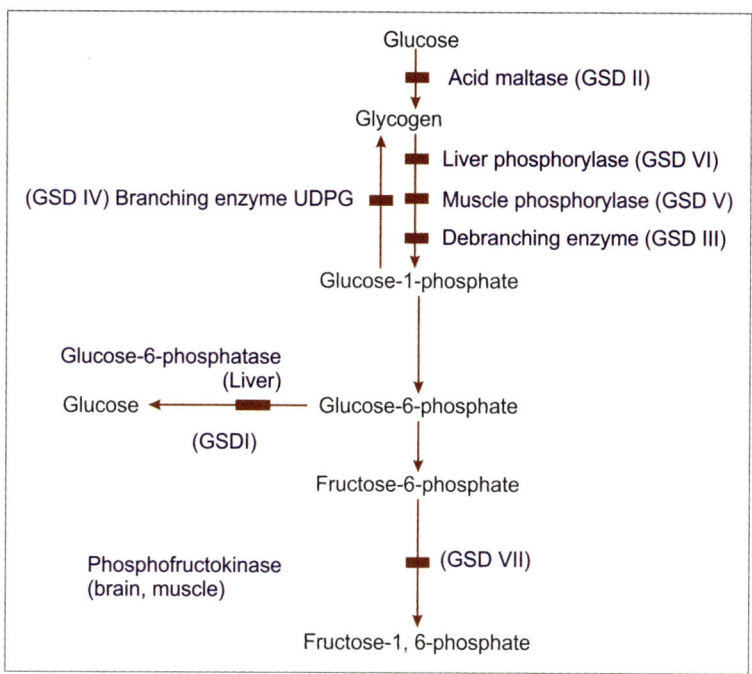

Figure 18.14: : Glycogen storage disorders mechanism. UDPG: Uridine diphosphate glucose

Q 55. Write the inheritance, etiology, genetic basis, clinical features and laboratory findings of glycogen storage disorder (GSD).

Ans. Glycogen storage diseases are inherited metabolic disorders caused by defective or deficient enzyme coded by genes result in storage of glycogen in liver and/or muscle tissues.

VARIOUS GLYCOGEN STORAGE DISORDERS WITH THEIR FEATURES				
Glycogen storage disorder	Inheri-tance	Candidate gene & enzyme deficiency	Clinical features	Laboratory findings
I. Primarily affecting liver				
von Gierke (GSD-I)	Auto-somal recessive (AR)	○ G6PC ○ Glucose-6-phosphatase	○ Doll-like face ○ Growth and pubertal retardation ○ Renal disease ○ Hepatomegaly	○ Hypoglycemia ○ Elevated blood lactate, cholesterol, triglyceride, and uric acid levels ○ Enzyme analysis in liver biopsy sample ○ Gene variant testing

Contd.

VARIOUS GLYCOGEN STORAGE DISORDERS WITH THEIR FEATURES *(Contd.)*

Glycogen storage disorder	Inheritance	Candidate gene & enzyme deficiency	Clinical features	Laboratory findings
Cori disease (GSD-III)	AR	o *AGL* o Amylo-1,6-glucosidase (liver and muscle debrancher deficiency)	o Hepatomegaly o Muscle weakness o Cardiac myopathy o Growth retardation	o Hypoglycemia o Hyperlipidemia o Elevated transaminase levels o Enzyme analysis in liver or muscle tissue o Genetic mutation
Anderson disease (GSD-IV)	AR	o *GBE* o Glycogen branching enzyme	o Growth retardation o Hypotonia o Hepatomegaly o Splenomegaly o Progressive cirrhosis (death usually before 5th year)	o Elevated transaminase levels o Enzyme analysis in white blood cells, fibroblasts o Genetic mutation
Hepatic phosphorylase (GSD-VI)	AR/X-linked	o *PYGL* o Hepatic phosphorylase deficiency	o Hepatomegaly o Failure to thrive	o Hypoglycemia o Increase in lipid levels, and ketones o Genetic mutation
II. Primarily affecting muscle				
Pompe disease (GSD-II)	AR	o *GAA* o Acid α-glucosidase (acid maltase)	o Heart failure o Muscle weakness o Floppy infant	o Increase in CPK, LDH o Enzyme assay—absent/decreased acid α-glucosidase o Genetic mutation
McArdle disease (GSD-V)	AR	o *PYGM* o Muscle phosphorylase	o Muscle cramps	o Increase CPK, muscle biopsy o Enzyme analysis in muscle tissue o Gene mutation
Tarui disease (GSD VII)	AR	o *PFKM* o Muscle phosphofructo kinase	o Muscle pain o Muscle weakness o Myoglobinuria o Rhabdomyolysis	o Enzyme deficiency in muscles and red blood cells o Gene mutation

CPK—Creatine phosphokinase; LDH—Lactate dehydrogenase

Q 56. Write the management of glycogen storage disorders.

Ans.

GENERAL MANAGEMENT
o Maintain normal blood glucose levels with glucose and uncooked corn-starch in type I and III.
o Avoid fructose and galactose in type 1 GSD.
o Type III, VI, VII: Give high proteins to activate gluconeogenesis and keto diet for better cardiac function and advise minimal exercise.
o Type V: Carbohydrate meals, creatine, vitamin B$_6$ and sucrose before exercise.
o Type VII: No meals before exercise. Statin drugs and anesthesia should be given carefully.
o Low fat intake and medium chain triglyceride should be given.
o Calcium and vitamin D supplementation.
o Clinical and biochemical parameter monitoring.

SPECIFIC MANAGEMENT
o Orthotopic liver transplantation.
o Bone marrow transplantation.
o Specific enzyme replacement therapy (ERT) with recombinant human acid α-glucosidase (alglucosidase-alfa—myozyme or lumizyme) is available for treatment of Pompe disease.
o Vitamin B$_6$ supplementation reduces exercise intolerance and muscle cramps in McArdle syndrome.

FATTY ACID OXIDATION DEFECTS
Sarah Bailur

Q 57. Write a note on classification of fatty acid oxidation defects.

Ans. Classification of fatty acid oxidation defects: In the human body various metabolites like glucose (in brain), fatty acids (in muscles), ketone bodies, lactate and glycerol are used as a source of energy in the various tissues. During prolonged periods of starvation and reduced caloric intake, the fatty acids are used as a fuel by brain, and other main tissues of body like cardiac, hepatic and skeletal muscles. These get metabolized in the mitochondria to produce energy. The defect in the mitochondrial β-oxidation pathway of fatty acids causes fatty acid disorders.

1. **Defects in β-oxidation cycle**
o Medium-chain acyl-coenzyme A dehydrogenase deficiency
o Very-long-chain acyl-coenzyme A dehydrogenase deficiency
o Short-chain acyl-coenzyme A dehydrogenase deficiency
o Long-chain 3-hydroxyacyl-CoA dehydrogenase/mitochondrial trifunctional protein deficiency
o Short-chain 3-hydroxyacyl-coenzyme A dehydrogenase deficiency
2. **Defects in carnitine cycle**
o Plasma membrane carnitine transport defect (primary carnitine deficiency)
o Carnitine palmitoyl transferase-IA deficiency
o Carnitine acylcarnitine translocase deficiency
o Carnitine palmitoyl transferase-II deficiency
3. **Defects in electron transfer pathway**
o Electron transfer flavoprotein and electron transfer flavoprotein dehydrogenase deficiencies (glutaric acidemia type 2, multiple acyl-coenzyme A dehydrogenation defects)
4. **Defects in ketone synthesis pathway**
o β-Hydroxy-β-methylglutaryl-coenzyme A synthase deficiency
o β-Hydroxy-β-methylglutaryl-coenzyme A lyase deficiency
5. **Defects in ketone body utilization**
o Succinyl-coenzyme A: 3-Ketoacid-coenzyme A transferase deficiency
o β-Ketothiolase deficiency

Q 58. Draw the normal fatty acid oxidation pathway.

Ans. The normal fatty acid oxidation pathway. (Figure 18.15)

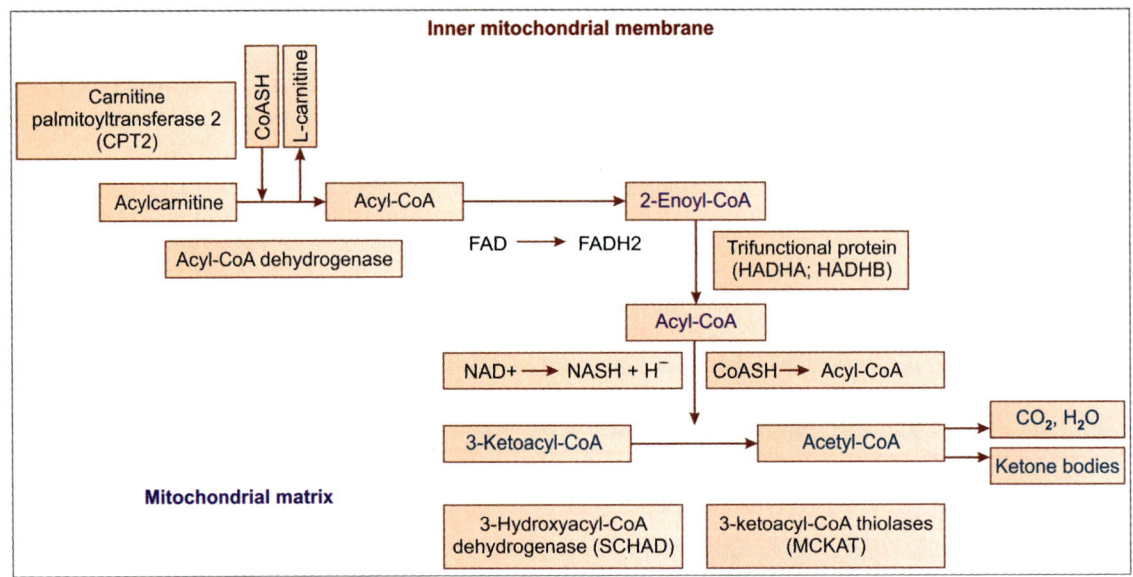

Figure 18.15: : Fatty acid oxidation pathway (FAO)
CPT I—Carnitine palmitoyl transferase I; CPT II—Carnitine palmitoyl transferase II; FADH—Flavin adenine dinucleotide; NADH—Nicotinamide adenine dinucleotide; CoASH—Coenzyme A

Q 59. Write the inheritance, etiology, genetic basis, clinical features and investigation findings of fatty acid disorders.

Ans.

Disorder	Inheritance	Gene, enzyme deficiency	Clinical features	Investigation findings
1. **Fatty acid oxidation defects**				Biochemical and next generation sequencing for gene defects
i. *Medium-chain acyl-coenzyme A dehydrogenase deficiency*	AR	○ *MCAD, ACADM* ○ Medium-chain acyl-coenzyme A dehydrogenase	○ Hypoglycemia ○ Hepatic encephalopathy ○ Unexpected death ○ Pre-eclampsia ○ HELLP syndrome	○ Normal or ↓ free carnitine ○ ↑ plasma acylglycine ○ Plasma C6–C10 free fatty acids ○ ↑ C8–C10 acylcarnitine
ii. *Very long-chain acyl-coenzyme A dehydrogenase deficiency*	AR	○ *VLCAD, ACADVL* ○ Very long-chain acyl-CoA dehydrogenase	○ Dilated cardiomyopathy ○ Arrhythmias ○ Hypoglycemia ○ Fatty liver ○ Late-onset, stress-induced rhabdomyolysis ○ Myopathy	○ Normal or ↓ free carnitine ○ ↑ plasma C14:1, C14 acylcarnitine ○ ↑ plasma C10–C16 free fatty acids

Contd.

Disorder	Inheritance	Gene, enzyme deficiency	Clinical features	Investigation findings
iii. *Short-chain acyl-coenzyme A*	AR	o *SCAD, ACADS* o Short-chain acyl-CoA dehydrogenase	o Clinical phenotype is unclear o Varies from normal to mid to severe signs and symptoms	o Normal or ↓ free carnitine o Elevated urine, ethylmalonic acid o Inconsistently abnormal acylcarnitine profile
iv. *Long-chain 3-hydroxyacyl-CoA*	AR	o *LCHAD, HADH-A* o Long-chain 3-hydroxyacyl-CoA dehydrogenase	o Pre-eclampsia o HELLP syndrome, and AFLP	o Normal or ↓ free carnitine o Increased ratio of acyl-free carnitine o ↑ free fatty acids o ↑ C16-OH and C18- OH carnitines
2. Defects in carnitine cycle				
i. **Carnitine palmitoyl transferase-I**	AR	o *CPT-IA* o Carnitine palmitoyl transferase-I	o Hepatic failure o Renal tubular defects o Sudden death o Pre-eclampsia o HELLP syndrome	o Normal or ↑ free carnitine o Normal acylcarnitines, acylglycine and urine organic acids
ii. **Carnitine palmitoyl transferase-II**	AR	o *CPT-II* o Carnitine palmitoyl transferase-II	o Early and late onset types symptoms of liver, brain, skeletal muscles, cardiac muscles o Cystic kidney o Adult form with acute rhabdomyolysis, myoglobinuria	o Normal or ↓ free carnitine o Abnormal acylcarnitine profile
3. Defects in electron transfer pathway				
ETF dehydrogenase	AR	o ETF-DH o ETF dehydrogenase	o Nonketotic fasting hypoglycemia o Congenital anomalies o Milder forms of liver, cardiac and skeletal muscle disorders	o Normal or ↓ free carnitine o Increased ratio of acyl-free carnitine o ↑ acylcarnitine, urine organic acid and acylglycines
4. Defects in ketone synthesis pathway				
i. **β-Hydroxy-β-methylglutaryl-coenzyme A synthase deficiency**	AR	o *HMGCS2* o β-Hydroxy-β-methylglutaryl-coenzyme A synthase deficiency	o Hypoketosis o Hypoglycemia o Rarely myopathy	o Elevated total plasma fatty acids o Genetic testing is preferred

Contd.

Disorder	Inheritance	Gene, enzyme deficiency	Clinical features	Investigation findings
ii. **β-Hydroxy-β-methylglutaryl-coenzyme A lyase deficiency**	AR	○ HMGCL ○ β-Hydroxy-β-methylglutaryl-coenzyme A lyase deficiency	○ Hypoketosis ○ Hypoglycemia ○ Rarely myopathy	○ Normal free carnitine ○ ↑C5-OH, and methylglutaryl- carnitine ○ Enzymes studies in fibroblasts may be diagnostic

HELLP syndrome: Hemolysis, elevated liver enzymes, low platelet count; AFLP: Acute fatty liver of pregnancy; AR: Autosomal recessive

Q 60. Write the management of fatty acid oxidation defects.

Ans.

MANAGEMENT OF COMMON FATTY ACID OXIDATION DEFECTS

Acute Episode: 10% dextrose and carnitine should be given. Proteins should be avoided.

Chronic management:

1. **Supportive:**
   - ○ Avoid prolonged fasting under any circumstance: Medical procedures, alcohol consumption.
   - ○ Treat infections.
   - ○ Provide caloric support in illness.
   - ○ Avoid prolonged exercise to prevent rhabdomyolysis
   - ○ Hyperhydration, alkalinization, analgesia, rest.

2. **Specific:**
   - ○ Diet: Ratio of medium chain triglycerides to long chain triglycerides varies by condition.
   - i. MCAD: Avoid medium-chain triglycerides (MCT). Rarely supplement uncooked cornstarch at night.
   - ii. VLCAD:
     - ○ Diet very low in long chain fat (10% of calories in severe VLCAD).
     - ○ Sufficient amounts of essential fatty acids.
     - ○ Add MCT 20% of calories, high carbohydrate intake.
   - iii. Supplements:
     - ○ Provide L-carnitine 100 mg/kg/day in acute episodes

   - ○ Riboflavin 100 mg/kg/day to activate the residual enzyme.
   - ○ Ketone bodies in electron transfer pathway defects.

3. **Surveillance:**
   - ○ Monitor cardiac function.
   - ○ Biochemical parameters.

MITOCHONDRIAL DISORDERS
CHAITANYA A. DATAR

Q 61. Write about the clinical features of common mitochondrial disorders.

Ans. Clinical features: Mitochondria vary from 10 to 1000 in each cell carries out the important function of generating energy for respiratory chain complex. So, the clinical features of mitochondrial impairment usually pertain systems with high energy requirement such as brain, muscle and eyes.

Though specific features vary according to the type of disorder, some general features involving multisystem are described in Figure 18.16.

DISEASE ACRONYMS FOR SOME MITOCHONDRIAL DISORDERS ARE SELF-EXPLANATORY OF THE CLINICAL INVOLVEMENT

Disease	Clinical features
Leigh syndrome	○ Early onset ○ Severe neurodegeneration ○ Visual loss ○ Seizure ○ Respiratory problem.

Contd.

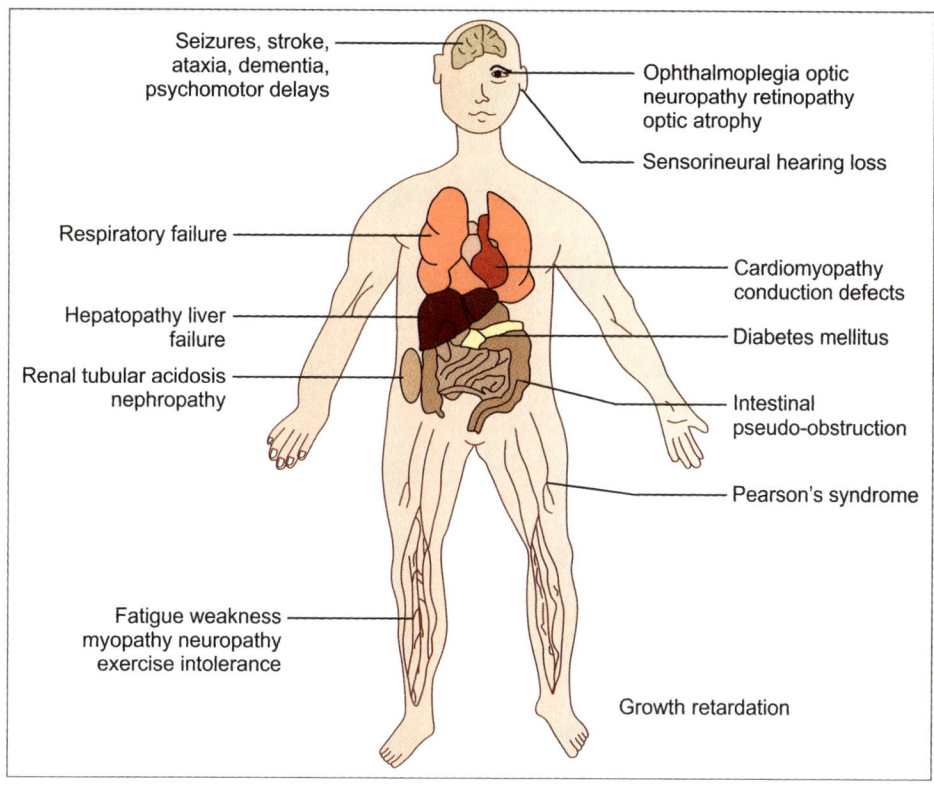

Seizures, stroke, ataxia, dementia, psychomotor delays

Ophthalmoplegia optic neuropathy retinopathy optic atrophy

Sensorineural hearing loss

Respiratory failure

Cardiomyopathy conduction defects

Hepatopathy liver failure

Diabetes mellitus

Renal tubular acidosis nephropathy

Intestinal pseudo-obstruction

Pearson's syndrome

Fatigue weakness myopathy neuropathy exercise intolerance

Growth retardation

Figure 18.16: : Specific features of mitochondrial disorders involving multisystem

DISEASE ACRONYMS FOR SOME MITOCHONDRIAL DISORDERS ARE SELF-EXPLANATORY OF THE CLINICAL INVOLVEMENT *(Contd.)*	
Disease	*Clinical features*
MELAS	o Mitochondrial encephalomyopathy o Lactic acidosis with stroke-like episodes o Diabetes mellitus o Hearing loss.
MERRF	o Mitochondrial encephalo-myopathy with ragged red fibers o Cognition problems o Ataxia o Hearing loss.
MNGIE	o Mitochondrial neurogastro-intestinal encephalomyopathy
NARP	o Neuropathy o Ataxia o Retinitis pigmentosa

CPEO	o Chronic progressive external ophthalmoplegia
LHON	o Leber hereditary optic neuropathy
KSS	o Kearns-Sayre syndrome, myopathy o Cardiomyopathy o Gait problem o Retinitis pigmentosa o Diabetes.
Mitochondrial DNA depletion	o Multiorgan dysfunction: Neuropathy, encephalopathy, myopathy, hepatopathy

Q 62. How will you make a diagnosis of common mitochondrial disorders?

Ans. Diagnosis of mitochondrial disorders is complex: Clinical features with multisystem involvement and with clinical variability among individuals can make the diagnosis challenging. So, there are various investigations to suspect and diagnose mitochondrial disorders:

BASIC BIOCHEMICAL INVESTIGATIONS

1. Complete hemogram, CPK levels, liver function tests, renal function test, serum electrolytes, arterial blood gas.

2. Ophthalmological and hearing assessment.

SPECIFIC BIOCHEMICAL INVESTIGATIONS

1. Lactate, pyruvate and lactate/pyruvate ratio in blood or CSF.

2. New analytes: (Not widely available) FGF21, GDF15, etc.

3. Tandem mass spectrometry: Alanine levels, acylcarnitine and carnitine profile, etc.

4. Urine gas chromatography to detect underlying fatty acid oxidation defects.

5. MR spectroscopy: Lactate peak in the brain.

6. MRI brain to see cerebral, cerebellar, white matter lesions. Basal ganglia and brainstem lesions are common in Leigh disease.

7. ECG, 2D Echocardiography, EEG, EMG/NCV, etc.

8. Muscle biopsy followed by histopathology, immunohistochemistry may be diagnostic in some cases, like ragged red fibers, abnormal segregation of mitochondria, etc.

9. Enzyme studies detect the malfunctioning complex among the respiratory chain.

DEFINITE DIAGNOSIS BY GENE STUDIES

- Exome-based sequencing for the nuclear DNA genes for over 90% mitochondrial disorders.
- If exome-based sequencing does not yield the mutation, the mitochondrial genome may have to be sequenced.
- Specific point mutations in mitochondrial DNA may be tested, e.g. for LHON, MERRF, etc.
- Deletion studies for large deletions of the mitochondrial genome.

Q 63. Write about the inheritance pattern, recurrence risk, genetic counseling, management and prenatal diagnosis for subsequent pregnancy of common mitochondrial disorders.

Ans.

Inheritance patterns	Examples	Mutation status of the gene in proband	Risk of recurrence in subsequent siblings
Mito-chondrial	Leigh syndrome mitochondrial complex deficiencies	~90% disorders occur due to mutations in nuclear genes (autosomal recessive inheritance)	Recurrence in sibs is 25%
	LHON	Only about 10% mitochondrial disorders follow matrilineal inheritance pattern.	Estimating the risks of recurrence for mito-chondrial DNA disorders is complex due to homo-plasmy/ hetero-plasmy.

Genetic counseling: Following all the general principles of counseling and respecting the psychosocial aspects of family, discuss the following with families during counseling:

- Need of genetic testing in the proband and mother, details of the disease like etiology, basic genetics, natural history, prognosis, management options.

- Need to determine the clinical status in the mother (affected/nonaffected/mildly affected) and siblings, to find out the degree of homoplasmy/heteroplasmy in the family, homoplasmy/heteroplasmy concept, inheritance pattern, complexity in estimating the recurrence risk based on the gene involved and clinical variability in future generation and prenatal testing should be explained to the family.

Before prenatal testing, family should be informed regarding:

- Prenatal procedure and prenatal test details.
- Likely benefits of early diagnosis.
- Appropriate support and preparedness if the result returns positive.

Prenatal diagnosis for mitochondrial disorders will not be possible when the mitochondrial diagnosis is confirmed by biochemical/radiological/muscle biopsy techniques.

- Gene-based prenatal testing can be offered for the couple's pregnancy on the chorionic villus sample collected at 12 weeks or amniotic fluid sample collected at 16 weeks of gestation after a gene-based diagnosis in the index child and couple carrier testing is done.
- If the result returns positive, post-test counseling must be carried out to discuss the result and its implications for the family and decision regarding continuation of pregnancy is left on the parents.

PEROXISOMAL DISORDERS
Sarah Bailur

Q 64. Write the inheritance, genetic basis and clinical features of peroxisomal disorders.

Ans. Common peroxisomal disorders: Peroxisome, a subcellular organelle, is present in all cells except mature erythrocytes. All the enzymes in peroxisomes cause incomplete oxidation of very long chain fatty acids which get completed in the mitochondria. The combined incidence of the other peroxisomal disorders is estimated to be 1 in 50,000 live births. They can be caused by mutations in any of the 16 genes involved in peroxisome assembly (PEX gene) and are categorized as:

- **Category I:** Peroxisomal biogenesis disorders (PBDs) where the basic defect is the failure to import 1 or more proteins into the organelle.
- **Category II:** Defects affect a single peroxisomal protein.

Disorder	Inheri-tance	Gene	Clinical features
Zellweger syndrome (ZS)	AR	*PEX 1, 2, 3, 5, 6, 10, 11b, 12, 13, 14, 16, 19, 26.*	- Facial (high forehead, unslanting palpebral fissures, hypoplastic supraorbital ridges, and epicanthal folds) - Brushfield spots - Cataract - Glaucoma - Growth failure - Hypotonia - Neonatal seizures - Infants rarely live more than a few months.
Neonatal ALD (NALD)	AR	*PEX1, 2, 3, 5, 6, 10, 11b, 12, 13, 14, 16, 19, 26*	- Less-prominent craniofacial features - Seizures - Psychomotor developmental delay - Development may regress after 3–5 years of age - Hepatomegaly - Pigmentary degeneration of the retina - Impaired hearing - Adrenocortical function is usually impaired.

Contd.

Disorder	Inheritance	Gene	Clinical Features
Infantile Refsum's disease (IRD)	AR	*PEX1, 2, 3, 5, 6, 10, 11b, 12, 13, 14, 16, 19, 26*	o Ataxia o Impaired cognition o Sensorineural hearing loss and pigmentary degeneration of the retina o Moderately dysmorphic features o Early hypotonia o Hepatomegaly o Arrhythmias o Coarse skin o Small 4th toe
Classic Refsum's disease (CRD)	AR	*PHYH, PEX7*	o Defective enzyme (phytanoyl-CoA oxidase) o Impaired vision from retinitis pigmentosa o Ichthyosis o Peripheral neuropathy o Ataxia and cardiac arrhythmias o Cognitive function is normal. o No congenital malformations. o Manifest during young adulthood.
Rhizomelic chondro-dysplasia puctata (RCDP)	AR	*PEX7*	o Short long bones o Contractures o Facial dysmorphism o Cataract o Developmental delay o Seizure o Growth failure o Congenial heart and kidney diseases.
Adreno-leuko-dystrophy (X-linked)	XLR	o *ABCD1* genecodes for a peroxisomal membrane protein (ALDP, the ALD protein). o Mutation is associated with the accumulation of saturated VLCFAs (very long chain fatty acids) and a progressive dysfunction of the adrenal cortex and central and peripheral nervous system, testes.	o Childhood cerebral form (4–8 yrs) o Adolescent ALD (10–21yrs slower progression) o Adrenomyeloneuropathy (late adolescence or adulthood) o Hyperactivity and impaired scholastic performance o Behaviour problems o Auditory loss o Vision disturbance o Ataxia o Seizures o Progressive paraparesis caused by long tract degeneration in the spinal cord.

Q 65. How will you investigate and manage peroxisomal disorders?

Ans. Basic investigations: Blood count, liver function test, renal function test, vision and hearing assessment, growth and development, neurological assessment.

Specific investigations:

1. Biochemical investigations

Investigation	ZS	NALD	IRD	CRD	ALD	RCDP
Plasma VLCFA: C26:0, C26:1, C24/C22, C26/C22 ratio	Increased	Increased	Increased	Increased	-	-
Plasma phytanic, pristanic, and pipecolic acids	Increased	Increased	Increased	Increased	-	Decreased
Red blood cell levels of plasmalogens	Decreased	Decreased	Decreased	Decreased	-	Decreased
Bile acids in plasma and urine	Increased	-	-	-	-	-
Adrenocorticotrophic hormone	-	-	-	-	Increased	-

2. Enzyme analysis in **fibroblasts.**
3. Magnetic resonance imaging brain
   - **In ZS:** Pachygyria, polymicrogyria and heterotopias
   - **NALD:** Demyelinating changes
   - **ALD:** Cerebral white matter lesions
   - **RCDP:** Cerebellar abnormality
   - **IRD and CRD:** Nerve conduction study and nerve biopsy (onion bulb thickening)
4. **X-ray:** RCDP: Punctate calcification at the proximal ends of long bones.
5. Molecular genetic **testing.**

Management of peroxisomal disorders

I. SUPPORTIVE TREATMENT

1. ZS, NALD, IRD, CRD, ALD, RCDP: Multidisciplinary early intervention, including physical and occupational therapy, hearing aids or cochlear implants, alternative communication, nutrition, and support for the parents.

2. X-linked ALD
   - Baclofen for the treatment of acute episodic painful muscle spasms
   - Soft and pureed foods, most patients eventually require a gastrostomy tube
   - Standard anticonvulsant medications.
   - Hydrocortisone for adrenal insufficiency.

II. SPECIFIC TREATMENT

1. **ZS:**
   - Institution of a phytanic acid-restricted diet can reverse the peripheral neuropathy and prevent the progression of the visual and central nervous system manifestations.
   - Oral bile acids for better liver function.
   - Fat soluble vitamins.
   - Citric acid for renal stones.
   - Docosahexaenoic acid and plasmalogens are under studies for symptomatic improvement.

2. **NALD, IRD and CRD:** Vitamin K, phytanic acid-restricted diet and anti-epilepticus.

3. **X-linked ALD**
   - Bone marrow transplantation
   - **Lorenzo's oil therapy:** Reduces VLCFA levels but no evidence of clinical improvement in symptomatic patients. It can be given to pre-symptomatic patients.

LYSOSOMAL STORAGE DISORDER
Siyaram Didel, Varuna Vyas, Kuldeep Singh

Q 66. Write a short note on epidemiology and pathophysiology of lysosomal storage disorders (LSD).

Ans. Lysosomal storage disorders are group of heterogeneous genetic metabolic disorder with individual incidence ranges from 0.2–1/100000 but all collective incidence ranges from 0–1/10000.

Pathophysiology: Lysosomes are small organelles in the cell which are composed of ATPase proton pump, lysosomal membrane proteins and approximately 50 hydrolytic enzymes acting only at 4.5–5 acidic pH of lysosome, involved in various metabolic pathway of cells. It is involved in disposal of all micro- and macro-molecules of extracellular and intracellular origin like amino acid, carbohydrate, nucleic acids and fatty acids

by various enzymes like glycosidase, lipase nuclease, phosphatase, protease, and sulfatase. Enzymes synthesis happens in the rough endoplasmic reticulum and finally these enzymes reach to lysosome after post-translational modification. The transport of these hydrolases enzymes to lysosome take place by some transporter enzymes (N-acetyl glucosamine 1-phosphotransferase) which are coded by different genes. Mutation in these genes leads to disruption of various lysosomal enzymatic activity (decrease or absent) pathways, causing accumulation of various intermediate toxic metabolites, which are responsible for clinical manifestation (Figure 18.17).

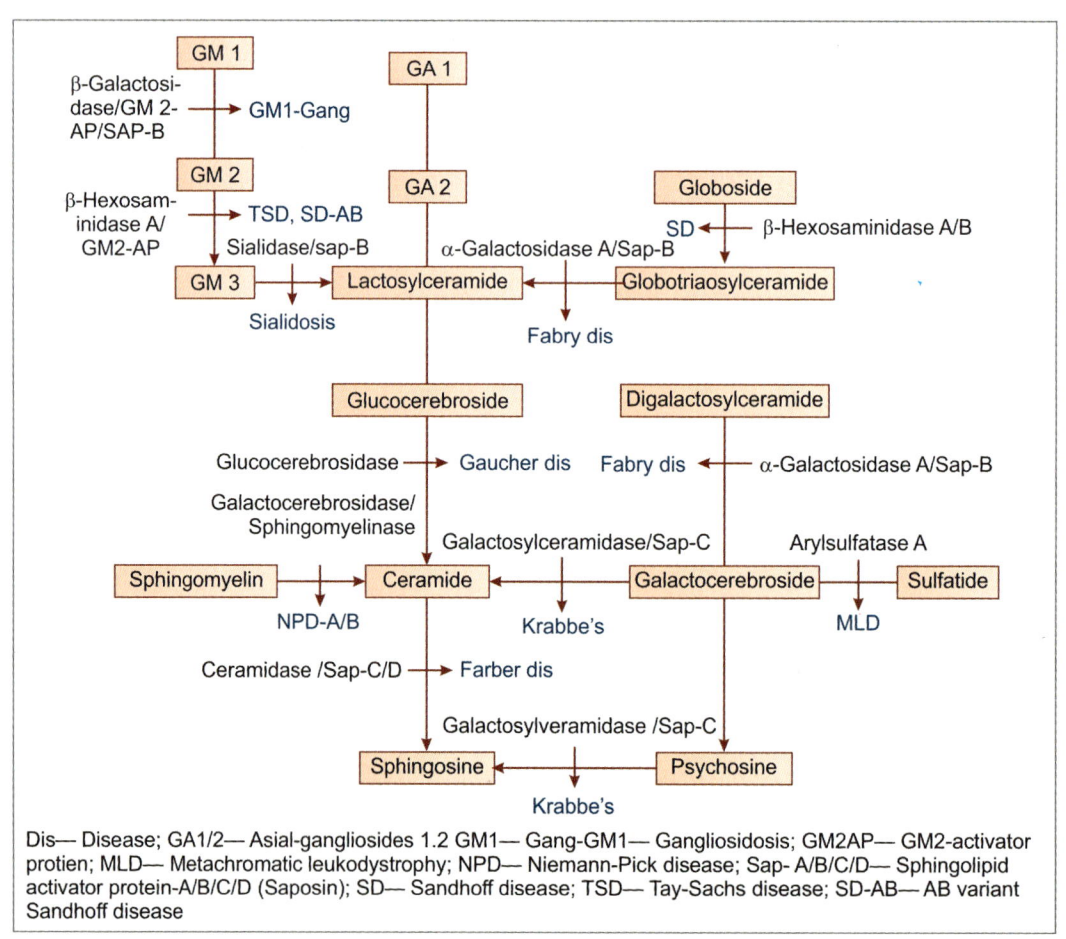

Dis— Disease; GA1/2— Asial-gangliosides 1.2 GM1— Gang-GM1— Gangliosidosis; GM2AP— GM2-activator protien; MLD— Metachromatic leukodystrophy; NPD— Niemann-Pick disease; Sap- A/B/C/D— Sphingolipid activator protein-A/B/C/D (Saposin); SD— Sandhoff disease; TSD— Tay-Sachs disease; SD-AB— AB variant Sandhoff disease

Figure 18.17: Various enzyme defects and affected substrate in different sphingolipidosis

Q 67. Draw a flowchart of organ spectrum in lysosomal storage disorders.
Ans.

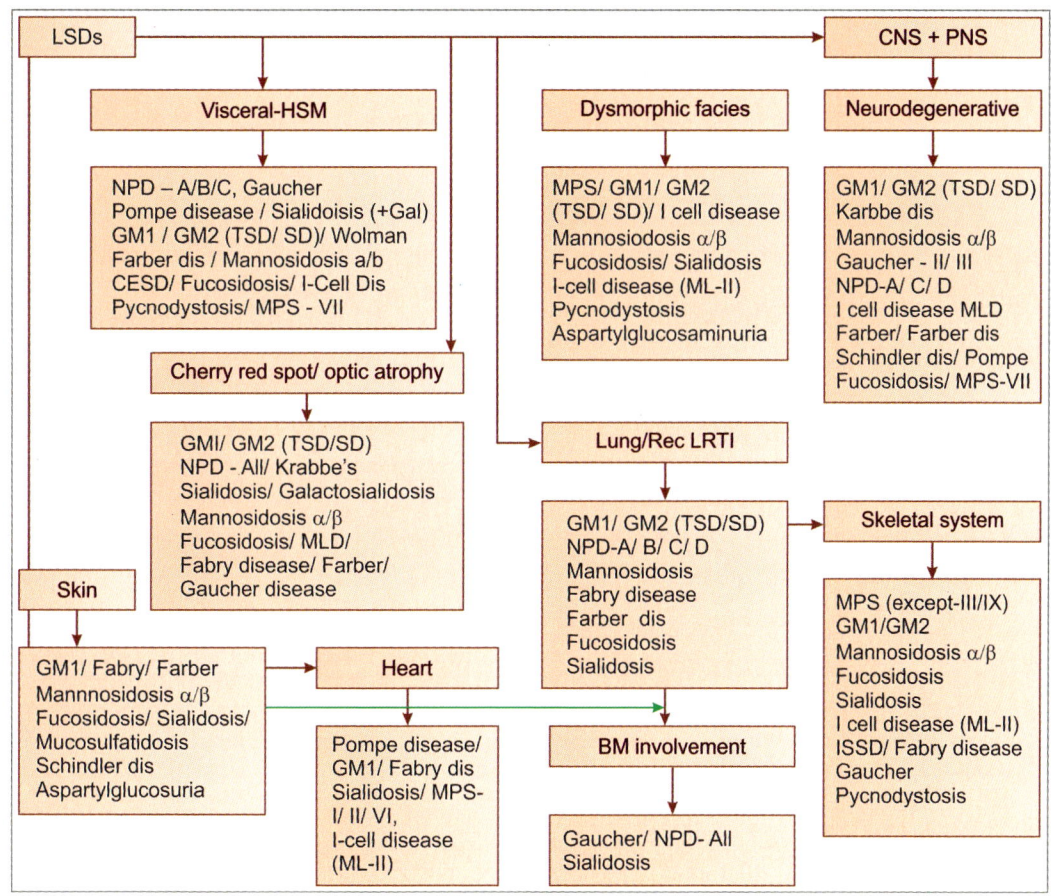

Figure 18.18: Organ spectrum in lysosomal storage disorders (LSD)
MPS—Mucopolysaccharidosis; GSD—Glycogen storage disorder; NCL—Neuronal ceroid lipofuscinosis; CESD—Cholesteryl ester storage disease ML—Mucolipidosis; ISSD—Infantile free sialic acid storage disease; dis—Disease

Q 68. Write the etiology, genetic basis and clinical features of mucopolysaccharidosis.
Ans.

MUCOPOLYSACCHARIDOSIS				
Primary substrate involved	Disorder with major organ involvement	Common types	Defective enzyme/ protein, gene defects	Specific features
Mucopoly-saccharides	Mucopoly—saccharidosis (MPS): All are autosomal recessive (AR) except MPS II.	**MPS-I** (H/S/HS) o Hurler (severe) o Scheie (mild)	o α-L-Iduronidase o *IDUA* gene	o Coarse facial features o Hepatosplenomegaly (HSM) o Hernia o Joint stiffness (arthrogryposis) o Skeletal dysplasia (dysostosis multiplexa)

Contd.

MUCOPOLYSACCHARIDOSIS (Contd.)

Primary substrate involved	Disorder with major organ involvement	Common types	Defective enzyme/ protein, gene defects	Specific features
				o Short stature o Heart disease o Mental retardation (MR) o Hearing loss o Corneal clouding.
	Predominant visceral, X-linked recessive (XLR).	**MPS-II** (Hunter syndrome)	o Iduronate-6-sulfatase o *IDS* gene	o Same as MPS I o No corneal clouding.
		MPS-VI (Maroteaux-lamy)	o N-acetyl galacto-samine 4-sulfatase o *ARSB* gene	o Same as MPS I o No mental retardation.
		MPS-VII (Sly)	o β-glucuronidase o GUSB gene	**Neonatal:** Non-immune hydrops (NIHF) **Infantile/adolescent** with or without o hydrops o cardiomegaly (valvular lesion and cardiomyopathy) o pulmonary insufficiency o obstructive sleep apnea, (similar to I/II with all other common problems of MPS) with variable spectrum.
	Predominant neuronal	**MPS-III** (Sanfilippo syndrome) (4 subtypes)	**A:** Sulphoglucosamine sulphohydrolase, *SGSH* gene	o Type A is most severe form. o Predominant neurological features o Psychomotor retardation o Behavioral problem o Hyperactivity o Seizures o Development delay o Language regression or delay o Sleep disturbance o Hearing and vision loss o Mildly dysmorphic face
			B: N-acetylgluco-saminidase, *NAGLU* gene	
			C: Heparan alpha-glucosaminide N-acetyltransferase, HGSNAT gene	
			D : N-acetylglucosamine -6 sulfatase, HTR3D gene	o Short stature o Skeletal abnormalities. o Cardiorespiratory diseases. o HSM, hernia. o Progress in continuum part of disease in all 4 types. o Average life expectancy 8–10 years.

Contd.

MUCOPOLYSACCHARIDOSIS *(Contd.)*				
Primary substrate involved	*Disorder with major organ involvement*	*Common types*	*Defective enzyme/ protein, gene defects*	*Specific features*
	Predominant Skeletal	**MPS-IV** (Morquio) A/B	○ Acetyl galactosamine 6-sulfatase, β galactosidases ○ *GALNS, GLB1* gene	○ Skeletal abnormalities in hip, knees, ankles and wrist ○ Bell-shaped chest ○ Spine deformity ○ Joint hyperflexibility ○ Coarse characteristic face ○ Cardiorespiratory problems ○ Neurological complication ○ Hearing, vision and dental problems. ○ Normal intelligence.
	Others	**MPS-IX** (Natowicz)	Hyaluronidase (HYAL1)	○ Intermittent painful joint due to nodular soft tissue swelling ○ Dysmorphism ○ Short stature ○ Preserved intelligence.

Q 69. Write the diagnosis and treatment of mucopolysaccharidosis.
Ans.

DIAGNOSIS AND TREATMENT OF MUCOPOLYSACCHARIDOSIS (MPS)				
Disease name	*Screening test*	*Confirmative test*	*Antenatal test*	*Any treatment if available*
MPS-I (H/S/ HS) Hurler (severe)/ Scheie (mild)	○ Urinary GAGs ○ (DS+HS)- I/II ○ DS-VI ○ **Skeletal X-rays:** Thick skull clavarium, bullet shaped metacarpals and phalanges, short iliac bones, oar-shaped ribs, anterior beaking of vertebrae, short ulna, spondyloepiphyseal dysplasia, femoral epiphysis dysplasia.	Enzyme assay in WBC/DBS genetic test.	Enzyme/ genetic test	ERT (laronidase (Aldurazyme)), HSCT
MPS-II (Hunter syndrome)				ERT (Idursulfase (Elap rase))
MPS-VI (Maroteaux- lamy)				ERT galsufase (Naglazyme)
MPS-VII (Sly)	○ Urine GAGs, Oligosaccharides, (HS+DS, CS). ○ PBF for Alder-Reilly granules (Also seen in MPS VI, Multiple sulphate deficiency)			BMT, ERT (r-GUS) with supportive palliative care

Contd.

DIAGNOSIS AND TREATMENT OF MUCOPOLYSACCHARIDOSIS (MPS) (Contd.)

Disease name	Screening test	Confirmative test	Antenatal test	Any treatment if available
MPS-III (Sanfilippo syndrome) (4 subtypes)	o Urinary GAGs (HS) Quantitative and qualitative o Skeletal survey	Enzyme assay inWBC/DBS Genetic test	Enzyme/ genetic test	Supportive/experimental gene/ERT/substrate reduction therapy
MPS-IV (Morquio) A/B	o Urine GAGs (KS) Quantitative and qualitative o Skeletal survey			ERT (elosulfase alfa) for MPS IVA
MPS-IX (Natowicz)	o Urine GAGs (KS) Quantitative and qualitative o Increased plasma hyaluronan			Supportive

GAG—Glycosaminoglycans; ERT—Enzyme replacement therapy; DS—Dermatan sulphate; HS—Heparan sulphate; CS—Chondroitin sulphate; KS—Keratan sulphate; WBC—White blood cell; DBS—Dried blood spot; HSCT—Haematopoietic stem cell therapy.

Q 70. Write the etiology, genetic basis and clinical features of sphingolipids.
Ans.

Primary substrate involved	Major disorders with inheritance pattern	Common types	Defective enzyme/ protein, gene defects	Specific features
Sphingo-lipids	Sphingo-lipidosis, **XLR**	Fabry disease	o α-Galacto-sidase A. o **GLA gene**	Characteristics can be divided into three age groups—up to 16 years, 17–30 years and beyond 30 years as continuum of disease. o **Autonomic nervous system:** Acroparesthesias, peripheral neuropathy, dyshidrosis. o **Skin:** Hypersensitive skin, angiokeratoma o **Eyes:** Corneal verticillata, corneal opacity o **Cardiovascular system:** Transient ischemia, cardiomyopathy, rhythm disorder o **Kidney:** Chronic kidney disease o **Pulmonary** system involvement o Typical facies, deafness o **Skeletal:** Osteopenia and scoliosis o Gastrointestinal problems o Most of these changes occurs due to deposition of fatty material and abnormal proliferation of cells (atypical manifestations: cryptogenic stroke, idiopathic left ventricular hypertrophy).

Contd.

Primary substrate involved	Major disorders with inheritance pattern	Common types	Defective enzyme/ protein, gene defects	Specific features
Sphingo-lipids	Sphingo-lipidosis, AR	**Gangliosi-dosis: GM1** Infantile (Type -1) Juvenile (Type-2) Adult (Type-3)	β-Galactosidase (GM1 ganglio-sides, oligo-saccharides, keratan sulphate (MPS) deposited) ○ *GLB1* gene	○ Heaptosplenomegaly (HSM) ○ Seizures ○ Coarse facial features ○ Dysostosis multiplex ○ Skeletal dysplasia ○ Walking difficulties ○ Angiokeratoma corporis diffusum ○ Mongolian spots ○ Hyperacusis ○ Blindness ○ Cherry red spot ○ Severe neuroregression ○ Recurrent lower respiratory tract infections (LRTI) ○ Cardiac failure (early onset–severe neuroregression, late onset–more affects other systems)
Sphingo-lipids	Sphingo-lipidosis	**GM2** Tay-Sachs/ B1 Variants	β-Hexosami-nidase A ○ *HEXA*	○ Coarse facies ○ Seizures ○ Mental retardation (MR) ○ Cherry red spot ○ Loss of vision ○ Motor deterioration ○ Startle response ○ Recurrent LRTI ○ Myoclonus ○ Rapidly die as per onset of age (onset–infantile/childhood/adulthood)
		Sandhoff/AB variants	β-Hexosami-nidase A/B (total) GM2A	Childhood to adulthood: ○ Neuroregression ○ MR ○ Paralysis ○ Seizures ○ Macrocephaly ○ Myoclonus ○ Doll-like facies ○ Blindness ○ Recurrent LRTI ○ HSM

Contd.

Primary substrate involved	Major disorders with inheritance pattern	Common types	Defective enzyme/ protein, gene defects	Specific features
Sphingo-lipids	Sphingo-lipidosis, AR	**Gaucher Disease Type-1:** Non-neuro-nopathic, most common form (80–90%)	o Acid-α-Gluco-cerebrosidase o GBA gene	o Onset infant to adult o HSM o Hypersplenism o Splenic infarct o Bony pain o Osteopenia o Growth failure o Pubertal delay o Varied severity o Bone marrow (BM) failure (anemia, thrombocytopenia)
		Type-II Acute infantile neuro-nopathic		o Severe neuroregression o MR o Seizures o Spasticity (Gaucher II) o Skeletal changes o Recurrent LRTI o Apnea o HSM (S>H) o Abnormal eye movements o BM failure o Feeding difficulty
		Type-III Chronic neuro-nopathic		o Slow progression o Milder than type-II o Rest is similar
Sphingo-lipids	Sphingo-lipidosis, AR	o Niemann-Pick disease A o (50%)	o Acid sphingo-myelinase (ASM) <5% o SMPD1 gene	o Infantile form—more common in Ashkenazi Jewish, symptomatic by second half of infancy o Neuroregression o Hypotonia o Low platelet o Abnormal lipid profile o Liver function test o Massive HSM (H>S) o Interstitial lung disease o Failure to thrive o Feeding difficulties o Cherry red spot o Die by 3 years of age due to recurrent respiratory tract infections.

Contd.

Primary substrate involved	Major disorders with inheritance pattern	Common types	Defective enzyme/ protein, gene defects	Specific features
		B	○ Acid sphingo-myelinase (ASM) <10% ○ *SMPD1 gene*	**Non-neuronopathic** ○ Juvenile and adult onset ○ Low platelet ○ Abnormal lipid profile ○ Mod-Massive HSM ○ Restrictive lung disease ○ Delayed bone age and puberty ○ Osteopenia and pathological fractures ○ Cherry red spot (25%) ○ Risk of coronary artery disease ○ Severe cases die due to liver failure, splenic rupture and respiratory problem.
		C D	○ Transport protein NPC1 or 2 ○ ***NPC1 gene*** ○ ***NPC2HE1 gene*** (NPC: Dystonic juvenile lipidosis) (NPD: Nova Scotia variant)	○ Hydrops ○ **Neonatal cholestasis** ○ Global developmental delay ○ Ataxia ○ Dystonia ○ Seizures ○ Vertical **supranuclear gaze palsy (VSGP)** ○ Progressive neurodegeneration (death of Purkinje cell) ○ 50% die during early infancy.
Sphingo-lipidosis	Ceramide, AR	Farber lipo-granulo-matosis: 4 types docu-mented, very rare	○ Acid-ceramidase (N-acyl sphingosine amidohydro-lase) ○ *ASAH1 gene*	○ Triad of clinical features include: 　◆ Progressive hoarseness 　◆ Subcutaneous nodules 　◆ Painful joint swelling ○ Lung infiltrate ○ Corneal clouding ○ HSM ○ Histiocytosis mostly fatal except in milder case.
Sphingo-lipidosis	Sulfatides (in oligodendro-cytes of white matter), AR	**Meta-chromatic leukodystro phy (sulfati-dosis)** (Infantile, late infantile, juvenile and adult form).	○ Arylsulfatase A ○ *ARSA* gene in 50% cases or Saposin B in some variants (PSAP gene)	○ Loss of oligodendrocytes and myelin ○ Neuroregression ○ MR ○ Ataxia ○ Spasticity ○ Gait abnormality ○ Seizures ○ Abnormal movement

Contd.

Primary substrate involved	Major disorders with inheritance pattern	Common types	Defective enzyme/protein, gene defects	Specific features
				o Rigidity o Peripheral neuropathy o Psychiatric manifestation o Loss of vision o Feeding difficulty o Heterogeneous course, depend upon age of onset, enzyme level, type of mutation o Death by age of 5 years to survival till adulthood
Sphingo-lipidosis	Sphingo-lipidosis, AR	Krabbe's disease	o Galacto-cerebrosidase (GALC) deficiency o GALC gene	**Infantile type:** o Excessive cry o Difficulty in feeding o Spasticity o Decorticate and opisthotonus posture o Axial hypotonia o Neuroregression o Peripheral neuropathy o Death between 8 months and 9 years **Later onset** o Delayed motor milestone o Behavior problems o Truncal hypotonia o Visual problems o Convulsions o Gait abnormalities o Rest symptoms similar to infantile type

Q 71. Write the diagnosis and treatment of sphingolipids.
Ans:

Disease	Screening test	Confirmative test	Antenatal test	Any treatment if available
Fabry	Tissue biopsy/urinary Gb3 (globotriasylceramide) (but not too specific)	Enzyme level/genetic test (*GLA* mutation)	Enzyme level/genetic study/dried blood spot	o Enzyme replacement therapy (ERT) (fabrazyme) agalsidase-α/β o Supportive care

Contd.

Disease	Screening test	Confirmative test	Antenatal test	Any treatment if available
Ganglio-sidosis: GM1, GM2	○ Urine screening for galactose containing oligosaccharides ○ Complete blood counts (CBC) ○ Vacuolation of lymphocytes. ○ Typical radiology like MPS ○ **Neuroimaging finding:** Grey matter, white matter, thalamus lesions. ○ Spectroscopy shows high N-acetyl aspartate and high myoinositol: creatine ratio.	Enzyme level/ genetic study (*GLB1* mutation)	Enzyme level/genetic study (*GLB1* mutation)	○ Miglustat (butyl-deoxynojirimycin, NB-DNJ) (a substrate inhibitor) may help in slow progression of juvenile/adult GM1. ○ Supportive treatment
Gaucher disease	**Basic investigation:** ○ **Complete hemogram:** Anemia, leukopenia and thrombocytopenia ○ Vitamin D, serum calcium, phosphorus, alkaline phosphate ○ Liver function test, coagulation profile ○ Iron profile ○ Ultrasound of abdomen ○ Cardiac evaluation ○ Radiograph femur (AP view demonstrates an Erlenmeyer flask appearance of the long bones) and spine (lateral view). ○ Bone density scans. ○ **Bone marrow:** Gaucher cells (foam cells/wrinkled tissue paper-large cell with eccentrically located nuclei and vacuolated cytoplasm engorged with gluco-cerebroside) ○ Elevation of serum tartrate resistant acid phosphatase level.	Enzyme level/ genetic study	Enzyme level/genetic study	○ ERT ○ Bone marrow transplantation ○ Substrate reduction therapy (Miglustat for adult) ○ Avoid splenec-tomy
Niemann-Pick disease A	Foam cells "NPD cells"	ASM level in cultural fibroblast of skin or other/*SMPD1* mutation	Enzyme level	No specific therapy, only supportive care (experimental-ERT, BMT, stem cell therapy, gene therapy)
B	**Foam cell and sea blue histiocytes**	Enzyme level/ mutation study		

Contd.

Disease	Screening test	Confirmative test	Antenatal test	Any treatment if available
C D	Skin fibroblast biopsy for cholesterol deposition/BM or liver	Mutation study for *NPC*-1 or *NPC*-2.		Miglustat (an iminosugar) with supportive therapy
Farber lipogranulo-matosis	Visual evoked potential/electro-encephalogram/repeated neuroimaging/tissue biopsy	Enzyme assay in white blood cells (WBC)/ genetic analysis.	Enzyme/ genetic analysis	BMT in experimental phase
MLD (Sulfati-dosis)	○ Urine—metachromatic granules, sulfatide, nerve conduction study ○ Neuroimaging ○ MRS	Enzyme assay in WBC/ *ARSA* gene study.	Enzyme or mutation study	○ Hematopoietic stem cell therapy in experimental phase. ○ Intrathecal enzyme replacement therapy and gene therapy are under trial. ○ No specific treatment, only supportive care.
Krabbe's disease	○ Newborn screening in asymptomatic infants ○ **Cerebrospinal fluid:** Increase protein. ○ **Neuroimaging:** Demyelination, periventricular white matter changes, deep gray matter changes ○ **MRI Spine:** Spinal nerve roots intensification ○ Visual evoked potential ○ Electroencephalogram ○ Brainstem ○ Brainstem evoked response audiometry	Enzyme assay in WBC/ *GALC* gene study.	Enzyme or mutation study	○ Before 6 months supportive and symptomatic treatment. ○ Hematopoietic stem cell therapy in experimental phase (in asymptomatic patient before 30 days of age) ○ Physiotherapy ○ Substrate reduction therapy, enzyme replacement therapy and chaperone are under trial.

Q 72. Write the etiology, genetic basis and clinical features of glycoproteinosis.
Ans.

Primary substrate involved	Major disorder	Common types	Defective enzyme/ protein, gene defects	Specific features
Glyco-proteins	Glyco-proteinosis	Mannosidosis-α I/II (Type III: Very severe, fatal in fetus)	o Acid α-manno-sidase o *MAN2B1*gene	Infantile form—severe form and milder juvenile form. o Neuroregression o Delayed speech o Motor retardation o MR o Skeletal changes o Kyphoscoliosis o Deafness o Ocular abnormality o Coarse facies o Persistent rhinorrhea and recurrent respiratory infections o Hydrocephalus o Spasticity o Hepatomegaly
		Mannosidosis-β	o Acid β-mannosidase o *MANBA* gene	o Same as mannosidosis-α and angiokeratomas o Behavioral problems o Peripheral neuropathy
		Fucosidosis	o α-L-Fucosidase o *FUCA1* gene	o Present in first year of life. o Same as mannosidosis.
		Galactosialidosis	o Cathepsin A (protective protein) o Combined deficiency of neuraminidase-1 (*NEU1*) and β-galactosidase (β-GAL) *CTSA* gene	o Early infantile form: Fetal hydrops. Hurler-like features, bone marrow shows foam cells and vacuolated lymphocytes, sialyloligosacchariduria. o Late infantile form: Juvenile/ adult
		Infantile sialidosis	o α-Neuraminidase o *NEU1* gene	o Hurler syndrome-like features o Cortical blindness o Spasticity o Neuroaxonal dystrophy.
		Pycnodysostosis	o Cathepsin K o *CTSK* gene	o Typical coarse facial features o Skeletal malformation: Osteosclerosis, brittle and fragile bone o Loose joint o Preserved IQ o Blue sclera

Contd.

Primary substrate involved	Major disorder	Common types	Defective enzyme/protein, gene defects	Specific features
				○ HSM and pituitary hypoplasia ○ Can be missed diagnosis as osteopetrosis
		Aspartylgluco-saminuria	○ Aspartyl-glycosamidase (AGU) ○ *AGA* gene	○ Psychomotor retardation ○ Delayed speech ○ Seizures ○ Recurrent fractures ○ Dysmorphic facies and hypermobile joint ○ Recurrent respiratory infections ○ Behavior problems ○ Lung, heart, and blood problems.

Q 73. Write the etiology, genetic basis and clinical features of other lysosomal storage disorders.

Ans.

Primary substrate involved	Major disorder with inheritance pattern	Common types	Defective enzyme/protein, gene defects	Specific features
Glycogen	Glycogen storage disease, AR	GSD-II (Pompe)	○ Acid-α-glucosidase ○ *GAA* gene	○ Varied clinical spectrum ○ Floppy infant ○ Cardiomegaly with life expectancy less than one year to life expectancy up to 60–70 years (other childhood/juvenile/adulthood (acid maltase deficiency) onset).
Combined defect	**Combined metabolites** neuronal ceroid lipofuscinosis	I-cell disease (mucolipidosis II)	○ Multiple enzyme deficiency (transfer protein-UDP-N-acetyl-glucosamine-1-phosphate transferase (GlcNAc-P transferase) activity).	○ **Coarse facial features** ○ Micrognathia, gingival hypertrophy and retroglossia ○ Feeding difficulty ○ Skeletal dysplasia ○ Severe short stature ○ Mental retardation ○ Neuroregression ○ Hernias ○ Sleep disorders ○ Cardiorespiratory problems

Contd.

Primary substrate involved	Major disorder with inheritance pattern	Common types	Defective enzyme/protein, gene defects	Specific features
			○ *GNPTAB* gene	○ Average life expectancy up to 7 years ○ Similar to Hurler but more severe
		Multiple sulfatase deficiency (Austin's disease/mucosulfatidosis) Other types: Late infantile and juvenile	Formylglycine–generating enzyme (FGE), SUMF1 gene	○ Onset 1–2 years of age ○ Typical skin, ichthyosis, dry skin ○ Mental retardation ○ Global developmental disorder ○ Deafness ○ Coarse facies ○ Organomegaly ○ Skeletal changes
		Neuronal ceroid lipofuscinosis (NCL-1, 14 types in total reported till now) four common form described—infantile, late infantile, juvenile and adult onset NCL	○ Multiple genes. ○ Ceroid lipofuscinosis neuronal protein	○ Varied phenotypic features ○ Myoclonic type of epilepsy ○ Progressive neurodegeneration ○ Behavioral problems ○ Psychomotor delay and ultimately death
Miscella-neous	---	Wolman disease (severest form)	○ Lysosomal acid lipase (LAL/LIPA) ○ LIPA gene	○ Abdomen distension ○ Hepatosplenomegaly ○ Forceful vomiting ○ Liver fibrosis ○ Malabsorption ○ Adrenal gland calcification ○ Atherosclerosis ○ Failure to thrive and even death
		Cystinosis	○ Cystinosin deficiency (transport protein) ○ CTNS gene (17p13)	○ Clinical features depend upon age of onset, have various form like nephropathic (infantile form) present like Fanconi syndrome. ○ Other intermediate and non-nephropathic cystinosis. ○ Adult/ocular or benign form

Q 74. Write the diagnosis and treatment of other lysosomal storage disorders.
Ans.

Disease	Screening test	Confirmative test	Antenatal test	Any treatment if available
GSD-II (Pompe)	Glucose 4 in urine, serum creatinine kinase, lactate dehydrogenase, liver function test	Enzyme assay/ mutation study	Enzyme assay/ mutation study	ERT rh-acid-α-glucosidase (Genozyme/ Myozyme)
I-cell disease (ML-II)	UDP-N-acetyl-glucosamine-1-phosphotransferase enzyme level in WBC (decreased) or in cultured fibroblasts (increase)	GNPTAB gene mutation (UDP-N-acetyl-glucoseamine-1-phospho-transferase)	Enzyme level or mutation study	No specific treatment and supportive care only
Multiple sulfatase deficiency (Austin's disease/ mucosulfatidosis)	Urine GAGs level	Enzyme assay/ genetic mutation	Enzyme assay/genetic mutation study	Supportive therapy
NCL-1 (total of 14 types reported till now)	Clinical features, skin biopsy, electro-encephalogram, neuroimaging.	Enzyme assay/ genetic mutation study	Enzyme assay/genetic mutation study	Symptomatic treatment
Wolman disease	Clinical features, abnormal lipid profile	Enzyme assay/ genetic mutation study	Enzyme assay/genetic mutation study	○ Kanuma (sebelipase alfa) and symptomatic ○ Diet low in cholesterol and cholesterol lowering drugs, mineralocorticoids and corticos-teroids, hemato-poietic stem cell therapy ○ Liver transplan-tation
Cystinosis	Urine for Fanconi syndrome/corneal crystal on slit lamp		Cystinosin level in serum/ mutation study	○ Symptomatic and supportive, cystine depleting treatment.

Q 75. Draw a flowchart to diagnose various lysosomal disorders.
Ans.

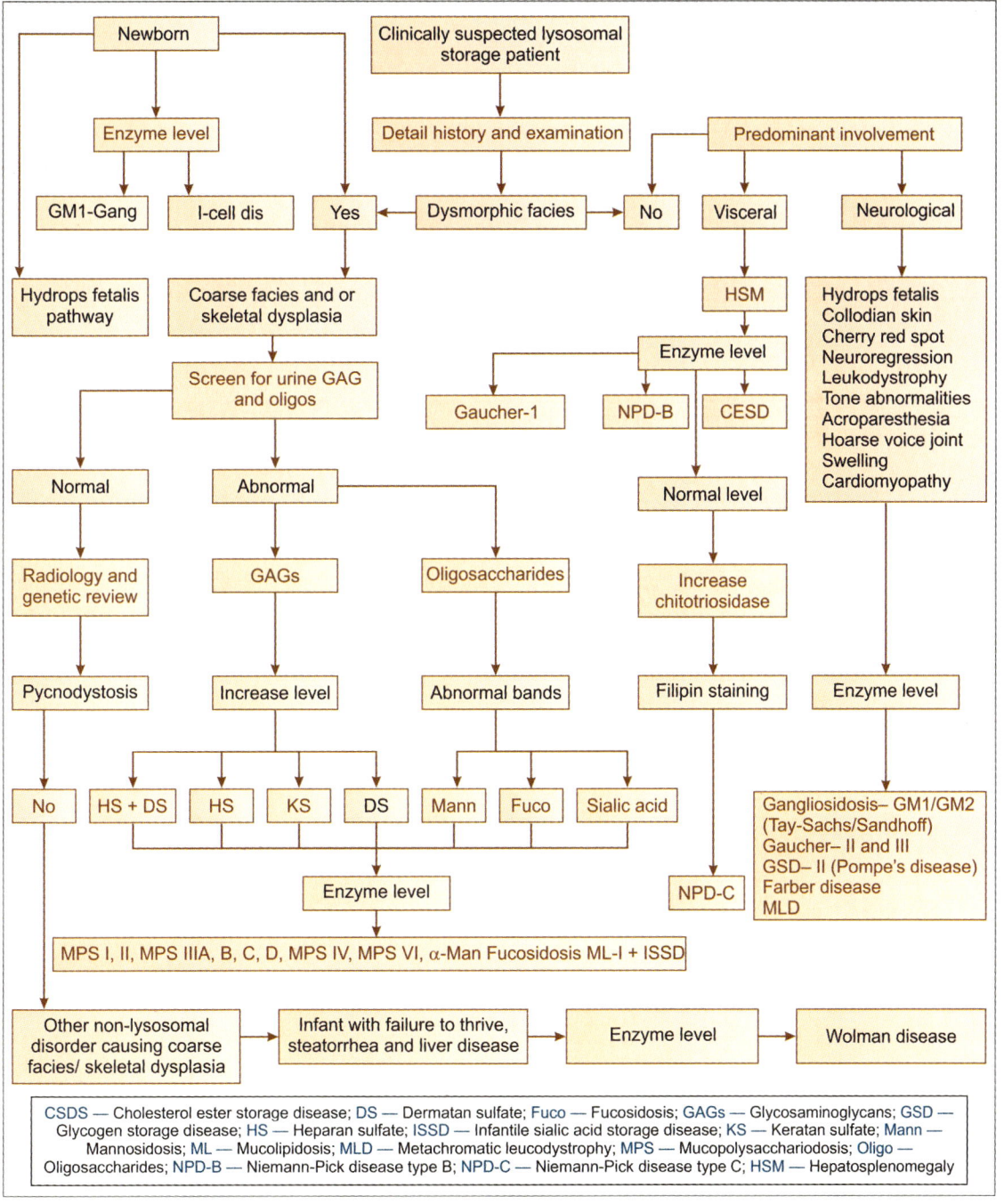

Figure 18.19: How to diagnose a suspected lysosomal storage patient?

Q 76. Write a short note about genetic counseling of a couple during their antenatal visit to you with family history of one affected child with lysosomal storage disorder (LSD).

Ans. LSDs are genetic disorders and inherited as autosomal recessive or X-linked recessive (Hunter syndrome and Fabry disease). These disorders may be inherited or due to *de novo* mutation in the indexed case. With confirming genetic diagnosis, parents can be counseled appropriately about details of the disease, prognosis, treatment option, prenatal diagnosis and pregnancy termination option if they want. Every effort must be done to confirm the diagnosis of indexed case and to counsel the parents about need of antenatal diagnosis for target mutation during future pregnancy for confirmation of affected pregnancy.

BIBLIOGRAPHY

1. Emery and Rimoin's Principles and Practice of Medical Genetics, 7th ed.
2. Fernandes J, Saudubray J, Berghe G., Inborn metabolic diseases, 5th edition, Germany, Springer, 2011.
3. Häberle J, Rubio V. Disorders of the Urea Cycle and Related Enzymes. In: J-M Saudubray, et al. eds. Inborn Metabolic Diseases, 6th Ed. Berlin Heidelberg: Springer-Verlag; 2016. p. 297–308.
4. Narayanan MP. "Lysosomal Storage Disorders: An Indian Perspective". Acta Scientific Pediatrics 3.2 (2020): 1–4.
5. Shchelochkov OA, Venditti CP. In: Kliegman RM, editor. Nelson Textbook of Pediatrics, 21st Ed. Philadelphia: Elsevier; 2020. p. 3128–3314.

Primary Immunodeficiency Disorders

Soma Santosh Kumar

Q 1. What are the hallmarks of primary immunodeficiency disorders (PID)?

Ans. Primary immunodeficiency disorders are a group of heterogenous inherited disorders that result from defect in immune system development and/or function resulting in a poor protective immune response. **The hallmarks of PID are:**

➽ Recurrent infections
➽ Development of autoimmunity
➽ Susceptibility to develop malignancies.

Q 2. What are the warning signs for suspecting PID?

Ans. Recurrent infections are the predominant clinical manifestation in patients. European Society of Immunodeficiencies has suggested 10 warning signs for suspicion of PID.

1. Four or more ear infections in one year.
2. Two or more serious sinus infections within a year.
3. Two or more months on antibiotics with little effect.
4. Two or more pneumonias within a year.
5. Failure to thrive.
6. Recurrent skin or organ abscesses.
7. Persistent oral thrush or elsewhere for one year.
8. Need for intravenous antibiotics for infections.
9. Two or more deep seated infections.
10. Family history of PID.

Q 3. How do you classify PID?

Ans. Primary immunodeficiencies can be classified as follows:

1. Cellular and humoral immunodeficiency.
2. Combined immunodeficiencies associated with syndromic features.
3. Mainly humoral deficiencies.
4. Disorders related to unregulated immune system.
5. Congenital abnormal phagocyte number, function or both.
6. Intrinsic and innate immunity disorders.
7. Autoinflammatory diseases.
8. Complement deficiencies.
9. Phenocopies of PID.

Q 4. Write the genetic basis of different primary immunodeficiency disorders.

Ans. Genetic basis of primary immunodeficiency disorders:

Category	Disorders	Genetic defect
Cellular and humoral immunodeficiency	○ Severe combined immunodeficiency (SCID) ○ Combined immunodeficiencies less severe than SCID-MHC I, II deficiency	○ T-B+:*IL2RG* (XL), *Jak3* (AR), *IL-7Rα* (AR), ○ T-B-:*ADA* (AR), *RAG1* (AR) ○ *MHCII*, *MAGT1V* (AR)

Contd.

Category	Disorders	Genetic defect
Combined immunodeficiencies associated with syndromic features	o Wiskott-Aldrich syndrome o Ataxia telangiectasia o DiGeorge syndrome o Hyper-IgE syndrome	o *WASP* (XL) o *ATM* (AR) o *TBX1* (AD) o *DOCK8* (AR)
Mainly humoral deficiencies	o X-linked agammaglobulinemia o Common variable immunodeficiency o Hyper-IgM deficiency o Selective IgA deficiency	o *Btk* (XL) o *ICOS, SH2DIA, DNMT3B* o *NEMO* (XL), *CD40* (AR, XL) o *CD79A* (AR)
Disorders of unregulated immune system	o Chediak-Higashi syndrome o Griscelli syndrome 2 o Familial HLH	o *LYST* (AR) o *RAB27A* (AR) o *PRF1, STX11* (AR)
Congenital abnormal phagocyte number, function or both	o Leukocyte adhesion defects o Shwachman-Diamond syndrome o Chronic granulomatous disease o Congenital neutropenia o Myeloperoxidase deficiency	o *LFA-1* (AR), *Mac-1, SBDS* (AR) o *CYBB, NCF1* (AR) o *G6PC3* (AR), *ELANE* (AD) o *MPO* (AR)
Intrinsic and innate immunity disorders	o Predisposition to invasive bacterial and viral infection. o Predisposition to parasitic and fungal infection o Mendelian susceptibility to myco-bacterial disease	o *TIRAP, IRAK4* (bacterial) (AR) o *UNC93B1, STAT1, IRF7* (viral) (AR) o *STAT1* (AR), *GOF* (AD) o *IFNGR1, IFNGR2* (AR)
Autoinflammatory disorders	o Familial Mediterranean fever o Muckle-Wells syndrome	o *MEFV* (AR, AD) o *NLPR3* (AD)
Complement deficiencies	o Deficiency of classical and lectin pathway components o Deficiency of alternate pathway components	o C1–9 gene defects, *MBL, MASP2* (AR)
Phenocopies of PID	o Cryopyrinopathy o Pulmonary alveolar proteinosis o Acquired angioedema	o *NLPR3* (AD) o Autoantibody to *GMCSF* (AD, AR, XLR) o Autoantibody to *C1* inhibitor (AD)

MHC—Major histocompatibility complex; HLH—Hemophagocytic lymphohistiocytosis; AR—Autosomal recessive; AD—Autosomal dominant; XLR—X-linked recessive

Q 5. What are the clinical manifestations of PID?

Ans. The clinical manifestations of **PID**:

	B cell deficiency	T cell deficiency	Complement deficiency	Phagocyte defects
Age of presentation	5–6 months after maternal transmitted immunoglobulins diminish	First 3 months of life	Any age	Early onset; usually first 3 months

Contd.

	B cell deficiency	T cell deficiency	Complement deficiency	Phagocyte defects
Microbial pattern	o Pneumococcus o H. influenzae o S. aureus o Enterovirus o Giardia	o Mycobacteria o CMV o EBV o RSV o VZV o Candida o P. jirovecii	o Pneumococcus o Neisseria	o Staphylococci o Klebsiella o Pseudomonas o Salmonella o Candida o Nocardia o Aspergillus o Serratia o Burkholderia
Clinical features	o Recurrent sinopulmonary infections o GI infections o Sepsis o Meningitis	o Failure to thrive o Gastroenteritis o Mucocutaneous candidiasis	o Recurrent skin, liver and lung abscesses o Cellulitis o Lymphadenitis o Mouth ulcers and gingivitis	o Recurrent meningitis o Systemic bacterial infections
Other features	o Autoimmunity o Lymphomas o Thymoma o Post-vaccination paralytic polio	o GVHD o Post-vaccination disseminated BCG	o Autoimmune disorders: SLE, vasculitis o Glomerulonephritis o Angioedema	o Prolonged attachment of umbilical cord o Poor wound healing

CMV—Cytomegalovirus; EBV—Epstein-Barr virus; RSV—Respiratory syncytial virus; VZV—Varicella zoster virus; GVHD—Graft versus host reaction; SLE—Systemic lupus erythematosus, BCG—Bacillus Calmette-Guérin

Q 6. Write the clinical features of most common PID.

Ans. Clinical features of most common PID disorders are mentioned below.

Category	Disease	Clinical features
Cellular and humoral immunodeficiency	SCID	o Presents in early infancy in first few months. o Recurrent diarrhea, pneumonia, otitis media, skin infections and sepsis. o Growth failure once infections sets in.
Combined immuno-deficiencies associated with syndromic features	Wiskott-Aldrich syndrome	o X-linked recessive o Recurrent eczema, thrombocytopenia (small defective platelets) leading to prolonged bleeding from wounds, recurrent infections.
	Ataxia telangiectasia	o Oculocutaneous telangiectasias that begin by 3–6 years o Chronic sinopulmonary infections o Progressive cerebellar ataxia o Increased risk of lymphoreticular malignancies.
	DiGeorge syndrome	o Dysmorphogenesis of 3rd and 4th pharyngeal pouches o Thymus hypoplasia/aplasia o Hypocalcemic seizures o Right-sided aortic arch

Contd.

Category	Disease	Clinical features
		○ Esophageal atresia ○ Conotruncal heart disease, hypertelorism, antimongoloid slant, mandibular hypoplasia, low set ears.
	Hyper-IgE syndrome (Job's syndrome)	○ Dermatological, respiratory, fungal infections ○ Dysmorphic face, dental, eye and skeletal abnormalities.
Mainly humoral deficiencies	X-linked/Bruton agammaglo-bulinemia	○ Defect in B-lymphocyte development, present after 6–9 months ○ Absent circulating B cells ○ Small to absent tonsils ○ No palpable lymph nodes ○ Recurrent sinopulmonary infections, commonly acquire infections with extracellular pyogenic organisms.
	Common variable immuno-deficiency	○ Hypogammaglobulinemia with phenotypically normal B cells ○ Normal tonsils ○ Recurrent sinopulmonary infections ○ Associated with sprue-like enteropathy, alopecia areata, hemolytic anemia, pernicious anemia, non-caseating sarcoid granulomas of lung and spleen.
	Selective IgA deficiency	○ Most common immunodeficiency ○ Recurrent respiratory, genitourinary and gastrointestinal infections ○ Intestinal giardiasis ○ Autoimmune diseases and malignancies.
Disorders of unregulated immune system	Chédiak-Higashi syndrome	○ Partial oculocutaneous albinism, silvery hair, solar sensitivity and photophobia ○ Mild bleeding diathesis ○ Peripheral neuropathy ○ Recurrent infection ○ Prone for HLH ○ Granules noted in nucleated cells on peripheral smear.
Congenital abnormal phagocyte number, function or both	Leukocyte adhesion defects	○ Recurrent bacterial infections ○ Delayed separation of umbilical cord, infection of cord stump ○ Gingivitis, periodontitis, typical signs of inflammation are absent, pus does not form, neutrophilic leukocytosis (>25,000 cells/mm^3)
	Shwachman-Diamond syndrome	○ Exocrine pancreatic insufficiency ○ Pancytopenia ○ Short stature ○ Metaphyseal dysplasia ○ Long bones tubulation ○ Short ribs.

Contd.

Category	Disease	Clinical features
	Chronic granulomatous disease	o Recurrent infections with catalase positive organisms o Recurrent pneumonia o Lymphadenitis o Hepatic abscesses o Granuloma formation being hallmark o Esophageal dysmotility o Pyloric outlet narrowing.
	Neutropenia	o Absolute neutrophil count <500 cells/mm^3 o Bacterial, viral infections o Mouth ulcers o Decrease in all cell lines and immunoglobulins o Liver dysfunction o Seizures.
SCID—Severe combined immunodeficiency; HLH—Hemophagocytic lymphohistiocytosis		

Q 7. How do we diagnose PID?

Ans. Diagnosis of PID can be made by:

➲ Clinical presentation

➲ Initial laboratory evaluation: A wide array of assay is available for evaluation of immune system.

The most useful first-line investigations include:

Investigation	Disease
Complete blood count	
Neutropenia	o Cyclical neutropenia o Kostmann syndrome
Lymphopenia	o Severe combined immunodeficiency o Wiskott-Aldrich syndrome o DiGeorge syndrome o Normal absolute lymphocyte count rules out T cell deficiency
Eosinophilia	o Hereditary angioedema o Hyper-IgE syndrome o Omenn syndrome
Thrombocytopenia	o Wiskott-Aldrich syndrome
Erythrocyte sedimentation rate	o Normal result indicates chronic bacterial or fungal infection unlikely
Peripheral smear	
Howell-Jolly bodies	o Asplenia
Neutrophils with large cytoplasmic granules	o Chédiak-Higashi syndrome
Absent granules in neutrophils	o Congenital specific granule deficiency

SCREENING AND ADVANCED TESTS

Type of deficiencies	Screening tests	Advanced tests
B cell deficiency	o Immunoglobulin levels of IgG, IgM, IgE, IgA o Specific antibody response: Measuring antibody titre to common vaccines such as protein (diphtheria, TT) and polysaccharide (Pneumococcus) antigens.	Flow cytometry: o Enumerate different lymphocyte subsets o B cell enumeration (CD19, CD20, CD21) o Brutons tyrosine kinase expression on monocytes (Btk) o Advanced B-cell phenotyping
T cell deficiency	o Absolute lymphocyte count: Compare with age-specific reference values o Delayed type of hypersensitivity (DTH) testing o HIV testing o Assessment of thymus	o Lymphocyte subset enumeration in peripheral blood (T, B and NK cells) o Functional assessment of T cells by proliferative responses to mitogens such as phytohemagglutinin (PHA), antigens and allogenic cells o HLA typing o Flow cytometry: CD132, CD154 estimation o Enzyme assays: ADA, PNP
Neutrophil and phagocyte deficiency	o WBC count, differential count, morphology o Estimation of absolute neutrophil count o Nitroblue tetrazolium reduction test (NBT)	o Flow cytometry: CD11, CD18, CD15 for LAD o Dihydrorhodamine assay for diagnosis of CGD o Enzyme assays (MPO, G6PD, NADPH oxidase) o Mutational analysis
Complement defects	o C3, C4 levels o CH50 activity	o Component assays o C3a, C4a, C5a activation assays

ADA—Adenosine deaminase; PNP—Purine nucleoside phosphorylase; LAD—Leukocyte adhesion defects; CGD—Chronic granulomatous disease; MPO—Myeloperoxidase; G6PD—Glucose-6-phosphate dehydrogenase; NADPH—Nicotinamide adenine dinucleotide phosphate; CGD—Chronic granulomatous disease; HLA—Human leucocyte antigen

Q 8. How will you manage PID?

Ans. Management of PID differs across the spectrum of severity and depends largely on the specific defect in question. Accurate diagnosis is essential for proper management, targeted pharmacotherapy and biologic use, and consideration of curative therapies such as bone marrow transplantation or gene therapy.

Management of antibody deficiencies:

A. **Intravenous immunoglobulins (IVIG):**
   - It contains pooled immunoglobulins (IgG) from over thousands of plasma donors.

   - *Dose*: 400 mg/kg every 28 days.

Indications:
   - X-linked agammaglobulinemia
   - Severe combined immunodeficiency
   - Common variable immunodeficiency (CVID)
   - Wiskott-Aldrich syndrome (WAS)
   - Hyper-IgE syndrome

B. **Supportive therapy:**
   - *Prophylactic antibiotics:* Antibody prophylaxis is standard of care in PID.
     - Use of prophylactic antimicrobials is intended to reduce the frequency and

severity of sinopulmonary infections caused by common bacteria.

- Antiviral and antifungal treatments may be necessary disorders.
  - *Pneumocystis carinii pneumonia*: Cotrimoxazole at 5 mg/kg/day of trimethoprim alternate day in a week
  - *Candida—oral thrush*: Fluconazole at 6 mg/kg/day
  - *Aspergillus:* Itraconazole 5 mg/kg/day once a day

  ꙮ *Diet:*
  - Low bacterial diet prevents diarrhea and sepsis.
  - Use of tap water for mouth care must be avoided to prevent risk of cryptosporidium diarrhea.
  - Hypoallergenic formula like soya-based diet will help prevent failure to thrive or loose tools.
  - Avoid salads and fresh fruits in children with neutrophil dysfunction.
  - Avoid canned foods.

C. **Treatment of infections:** Bacterial infections are the most common ones. Source of infection is usually child's own body.
  - ꙮ Streptococcus from throat, Staphylococci from nostrils and gram-negative bacteria from GIT are commonly seen and need to be treated with appropriate antibiotics based on local antibiotic policy.
  - ꙮ *Complement deficiency:* Children with complement deficiency needs penicillin or cephalosporins when they present with fever.
  - ꙮ *SCID:* Children are prone for CMV, pneumocystis, disseminated BCG infection. Ganciclovir, high dose cotrimoxazole or antitubercular drugs will help the child.

D. **Definitive therapy:** Hematopoietic stem cell transplantation is the only curative option for children with immunodeficiency. HSCT aims to give stable donor stem cell engraftment to help regain full immune system.

a. *Hematopoietic stem cell transplant (HSCT):* Early diagnosis and management are important factors influencing outcome of HSCT.
  - ꙮ *Indications:*
    1. *SCID*: Severe combined immunodeficiency
    2. Phagocytic cell disorders: CGD, LAD
    3. *T Cell immunodeficiency:* CD40 ligand deficiency, Wiskott-Aldrich syndrome, X-linked lymphoproliferative disorder.
    4. *Severe immune dysregulation:* Familial HLH, Chédiak-Higashi syndrome, Griscelli syndrome.
  - ꙮ *Complications of HSCT*:
    - *Infections:* Viral, bacterial, fungal or parasitic.
    - *Acute GVHD:* It occurs due to immune system of donor reacting against recipient tissues like skin, liver and GIT manifesting as rashes, jaundice and diarrhea.
    - *Chronic GVHD:* It occurs after 100 days. It manifests as dry skin patches, dry oral mucosal lesions, diarrhea and malabsorption.
    - *Sinusoidal obstruction syndrome:* It occurs due to fibrosis of smaller blood vessels in liver and manifests as jaundice, weight gain, and abdominal distention.
    - *Graft rejection*
    - *Thrombotic microangiopathy:* It manifests as anemia, thrombocytopenia and renal failure

b. *Gene therapy* is feasible and effective in severe forms of PID that are limited to hematopoietic cell lineages.
  - ꙮ *Indications:*
    - SCID
    - Wiskott-Aldrich syndrome
    - Chronic granulomatous disease

c. *Enzyme replacement:*
  - ꙮ Adenosine deaminase (ADA)

deficiency accounts for 20% children with SCID and can be treated via enzyme replacement with recombinant ADA stabilized with polyethylene glycol (PEG-ADA) which is administered once a week. The disadvantage is huge cost and requirement of lifelong infusions.

- ○ Rare defects in B_{12}/folate intracellular metabolism associated with combined immunodeficiency needs to be treated with lifelong B_{12} or folate supplementation therapy.

d. *Thymic transplantation:* Transplantation of thymic tissue has been successfully performed in children with DiGeorge syndrome.

BIBLIOGRAPHY

1. Buckley RH. Evaluation of suspected immuno-deficiency. In: Kliegman, Stanton, St Geme, (eds). Nelson textbook of pediatrics, 1st South Asian edition, Vol 1, New Delhi:Elseiver: 2016. p.999–1005.

2. Manisha M. PG Textbook of pediatrics: Primary immunodeficiency disorders, Vol 1, 1st edition, Delhi, Jaypee Brothers Medical Publishers (P) Ltd.:2015.p.170–177.

Reproductive Genetics

Seema Thakur

Q 1. What are the various common fetal abnormalities found on prenatal ultrasound (USG)?

Ans. Fetal abnormalities on prenatal ultrasound are seen in 5–10% of cases during antenatal period. These can be isolated or multiple and can happen either due to various genetic or non-genetic causes. These include:

- Major anomalies
- Minor malformations
- Soft markers
- Abnormalities of fetal growth (small fetus in Russell-Silver or Smith-Lemli-Opitz syndrome)
- Fetal macrosomia in Beckwith-Wiedemann syndrome
- Amniotic fluid abnormalities (polyhydramnios in Bartter syndrome or oligohydramnios in renal diseases).

VARIOUS TYPES OF COMMON MAJOR AND MINOR FETAL ANOMALIES

Anomaly	Etiology
Ventriculomegaly isolated (Figure 20.1) or associated (neural tube defect NTD, cardiac defects)	Infections, chromosomal (10% trisomy 13,21) or single gene disorders (Lissencephaly or X-linked aqueductal stenosis, Meckel-Gruber syndrome)
Neural tube defects: isolated (Figure 20.2) or associated	Folic acid deficiency, maternal diabetes, Meckel-Gruber syndrome trisomy13,18
Dandy-Walker anomaly	Trisomy, Meckel-Gruber syndrome, orofacial digital syndrome
Congenital diaphragmatic hernia	Trisomy 18,13, Tetrasomy 12p, Donnai-Barrow syndrome, Fryns syndrome.
Cardiac malformations—isolated or associated	Acquired, Down syndrome, Noonan syndrome.
Cleft lip and palate (multifactorial)	Acquired, Trisomy 13, DiGeorge syndrome, Stickler syndrome.
Club foot	Acquired, aneuploidies, skeletal dysplasias.
Multicystic kidney disease	Trisomy 13, Meckel-Gruber syndrome.
Cystic hygroma (Figure 20.3)	Turner syndrome in 50% cases, Down syndrome, Noonan syndrome, multiple-pterygium syndrome, Fryns syndrome, skeletal dysplasia.
Arthrogryposis	Trisomy 18, connective tissue disorder, skeletal dysplasia.

Radial ray defects	Trisomy 18, TAR syndrome, Fanconi syndrome, VACTERL.
Overlapping of fingers	Trisomy 18, distal arthrogryposis
Hydrops fetalis	Blood group incompatibility, intrauterine infections, aneuploidies, Noonan syndrome, cardiac malformations, alpha thalassemia, lysosomal storage disorders, etc.
Preauricular tag	Isolated or as a syndrome like Goldenhar syndrome, first

	and second branchial arch syndrome.
Polydactyly	Isolated or part of the syndrome like Trisomy 13, Pallister-Hall syndrome, orofaciodigital syndrome.
Sandal gap	Isolated or associated syndrome like Down syndrome.
Simian crease	Isolated or Down syndrome, Patau syndrome, Noonan syndrome, etc.

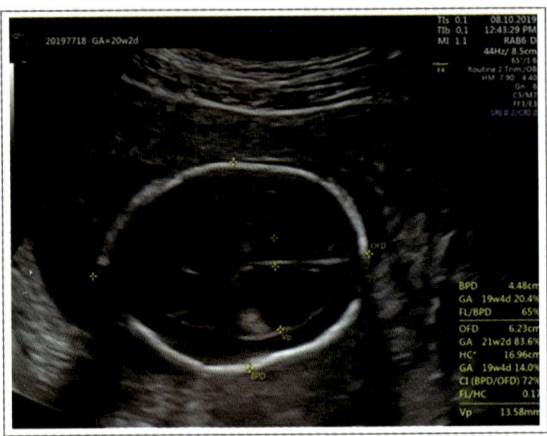

Figure 20.1: Ventriculomegaly in a fetus with NTD (*Courtesy*: Dr Rachna Gupta, Sunheri Devi Hospital)

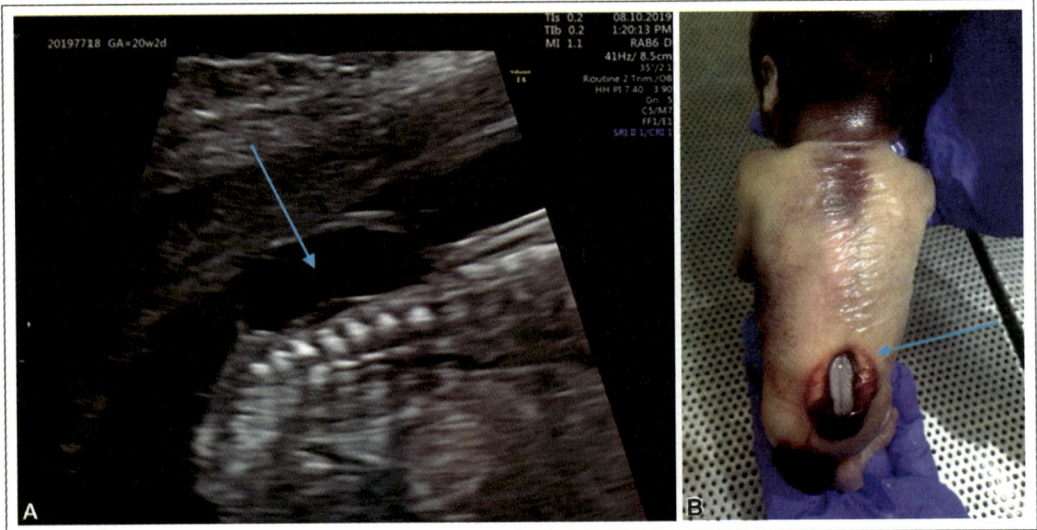

Figure 20.2: : (A) USG showing cystic swelling at lumbosacral area—meningomyelocele (*Courtesy*: Dr Rachna Gupta, Sunheri Devi Hospital); (B) Fetus with open NTD after termination

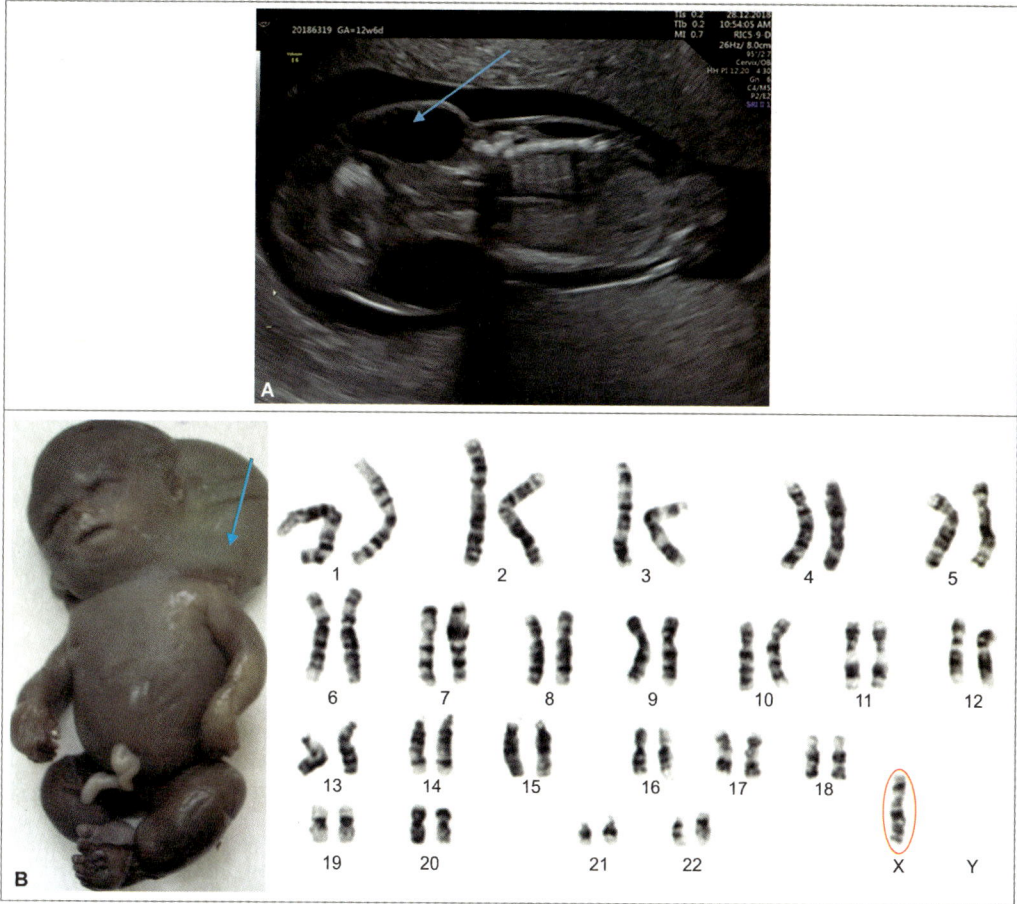

Figure 20.3: (A) USG showing cystic hygroma; (B) 19 weeks fetus with cystic hygroma karyotype showing 45X

Q 2. Write about the clinical significance of major and minor antenatal sonographic anomalies.

Ans. Clinical significance of major and minor anomalies depends upon whether it is isolated or multiple.

- ➲ Isolated abnormality can be non-genetic also but multiple major or minor anomalies points toward possibility of genetic cause.
- ➲ One major or two minor anomalies have a relatively poor prognosis.
- ➲ Significance depends upon whether the prognosis is uniformly poor (like for anencephaly, holoprosencephaly), or likelihood ratio is positive for poor prognosis as in Dandy-Walker malformation and bilateral multicystic kidney or prognosis is

variable as in mild ventriculomegaly and congenital diaphragmatic hernia.

- ➲ Antenatal abnormal USG guides to take detailed history and examination. Detailed 3D USG guides to take decision to get prenatal testing to know the etiology and prognosis to continue pregnancy or termination and need of fetal autopsy and the recurrence risk and help in genetic counseling of the couple.

Q 3. How will you counsel and conduct the management of a couple who has been diagnosed with abnormal sonographic report?

Ans. Genetic counseling and management of the couple with fetal anomalies detected on ultrasound (Figure 20.4) is conducted as follows:

Whenever an anomaly is detected on ultrasound, we must counsel about 2 issues mainly:

1. Counseling regarding prognosis.
2. Counseling regarding recurrence risk depends upon etiological diagnosis and whether it is isolated or associated anomaly (*see* Appendix Tables 8 and 9) .

Counseling regarding prognosis	Counseling regarding recurrence risk
Depends upon these factors:	**Depends on etiology:**
o Type of anomaly	o *Aneuploidies* involve trisomy or monosomy with sporadic recurrence risk.
o Severity of the anomaly	
o Associated malformations	o *Structural malformations: De novo* or inherited with high recurrence risk if parents also have balanced translocation
o Gestational age	
o Availability of treatment	
o Precious pregnancy	
o Social factors	o *Single gene disorder:* Depends upon the gene inheritance pattern.
o Amniocentesis/ CVS-FISH/culture/ Microarray 750 K report.	

Management for antenatal USG detected anomaly (Figure 20.4)

Q 4. What are the various common fetal soft markers found on prenatal ultrasound? Write about their clinical significance.

Ans. A soft marker is a common finding on ultrasound examination. These are not structural anomalies but may be indicators of an increased risk for aneuploidy. The presence of multiple soft markers increases the risk for certain aneuploidies, while risk is relatively small when only an isolated soft marker is detected.

The common first trimester and second trimester soft markers include (Figures 20.5 and 20.6):

- Increased nuchal translucency
- Absent nasal bone
- Pyelectasis
- Shortened long bones (humerus, femur)
- Echogenic intracardiac focus
- Choroid plexus cysts
- Echogenic bowel
- Aberrant right subclavian artery
- Cystic hygroma.

Clinical significance:

- Isolated soft markers are identified in 11 to 17% of normal fetuses.
- **Clinical significance** of soft marker depends upon its number, positive or negative likely hood ratio of the marker and associated risk with maternal age and positive antenatal screening.

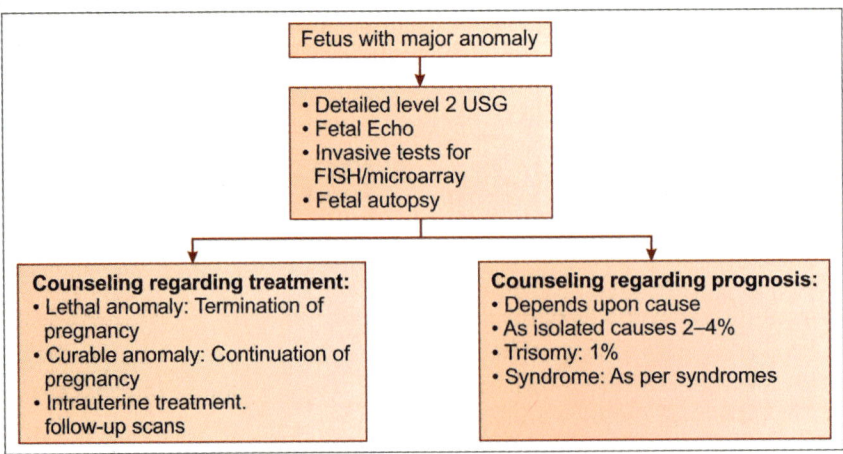

Figure 20.4: Management algorithm for antenatal USG detected anomaly (*see* Appendix Table 8)

- After the detection of anyone of the markers, all other markers or defects associated with aneuploidy should be excluded.
- In most of the isolated markers, there is only a small risk for trisomy 21, but with ventriculomegaly, nuchal fold thickness and aberrant right subclavian artery there is a 3–4-fold increase in risk and with hypoplastic nasal bone a 6–7-fold increase in risk will be there.
- Some isolated soft markers, particularly nuchal translucency, absent nasal bone, and echogenic bowel are more strongly associated with fetal aneuploidy than other soft markers (e.g. pyelectasis).
- Some soft markers in euploid fetuses are associated with disorders other than aneuploidy (e.g. echogenic bowel and cystic fibrosis, nuchal translucency and congenital heart disease in Noonan syndrome), may require additional evaluation, including invasive diagnostic testing.
- A detailed evaluation of fetal anatomy and likelihood ratio of soft markers should be analysed whenever one or more soft markers have been identified. This is to make decision about further need of prenatal genetic testing to know the etiology which will help in analyzing the prognosis, to make decision to continue pregnancy or to terminate and in indicating need of fetal autopsy, in understanding recurrence risk and help in genetic counseling.

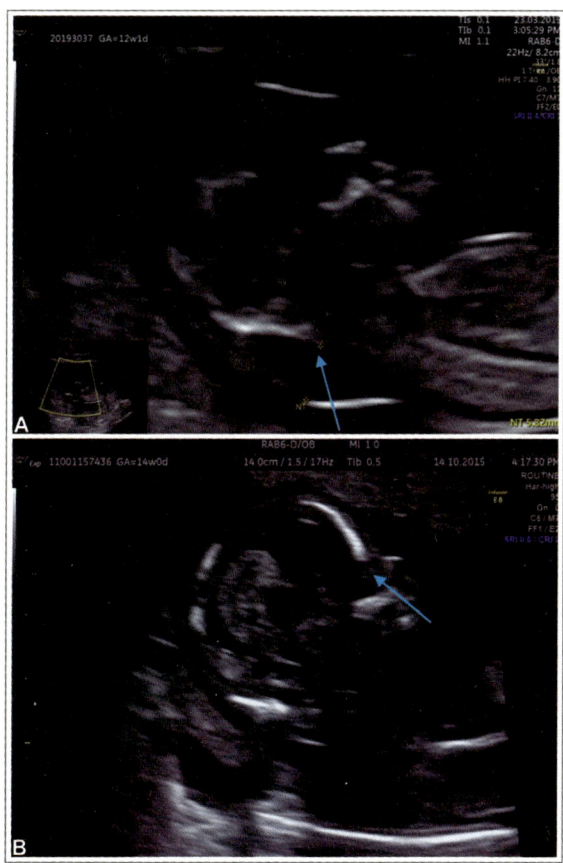

Figure 20.5: First trimester markers of aneuploidy. (A) Increased NT—3.2 mm; (B) Nasal bone

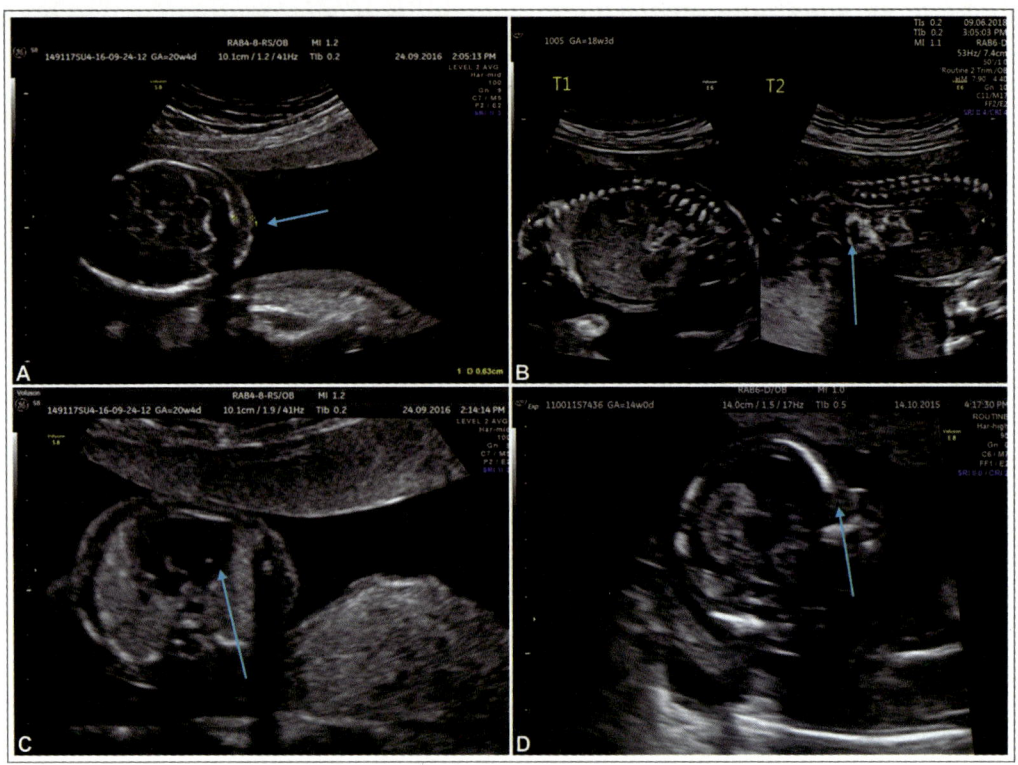

Figure 20.6: USG showing second trimester markers of aneuploidy. (A) Increased NFT 7.2 mm; (B) Echogenic bowel; (C) Echogenic focus; (D) Absent nasal bone
(*USG Pic Courtesy:* Dr Savita Dagar, Venkateshwar Hospital)

Management of isolated soft marker (Figure 20.7)

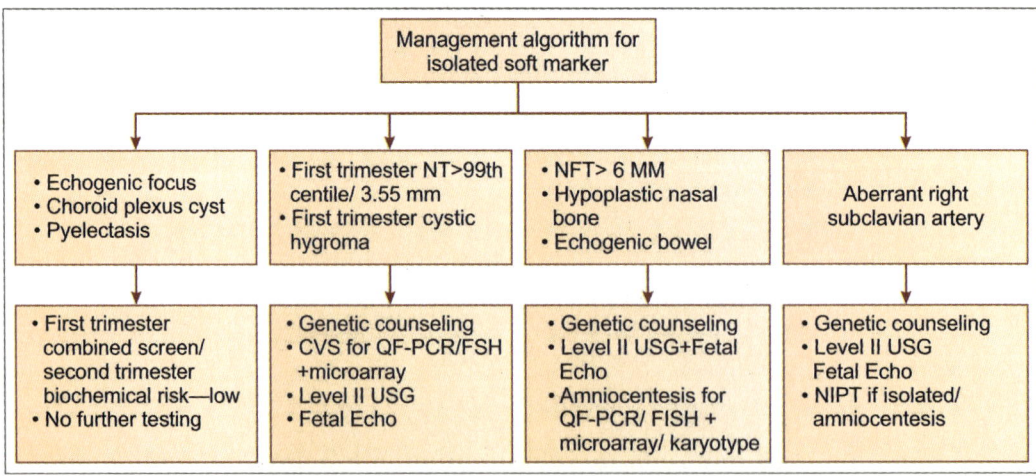

Figure 20.7: Management of isolated soft marker (*see* Appendix Table 7 based on likelihood ratio also). NT—Nuchal fold thickness; CVS—Chronic villi sampling; QF-PCR—Quantitative fluorescent polymerase chain reaction; FISH—Fluorescent *in situ* hybridization, USG—Ultrasonography; Echo—Echocardiography, NIPT—noninvasive prenatal testing

Q 5. Define infertility. What are the causes of female infertility?

Ans. According to World Health Organization (WHO), infertility is the inability to conceive after 1 year of unprotected sexual intercourse. It affects 15% of couples.

- Male infertility: 40%
- Female infertility: 40%
- Both: 20%

Female infertility causes can be either primary or secondary.

Primary causes: Female infertility could be due to abnormal germ cells. The common causes are ovarian and ovulation, premature ovarian failure, polycystic ovary disease.

Secondary causes: Female infertility could also be due to abnormality of reproductive structures and genetic causes.

- *Cervical:* Stenosis.
- *Uterine:* Congenital or acquired defects (endometriosis and leiomyomas).
- *Tubal:* Tubal block.
- *Endocrine causes:* Steroid synthesis defect. (CYP 17, CYP 21, CYP21A2 mutations).
- *Metabolic:* Galactosemia and mitochondrial defects.
- *Genetic:*
  - *Chromosomal abnormalities:* Turner syndrome, fragile X syndrome.
  - Microdeletion and duplications lead to premature ovarian failure.

- *Single gene disorders:* Sickle cell anemia, Perrault syndrome disorders or sex development disorders (*DAX1, SRY, SOX 9, AMH, WT1, WNT4*) and Kallmann syndrome.
- *Multifactorial:* Polycystic ovarian disease.

Q 6. What are the causes of male infertility?

Ans. Male infertility can result from several causes that include (EAU {European Association of Urology} guideline on male infertility):

Primary: Abnormal semen and spermatogenesis.

Secondary:
- *Idiopathic:* Semen analysis normal.
- Mechanic urogenital obstruction (vas deferens, ductal system, etc.)
- Physical trauma
- Infection
- Lifestyle (obesity, psychological problems, age, exercise, drugs, smoking)
- Varicocele
- Endocrine disorders
- *Metabolic:* Galactosemia and mitochondrial defects
- Malignity
- Cryptorchidism
- *Genetic causes:* Common chromosomal and genomic variations are shown in Figure 20.8.

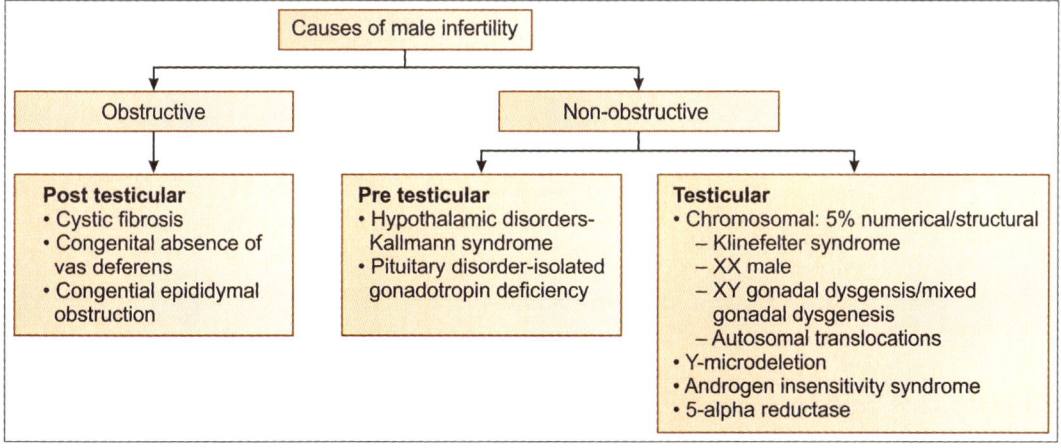

Figure 20.8: Causes of male infertility

- *Other causes:* 47 XYY, aneuploidies, Robertsonian translocation, sickle cell disease, Kartagener syndrome, Thalassemia and Fanconi anemia, Y microdeletion involving AZF sites AZFa, AZFb, and AZFc in 10–15% and Klinefelter constitutes in 14%.

Q 7. How will you investigate a case of infertility?

Ans. Following is the approach to a case of infertility:

1. **History:**
   A. *History from a female partner:*
      - Duration of infertility, medical reports, any infertility treatment done, menstrual history, sexual history, secondary sex characters and obstetric history.
      - *History of androgen excess:* Hirsutism.
      - *Surgical history:* Pelvic or abdominal surgery.
      - *Family history:* Infertility, birth defects, genetic mutations, or mental retardation.
      - History of consanguinity.
      - *Personal history:* History of drug abuse, exposure to chemotherapy or radiation, or excessive stress.
      - History related to any obvious syndrome or genetic cause.
   B. *History from male partner:*
      - Medical history and history of puberty onset.
      - Any history of surgery or trauma
      - Sexual history.
      - Personal history of drug abuse, exposure to chemotherapy or radiation.
      - History related to any obvious syndrome or genetic cause.
      - Family history of genetic diseases, e.g. cystic fibrosis, family history of male infertility.
      - Assessment of medical reports.
2. **Physical examination:**
   A. Body mass index (BMI)
   B. Female examination:

   - Secondary sex characters, e.g. breast development, axillary hair, etc.
   - Goiter, galactorrhea, hirsutism.
   - Pelvic examination for examination of vagina, cervix and uterus.
   C. *Male examination:* Degree of virilization, gynecomastia, focal neurologic findings (anosmia, visual field impairments, and assessment of the genitalia for undescended testes, varicocele.
   D. Signs related to any obvious syndrome (Turner or fragile X) or genetic cause.
1. **Investigation: Male: Table 20.2** shows evaluation and management of infertile male partner.
   A. **Husband's seminal fluid examination include** (Table 20.1)
      - Sperm concentration, appearance, mobility.

TABLE 20.1: WHO criterion of accepted reference Value for semen parameters—5th percentile	
Volume:	1.5 mL
pH:	>7.2
Sperm concentration:	15 million/mL
Total sperm number:	39 million spermatozoa per ejaculate
Morphology: Vitality:	4% normal 58% live
Total motility:	40%
Progressive motility: Sperm agglutination:	32% Absent

   - If the results are normal according to WHO criteria, one test is sufficient.
   - If the results are abnormal in at least two tests, further andrological investigation is indicated. It is important to differentiate between the following:
      a. *Oligozoospermia:* <15 million spermatozoa/mL
      b. *Asthenozoospermia:* <32% progressive motile spermatozoa.
      c. *Teratozoospermia:* <4% normal forms.

○ Often, all three anomalies occur simultaneously, which is defined as oligo-astheno-teratozoospermia (OAT) syndrome.

○ As in azoospermia, in extreme cases of oligozoospermia (spermatozoa <1 million/mL), there is an increased incidence of obstruction of the male genital tract and genetic abnormalities.

B. **Endocrine:** Serum follicular stimulating hormone, leutinizing hormone and testosterone levels.

C. **Karyotypes** to see numerical and structural chromosome anomalies.

D. **Y-microdeletion** testing is done in following conditions (Figure 20.9).

○ All men with non-obstructive azoospermia

○ Severe oligospermia (< 5–10 million)

E. **Specific molecular genetic tests** based on the underlying etiological syndrome or clinically suspected etiology like KAL1 gene analysis.

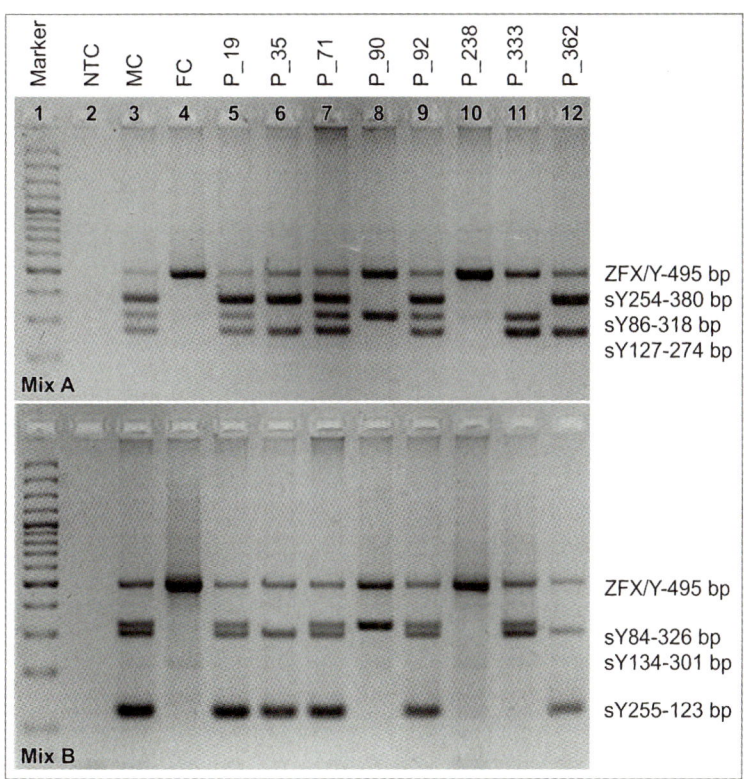

Figure 20.9: Agarose gel electrophoresis showing Af. Fa, b & cY- microdeletions. Mix A: sY254 (cl), sY86 (a2),sY127(bl); Mix B: sY84(al), sY134(b2), sY255(c2). Lane 1 is the DNA marker. Lane 2 is non-template control. Lane 3 is normal male control. Lane 4 is normal female control. Lanes 5, 7 and 9 are normal. Lane 6 and 12 are AZFa deletion. Lane 8 is AZFb & c deletion. Lane 10 is AZFa,b& c deletion and Lane 11 is Af. Fc deletion (Dutta UR, Suttur MS, Venugopal VS, et al. Cytogenetic and molecular study of 370 infertile men in South India highlighting the importance of copy number variations by multiplex ligation-dependent probe amplification. Andrologia. 2020;00:e13761. https://doi. org/10.1111/ and.13761). Y-microdeletion testing: Gel photograph showing deletion in the AZFc region (sY255–126 base pairs) in lanes 4, 6, 8, 10)

TABLE 20.2: Evaluation and management of infertile male partner

Etiology	First line investigations	Second line investigations	Management
Oligospermia/ azoospermia	Husband seminal fluid examination (HSF)	Genetic tests if azoospermia/ oligospermia	o Genetic counseling o Referral to urologist o ICSI/TESE/donor sperm
Hypergonadotropic hypogonadism	FSH, LH, serum testosterone	Karyotype in hypergonadotropic hypogonadism	o Genetic counseling in case of abnormal karyotype o Referral to urologist o Referral to endocrinologist o ICSI/TESE/donor sperm
Hypogonadotropic hypogonadism	FSH, LH, testosterone	MRI brain, fundus examination in hypogonadotropic hypogonadism	o Referral to endocrinologist
Obstructive azoospermia	HSF examination	CFTR gene analysis	o Genetic counseling o Referral to urologist

FSH—Follicular stimulating hormone; LH—Luteinizing hormone; ICSI—Intracytoplasmic sperm injection; TESE—Testicular sperm extraction; MRI—Magnetic resonance imaging

Female evaluation and management (Table 20.3)

TABLE 20.3: Evaluation and management of female partner in infertility

Etiology	Investigations	Management
Ovarian reserve	o Anti-müllerian hormone o FSH o LH o Serum estradiol o USG for antral follicle count	IVF
Ovulatory dysfunction	o Serum progesterone on D21 o USG for PCOD o TSH o Prolactin	Ovulation induction
Tubal/uterine factor	o HSG/3DUSG/hysteroscopy	Surgery as per cause, IVF
Genetic causes	o Karyotype, FMR1 gene o Specific molecular genetic tests based on the underlying etiological syndrome or clinically suspected etiology.	Genetic counseling

IVF—In vitro fertilization; USG—Ultrasound; PCOD—Polycystic ovarian disease; TSH—Thyroid stimulating hormone; HSG—Hysterosalpingography

Q 8. What are the causes of recurrent abortions?

Ans. Recurrent miscarriage: Incidence of recurrent spontaneous abortion (RSA) is 1–2%. Spontaneous abortion is the pregnancy loss before 20 weeks (10–20%) and any loss after 20 weeks is defined as intrauterine fetal death.

Definition of **recurrent miscarriage** varies by different society guidelines:

- ⮑ Three or more consecutive abortions before 20 weeks of pregnancy (RCOG, 2011)
- ⮑ Two or more clinically recognized pregnancy confirmed by USG/histo-pathology (ASRM, 2012), especially if:
  a. maternal age >35
  b. history of subfertility
  c. young mother, family history of miscarriages present.

Causes of **RSA** are as shown below:

1. **Immunological (15–20%):**
   1. Antiphospholipid antibody
   2. Anticardiolipin antibody: IgG and IgM
   3. Lupus anticoagulant
   4. Anti-B$_2$ glycoprotein- IgG and IgM
   5. Antinuclear and antithyroid antibodies.
   6. HLA-B, C, G related RSA need further confirmation.
2. **Endocrine (8–12%):**
   1. Luteal phase deficiency
   2. Untreated hypothyroidism
   3. Abnormal glucose metabolism
   4. Hyperprolactinemia
   5. Diminished ovarian reserve.
3. **Anatomical (8–10%):**
   1. Congenital malformations of the reproductive tract
   2. Intrauterine adhesions
   3. Intrauterine masses, including fibroids or polyps
   4. Incompetent cervix.
4. **Thrombophilia:** Responsible for more than half of maternal venous thromboembolisms. Major causes of thrombophilia are:
   - ⮑ Factor V Leiden mutation
   - ⮑ Prothrombin G20210A gene mutation
   - ⮑ Antithrombin activity

- ⮑ Protein S activity
- ⮑ Protein C activity
5. **Intrauterine infections** (0.5–1.5%)
6. **Genetic (5%):** These are either:
   a. *Chromosomal causes:*
      - ⮑ *Parental chromosomal disorders:* Common rearrangements are reciprocal translocation, Robertsonian translocation and inversion.
      - ⮑ *Balanced translocation carriers* occur in 3–5% of couples with RSA as opposed to 0.7% in the general population (Figure 20.10).
   b. *Single gene disorder:*
      - ⮑ Multiple genes (*ApoE, TNFα, p53,* etc.) are responsible for RSA which need further studies for definite evidence.
      - ⮑ *Unexplained:* 30–40%.

Q 9. How do you manage a case with recurrent abortions?

Ans. In clinical practice, we generally start the work after 2 miscarriages as risk of loss after 2 abortions (24–29%) is only slightly lower than the loss after 3 abortions (31–33%).

Approach to a case of RSA:

1. **History:** Detailed medical history for endocrine dysfunction, hemorrhagic disorder, galactorrhea, autoimmune disorders such as skin rash, joint pain, history of thrombosis, menstrual, obstetric and family history of RSA, mental retardation, consanguinity and medical records should be assessed.
2. **Examination:** Physical examination should include a general physical assessment with attention to signs of endocrinopathy (e.g. hirsutism, galactorrhea) and pelvic organ abnormalities (e.g. uterine malformation, cervical laceration).

Counseling for recurrent abortion at first visit:

1. Recurrent miscarriages are noted in 1–2% of couples.
2. Diagnostic work up is advised for etiological diagnosis for appropriate management (Tables 20.4 and 20.5).

3. The reason can be identified in about 50–60% cases and appropriate guidance as per diagnosis can be done.

4. In cases of unexplained recurrent abortion cases, success rate is about 70–75% without any treatment.

TABLE 20.4: First level of investigation and management

Etiology	Investigation	Management
Genetic	o Karyotype of both partners for balanced re-arrangements (Figure 20.10) o Carrier screening for more than 3 abortions.	o Genetic counseling o Donor gametes o Preimplantation genetic diagnosis
Anatomical	o HSG/hysteroscopy/3D USG	o Septum transaction o Adhesiolysis
Endocrine	o Day: 21, progesterone o TSH o TPO antibody o Blood sugar or HbA1c o If galactorrhea (PCOD)	o Progesterone o Levothyroxine o Bromocriptine o Metformin
Autoimmune work-up	o Anticardiolipin antibody: IgG and IgM o Anti-B$_2$ glycoprotein: IgG and IgM o Lupus anticoagulant	o Aspirin o Low molecular-weight heparin
TPO : Thyroid peroxidase		

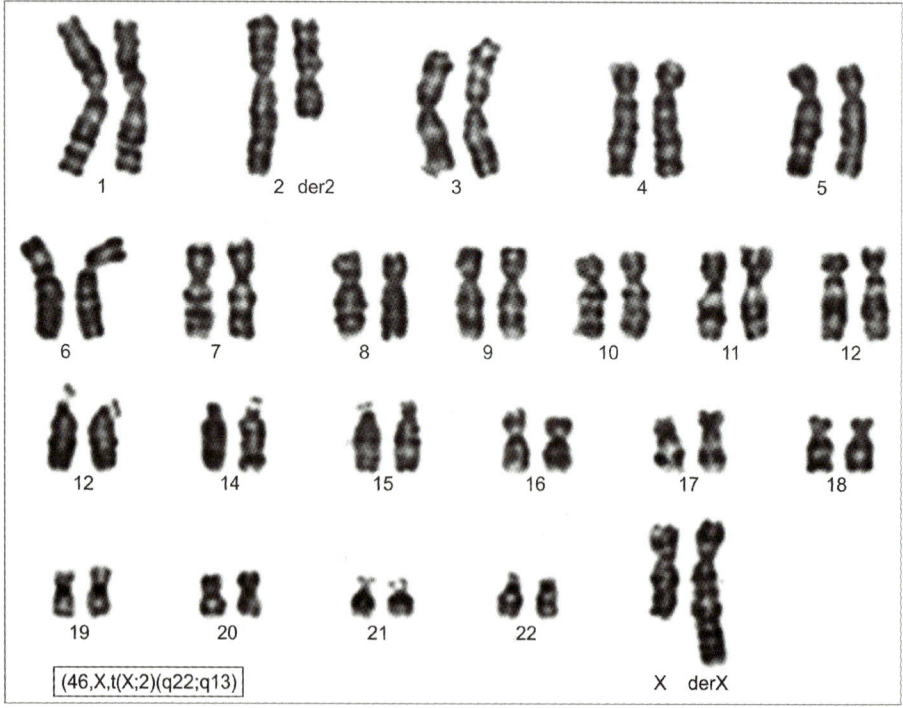

(46,X,t(X;2)(q22;q13)

Figure 20.10: : Balanced reciprocal translocation involving chromosomes X and 2 with a karyotype of 46,X,t(X;2)(q22;q13) (*Source:* Usha R. Dutta, Diagnostics Division, Centre for DNA Fingerprinting and Diagnostics, Inner Ring Road, Uppal, Hyderabad 500 039)

TABLE 20.5: Second level of Investigation and Management

Etiology	Investigations	Management
Auto-immune	○ Anti-nuclear antibody by immuno-fluorescence	If positive, referral to immunologist for immuno-therapy opinion.
Thrombo-philia	○ Factor V Leiden ○ Prothrombin gene mutation ○ Antithrombin III/protein C/protein S	Heparin prophylaxis
Genetic	○ Test for products of conception	Genetic counseling

Test for products of conception: Karyotype, microarray and target gene mutation testing can be done on products of conception. It should be done after second or third abortion.

⊃ Less than 12 weeks samples are taken before suction, by dilatation and curettage, in medium/sterile normal saline (NS) with added gentamicin (50 µg/ml) and heparin.

⊃ **After 12 weeks:**
  i. Cord blood in heparin/EDTA vacutainer
  ii. Placenta, fetal skin in media or sterile NS. Add a drop of gentamicin and heparin.

Conclusion: Early pregnancy loss is a frustrating entity for both patients and providers. Possibility of successful pregnancy outcome highly depends on etiology, maternal age and number of prior losses. Counseling with empathy to give hope and patience, tender love and care are most important. In unexplained cases of recurrent abortions, success rate is 65–75% even without any treatment.

BIBLIOGRAPHY

1. Emery and Rimoin's Principles and Practice of Medical genetics, 7th edition.
2. GeneReviews® [Internet]. Seattle (WA): University of Washington, Seattle; 1993–2020. Available from: https://www.ncbi.nlm.nih.gov/books/NBK1116/.
3. Genetic Clinics, IAMG.

Chapter

21

Genodermatosis

Irene Mathews, Jerene Mathews

Q 1. Write the classification of various inherited human pigmentation disorders.

Ans. Human pigmentation disorders can be inherited or acquired. Inherited disorders are categorized based on the level of depigmentation as follows:

A. **Inherited disorders with localized hypopigmentation:**
- Depigmentation (total pigment loss)
  1. Piebaldism
  2. Waardenburg syndrome.
- Hypopigmentation (partial loss of pigment)
  1. Nevus anemicus (due to vasocons-triction: no true loss of pigment)
  2. Nevus depigmentosus, hypomela-nosis of Ito (pigmentary mosaicism), chimerism
  3. Hypomelanotic macules of tuberous sclerosis
  4. Incontinentia pigmenti (4th stage)
  5. Guttate hypopigmentation in Darier disease

These could be **differentiated** from the **acquired** cases like **vitiligo** by:
- Congenital onset
- No extension of lesions, grows propor-tionately with the body
- Association with other extracutaneous features like deafness
- Lack of specific features of vitiligo like trichrome sign, presence of specific markers like midline location in piebaldism.

Other **rare acquired** conditions which are thought to be autoimmune responses against melanocytes in skin, hair follicle, eye and inner ear to be differentiated are:
- *Alezzandrini syndrome:* Adults develop unilateral retinal pigment degeneration and retinal detachment followed by ipsilateral facial vitiligo and poliosis alignment with deafness.
- *Vogt-Koyanagi-Harada syndrome:* Adults develop uveitis, deafness, aseptic meningitis, vitiligo, poliosis and alopecia.

B. **Inherited disorders with generalized hypopigmentation:**
- Chédiak-Higashi syndrome (CHS)
- Griscelli syndrome

Both cause silver color to hair (silvery hair syndromes). Some of these disorders are related to loss of function of genes needed for formation, transport or functioning of lysosomes and lysosome related organelles (LROs) like melanosomes, lysosomes in granulocytes, lytic granules in T-cytotoxic and NK-cells, dense core granules in platelets. Involvement of these tissues causes:
- Pigment dilution of skin, hair, eyes.
- Immunodeficiency (phagocyte/T-cell/NK-cell defects).
- Platelet dysfunction and bleeding tendency.

Q 2. **Describe the inheritance, genetic basis and clinical features of human pigmentation disorders.**

Ans. **Genetic disorders with hypopigmentation:** Genetic basis and clinical features

Disorder	Inheritance	Genetic basis	Clinical features
Piebaldism	AD	o **KIT** gene mutations o Gene codes for receptor c-kit (receptor is a dimer) on melanocyte surface. o Normal c-kit is needed for melanocyte migration from neural crest. o Dominant negative effect due to loss of function mutation in one allele leads to localized absence of melanocytes in skin.	o Depigmented macules in midline of anterior trunk, midfrontal scalp, midforehead, mid-extremities. o White forelock o Normal/hyperpigmented macules within the lesions o Deafness very rare
Waardenburg syndrome	AD WS4- AR	o WS1-*PAX3* o WS2-*MITF* o WS3-*PAX3* o WS4-*EDNRB* Defect of melanocyte migration and survival during embryogenesis to skin, inner ear, eye (tissue affected).	o **WS1:** White forelock and/or depigmented macule on skin, dystopia canthorum, heterochromia iridis, sensorineural hearing loss (SNHL). o **WS2:** No facial dysmorphism, heterochromia iridis and SNHL. o **WS3:** WS1 features with musculoskeletal defects. o **WS4:** White forelock with Hirschsprung's disease (Shah-Waardenburg).
Tietze syndrome	AD	**MITF (same as WS2)**	o Like a severe form of WS2, but with diffused hypopigmentation of skin, hair, eye. o Complete deafness (albinism-deafness syndrome of Tietze)
Chédiak-Higashi syndrome	AR	o **CHS1/LYST gene**—both alleles cause loss of function o Gene codes lysosomal trafficking regulator which transfers material into lysosomes. o Defective gene causes defective phagolysosomes—giant membrane bound organelles which affects phagocytes, T/NK-cells, platelets, melanocytes.	o Diffuse hypopigmented skin, silvery hair, eye affected o Primary immunodeficiency (usually pyogenic infections) o HLH (hemophagocytic lymphohistiocytosis) in accelerated phase o Death in first few years o Bleeding tendency o Milder cases which survive develop progressive neurodegeneration.
Hermansky-Pudlak syndromes (HPS)	AR	o Deficiency of BLOC (biosynthesis of lysosome related organelle complex) proteins needed for assembly and functioning of lysosomes and	o Bleeding tendency o Pigment dilution of skin, hair, eyes o **HPS2:** Primary immunodeficiency

Contd.

Disorder	Inheritance	Genetic basis	Clinical features

		lysosome related organelles (LROs) found in melanosome and other cells and organs.
		○ HPS 1–10. 10 genes encoding components of
		  • HPS1 (75%), 4-BLOC-3 complex
		  • HPS2-AP3B1 of AP3 protein
		  • HPS3,5,6-BLOC2 complex
		  • HPS7,8,9,10-BLOC1 complex
			○ **HPS 1,4:** Pulmonary fibrosis, granulomatous colitis

Griscelli syndrome	AR	Defect of proteins needed for transfer of melanosome from melanocyte to keratinocyte. ○ Type 1: Myosin 5A ○ Type 2: RAB27A ○ Type 3: Melanophilin (MLPH)	All subtypes have pigment dilution of skin with silvery hair. ○ Type 1: Progressive neurodegeneration ○ Type 2: Primary immunodeficiency, HLH ○ Type 3: No other manifestations
Oculocutaneous albinism (OCA)	AR XLR	**OCA 1–7** Deficiency of enzymes/proteins needed for melanin synthesis ○ Type 1A: TYR gene, tyrosinase-total loss ○ Type 1B: *TYR* gene, tyrosinase-partial loss ○ Type 2: *OCA2* gene, MC1R-P-protein ○ Type 3: *TYRP1* ○ Type 4: *SLC45A2* coding MATP (membrane associated transporter protein) ○ Type 5: 4q24 chromosome mutation ○ Type 6: *SLC24A5* gene ○ Type 7: *C10orf11* gene.	**OCA1A** ○ Complete absence of pigment ○ Milky white skin, red iris, white hair ○ Not freckle or get pigmented nevi. **Other subtypes:** ○ Skin, eyes and hair lighter than family ○ Develop more pigmentation of skin, hair as they age ○ Gets freckles and pigmented nevi ○ Isolated ocular albinism

AR—Autosomal recessive; AD—Autosomal dominant; XLR—X-linked recessive, HLH—Hemophagocytic lymphohistiocytosis

Q 3. Write the diagnosis of various human pigmentation disorders.

Ans. Diagnosis:

⮑ Conditions with localized pigmentation are usually **diagnosed clinically**.

⮑ Along with clinical diagnosis, other useful investigations needed in case of diffuse hypopigmentation of skin and hair ± eyes are (Figure 21.3)

1. **Hair microscopy** shows pigment granule clumping.

   ⮑ Chédiak-Higashi syndrome (CHS)—fine, unevenly distributed clumps.

   ⮑ Griscelli syndrome—coarse, irregularly distributed clumps (Figure 21.1).

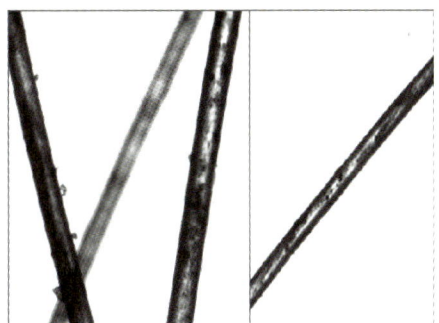

Figure 21.1: Irregular coarse clumping of pigment granules in an infant with pigment dilution of skin and hair with recurrent major infections including bacterial meningitis-suspected Griscelli syndrome type 2

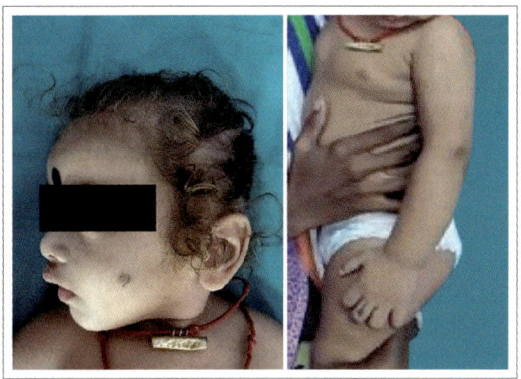

Figure 21.2: Infant presenting with pigment dilution of skin, hair and eyes found to have phenylketonuria. Infant was significantly fairer than the family members; including the mother who is holding the child

2. **Peripheral blood smear:**
   - Chédiak-Higashi syndrome **(CHS)**: Giant neutrophil granules
   - Hermansky-Pudlak syndromes (HPS2) may have neutropenia.
3. **Platelet function tests:** Abnormal in CHS, HPS.
4. **Tandem mass spectrometry (TMS), high performance liquid chromatography (HPLC):** IEMs need to be ruled out in neonates/infants presenting with pigment dilution for early intervention (Figure 21.2).

5. **Skin biopsy:**
   - *Griscelli syndrome:* Melanocytes 'stuffed' with many normal looking melanosomes, 'giant' melanosomes within melanocytes.
6. **Ophthalmology examination:** Photophobia, nystagmus, reduced vision, pale iris and retinal diseases where pigment loss affects eye as well.
7. **Confirmation by genetic analysis.**

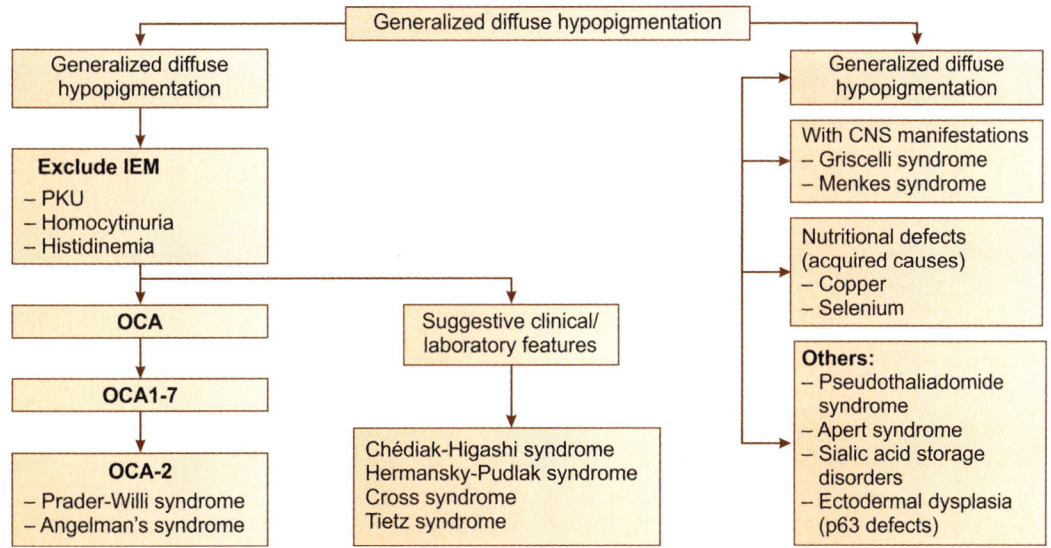

Figure 21.3: Approach to genetic disorders with diffuse hypopigmentation

PKU—Phenylketonuria, OCA—Oculocutaneous albinism, CNS—Central nervous system, IEM—Inborn error of metabolism

Q 4. Discuss treatment options of various human pigmentation disorders.

Ans. Treatment options for human pigmentation disorders are as follows:

1. **Piebaldism, Waardenburg syndrome:** The management is primarily supportive.
   - For hypopigmentation of skin and hair, cosmetic camouflage/hair dye may be used.
   - Split-skin grafts or cell grafts.
   - Management for hearing impairment (hearing aids, cochlear implant).

2. **Oculocutaneous albinism (OCA):** Treatment is supportive.
   - Photoprotection to prevent sunburns and skin malignancies (clothing, hats, sunscreens).
   - Dermatology surveillance for skin malignancies (especially in OCA1A).
   - Dark goggles for photophobia, disability management for low vision.
   - Genetic diagnosis is rarely undertaken in clinical settings unless severe disease (like OCA1A) merits prenatal counseling.

3. **Experimental therapies: L-DOPA** tried for vision improvement (no benefit noted), **Nitisinone** (tyrosine degradation inhibitor) has produced pigmentation of skin in albino mice.

4. **Tietze syndrome (deafness-albinism):**
   - Supportive management as in OCA (see above).
   - Disability management for hearing impairment.

5. **Griscelli syndrome type 1:**
   - Only supportive measures.

6. **CHS and Type 2 Griscelli syndrome:**
   - They have primary immunodeficiencies.
   - Need to have protective isolation, avoidance of live vaccines.
   - Prophylactic antibiotics.
   - Hematopoietic stem cell transplant (**HSCT**), corrects immunodeficiency and prevents or treats hemophagocytic lymphohistiocytosis (**HLH**) (after immunochemotherapy).

   - HSCT does not alter skin findings or course of neurodegeneration.
   - Prognosis is better if **HSCT** is undertaken prior to onset of **HLH**.

7. **Griscelli syndrome type 3:** Only photo-protection of skin needed.

8. **Hermansky-Pudlak syndrome:** Only supportive therapy is available.
   - Surveillance for pulmonary fibrosis in adulthood and rare cardiomyopathy and renal disease.
   - Prophylactic antibiotics and management of infections (immunodeficiency).
   - Supportive management of any major bleeding episodes (platelet transfusions).
   - Photoprotection of skin and eye, low-vision aids.

Q 5. Write the genetic classification of ectodermal dysplasia (ED).

Ans. Group of inherited disorders which have developmental abnormalities of two or more are of the following: Hair, nail, teeth, sweat glands and other ectodermal structures like central nervous system, eye, lacrimal apparatus, external ear, nose, mouth pituitary, thyroid, mammary gland, thymus, adrenal medulla, melanocytes.

There are various genetic EDs but the most common one is **XLR-hypohidrotic ED.**

Genetic basis	Disorders included
Ectodys-plasmin/ NF-κB pathway defects	○ **XLR/AD/AR-hypohidrotic ED** (XLR-Christ-Siemen-Touraine syndrome) ○ XLR hypohidrotic ED with immunodeficiency ○ XLR hypohidrotic ED with immunodeficiency, osteo-petrosis and lymphedema ○ Incontinentia pigmenti ○ AD hypohidrotic ED with severe and unique T-cell deficiency
P63 trans-cription factor defects	○ AEC syndrome (Hay-Wells syndrome) ○ EEC syndrome ○ ADULT syndrome

Contd.

Genetic basis	Disorders included
	○ LMS ○ Non-syndromic split-foot/split-hand syndrome
Defects in other transcription factors	○ Tricho-dento-osseous syndrome ○ Tricho-rhino-phalangeal syndrome
Wnt-β catenin pathway defects	○ Odonto-onychodermal dysplasia ○ Schopf-Schulz-Passarge syndrome
Connexin defects	Oculodental-digital dysplasia Clouston syndrome
Defects of adhesion molecules and cytoskeleton	○ Ectodermal dysplasia with skin fragility (plakophilin defect) ○ Pure hair-nail type ED (KRT85)

NF-κB—Nuclear factor κB; XLR—X-linked recessive; AD—Autosomal dominant; AR—Autosomal recessive; ED—Ectodermal dysplasia; AEC—Ankyloblepharon-ectodermal dysplasia-clefting; EEC—Ectrodactyly-ectodermal dysplasia-clefting; ADULT—Acro-dermato-ungual-tooth syndrome; LMS—Limb mammary syndrome

Q 6. Write down the clinical features of various ectodermal dysplasia (ED).

Ans. The clinical features of various ectodermal dysplasia (ED) are:

Ectodermal dysplasia class	Clinical features
Ectodysplasin/NF-κB pathway defects ○ Classical-XLR hypohidrotic ED/Christ-Siemen-Touraine syndrome ○ EDA1 mutation—loss of function (Ectodysplasin A)	**Males:** ○ Hypohidrosis and hyperthermia ○ Hypotrichosis ○ Hypodontia (Figure 21.4) ○ Normal nails ○ Facial dysmorphism ○ Athelia ○ Reduced mucus in respiratory and GIT mucosa **Variable severity in women based on skewed lyonization** (Figure 21.4) ○ Teeth defects prominent ○ Mosaic pattern of sweating deficits (starch-iodine test) ○ Breast asymmetry or athelia
P63 transcription factor defects	**AEC syndrome** ○ Ankyloblepharon filiforme adnatum ○ Collodion membrane, erythroderma, skin fragility, blistering, erosions in neonate.

Contd.

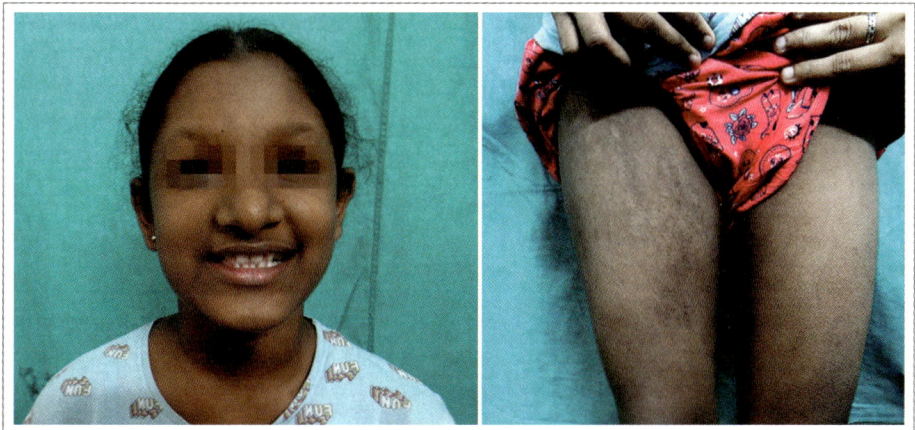

Figure 21.4: Adolescent girl with mosaic form of XLR—hypohidrotic ectodermal dysplasia

Ectodermal dysplasia class	Clinical features
	o Hypotrichosis, hair fragility o Hypodontia with cleft palate lip o Nail dystrophy/anonychia o Variable reduction in sweating, no hyperthermia o Chronic scalp erosions with granulation, scarring o Facial dysmorphism o Lacrimal duct obstruction o Athelia or supernumerary nipples o Hypopigmentation of skin **EEC syndrome** o Hypotrichosis o Hypodontia with cleft palate ± lip o Nail dystrophy/anonychia-lobster claw hand, feet (ectrodactyly) o Variable reduction in sweating, no hyperthermia o Genitourinary abnormalities (megaureter), endocrine deficits (pituitary/thyroid)
Wnt-β catenin pathway defects o Wnt10A loss of function mutations	Odonto-onychodermal dysplasia and Schopf-Schulz-Passarge syndrome **Common features:** o Severe oligodontia o Nail dystrophy/ anonychia o Hypotrichosis o Normal sweating with hyperhidrosis of palms, soles o Palmoplantar keratoderma

Contd.

Ectodermal dysplasia class	Clinical features
	Specific features: o Odonto-onychodermal dysplasia: Smooth tongue o Schopf-Schulz-Passarge syndrome: Eyelid cysts adnexal tumors
Connexin defects o GJB6/Connexin 30 o Dominant negative mutation	**Clouston syndrome** o Diffuse palmoplantar keratoderma, nail thickening o Oral leukokeratosis o Hypotrichosis o Teeth, sweating will be normal

Q 7. How will you make a diagnosis of ectodermal dysplasia?

Ans. Establishing the diagnosis:

1. **Clinical diagnosis:**
   ⮞ The diagnosis of ectodermal dysplasia is primarily clinically based.

2. **Investigations along with multidisciplinary assessments:**
   ⮞ Starch-iodine tests to assess sweating.
   ⮞ Ortho-pant-tomogram, dental consultation.
   ⮞ Hair shaft microscopy.
   ⮞ Endocrine—thyroid function test, serum cortisol, growth hormone (especially in P63 defects).
   ⮞ Ophthalmology examination in cases with ankyloblepharon/lacrimal duct atresia.
   ⮞ Ultrasonograph of abdomen/pelvis-especially in P63 defects with genito-urinary defects like megaureter.
   ⮞ Developmental assessment, neurological examination.
   ⮞ Growth and nutritional assessment—especially in those with teeth defects and palatal clefting.
   ⮞ Speech therapy as needed.
   ⮞ Surgical repair of palatal clefting, limb defects.

When the diagnosis is not clear clinically or if prenatal diagnosis is planned, genetic testing may be done.

Q 8. How will you do treatment of ectodermal dysplasia?

Ans. The management is primarily multidisciplinary and supportive. To prevent psychosocial effects and dental and facial abnormalities, treatments should start early.

1. **Treatment of severe anhidrosis or hypohidrosis resulting in hyperthermia**
   - Avoid exertion in hot weather.
   - Plenty of oral fluids.
   - Cold compresses or sprays, fan.

2. **Hypotrichosis**
   - Cosmetic camouflage—wigs/weaves.

3. **Hypodontia**
   - Affect nutrition, speech, cosmesis.
   - Artificial denture.
   - Speech therapy.

4. **Nail dystrophy**
   - Management of thick painful nails in pachyonychia congenita/Clouston syndrome.
   - Surgical or chemical nail plate removal if need.

5. **Surgical correction** or **prosthesis** with limb anomalies, rehabilitation.

6. **Cleft palate ±lip**
   - Feeding assistance in neonate, infant.
   - Treatment of recurrent upper respiratory infections (URI).
   - Surgical correction.
   - Speech therapy.

7. **AEC syndrome**
   - Neonatal erythroderma, blistering: asepsis, fluid and electrolyte management, prevent hypothermia.
   - Lysis of eyelid adhesions if not resolved spontaneously.
   - Lacrimal duct obstruction: Massage, probing, surgical correction.

- Topical steroids for granulating chronic erosions, skin grafts.
- Photoprotection if significant hypopigmented skin.
- Assess for genitourinary anomalies like megaureter.
- Assess and treat endocrinopathies—hypopituitarism, hypothyroidism.

8. **Reduced mucus secretion in ectodysplasin pathway defects**
   - *ENT consultation:* Saline drops for nasal crusting, treat recurrent URI.
   - Supportive treatment for gastroesophageal reflux disease, constipation.
   - *Recent therapy:* EDA-A1 recombinant fusion protein having receptor binding domain of IgG1 has been tried for the treatment of hypohidrotic ectodermal dysplasia.

Q 9. What is epidermolysis bullosa congenita?

Ans. A group of genetic disorders which are associated with blistering of skin and mucous membranes following trivial mechanical trauma.

The increased fragility of the epidermis in these disorders results from defects in protein that are important for keratinocyte integrity, keratinocyte adhesion or adhesion at the dermoepidermal junction.

Q 10. How is epidermolysis bullosa (EB) congenita classified?

Ans. EB is divided into 4 types based on the level of ultrastructural split (Figure 21.5)

- Epidermolysis bullosa **Simplex** (EBS) (level of basal and suprabasal keratinocytes)
- **Junctional** epidermolysis bullosa (JEB) (level of lamina lucida)
- **Dystrophic** epidermolysis bullosa (DEB) (below lamina densa)
- **Kindler** syndrome (KS) (variable level of split)

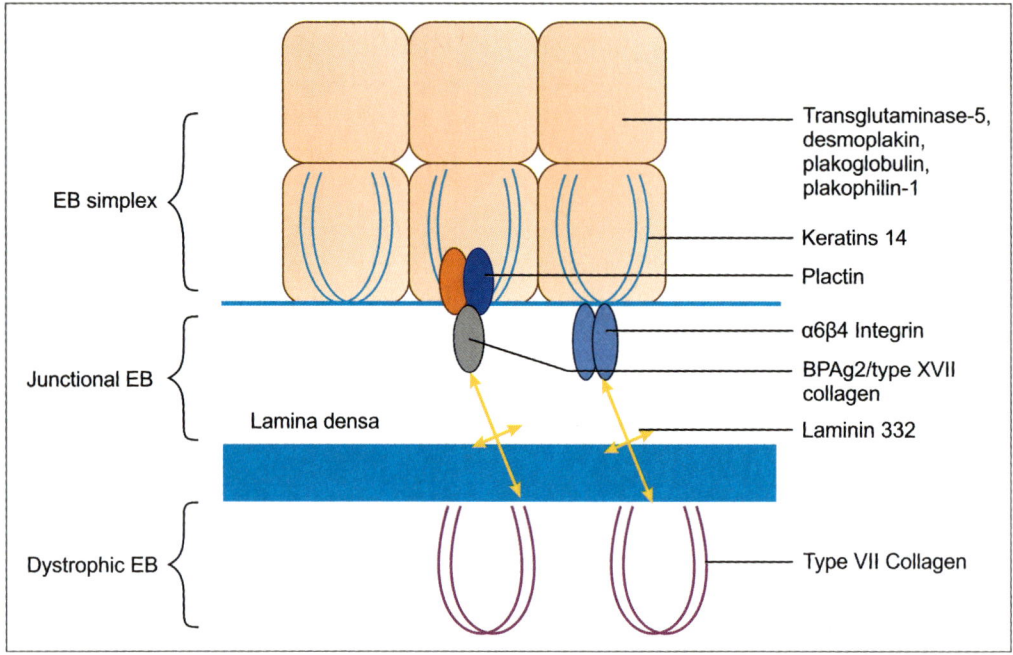

Figure 21.5: Level of split and proteins affected in major EB types

Q 11. Enumerate the major types of epidermolysis bullosa and their genetic basis.

Ans. There are four major types and over 18 subtypes of EBS:

○ **Epidermolysis bullosa simplex (EBS):** Autosomal dominant (*KRT5*, *KRT14*), rarely recessive (*EXPH5*, *TGM5*)

○ **Junctional epidermolysis bullosa (JEB):** Autosomal recessive (*COL17A1*, *ITGB4*, *LAMA3*, *LAMB3*, *LAMC2*)

○ **Dystrophic epidermolysis bullosa (DEB):** Autosomal dominant (DDEB) and recessive forms (RDEB: *COL7A1*).

○ **Kindler syndrome:** Autosomal recessive (*FERMT1*).

Type of EB	Subtype	Protein affected
EB simplex-suprabasal	○ Acral peeling skin syndrome ○ EB simplex superficialis ○ Severe acantholytic EB	○ Transglutaminase-5 ○ Unknown ○ Desmoplakin, plakoglobin
EB simplex-basal	○ Localized (Weber-Cockayne) ○ Generalized intermediate (Koebner) ○ Generalized severe (Dowling-Meara) ○ EBS with mottled pigmentation ○ EBS, Ogna ○ EBS with muscular dystrophy ○ EBS with pyloric atresia	○ Keratin 5 and 14 ○ Keratin 5 and 14 ○ Keratin 5 and 14 ○ Keratin 5 ○ Plectin ○ Plectin ○ Plectin

Contd.

Type of EB	Subtype	Protein affected
Junctional EB	o Generalized, severe o Generalized, intermediate o Generalized, late-onset o Generalized, with pyloric atresia o Generalized, respiratory and renal involvement o Localized	o Laminin 332 o Laminin 332, type XVII collagen o Type XVII collagen o α6β4 integrin o α3 integrin o Laminin 332, type XVII collagen, α6β4 integrin
	o Localized, inversa o Laryngo-onycho-cutaneous syndrome	o Laminin 332 o Laminin α3a
Dystrophic EB	o Dominant: Generalized, acral, pre-tibial, pruriginosa, bullous dermolysis of newborn. o Recessive: Generalized severe, generalized intermediate, inversa, localized, pre-tibial, pruriginosa, bullous dermolysis of newborn.	o Type VII collagen
Kindler syndrome		o Kindlin-1

Q 12. Describe the salient clinical features of the major types of epidermolysis bullosa (EB).
Ans. Salient clinical features of the major types of EB are described below.

Type of EB	Clinical features
EB simplex	**Localized EBS:** o Onset is after child starts to walk. o **Blisters** induced by rubbing of skin, due to friction from footwear o Worsened by warm weather o No scarring o Milia are absent/transient o Nails and mucosa are spared. **EBS, generalized intermediate:** o At birth or early infancy o **Blisters** induced by sites of rubbing, trauma or handling of neonate, improves with age o Nail and mucosae are usually spared. **EBS, generalized severe:** o Extreme fragile skin o Blistering without an obvious provocation. o Herpetiform blisters (annular or arcuate), erythematous border o Palmoplantar keratoderma, focal/diffuse with flexion deformity o Thickened nails

Contd.

Type of EB	Clinical features
	o Severe oral and esophageal blistering and poor feeding o Hoarse cry due to laryngeal involvement o Death due to sepsis in infancy o Blistering decreases with age o Pyloric atresia and Muscular dystrophy—in mutations of plectin.
Junctional EB (Figure 21.6)	o Death can occur in infancy, especially with generalized severe type. o Blistering starts in neonatal period. o In infancy, blisters heal rapidly without scarring. o Periungual erosions and nail loss o Hoarse cry, asphyxia due to laryngeal involvement o After infancy, chronic ulcers seen peri-orificially and periungually (mouth, nose, perineum, buttocks) o **Enamel hypoplasia** and dental caries o Oral mucosal involvement. o Corneal and conjunctival erosions (also in RDEB). o Dilated cardiomyopathy o Growth failure, delayed sexual maturation, anemia o Pyloric atresia—mutations of $\alpha6\beta4$ integrin o Respiratory and renal involvement—in $\alpha3$ integrin mutation.
Dystrophic EB (Figures 21.7 and 21.8)	o Deeper level of blister o Great variability between subtypes o Onset: Neonate to adulthood o **Blistering due to knocks and blows:** Dorsum of hands and feet, elbows and knees and persistent rubbing of clothes: Neck, axilla and waist o Heal with **atrophic scars and milia, contractures ++** o Hypopigmented papular lesions in a grouped pattern over the trunk (albopapuloid lesions): In any form of DEB o **Enamel hypoplasia** and dental caries o Oral mucosal involvement o Growth failure, delayed sexual maturation, anemia o Recessive DEB: Ectropion, corneal and conjunctival erosions. o Dilated cardiomyopathy
Kindler syndrome	o Acral blistering in neonate o Photosensitivity, progressive atrophy and poikiloderma o Palmoplantar keratoderma o Gingivitis and periodontitis o Keratoconjunctivitis and ectropion

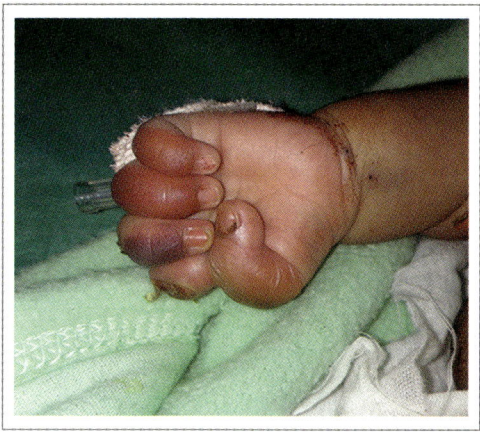

Figure 21.6: Periungual erosions in an infant with junctional EB

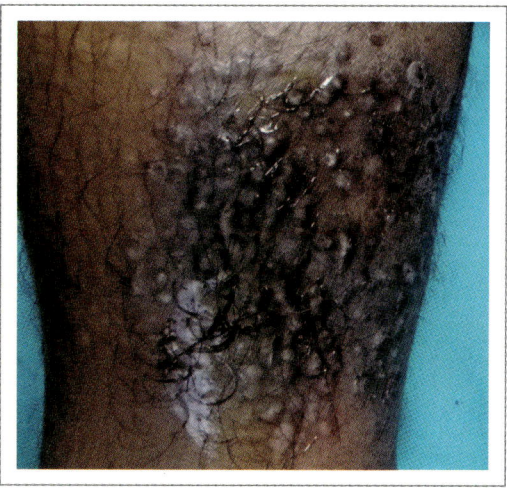

Figure 21.8: Dominant dystrophic EB, generalized type, presenting with extensive erosions which heal with milia and scarring. Images show scarring over the knees, shins

Q 13. How is EB diagnosed?
Ans. Diagnosis of suspected EB (Figure 21.9):
- **Skin biopsy and immunofluorescence (antigen mapping):** Biopsy of non-lesional rubbed skin to identify level of blistering.
- **Transmission electron microscopy (TEM):** To see the basement membrane structures like anchoring fibrils, tissue cleavage plane, keratin filaments.
- **Genetic diagnosis:** Next-generation sequencing, Sanger sequencing.

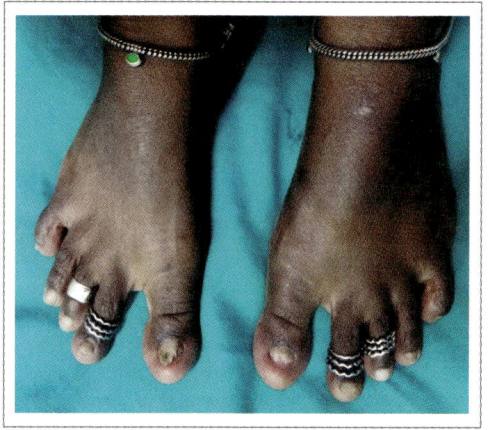

Figure 21.7: Dominant dystrophic EB, localized type, presenting with dystrophy of toenails

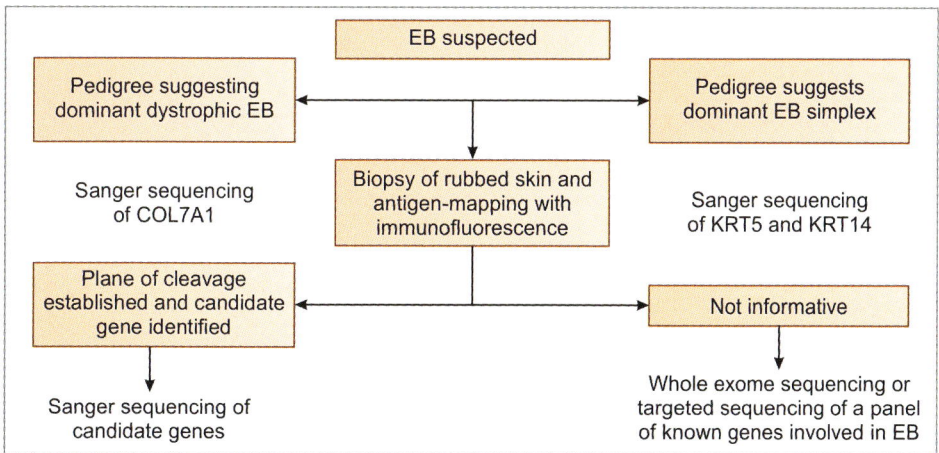

Figure 21.9: Diagnosis of suspected EB

Q 14. How are the skin lesions of EB managed?

Ans. The management is primarily supportive:

i. Minimize trauma—careful handling of newborn babies.
   - Soft clothes, padding over areas susceptible to friction, especially elbows and knees as child learns to walk
   - Well-fitted supportive shoes
ii. Reduce heat and humidity
iii. Care of blisters and erosions—
   - Blisters must be drained with aseptic precautions
   - Dressing of erosions with non-adherent dressing and an absorbent layer over it to absorb exudates. Non-adherent dressings include paraffin-impregnated gauze, silicone-based dressings and lipidocolloid.
   - Infections can be managed with topical silver sulphadiazine, silver–impregnated dressings and antibiotics as needed.
   - Excessive granulation tissue can be managed with potent topical steroids, electrocautery and skin grafting.
iv. Pain management with NSAIDs or opiates
v. Fluid and electrolyte balance, nutritional support, calcium, vitamin D, zinc and iron supplementation.
vi. Surveillance is done by eye examination, cardiac, dental, pediatrician involvement.
vii. Psychological support.
viii. Gene therapy: SiRNA for dominat negative mutations, e.g. KRT5 in EB simplex, genomic editing, intradermal allogenic fibroblasts, bone marrow stem cell therapy are under trial.

Q 15. How are inherited ichthyosis classified?

Ans. Inherited ichthyosis is a Mendelian disorder of cornification (**MeDOC**) which is characterized by generalized scaling or hyperkeratosis of skin.

Classification depends on the presence of organ-involvement other than skin and its appendages (Table 21.1). These can be:
- Non-syndromic
- Syndromic

TABLE 21.1: Clinicogenetic classification of non-syndromic ichthyosis		
Ichthyosis	*Inheritance*	*Genes involved*
Common ichthyosis: 1. Ichthyosis vulgaris 2. non-syndromic X-linked recessive ichthyosis (XLRI)	1. Autosomal semidominant 2. X-linked recessive	1. Filaggrin (FLG) 2. Steroid sulphates, deletions (STS)
Autosomal recessive congenital ichthyosis (ARCI): **Major types** 1. Lamellar ichthyosis and Non-bullous ichthyosiform erythroderma (NBIE) 2. Harlequin ichthyosis **Minor types:** 1. Self-healing collodion baby 2. Bathing suit ichthyosis	Autosomal recessive	**Lamellar ichthyosis and NBIE:** ○ Transglutaminase-1, missense mutations (*TGM*1) ○ Lipoxygenases (*ALOX12B, ALOXE3*) ○ Ichthyin (*NIPAL4*) ○ ATP-binding cassette transporter 12 (*ABCA12*) ○ Cytochrome P450 (*CYP4F22*) ○ Acid lipase (*LIPN*) ○ Ceramide synthase 3 (CERS3) ○ Patatin-like phospholipase (PNPLA1)

Contd.

TABLE 21.1: Clinicogenetic classification of non-syndromic ichthyosis *(Contd.)*		
Ichthyosis	*Inheritance*	*Genes involved*
		Harlequin ichthyosis: ○ *ABCA12*, nonsense or frameshift mutations **Self-healing collodion baby:** ○ TGM1, ALOX12B, ALOXE3 **Bathing suit ichthyosis:** ○ TGM1, temperature-sensitive mutations

Keratinopathic ichthyosis
1. Epidermolytic ichthyosis/bullous ichthyosiform erythroderma (BIE)
2. Superficial epidermolytic ichthyosiform/ichthyosis bullosa of siemens
3. Variants:
  a. Ichthyosis with confetti/ congenital reticular ichthyosiform erythroderma
  b. Ichthyosis of Curth-Macklin
  c. Autosomal recessive epidermolytic ichthyosis
	Autosomal dominant except for one variant, autosomal recessive epidermolytic ichthyosis	**Keratins**
		1. **Epidermolytic ichthyosis/BIE:** KRT1 or KRT10: Keratin 1 mutations are associated with palmoplantar involvement.
		2. **Superficial epidermolytic ichthyosiform/ichthyosis bullosa of siemens:** *KRT2*
		3. **Variants:**
		  a. *KRT10* or *KRT1*
		  b. *KRT1*
		  c. *KRT10*

Other non-syndromic ichthyosis: 1. Loricrin keratoderma 2. Erythrokeratoderma variabilis	1. Autosomal dominant 2. Autosomal dominant	1. Loricrin (LOR) 2. Gap-junction beta (GJB3, GJB4)

Q 16. Describe the clinical features of the ichthyosis vulgaris and non-syndromic X-linked recessive ichthyosis (XLRI).

Ans. Features of ichthyosis vulgaris and XLRI are described below.

	Ichthyosis vulgaris	*X-linked recessive ichthyosis (XLRI)*
Sex predilection	Males and females equally affected	Only males are affected
Onset	3 months—within the first year of life.	Delayed onset at 2–6 months of age or scaling/erythroderma/mild collodion at birth
Type of scales	○ Small, white scales ○ Larger, polygonal on shins	Dark brown, polygonal scales
Distribution of scales	○ Generalized with accentuated on extensors of limbs and trunk. ○ Sparing of flexures and face.	○ Face: Pre and retroauricular areas ○ Lateral aspect of neck ('dirty neck') ○ Trunk ○ Limbs ○ Cubital and popliteal fossa
Palms and soles	Hyperlinearity	Normal

Contd.

	Ichthyosis vulgaris	X-linked recessive ichthyosis (XLRI)
Associated features	Atopy	o Corneal opacities o Cryptorchidism (5–20%) o Contiguous gene deletion syndromes—short stature, Kallmann syndrome, chondrodysplasia punctata, behavioral disorders, mental retardation, retinitis pigmentosa o Carrier females—corneal opacities, prolonged labor and occasionally ichthyosis.
Histopathology of skin	Attenuated or absent granular layer in heterozygous and homozygous individual respectively	Normal thickness of granular layer.

Q 17. Describe the phenotypes of autosomal recessive congenital ichthyosis (ARCI).

Ans. Phenotypes of ARCI:

1. **Lamellar ichthyosis (LI)/congenital ichthyosiform erythroderma (CIE):** (Figure 21.10)
   - Whole body is affected including face and flexures.
   - Lamellar ichthyosis (LI) has large, dark, plate-like scales: Underlying erythema may be difficult to see.
   - Congenital ichthyosiform erythroderma (CIE): Generalized erythema with fine, white scales: Shins have larger scales.
   - Intermediate phenotypes of LI/CIE also seen with varying erythema and scale-size.
   - Nail dystrophy.
   - Palmoplantar keratoderma.
   - Scarring alopecia at the periphery of scalp.
   - Hypohidrosis.
2. **Bathing suit ichthyosis:** Lamellar-like scales involving trunk and sparing limbs.
3. **Harlequin ichthyosis:**
   - Neonate encased in large, thick, plate-like scales with deep-red fissures
   - Severe ectropion, eclabium
   - Deformed digits, ears, nose
   - Minimal hair growth
   - Constricting bands on limbs
   - Death in neonatal period.

- Few may survive with good neonatal care—severe CIE-like phenotype.

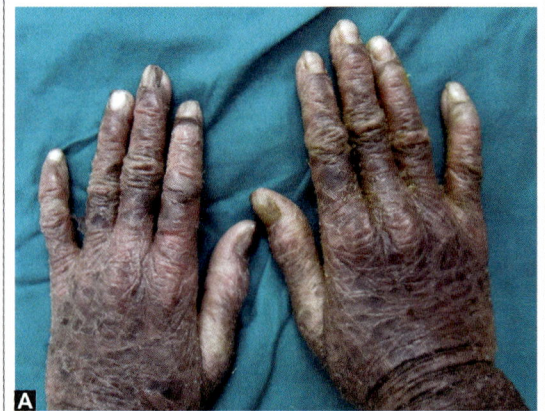

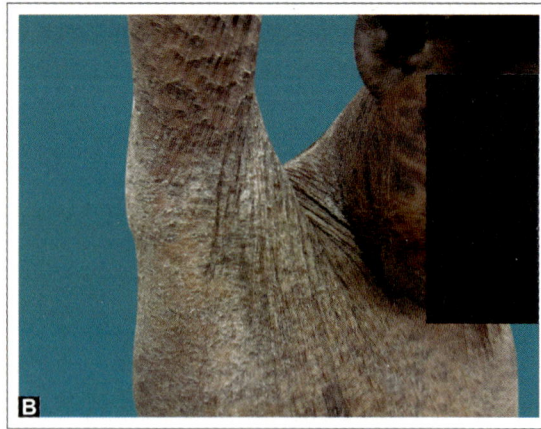

Figure 21.10: Lamellar ichthyosis (A) Mild flexion deformity of little fingers and nail dystrophy; (B) Involvement of axilla

Q 18. How do you classify syndromic ichthyosis?
Ans. **Classification of syndromic ichthyosis:**

	Ichthyosis	Inheritance	Genes involved
X-linked			
	Syndromic X-linked recessive ichthyosis (XLRI)	X-linked recessive	Deletions in STS, contiguous gene deletions
	Ichthyosis follicularis alopecia photophobia (IFAP)	X-linked dominant	MBTPS2
	Conradi-Hünermann-Happle syndrome	X-linked dominant	Emopamil-binding protein (EBP)
Autosomal			
1. **Prominent hair abnormalities**	Netherton syndrome	AR	SPINK5
	Ichthyosis hypotrichosis syndrome	AR	ST14
	Ichthyosis hypotrichosis sclerosing cholangitis syndrome	AR	CLDN1
	Trichothiodystrophy	AR	ERCC2, ERCC3, GTF2H5
2. **Prominent neurologic signs**	Sjögren-Larsson syndrome	AR	ALDH3A2 (Fatty aldehyde dehydrogenase deficiency)
	Refsum syndrome	AR	PHYH (phytanoyl-CoA hydroxylase)
	Gaucher syndrome type 2	AR	GBA (glucocerebrosidase)
	Multiple sulfatase deficiency	AR	SUMF1
	MEDNIK syndrome	AR	AP1S1
	CEDNIK syndrome	AR	SNAP29
3. **Fatal diseases course**	Gaucher syndrome type 2	AR	GBA (glucocerebrosidase)
	Multiple sulfatase deficiency	AR	SUMF1
	CEDNIK syndrome	AR	SNAP29
	ARC syndrome	AR	VPS33B
4. **Other associated signs**	Neutral lipid storage disorder/Chanarin-Dorfman syndrome	AR	ABHD5
	Keratitis ichthyosis and deafness (KID) syndrome	AD	GJB2
	Ichthyosis prematurity syndrome (IPS)	AR	SLC27A4
AD—Autosomal dominant; AR—Autosomal recessive			

Q 19. What is a collodion baby? What are the possible outcomes in a collodion baby?

Ans. It is a neonatal presentation of ichthyosis in which the newborn is encased in a tight, fissured and shiny membrane that looks like a cellophane sheet. Normal skin markings are absent. It can cause ectropion, eclabium, deformed nose and ears, and constricting bands on digits.

- The membrane sheds usually by 1 month revealing the underlying phenotype. (Figure 21.11)
- Most common outcome (80%) is an autosomal recessive congenital ichthyosis (ARCI) phenotype: Lamellar ichthyosis or congenital ichthyosiform erythroderma.
- 10% will eventually have mildest form of ARCI (self-healing collodion baby)
- 10% will have syndromic ichthyosis
    i. Neutral lipid storage disorder
    ii. Conradi-Hünermann syndrome (blaschkoid collodion)
    iii. Trichothiodystrophy
    iv. Sjögren-Larsson syndrome
    v. Gaucher syndrome type 2
    vi. Loricrin keratoderma
    vii. Netherton syndrome

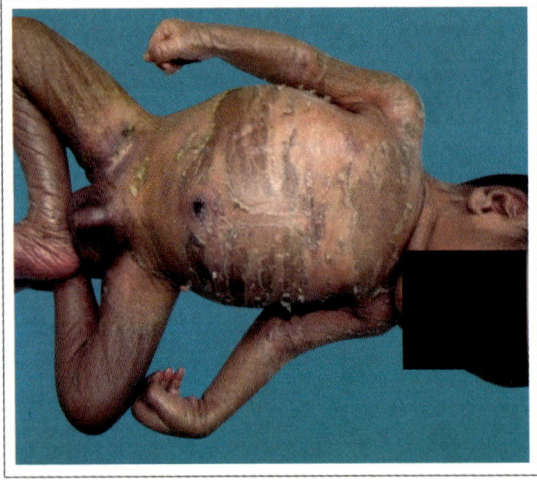

Figure 21.11: Neonate with a collodion membrane that is being shed.

Q 20. What are the different dermatological presentations in various ichthyosis forms during neonatal period other than collodion baby?

Ans. Different dermatological presentations in various ichthyosis is as follows:

Dermatological presentations	Ichthyosis
Normal skin (delayed onset ichthyosis)	○ Ichthyosis vulgaris ○ Some cases of syndromic X-linked recessive ichthyosis (XLRI) ○ Refsum disease (adult-onset) ○ Superficial epidermolytic ichthyosis ○ Erythrokeratoderma variabilis
Large, thick and constrictive scales	○ Harlequin ichthyosis
Blistering, with/without hyperkeratosis	○ Keratinopathic ichthyosis
Erythroderma	○ Congenital ichthyosiform erythroderma ○ Netherton syndrome ○ Keratitis ichthyosis and deafness (KID) syndrome
Excessive vernix	○ Ichthyosis prematurity syndrome
Erythema and scales in a blaschkoid distribution	○ Conradi-Hünermann-Happle syndrome ○ Inflammatory linear verrucous epidermal nevus (ILVEN)
Transient erythematous patches	○ Erythrokeratoderma variabilis

Q 21. What are the clinical manifestations of the common syndromic ichthyosis?

Ans. Clinical manifestations of common syndromic ichthyosis:

Ichthyosis	Clinical features
Netherton syndrome	o Erythroderma, ichthyosis linearis circumflexa o Brittle hair (trichorrhexis invaginata or 'bamboo' hair) o Atopy o Recurrent skin infections o Growth failure
Trichothio-dystrophy	o Ichthyosis (LI/CIE like) o Short stature o Mental retardation o Brittle hair ('tiger-tail' in polarized light) o Photosensitivity
Ichthyosis follicularis alopecia photophobia (IFAP)	o Congenital atrichia o Follicular hyperkeratosis o Keratitis and photophobia o Seizures, developmental delay
Conradi-Hünermann-Happle syndrome	o Blaschkoid ichthyosis o Chondrodysplasia punctata (short stature, short limbs) o Sectorial cataract o Deafness
Sjögren-Larsson syndrome	o Congenital ichthyosis, intense pruritus, periumbilical hyperkeratosis and radiating furrows o Mental retardation o Spastic paraparesis o Short stature
Refsum disease	o Ichthyosis vulgaris-like skin disease, late-onset in adult-life o Cerebellar ataxia, sensory-neural deafness, retinitis pigmentosa, peripheral neuropathy o Skeletal abnormalities.
Gaucher syndrome type 2	o Collodion membrane o Severe neurological compromise, hypertonia o Thrombocytopenia o Hepatomegaly o Perinatal death
Neutral lipid storage disorder/ Chanarin	o CIE-like presentation o Short stature o Mild mental retardation o Myopathy
Dorfman syndrome	o Sensorineural deafness o Nuclear cataracts o Hepatosplenomegaly
Ichthyosis prematurity syndrome (IPS)	o Generalized hyperkeratosis severe at birth and then improves o Vernix-like scaling o Prematurity and neonatal respiratory distress may be fatal at this time. On survival, may later develop atopy: Asthma and eosinophilia.

Q 22. How do follow-up investigations contribute to diagnosis in a patient with inherited ichthyosis?

Ans.

A. Clinical history and examination

B. Laboratory investigations.

➲ **Peripheral smear:** Lipid droplets are found within leukocytes (Jordans' anomaly) in neutral lipid storage disorder and can be seen as cytoplasmic vacuoles that stain with lipid stains like Oil red O.

➲ **USG abdomen:** Hepatosplenomegaly in neutral lipid storage disorder and Gaucher syndrome type 2.

➲ **Ocular examination:**

▪ *Syndromic X-linked recessive ichthyosis (XLRI):* Corneal opacities, more frequently in adult patients and female carriers

▪ *Sjögren-Larsson syndrome:* Glistening white spots in the fovea

▪ *Conradi-Hünermann-Happle syndrome:* Sectorial cataract, microcornea, microphthalmia

▪ *Refsum disease:* Retinitis pigmentosa

▪ *Neutral lipid storage disorder:* Nuclear cataract, nystagmus strabismus

▪ *KID syndrome:* Vascularizing keratitis

➲ **Skin biopsy:**

▪ *Ichthyosis vulgaris:* Attenuated granular layer is seen in heterozygotes and absent granular layer in homozygotes. The keratohyalin granules contain profilaggrin which is reduced or absent in ichthyosis vulgaris.

- *Epidermolytic ichthyosis (BIE):* Epidermolytic hyperkeratosis
- *Superficial epidermolytic ichthyosis:* Epidermolytic hyperkeratosis only in the superficial layers of the epidermis
- *Neutral lipid storage disorder:* Lipid droplets in the cytoplasm of the basal keratinocytes, stain with Oil red O in frozen sections.

⮑ **Immunohistochemistry:** To detect antibodies against antigen TGase1 or TGase1 enzyme activity in lamellar ichthyosis.

⮑ **Electrophoresis, STS activity** in fibroblasts or leucocytes in X-linked recessive ichthyosis.

⮑ **Molecular genetic testing.**

Q 23. Describe the management of ichthyosis.

Ans. Management is supportive and aimed at:
  i. Improving hydration of skin.
  ii. Treating and preventing complications, especially in severe forms of ichthyosis.

Management of complications due to poor barrier function of skin:
  i. Maintain the body temperature.
  ii. Fluid and electrolyte balance: Hypernatremic dehydration in neonate and infant.
  iii. **Infections:**
   ⮑ Fissures provide entry points for bacteria, neonatal sepsis
   ⮑ Herpes simplex and varicella can disseminate
   ⮑ Extensive dermatophytosis
   ⮑ Antibiotics can be given.
  iv. **Effects of tight skin:** Surgical release of bands, early institution of oral retinoids, taping of eyelids at night and ocular lubricants.
  v. **Growth failure:** Additional calories and protein, supplementation of vitamin D, oral iron, folate.

vi. **Improving hydration and appearance of skin:**
   ⮑ Application of bland emollients like petrolatum 3 or more times a day, especially after a bath.
   ⮑ Humectants like urea and keratolytics like salicylic acid can be used over limited areas. Possibility of systemic absorption and toxicity must be kept in mind, especially with children.
   ⮑ Retinoids:
    - Topical or oral
    - Reduce thickness of stratum corneum
    - May worsen epidermal fragility in some conditions
     Example: Epidermolytic ichthyosis, Netherton syndrome.

vii. **Surveillance for skin malignancies.**

Q 24. How will you conduct the genetic counseling and prenatal diagnosis for genodermatosis?

Ans. Genetic counseling: Discuss the following with families undergoing prenatal fetal testing for genodermatosis disorders:

⮑ Details of the disease like etiology, genetic basis, natural history, prognosis, management options, inheritance pattern, recurrence risk in future generation.

⮑ Need and details of genetic testing in proband by targeted gene panel or clinical exome analysis and target gene mutation in parents and prenatal sample based on the pattern of inheritance.

⮑ Once a pathogenic variant is identified, targeted sequencing in fetal cells by chorionic villi sampling/amniocentesis may be attempted for prenatal diagnosis. This may be considered for diseases with high morbidity and mortality.

⮑ Likely benefits of early diagnosis and preparedness if the result returns positive.

BIBLIOGRAPHY

1. Griffiths C, Barker J, Bleiker T, Chalmers R, Creamer D eds. Rook's Textbook of Dermatology. 9th edition. Chichester, West Sussex ; Hoboken, NJ: Wiley-Blackwell; 2016. 71.1–71.30.

2. Morice-Picard F, Taïeb A Albinism. In: P Hoeger, V Kinsler, A Yan, J Harper, A Oranje, C Bodemer, M Larralde, D Luk, V Mendiratta and D Purvis, (eds). Harper's Textbook of Pediatric Dermatology. 4th Ed. India:Wiley-Blackwell; 2019. p. 1486–91

3. O'Connor C, Asai Y, Irvine AD. Ectodermal dysplasias. In: P Hoeger, V Kinsler, A Yan, J Harper, A Oranje, C Bodemer, M Larralde, D Luk, V Mendiratta and D Purvis, (eds). Harper's Textbook of Pediatric Dermatology. 4th Ed. India:Wiley-Blackwell; 2019. p. 1629–705.

Cancer Genetics

Aruna Priya Kamireddy, Komal Uppal

Q 1. Define proto-oncogenes and tumor suppressor genes.

Ans. Proto-oncogenes:

- The protein coding genes which aid in normal cell growth like promoting cell division, inhibit cell differentiation and prevent apoptosis under normal conditions.
- A gain-of-function mutation like point mutations, gene amplifications, chromosomal translocation or may be external factors like viral infections, radiation, smoke and environmental toxins, etc. leads to uninterrupted cell growth that eventually lead to cancer.
- Examples:
  - *Ras* gene (colon, pancreas, urinary bladder cancer)
  - *BCR-ABL* (chronic myeloid leukemia)
  - *Myc* (Burkitt lymphoma)
  - *Neu* (ovary, breast)
  - *EGFR* (gliomas)
  - *HER2* gene (breast cancer).

Tumor suppressor genes:

- Protein coding genes that are involved in cell control functions like DNA damage repair, inhibiting cell division, promoting apoptosis and suppression of metastasis.
- They act at specific checkpoints controlling the cell cycle from progressing into next stage.

- Loss of function mutations due to deletions, nonsense mutations, frameshift mutations or insertions may lose their function, leads to initiation of cancer.
- Examples:
  - *TP53* gene
  - *APC*
  - *VHL*
  - *BRCA1*
  - *BRCA2*
  - *Rb* gene.

Q 2. Write a note on genetic basis of leukemia. Why is genetic information of these hematological malignancies needed for a physician?

Ans.

- Leukemia is malignant proliferation of myeloid and lymphoid series of hemato-poietic stem cells, accounting for almost 1 out of 3 cancers.
- Acute lymphocytic leukemia (ALL) is more common in children and acute myeloid leukemia (AML) is more common in adolescent age.
- Chronic myeloid (CML) and lymphocytic leukemias (CLL) are more common in adults.
- The various chromosomal rearrangements, deletions, hyper or hypoploidy or mutations in various genes {Li-Fraumeni syndrome (TP53)} leads to loss of key gene functions from a specific cell leading to proliferation of the malignant cells.

Genetic basis of leukemias

Type of leuke-mias	Genetic abnormality of good prognosis	Genetic abnormality of poor prognosis
ALL	o t(12:21) o Hyperploidy (>50)	o t(9;22) o t(4;11) o t(1;19) o Hypoploidy
AML	o t(8;21) o t(15;17) o inv(16)	o -7/del(7p) o -5/del(5q) o Gain of chromosomes 8 and 9
CLL	o del13q o Trisomy12	o del17p o del11q
CML	o Ph chromosome+	o trisomy8 o del22q

Diagnostic tests

- **Cytogenetic test:** Karyotype and fluorescent *in situ* (FISH).
- **Molecular test:** Polymerase chain reaction (PCR), real time PCR, causative gene analysis.

Need for physicians to know of hematological cancers like leukemia genetics

- Generally, all the hematological cancers occur sporadically but they can be a part of hereditary cancer syndromes also.
- In sporadic cases, the basic knowledge of the genetics of leukemia will help the physician in getting definitive diagnosis, its prognosis, recurrence risk (low), predicting the survival and will help in mutation-based treatment of the disease.
  Example: AML: t(15;17), ATRT (All-transretinoic acid) and CML Ph chromosome positive: Imatinib can be given.
- **In hereditary cancer syndrome,** it will help in providing information regarding underlying genetic predisposition, nature of the disease, diagnostic tests, management and surveillance of the proband, and family relatives, recurrence risk and geneticist consultation to family.

Q 3. Write a note on genetic basis of retino-blastoma and why it is important for a pediatrician to know the genetics of retinoblastoma.

Ans.

- Retinoblastoma (RB) is the most common intraocular cancer. It usually develops in children below the age of 5 years and is often curable when diagnosed early.
- The most common presentation is a white colored reflection from the retina of the eye (leukocoria) and strabismus.

Genetic basis:

- It can be sporadic (60%) affecting single eye (unilateral) or hereditary (40%) affecting both the eyes (bilateral). 15% of unilateral tumors can also be hereditary. It occurs generally below 3 years of age (it can be detected from birth to 7 years of age).
- RB results due to loss of function mutations, missense, nonsense or point mutation mutations in the RB1 gene located on chromosome 13, a tumor suppressor gene (Knudson's hypothesis, Figure 22.1).
- 5% of cases may result due to deletions involving RB1 locus, which transforms the primitive retinal cells into malignant. These can be detected by molecular genetic testing.
- In hereditary type, the affected children inherit it from the parent who may or may not be affected and it may be due to *de novo* germline mutation.

Knudson's hypothesis or two hit-hypothesis:

- Most children develop retinoblastoma as a sporadic event, where one copy gets mutated initially considered first hit followed by a second hit which completely turns the cell cancerous. This is called "two hit" hypothesis or Knudson hypothesis.
- In inherited cases, they inherit one mutation from the parents and acquire the second mutation during their lifetime. But it does not happen always.
- Penetrance of retinoblastoma is not 100%.
- Though it is inherited as autosomal dominant pattern but both hits make the gene recessive at molecular level.

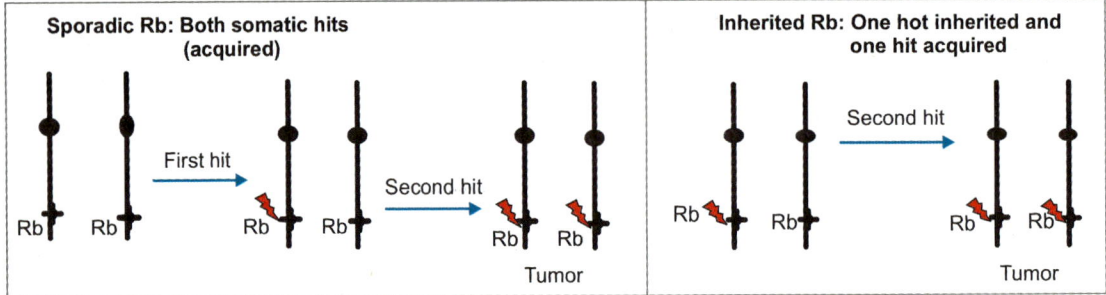

Figure 22.1: Knudson hypothesis or two-hit hypothesis

Need for the pediatrician to know about retinoblastoma:

- The pediatrician needs to know about the genetics of RB because the hereditary and sporadic cancer needs to be distinguished clearly as this differs in the severity and needs a different approach.
- To give information to the family about the type, nature, prognosis, management, surveillance of the proband for second eye examination, inheritance pattern, recurrence risk (50% if inherited and < 1% *de novo*) in the siblings and offspring of proband, prenatal diagnostic options and the fact that the affected children have increased risk for other tumors in the first few years of life.
- To survey the individuals with RB1 germline predisposition who also have a high lifetime risk of developing second primary malignancies, especially osteosarcomas, soft-tissue sarcomas, and melanomas.

Q 4. Write down features which are suggestive of inherited cancer susceptibility syndrome in a family.

Ans. Features which are suggestive of an inherited cancer susceptibility syndrome in a family are:

- More first or second-degree relatives having same cancer.
- Many of the close related family members having related cancers like breast and ovary.
- Rare cancer in two family members.
- Early onset of cancer (< 50 years of age).
- Bilateral or multisystem involvement.

- Features of a syndrome having cancer susceptibility like neurofibromatosis.

Q 5. Write the characteristics of some hereditary cancer syndromes.

Ans.

Hereditary cancer syndrome	Gene, inheritance	Other associated cancer
Familial breast +/– ovary cancer prostate	o BRCA1 o BRCA2 AD	o Breast o Ovary o Colon
Familial adenomatous polyposis	o APC AD	o Colorectal o Thyroid
Lynch syndrome	o hMLH1 o hMSH2 o hMSH6 o hPMS1 o hPMS2 AD	o Colorectal o Uterine o Ovary o Stomach o Small gut o Liver
Turcot syndrome	o APC o hMLH1 o hMSH2 AD	o Colon o Rectum o Brain
Peutz-Jeghers syndrome	o STK11 AD	o Stomach o Intestine o Breast o Uterus o Gonadal
Cowden (PTEN) syndrome	o PTEN AD	o Breast (females) o Testes o Papillary thyroid carcinoma

Contd.

Hereditary cancer syndrome	Gene, inheritance	Other associated cancer
Li-Fraumeni syndrome	o TP53 AD	o Breast o Brain o Adrenal o Hematological cancer o Sarcoma
Familial retino-blastoma	o RB AD	o Retinoblastoma
Multiple endocrine neoplasia (MEN)		
MEN1	o MEN1 AD	MEN 1: o Pituitary o Parathyroid o Pancreas

		o Thyroid o Adrenal
MEN2	o RET AD	MEN 2: o Medullary thyroid o Pheochro-mocytoma
Gorlin syndrome	o PTCH AD	o Basal cell carcinoma o Medullo-blastoma o Dental keratocyst o Ovary fibromas
von Hippel-Lindau disease	o VHL AD	o Brain o Kidney o Pancreas o Adrenal
AD: Autosomal dominant		

Q 6. What are the suggested screening tests recommended for various hereditary cancer syndromes?

Ans.

Cancer	Screening test	Periodicity	Age of starting (Year of age)
Breast/ovary cancer	o Mammography, ultrasound	Yearly once	o 40–50 (in average risk)
	o Doppler abdomen	–	o 35
	o CA 125	–	
Familial adenomatous polyposis	o Retinal examination	–	o Early childhood
	o Colonoscopy and sigmoidoscopy	o Yearly once	o 12
	o Endoscopy	o Once in 3 years	o 20
	o Neck ultrasound for thyroid	o Yearly once	o 20
Lynch syndrome	o Colonoscopy	o Once in 2–3 years	o At 25 years of age or 5 years before the age when cancer syndrome diagnosed earliest in the family member (not clear)
	o Ultrasound abdomen	o Yearly once	o 35
	o Mammography	o Yearly once	o 40–50
Cowden (PTEN) syndrome	o Magnetic resonance imaging	o Yearly once	o 30
	o Mammograph	o Yearly once	o 40
	o Ultrasound neck	o Yearly once	o 16

Contd.

Cancer	Screening test	Periodicity	Age of starting (Year of age)
	o Ultrasound abdomen	o Yearly once	o 40
	o Colonoscopy	–	o 35 and 55
Li-Fraumeni syndrome	o Magnetic resonance imaging	o Yearly once	o 20–25
	o Colonoscopy	o Once in 2–3 years	o 25
Familial retino-blastoma	o Retinal examination	o Frequently	o Birth
MEN 1	o Calcium; parathyroid, pituitary and pancreatic hormones	o Yearly once	o 8–50
MEN 2	o Calcium, parathyroid hormone, phosphorus, ultrasound neck	o Yearly once	o 10
	o Vanillyl mandelic acid in urine, calcitonin test	o Yearly once	
Gorlin syndrome	Clinical and dental examination	6–12 months	o 10 for medulloblastoma since 1st year of life.
von Hippel-Lindau disease	o Retinal examination	o Yearly once	o 5
	o Magnetic resonance imaging brain	o Once in 3 years	o 15
	o Ultrasound abdomen	o Yearly once	o 20
	o Vanillyl mandelic acid in urine	o Yearly once	o 10

Q 7. Write a note on etiological factors and genetic basis of breast cancer.

Ans. Breast cancer, a common cancer in women, accounts for 1 in 12 women characterized by:

- A lump
- Change in shape of the breast
- Discharge from the breast
- Alter overlying skin color or texture
- Depression in the breast
- Inverted nipples.

Breast symptoms can also be related with:

1. **Benign disease** like mastitis or fibro-adenoma
2. **Can be a clue to underlying malignancy** (ductal or lobular carcinoma) associated with other primary conditions like Paget's disease, inflammatory breast cancer or phyllode tumor.

When any of the clinical features points toward carcinoma, it is diagnosed by breast tissue biopsy and based on the invasiveness it is categorized into 5 stages. Molecular genetic testing is done to know the etiological variant. It is treated by various modalities like surgery, radiotherapy, chemotherapy or mutation-based therapy like tamoxifen in triple positive (HER2, oestrogen and progesterone receptor) and PARP inhibitors (poly ADP ribose polymerase) in triple negative. Prophylactic treatment is also given for various other associated complications like oophorectomy in case of *BRCA1/2* mutation.

The breast cancer can be sporadic (90%) or hereditary (5–10%) and is caused by various nongenetic and genetic factors like:

NONGENETIC FACTORS
○ Obesity
○ Age
○ Alcohol, tobacco
○ Lack of physical activity
○ Hormonal therapy, contraceptive pills radiation exposure
○ Chemicals like aromatic or organic compounds early-onset menstruation
○ Late-age pregnancies
○ Females not breastfed their children
○ Past and family history of breast cancer
○ Associated with syndrome like Klinefelter syndrome.

Genetic factors: Hereditary cancer constitutes 5–10% of the total cases of breast cancer. These can be either autosomal dominant (AD) or recessive. **The following genes are involved in hereditary breast cancers**.

a. **BRCA1 (46–87%) and BRCA2 (38–84%) genes having following features:**
  ○ Autosomal dominant (AD)
  ○ It can be suspected in families with occurrence before 50 years of age
  ○ Unilateral or bilateral
  ○ 2–3 members having similar history.
  ○ Associated ovarian cancer
  ○ Triple negative (HER2, estrogen and progesterone receptor gene)
  ○ Affected male
  ○ Identified mutation in family.
  Females with *BRCA1/2* have risk of 87% and males have risk of 20% to develop cancer. *BRCA1* mutation has risk of developing ovarian cancer of 20–60%. *BRCA2* mutation is more responsible for male breast cancer (6–10%), pancreas (2–7%), prostate cancer (15–20%) and melanoma.

b. **Other genes:** *HER2*, c-*MYC*, *RAS*, estrogen and progesterone receptor genes, cell cyclins D1 and E, *Rb*, *TP53*, *PTEN*, *CDH1*, *CHEK2*, *ATM*, *STK11*, *PALB2*, *BLM*, *WRN*, *RAD51C*, Lynch syndrome genes.
c. Associated with syndrome like Klinefelter syndrome.
d. Racial factors.

Genetic Mechanism

○ Breast cancer shows variable genetic and environmental interactions.
○ These genetic mutations along with associated environmental factors switch on P13K/AKT, RAS/MEK/ERK pathway permanently which interferes with the normal programmed cell death. Various growth factors and estrogen receptor mutations cause overexpression of adipose tissue in breast tissue which in turn causes cell proliferation and malignancy.
○ *BRCA1/2* causes DNA repair defect and mismatch repair leading to cancer.

Q 8. What is the recurrence risk of hereditary breast cancer with BRCA1/2 in siblings and other family members of the proband?

Ans. The recurrence risk of hereditary breast cancer with BRCA1/2 in siblings: 50% if one of the parents of proband has *BRCA1/2* germline mutation. Risk of developing cancer depends upon the peneterance of the variant, age and gender of the individual at risk.

The recurrence risk in other family members of the proband depends upon the mutation status of the parents of proband and pedigree analysis.

Q 9. Write about recommendations on breast cancer screening for women with personal history of breast cancer.

Ans. According to National Institute of Health and Care Excellence (NICE) guidelines, recommendations on breast cancer screening for women with personal history of breast cancer are as follows:

Age (in years)	High-risk: BRCA1/2 positive, TP53 negative	No testing but chance is greater than 30% for TP53 carrier	TP53 positive
20–69	o Annual MRI	Annual MRI	Annual MRI
30–49	o No mammography o Annual MRI	–	–
50–69	o Annual mammography o MRI if breast tissue is dense	–	–
70	o Mammography as part of the population screening program	–	–

Surveillance for individuals who are at moderate risk:

Females:
- *Self-examination:* Monthly once.
- *Clinical examination:* At 25 years of age, every 6–12 months.
- *MRI breast:* At 25–30 years of age, once in a year.
- *Mammography:* At 30 years of age, once in a year.
- *Transvaginal ultrasound and serum CA 125:* At 35 years of age.

Males:
- *Self and clinical examination:* Monthly once, started at 35 years of age.
- *Prostate examination:* At 45 years of age, once in a year.

Q 10. Write about recommendations on breast cancer screening for women with no personal history of breast cancer.

Ans. According to NICE guidelines following are the recommendations on breast cancer screening for women with no personal history of breast cancer:

Age	Moderate risk	High-risk					
		High-risk of breast cancer but with a 30% or lower chance of being a BRCA or TP53 carrier	Not tested but chance is greater than 30% for BRCA carrier	BRCA1 or BRCA2 mutation identified	Not tested but chance is greater than 30% for TP53 carrier	TP53 mutation is identified
20–29	No mammography or MRI	No mammography or MRI	No mammography or MRI	No mammography or MRI	o No mammography o Suggest MRI yearly once	o Do not suggest mammography o Suggest MRI yearly once

Contd.

Age	Moderate risk	High-risk				
30–39	No	Mammography yearly once but no MRI	MRI and consider mammography yearly once	MRI and consider mammography yearly once	○ No mammography but MRI yearly once	○ No mammography but MRI yearly once
40–49	Mammography yearly once but no MRI	Mammography yearly once but no MRI	Mammography and MRI, yearly once		○ No mammography but MRI yearly once	○ No mammography but MRI yearly once
50–59		Mammography yearly once but no MRI	Mammography yearly once, no MRI until dense breast signs present		○ Mammography according to general population guidelines	○ No mammography
				No MRI until dense breast signs present	○ Recommend MRI yearly once	
60–69		Mammography according to general population guidelines	Mammography according to general population guidelines		○ Mammography as part of the population screening program	○ Do not offer mammography
No MRI	No MRI	No MRI until dense breast signs present	No MRI until dense breast signs present	No MRI until dense breast signs present	○ MRI yearly once	
70+						○ No mammography

Q 11. Write about recommendations on breast cancer screening for women with no personal history of breast cancer.

Ans. According to NICE guidelines following are the recommendations on breast cancer screening for women with no personal history of breast cancer:

Age	Moderate risk	High-risk	Not tested but chance is greater than 30% for BRCA carrier	BRCA1 or BRCA2 mutation identified	Not tested but chance is greater than 30% for TP53 carrier	TP53 mutation is identified
		High-risk of breast cancer but with a 30% or lower chance of being a BRCA or TP53 carrier				
20–29	No mammography or MRI	No mammography or MRI	No mammography or MRI	No mammography or MRI	o No mammography o Suggest MRI yearly once	o Do not suggest mammography o Suggest MRI yearly once
30–39	No	Mammography yearly once but no MRI	MRI and consider mammography yearly once	MRI and consider mammography yearly once	o No mammography but MRI yearly once	o No mammography but MRI yearly once
40–49		Mammography yearly once but no MRI	Mammography and MRI, yearly once		o No mammography but MRI yearly once	o No mammography but MRI yearly once
50–59		Mammography yearly once but no MRI	Mammography yearly once, no MRI until dense breast signs present		o Mammography according to general population guidelines	o No mammography
				No MRI until dense breast signs present	o Recommend MRI yearly once	
60–69	No MRI	Mammography according to general population guidelines	Mammography according to general population guidelines		o Mammography as part of the population screening program	o Do not offer mammography
70+	No MRI	No MRI until dense breast signs present	No MRI until dense breast signs present	No MRI until dense breast signs present	o MRI yearly once	o No mammography

MRI: Magnetic resonance imaging

BIBLIOGRAPHY

1. AlAli A, Kletke S, Gallie B, Lam WC. Retinoblastoma for pediatric ophthalmologists. The Asia-Pacific Journal of Ophthalmology. 2018 May 1; 7(3):160–8.
2. Emery and Rimoin's Principles and Practice of Medical genetics, 7th edition.
3. Malkin D, Nichols KE, Zelley K, Schiffman JD. Predisposition to pediatric and hematologic cancers: a moving target. American Society of Clinical Oncology Educational Book. 2014; 34(1):e44–55.
4. Thompson and Thompson. Genetics in Medicine, 8th Edition.

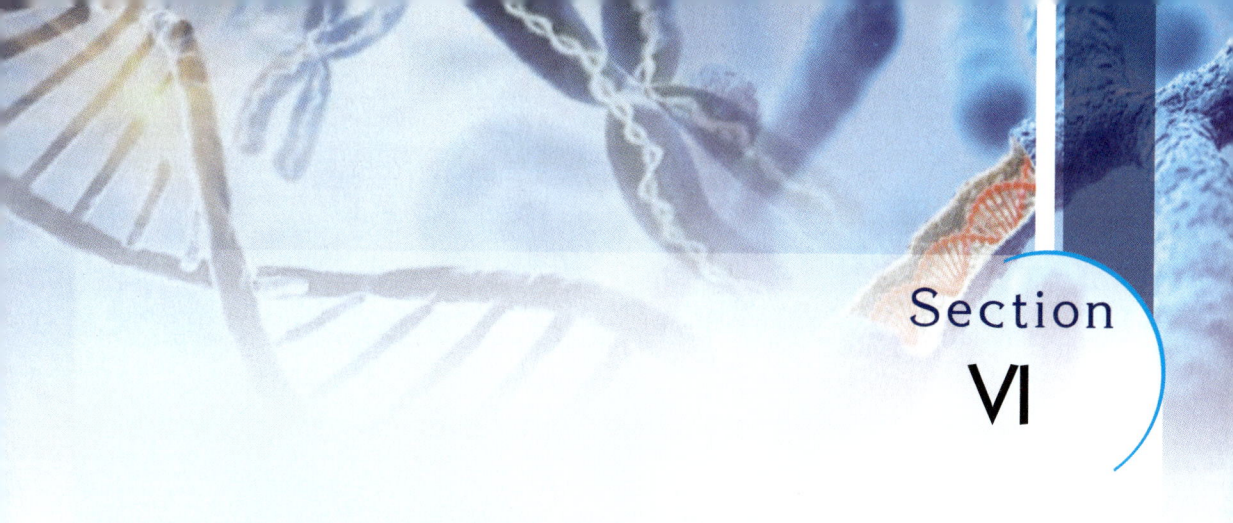

Recent Advances in Genetics

- Recent Advances in Diagnostic and Therapeutic Genetics

Recent Advances in Diagnostic and Therapeutic Genetics

Prajnya Ranganath, Risha Nahar Lulla, T Karthik Bharadwaj

RECENT ADVANCES IN DIAGNOSTIC GENETICS
PRAJNYA RANGANATH, RISHA NAHAR LULLA, T KARTHIK BHARADWAJ

Q 1. Write a brief note on noninvasive prenatal testing (NIPT), its procedure, clinical indications and applications.

Ans. Noninvasive prenatal testing (NIPT) is the method of looking for genetic abnormalities in the fetus, by studying the fetal genetic material obtained from the mother's blood rather than through invasive fetal sampling procedures.

Procedure: NIPT includes cell-based and cell-free methods. The most popular technique involves study of the circulating cell-free fetal DNA (cffDNA) obtained from the maternal plasma. cffDNA derived from apoptosis of trophoblasts, starts appearing in the maternal circulation by around 7 weeks of gestation, and becomes readily detectable by around 9 to 10 weeks gestation, by which time it accounts for around 5–10% of the total cell-free DNA in the maternal plasma.

Approaches: Two different **approaches** based on next-generation sequencing are used for detection of common numerical chromosomal aberrations.

- In the **counting-based approach,** millions of sequences generated by massive parallel sequencing of the cell-free DNA are aligned against the reference human genome and reads are counted to determine the chromosomal ploidy status.
- In the **SNP genotyping approach,** the pattern of single nucleotide polymorphisms (SNPs) in the fetus is compared to the maternal SNP genotype to detect fetal aneuploidy.

Clinical Indications of NIPT:

- Elderly mother >35 years of age
- Parents are carriers for balanced rearrangements
- Previous child affected with aneuploidy
- Abnormal ultrasound findings and prenatal screening reports.

Clinical Application of NIPT:

- The most common application of NIPT currently is for the prenatal detection of common chromosomal aneuploidies (i.e. trisomy of chromosomes 21, 13 and 18, monosomy of chromosome X, and other sex chromosome aneuploidies).
- The other less commonly used applications of NIPT include detection of fetal chromosomal microdeletions.
- For fetal RhD genotyping in an Rh-negative mother with an Rh-positive husband, and to determine the fetal sex (not permitted in India).
- Standardization of NIPT for prenatal testing for monogenic disorders is also currently underway.

Q 2. Write a brief note on advantages and limitations of noninvasive prenatal testing (NIPT).

Ans.

ADVANTAGES OF NIPT
○ It is noninvasive in nature and consequently poses no risk for procedure-related miscarriages.
○ The detection rate of NIPT is >99% and false positive rate is <0.1% for trisomy 21, because of which it is being offered to prenatal women with increased risk of fetal Down syndrome.

LIMITATIONS OF NIPT
○ The test may be non-informative, requiring a redraw if the fetal DNA fraction sample is less than 4%.
○ The problem of confined placental mosaicism can give false positive result. So, invasive fetal sampling and chromosomal analysis must be done for confirmation.
○ NIPT being used in some centers for common chromosomal aneuploidies, even in low-risk prenatal women, raises the issue of much higher costs at present.

Q 3. Write a note on pre-implantation genetic screening (PGS) testing and pre-implantation genetic diagnosis (PGD) testing and their limitations. Mention a few clinical conditions in which PGD can be done.

Ans. Preimplantation genetic testing is performed prior (preimplantation) to embryo (a fertilized egg) transfer during the process of *in vitro* fertilization (IVF) technique. An embryo biopsy is done to remove about 3–8 cells from each day-5 embryo (a blastocyst). Then these cells are sent to a lab for testing. The embryo is usually frozen and implanted later. Genetic testing of the embryos is broken down into two categories:

1. **Preimplantation genetic screening (PGS)**
2. **Preimplantation genetic diagnosis (PGD)**

Although sometimes these terms may be used interchangeably, they are in fact different. The goal of both, however, is to increase the chance of selecting a healthy embryo that will develop into a healthy baby.

1. **PGS** analyses biopsied cells from the embryo to screen for and identify any potential chromosomal abnormalities when there are no known potentially inherited disorders. This is known to be better for couples who have a history of miscarriages or failed IVF cycles due to unknown etiology.

2. **PGD,** on the other hand, uses the same process to detect a specific disorder (using a special created probe) that has a high probability of being passed down from parents to their offspring. Hence, PGD can only be run if the partners are carriers of a genetic disorder, and the causative mutation is known for both. PGD can be done in several clinical scenarios such as:

   ○ Single gene disorders including thalassemia and cystic fibrosis
   ○ Sex-linked disorders such as fragile X syndrome and Duchenne muscular dystrophy
   ○ To find matching stem cells for siblings in need of a bone marrow transplant.

Drawbacks of preimplantation genetic testing:

○ It is a costly procedure.
○ The damage to the embryo caused due to the removal of cells and freezing is uncertain and warrants further studies.
○ The genetic testing process can sometimes fail due to various reasons and resampling of cells from same embryo is difficult.
○ Mosaicism does not accurately reflect the genetic status of the embryo.

Q 4. Define pharmacogenomics and write a brief note on the role of pharmacogenomics in medicine.

Ans. Pharmacogenomics is the study of how genes affect an individual's response to drugs. It combines pharmacology along with the study of genes and their functions to help develop effective, safe medications and doses that may be tailored to an individual's genetic makeup. When studying drug action in individuals, researchers focus on two major determinants:

1. Amount of drug needed to reach its target in the body, i.e. pharmacokinetics
2. Level of response to drug by target cells in the body, i.e. pharmacodynamics.

Both are critical considerations in the field of pharmacogenomics.

There are four categories for drug metabolism based on that dose or drug has to be changed:

1. **Poor metabolizer:** Alternative drug has to be prescribed.
2. **Intermediate metaboliser:** Dose of drug has to be decreased.
3. **Extensive metabolizer:** Same dose to be continued.
4. **Ultra metabolizer:** Dose of drug has to be increased.

Many drugs are currently prescribed with the ideology of one-size-fits-all. However, several drugs do not work with the same efficiency for everyone. Some individuals will benefit from a medication, few will not respond at all, and others will experience unfavorable adverse drug reactions (ADRs). A significant cause of hospitalizations and deaths are due to ADRs. With the knowledge gained from the Human Genome Project, researchers are learning how inherited differences in genes affect the body's response to medications. These genetic differences are now used to predict whether a drug will be effective for a particular person, prediction of optimum dosage, and to help prevent ADRs.

Examples of conditions that affect a person's response to certain drugs include isoniazid (autosomal recessive mutation), slow metabolism, G6PD disorder, warfarin sensitivity/resistance, clopidogrel resistance, Stevens-Johnson syndrome/toxic epidermal necrolysis and thiopurine S-methyltransferase deficiency among others.

Q 5. What do you mean by personalized medicine? Write about the role of genomic information in personalized medicine.

Ans. Personalized medicine is the tailoring of medical treatment to the individual characteristics of each patient. The approach relies on our understanding of how a person's unique molecular and genetic profile makes them susceptible to certain diseases and drugs. According to recent updates by the Food and Drug Administration, USA, there are 406 pharmacogenomic biomarkers in drug labeling.

Personalized medicine is impacting patient care in many diseases. For example:

⊃ **Trastuzumab for breast cancer:** Patients with HER2 positive tumors treated with trastuzumab showed reduced recurrence by 52% in combination with chemotherapy.

⊃ Vemurafenib for melanoma only works in the treatment of patients whose cancer tests positive for the V600E BRAF mutation.

⊃ Sulfonylurea in HNF1A mutation.

⊃ B*5701 mutation causes hypersensitivity due to abacavir used in human immunodeficiency virus.

Q 6. What is the scope of whole genome sequencing (WGS) as a clinical diagnostic test in future?

Ans. After the advent of next generation sequencing and with growing insights into the importance of non-coding regions of the genome in determining the phenotype of a patient, we are staring at a 100-dollar genome, which would soon become a reality to test all kinds of genetic diseases in future like:

⊃ **Neonatal diagnosis:** Rapid WGS has been recently used for diagnosis of sepsis in infected neonates in addition to investigating the possibility of a coexisting/stand alone genetic disorder in sick neonates and to intervene early.

⊃ **Cell-free fetal DNA analysis:** WGS approaches from cell-free fetal DNA in maternal plasma have been successfully used for noninvasive prenatal diagnosis of not only trisomies but also microdeletion syndromes and in some cases single gene disorders too.

- **Prenatal diagnosis:** Though chromosomal microarray is still the first line investigation of choice in fetuses with malformations detected prenatally, many recent papers have demonstrated the utility of WES as well. WGS which can replace both of the above technically would be investigation of choice in near future.
- **Neurodevelopmental disorders:** In the future, WGS will be the only test to identify various simple variants to complex variants across the whole genetic material responsible for unidentified neurodevelopmental disorders.
- **Newborn screening:** The data generated by newborn screening done by WGS would be stored and subsequently utilized during various stages in a person's life including evaluations during hospital admissions, pharmacogenomics, premarital carrier screening, etc. in addition to recognition of treatable/potentially treatable disorders at birth.
- **Products of conception and fetal autopsies:** For etiological identification.
- **Personalized medicine based on genomes:** WGS may soon become a diagnostic clinical tool to diagnose various mutations across the whole genome of a person.

Q 7. Write a note on functional studies of human genome.

Ans. Functional studies of human genome

Due to the advent of NGS at low cost, generating genomic information of an individual has become easier than ever before. However, understanding the functional implications of the variations detected has become a major roadblock. Many technologies have been developed in the recent years to enable high throughput screening of functional implications of the variations. These can be divided into:

1. **Technologies looking into regulatory mechanisms at the DNA level:**
   - **ChIP Seq:** Chromatin immuno-precipitation uses antibodies against specific targets like histones, methylated sequences, transcription factors, etc. to study the chromatin organization and regulation at genomic scale.
   - **Bisulphite sequencing** relies on the principle of conversion of unmethylated cytosine to uracil on exposure to bisulphite, to recognize methylation patterns across the genome.
   - **Conformation sequencing strategies** (3C/4C/5C/HiC): Using various crosslinking strategies, the proximally ligated segments of DNA are sequenced to understand spatial organization of the chromatin, that are called topologically associated domains.
   - **Long range sequencing technologies** like nanopore sequencing to recognize base modifications and to study epigenomics with more sensitivity.

2. **Transcriptomic studies identify the relation between genomic variants and the gene expression:**
   - **RNAseq:** RNA sequencing to study the transcriptomes, sequencing of long non-coding RNA and micro RNAs.
   - **Single cell RNA sequencing** relies on molecular barcoding of transcripts from individual cells to identify expression profile at single cell.
   - **Spatial transcriptomics:** To study expression profiles of physically related cells on a histological section.

3. **Proteomics**
   - **Mass spectrometry:** Used for large-scale protein identification and also for high throughput affinity detection assays.

4. **Metabolomics:** Used to study the metabolites which can be the initial, intermediate or end product of a metabolic reaction either at cellular or tissue level and can assess directly the cell function of an organism.

5. **CRISPR technologies** or creating targeted functional knockdowns using anti-sense oligonucleotides, siRNAs or other RNA interference technologies to study implications of loss of function mutations.

The ENCODE (encyclopedia of DNA elements) project to identify functional elements of the genome and the GTEx (genotype tissue expression) project which aims to understand transcriptomes in various tissues are two international consortia deserving a special mention.

Q 8. Write a note on direct consumer testing.

Ans. Genetic tests that are marketed directly to consumers without the involvement of a healthcare provider are commonly referred to as direct-to-consumer tests (DTC) (recreational genetic tests or personal genomic tests). These tests generally require the customer to collect a specimen, such as saliva, buccal swab or urine, and send it to the company for testing and analysis.

DTC testing is expanding the number of people who can get genetic testing to know their genomic variants. Some of these genetic variants can be used to diagnose a rare disease, provide information about a person's risk of developing disease, or other types of information. Some variants have clinical significance and may give consumers insight into monitoring their own health, or about potential disease or conditions.

To keep in mind, not all direct-to-consumer tests are genetic tests, though the majority in the market today are. Some measure other things, such as levels of proteins in your body, levels of toxins in urine, or levels and types of bacterial flora (referred to as a "microbiome").

DTC genetic tests provide only partial information about an individual's health. Other genetic variants, environmental factors, lifestyle choices, and family medical and personal history will also affect the likelihood of developing many disorders. These factors would be discussed during a consultation with a doctor or genetic counselor, but in many cases, they are not addressed when using at-home genetic tests. The different DTC tests that are available in the market will differ widely in their selection of genetic markers, types of health conditions included and will also have variable analytical and clinical validity—the consumer needs to be aware of these as a part of informed decision-making process prior to testing. Now in the genetic field CD-GT (consumer directed genetic testing) where the patients ask the clinicians for specific genetic testing to be done for them. But there are lot of challenges related to the results, interpretation of reports and difficult questions asked by the patients in elation these tests.

Q 9. Describe the role of artificial intelligence in genetics.

Ans. Artificial intelligence (AI) is the development of computer systems that can perform tasks by simulating human intelligence. AI systems heavily rely on the methods of natural language processing (NLP), machine learning (ML), deep learning algorithms, speech recognition and graphics processing units that power their training. These advances in AI have led to a recent and rapidly increasing interest in medical AI applications, including clinical genomics.

- These AI systems are trained on external health data that have usually been interpreted by humans, e.g. clinical images that have been labeled and interpreted by a clinical expert.
- The AI system then learns to execute the interpretation task on new health data of the same type, which in clinical diagnostics is often the identification or forecasting of a disease state.
- To tackle the vast amount of genomic and clinical data that must be analyzed, many researchers are implementing machine learning techniques to bring down costs.
- In genomic sequencing and diagnostics, deep learning is used to process large and complex genomic and clinical datasets for specific tasks such as variant calling/prioritization, genome annotation, variant classification, and phenotype-to-genotype correspondence.
- AI-based computer vision approaches are poised to revolutionize image-based diagnostics such as medical imaging/scans, dysmorphology analytics tools (London Medical Database).

⌁ There is future potential of AI in personalized medicine applications, especially for risk prediction in common complex diseases, rapid high throughput genomic reporting for patients in intensive care units.

However, the challenges, limitations, and biases must be carefully addressed for the successful deployment of AI in medical genetics.

RECENT ADVANCES IN THERAPEUTIC GENETICS
PRAJNYA RANGANATH

Q 10. Write a note on recent therapeutic advances in the treatment of hemo-globinopathies.

Ans. Numerous therapeutic trials which have been approved, are ongoing for hemoglo-binopathies beta thalassemia and sickle cell disease (SCD) include:

i. **Modulators of erythropoiesis:** Luspatercept (in phase III clinical trials) acts via the TGF-β (transforming growth factor beta) signalling pathway and ruxolitinib (in phase II trials) cause JAK2 (janus kinase 2) inhibition, promote the differentiation and maturation of late-stage erythrocyte precursors.

ii. **Iron-overload reducing agents:** Hepcidin mimetics (e.g. PTG-300) and ferroportin inhibitors (e.g. S142).

iii. **Agents to increase HbF:** Apart from hydroxyurea approved by FDA, other HbF-enhancing drugs under investigation include LSD-1 (lysine specific demethylase 1) inhibitors, HDAC (histone deacetylase) inhibitors and thalidomide inhibitors.

iv. **Inhibitors of HbS polymerization:** Agent Voxelotor binds reversibly to Hb by covalent bond and inhibits HbS polymerization . It is granted approval by FDA for SCD patients older than 12 years with only mild side effects such as headache, fever, diarrhea and nausea.

v. **Agents that reduce RBC adhesion to endothelium:** Phase III trials are ongoing for crizanlizumab, an antibody which acts against the adhesion molecule P-selectin to improve blood flow in SCD patients.

vi. **Gene therapy** (called Zynteglo) with autologous CD34+ cells transduced with a lentiviral vector containing the genetically modified beta globin gene has been approved in Europe for beta thalassemia patients older than 12 years with side effects like infusion-related reactions, thrombocytopenia, nausea, headache, and hypocalcemia.

vii. **CRISPR-Cas9 gene editing** to correct the defective beta globin gene.

viii. **BCL11A inactivators** to reactivate gamma-globin production and increase fetal hemoglobin (HbF) levels.

Q 11. Write a note on recent therapeutic advances in the treatment of cystic fibrosis.

Ans. Mutations in the *CFTR* gene lead to absence or reduction in functioning of the cystic fibrosis transmembrane conductance regulator (CFTR) protein, which results in abnormal mucus secretion and damage to multiple organs. The therapies which have been recently approved or are being investigated for cystic fibrosis include:

i. **CFTR modulators:** FDA approved ivacaftor (CFTR potentiator which enhances the movement of the chloride ions through the channel pore) and lumacaftor (which acts as a chaperone for CFTR protein folding and improves trafficking of CFTR proteins to the cell surface). Depending on the *CFTR* gene mutations, e.g. for patients with the common F508del mutation, ivacaftor + lumacaftor combination is used. Adverse effects, such as nausea, diarrhea, dyspnea, and nasopharyngitis (<10%), altered liver functions and hepatic encephalopathy (<1%) may also occur. Triple combination CFTR modulators (elexacaftor + tezacaftor + ivacaftor) are under phase III clinical trials.

ii. **Dornase alfa:** This is a recombinant human deoxyribonuclease enzyme which reduces the viscidity of the mucus and helps in better clearance of secretions from the airways.

iii. **CFTR mutation-specific correctors:** VX-661 are small-molecule therapies to increase the quantity of functional CFTR protein with specific *CFTR* pathogenic variants.

iv. **Alternate ion channel regulation:** To restore airway surface liquid.

v. **Gene therapy:** This is in early clinical trials.

Q 12. Write a note on recent therapeutic advances in the treatment of Duchenne muscular dystrophy.

Ans. Duchenne muscular dystrophy (DMD) is a relatively common genetic disorder. Many treatment strategies for DMD are in various experimental stages at present. The important ones are as:

1. **Pharmacologic agents:**
   i. *Ataluren (PTC124) stop codon read through agents:* These agents misread the RNA and allow alternative amino acids to be inserted at the site of the mutated premature stop codon, thereby allowing continuation of translation into a functional (albeit partially functional) protein (phase III trials).

   ii. *Utrophin upregulating agents:* These increase the expression of utrophin, a muscle sarcolemmal protein similar to dystrophin. Utrophin, if upregulated, can partially compensate for absence of dystrophin (phase I trials).

   iii. *Myostatin and histone deacetylase inhibitors* suppress muscle degeneration and improve skeletal muscle mass in animal models but have not shown significant benefits.

2. **Gene modification:**
   i. *Antisense oligonucleotides (AONs):* Exon skipping involves blocking of transcription and prevention of translation of only the mutated portion of the mutated *DMD* gene with AONs.

The rest of the mRNA is allowed to undergoes translation into a functional protein. **Eteplirsen** for exon 51-skipping and golodirsen for exon 53-skipping have been approved by FDA showing less severe side effects, such as headache, fever, falls, nausea, vomiting, cough and abdominal pain especially for golodirsen.

   ii. *Gene editing:* Correction of the defective gene with the CRISPR-Cas9 system has been found to be effective in cell lines and animal models and clinical trials are going to commence shortly.

3. **Gene transfer:** Recombinant adeno-associated viral vectors (rAAV) have been used for transfer of the normal gene into patients. As the entire *DMD* gene is large, mini and microdystrophin constructs containing only sequences which code for important functional domains have been tried. Phase I trial has been completed.

4. **Cell therapy** by transferring myoblasts from a normal person into a DMD patient, has not been found to be beneficial in early clinical trials.

Q 13. Write a note on recent therapeutic advances in the treatment of spinal muscular atrophy (SMA).

Ans. Spinal muscular atrophy (SMA) is an autosomal recessive disorder caused by mutations in the SMN1 (survival of motor neuron 1) gene. In addition to physical rehabilitation and supportive care, some new available targeted therapies now can be classified as:

1. **SMN2-targeted approaches** aim to promote translation of SMN2 to increase functional protein to compensate for reduced or absent expression of SMN1 in SMA patients. For example, antisense oligonucleotides, i.e. short single stranded RNA molecules, which bind to complementary sequences in the SMN2 transcript and alter its splicing, results in generation of more full-length transcripts involving exon 7.

Drugs recently discovered which can be used for SMA therapy:

- *Nusinersen* (marketed as Spinraza), given intrathecally, is one such ASO therapy approved by FDA for all subtypes of SMA, and has been reported to lead to significant improvement in motor function. Side effects like fever, constipation, vomiting, lower respiratory infection, back pain and post-lumbar puncture headache are known to occur in very low proportion.
- *Risdiplam* and *Branaplam* are two other oral splicing modifiers under clinical trials.

2. **SMN-independent approaches** are based on the use of agents to increase muscle strength in patients with SMA (phase II trials).
   - *Reldesemtiv,* a tropinin complex activator which slows the rate of calcium release from the regulatory troponin complex of fast skeletal muscle fibers.
   - *SRK-015,* a myostatin inhibitor.
3. **Gene transfer therapy, Zolgensma,** recently approved by FDA is delivered using the adeno-associated virus serotype 9 (AAV9) vector in SMA type I patients. It is given intravenously as a single dose and has been reported to result in significant improvement in motor milestones and to prolong survival without ventilator-dependence. Elevation of liver enzymes and vomiting are the two most common adverse effects. It is, however, very expensive.

Q 14. Write a note on recent therapeutic advances in the treatment of Marfan syndrome.

Ans. Marfan syndrome is a genetic connective tissue disorder and aortic aneurysm and aortic dissection are the major cause for the mortality. Newer therapeutic strategies for Marfan syndrome mainly to prevent aortic remodelling in affected patients in addition to beta blockers such as propranolol and atenolol are:

- **Angiotensin II receptor blocker (ARB):** The aortic root dilatation in Marfan syndrome results from excess activation of trans-forming growth factor beta (TGFβ), a cytokine involved in cellular proliferation, migration and programmed cell death. The angiotensin II receptor blocker (ARB) Losartan decreases TGFβ signalling as well as reduce hemodynamic stress and thereby prevents or slows down aortic root dilatation and aortic wall changes. Many prospective trials have suggested that the combination of beta blockers and losartan affords better protection against aortic complications than beta blockers alone in both children and adults with Marfan syndrome.

- **Doxycycline and statins:** Study of the role of matrix metalloproteinase inhibition with doxycycline and of statins such as pravastatin, in reducing and delaying aortic root dilatation is undergoing.

- **Induced pluripotent stem cell (iPSC)-derived vascular models** of Marfan syndrome are being designed to study the pathogenesis of aortic aneurysms and identify newer therapeutic targets.

Q 15. Write a note on RNA modification therapy.

Ans. RNA-modification therapeutic strategies targeting the messenger RNA (mRNA), can be categorized based on the mechanism of action as follows:

1. **Inhibition of mRNA translation with antisense oligonucleotides (ASOs):** ASOs, short single stranded sequences (13 to 25 nucleotides) are chemically modified to increase their efficiency, cellular uptake and intracellular stability. ASOs inhibit gene expression by altering mRNA splicing, arresting mRNA translation, and inducing degradation of mRNA through RNase H.

USE OF ASOs

- Can be used for 'exon skipping', where the translation of only the mutated portion of the mRNA that cause shift in the reading frame is blocked, and the rest of the mRNA is allowed to undergo translation into a functional protein.

o The FDA approved ASO-based therapies include
   a. Nusinersen for spinal muscular atrophy
   b. Eteplirsen for exon 51-skipping and golo-dirsen for exon 53-skipping for Duchenne muscular dystrophy
   c. Inotersen for hereditary transthyretin-related amyloidosis.

2. **RNA interference (RNAi) using small interfering RNAs (siRNAs) or short hairpin RNAs (shRNAs):** RNA interference (RNAi) uses short double-stranded RNA molecules, made up of around 21 to 23 nucleotides, called siRNAs or shRNAs and microRNAs, to silence the expression of genes by degrading the mRNAs and thereby preventing their translation.
   Example: Two siRNA-based therapies approved by FDA:
   a. Patisiran for hereditary transthyretin-related amyloidosis
   b. Givosiran for acute hepatic porphyria.
3. **RNA cleavage with ribozymes:** Ribozymes enzymes, siRNAs and shRNAs catalyse RNA cleavage and can be delivered to the target cells directly in RNA form or in transcribed form from 'therapeutic genes' delivered through viral vectors. For studying their efficacy for treatment of viral infections such as human immuno-deficiency virus and hepatitis C virus, certain genetic disorders and some cancers, clinical trials are ongoing.

Q 16. Write a note on CRISPR-Cas9 techno-logy.

Ans. CRISPR-Cas9 technology: The CRISPR loci consist of 21–47 nucleotides long, clustered, direct palindromic repeats. At present, CRISPR-Cas9 is the most extensively studied genome-editing technique. It is based on the bacterial immune mechanism of RNA-directed DNA cleavage.

- **It is made up of two components:** Cas9 and single guide RNA sequence (sgRNA).
- sgRNA consists of a custom-designed short sequence called CRISPR RNA (crRNA) fused to the trans-activating crRNA (tracrRNA) sequence.
- The crRNA sequence is complementary to a 20 bp-long sequence in the target DNA, while the tracrRNA acts as a scaffold linking the crRNA to Cas9.
- Cas9 is a DNA endonuclease which contains the HNH domain and RucV-like domain.
- The HNH domain cuts the target DNA strand complementary to crRNA, while the RucV-like domain cleaves the opposite strand of the target DNA, thereby creating a double-strand break at this site.
- Thus, sgRNA directs the Cas9 endonuclease system to the specific target genomic locus, following which Cas9 nuclease generates a DSB at the target site (Figure 23.1).

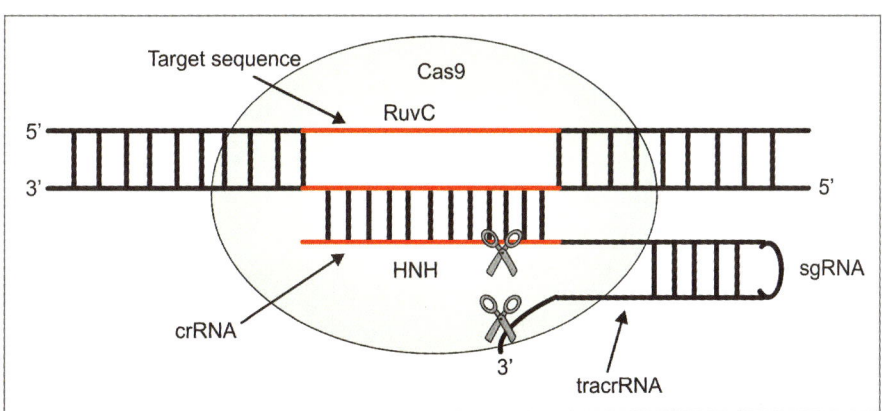

Figure 23.1: : Schematic representation of the CRISPR-Cas9 gene editing system

⟳ The DSB is further repaired through the NHEJ or HDR mechanism, which are separated by interspersed nucleotide sequences called spacers. The spacer sequences are transcribed into CRISPR RNA (crRNA), which bind to tracrRNA to direct sequence-specific DNA breaks by the Cas9 protein.

Q 17. What do you mean by 'three-parent baby' and for which genetic disorder can this technology be used to circumvent the problem of transmission of disease to future generation?

Ans. 'Three-parent baby' is an assisted reproductive technique that involves three gametes. The nuclear DNA is taken from the prospective parents (from the male and female partner) and the mitochondrial DNA is taken from a donor oocyte. This method, also referred to as 'mitochondrial transfer' has been developed to permit women affected by mitochondrial diseases and/or who are carriers for mitochondrial genome mutations, to have genetically related children that do not inherit these diseases. Mitochondrial genome mutations are transmitted by an affected mother to all her offspring through mitochondria in the oocyte cytoplasm.

The three main mitochondrial replacement techniques used are:

a. In the **pronuclear transfer technique,** two zygotes are created *in vitro*, one with the prospective parents' sperm and oocyte and the other one with a donated oocyte and the father's sperm. After the sperm has fertilized the oocyte, the nuclear material of both parents is enclosed in different membranes that are called the male and female pronuclei. At day one in the development, and prior to their fusion, the two pronuclei are removed from both zygotes and the intending parents' pronuclei are transferred to the enucleated cell produced with the donor's oocyte. Thus, the resulting embryo gets the nuclear genes of the parents and only the mitochondrial genes of the donor.

b. The **maternal spindle transfer technique** is similar to pronuclear transfer but uses unfertilized eggs instead of the early-stage embryos.

c. In **polar body transfer,** a polar body from the mother is used instead of nuclear material extracted from her oocyte.

This therapy is legally permitted in the United Kingdom but owing to the ethical challenges it has not yet been approved for clinical use in many countries across the world.

Q 18. Write a note on recent advances *in utero* stem cell therapy.

Ans. *In utero* stem cell transplantation (IUSCT) is a fetal therapeutic modality aimed at correcting prenatally detected genetic disorders.

***In utero* stem cell therapy (IUSCT):** Apart from early correction of the genetic disorder, the rationale behind IUSCT is that it has numerous therapeutic advantages and the immature immune system of the developing fetus does not elicit an immune response to allogenic cells. This facilitates better acceptance and engraftment of the donor cells, removes the need for use of prior myeloablative therapy and its related toxicity and complications, and also helps the baby to develop donor-specific tolerance, so that postnatally if required, further stem cell transplantation can be done from the same donor, with minimal immunosuppression.

Procedure: IUSCT involves administering the stem cells through the umbilical vein of the fetus (intravascular route) or into the fetal peritoneum (intraperitoneal route), usually between 16 and 26 weeks of gestation, with the intravascular route showing better cell engraftment in human experiments.

APPLICATIONS OF IUSCT

○ *In utero* hematopoietic SCT has been tried in humans to treat some genetic disorders including hemoglobinopathies, primary immunodeficiencies and inborn errors of metabolism.

○ *In utero* mesenchymal SCT has also been tried for osteogenesis imperfecta (OI).

○ IUSCT has shown very promising results in mouse model than in human experiments except only in a few disorders mentioned above with a low level of engraftment.

Q 19. Write a note on *in utero* gene therapy.

Ans. Like IUSCT, *in utero* gene therapy (IUGT) is also a fetal therapeutic modality aimed at correcting prenatally detected genetic disorders.

Procedure: It involves ultrasound-guided prenatal transfer of the normal gene or corrected gene via injection into the umbilical vein or the concerned fetal organ to enable normal production of the deficient gene product before the onset of irreversible organ damage. The immaturity of the fetal immune system and the small size of fetus are expected to improve the uptake of the transgene and enable its integration into a large proportion of cells.

APPLICATIONS OF IUGT

○ IUGT experiments have been performed in animal models for various metabolic, central nervous system and musculoskeletal disorders. However, most studies have shown only transient expression of the transgene and have not shown sustained benefit.

○ Human IUGT is not currently approved because of ethical concerns and the potential for teratogenic effects.

BIBLIOGRAPHY

1. ACOG Committee Opinion (2020). Preimplantation Genetic Testing, No. 799. American College of Obstetricians and Gynecology. Available online at https://www.acog.org/clinical/clinical-guidance/committee-opinion/articles/2020/03/preimplantation-genetic-testing

2. Adams J. (2008) Pharmacogenomics and personalized medicine. Nature Education 1(1):194

3. Crooke ST, Witztum JL, Bennett CF, Baker BF. RNA-Targeted Therapeutics. Cell Metab. 2018; 27:714–39.

4. Dougherty MP, Dolitsky S, Chattopadhyay R, Sauer MV. Mitochondrial replacement therapy. Curr Opin Obstet Gynecol. 2018; 30:217–22.

5. GeneReviews® [Internet]. Seattle (WA): University of Washington, Seattle; 1993–2020. Available from: https://www.ncbi.nlm.nih.gov/books/NBK1377/

6. Genetics home reference. What are the benefits and risks of direct-to-consumer genetic testing? (2020). Last accessed on 16 June 2020. Available online at https://ghr.nlm.nih.gov/primer/dtcgenetictesting/dtcrisksbenefits

7. Gil MM, Quezada MS, Revello R, Akolekar R, Nicolaides KH. Analysis of cell-free DNA in maternal blood in screening for fetal aneuploidies: updated meta-analysis. Ultrasound Obstet Gynecol 2015; 45:249–66.

8. Loukogeorgakis SP, Flake AW. *In Utero* Stem Cell and Gene Therapy: Current Status and Future Perspectives. Eur J Pediatr Surg 2014; 24:237–45.

9. Messina S. New Directions for SMA Therapy. J Clin Med 2018;7(9):251.

10. Rafeeq MM, Murad HAS. Cystic fibrosis: current therapeutic targets and future approaches. J Transl Med 2017;15:84.

11. Sennaar K (2019). Machine Learning in Genomics—Current Efforts and Future Applications. Last accessed on 20 June 2020. Available online at; https://emerj.com/ai-sector-overviews/machine-learning-in-genomics- applications/

12. Shieh PB. Emerging Strategies in the Treatment of Duchenne Muscular Dystrophy. Neurotherapeutics. 2018; 15:840–8.

Glossary

Yashodhara Bhattacharya

1. **Allele:** Different alternative forms of a gene found at the same locus of homologous chromosomes.
2. **Amplicon:** It is a part of DNA or RNA formed as a result of a multiplication (amplification) during a natural or artificial replication.
3. **Aneuploid:** A number of chromosomes in a cell which is not a multiple of a haploid number.
4. **Anticipation:** Autosomal dominant diseases have an ability to manifest at an earlier age and with greater severity in the next generations.
5. **Association:** The occurrence of a particular allele more frequently in a given population than can be attributed to chance.
6. **Autonomy:** It is defined in medical ethics as the informed and uncoerced decision made by a rational individual.
7. **Autosomal dominant:** It is a pattern of inheritance wherein genes on a non-sex chromosome manifest in a heterozygous state.
8. **Autosomal recessive:** A pattern of inheritance wherein a gene on a non-sex chromosome is able to manifest in a homozygous state.
9. **Autosome:** They are any of the 22 non-sex chromosomes.
10. **Balanced translocation:** When there is an exchange of chromosomal material wherein the net material is balanced and there is no loss or gain in genetic material.
11. **Barr body:** The compacted inactive X-chromosome seen in some cells of females.
12. **Candidate gene:** A specific gene causing a particular genetic condition.
13. **Cell-free fetal DNA:** Is the DNA from the growing fetus (derived from the placental-trophoblast tissue) which enters the maternal blood circulation.
14. **Chimera:** An individual having two different genotypic population of cells.
15. **Chromosomes:** Are thread-like structures composed of DNA packaged with chromatin present in the nucleus of the cell, carries the genetic information.
16. **Co-dominance:** When two dominant alleles express together in an individual.
17. **Codon:** It is a sequence of three nucleotides in an mRNA which codes for an amino acid or lead to chain termination.
18. **Compound heterozygote:** An individual who is affected with an autosomal recessive genetic disorder with two different mutations in same gene.
19. **Congenital:** Any abnormality present in an individual from birth.
20. **Consanguineous:** The mating of two individuals who are from the same family having a common ancestor.
21. **Consultant:** The individual who first approaches for genetic counseling.
22. **DNA probes:** A fluorescent labeled oligonucleotide sequence used for detection of a particular segment or gene in the DNA.

23. **Dominant:** A particular trait which is able to manifest in a heterozygous individual.

24. **Duplication:** It is the presence double copy for DNA or chromosome in an individual.

25. **Epigenetic:** Changes in the expression of a gene without change in the sequence of DNA.

26. **Euchromatin:** Regions of a DNA which are active and expressed make the functional proteins.

27. **Exome:** The region of the genome which is made up of exons.

28. **Exon:** It is the region of the gene which is not removed by splicing and takes part in the formation mature protein.

29. **First degree relatives:** Individuals in a family with the closest genetic relations—mother, father, siblings. Such individuals share an average of 50% of their DNA.

30. **Genetic susceptibility:** The tendency of an individual to a genetic condition which is caused due to the effects of multiple genes.

31. **Genocopy:** When different genetic variations are responsible for the same phenotype.

32. **Genome:** The whole genetic material present in an individual including coding and non-coding sections of the DNA.

33. **Genomic DNA:** The complete DNA material which is present in the chromosomes.

34. **Genomic imprinting:** Differential expression of genes depending upon whether the allele has been inherited from the mother or the father of the individual.

35. **Genotype:** The genetic constitution of a particular individual.

36. **Genotype-phenotype correlation:** It is the correlation of a mutation in a specific gene and the corresponding phenotype in the individual.

37. **Germ cells:** Those cells which transmit genetic information to the next generation.

38. **Germline mosaicism:** When two different population of cells with different genotypes is present in the gametes or gonadal tissue.

39. **Germline mutation:** Mutation present in the DNA of the gametes.

40. **Haplotype:** A group of genes which are inherited together from a single parent.

41. **Hb Bart's:** It is a tetramer of γ-globulin seen in the severe form of α-thalassemia. It is known to cause hydrops fetalis.

42. **Heme:** It is the iron-containing part of hemoglobin.

43. **Hemizygous:** It a trait which is seen expressed in males caused due to a gene on the X chromosome as males have only one copy of the X-linked genes.

44. **Hereditary persistence of Fetal Hb (HPFH):** It is the continuation of the production of fetal hemoglobin in an individual up to adult life.

45. **Heritability:** It is a proportion of total variation of a phenotype in a population attributed to genetic etiology.

46. **Heterochromatin:** Regions of the chromosome which are genetically inactive or are not expressed.

47. **Heterogeneity:** It is the phenomenon which has more than one cause for a single disease.

48. **Heteroplasmy:** The mitochondria of an individual consisting of different types of DNA normal and mutated.

49. **Heterozygote carrier:** An individual carrying two different alleles on a particular gene locus on homologous chromosomes.

50. **Homologous chromosomes:** Chromosomes which pair during the meiosis phase of the cell cycle and bear similar gene loci.

51. **Homoplasmy:** When the total number mitochondria in an individual consists of a single type of DNA.

52. **Homozygous:** The state of having two identical alleles of a gene on a particular locus on a pair of homologous chromosomes.

53. **Housekeeping genes:** Those genes which express proteins to all cells equally.

54. **Human Genome Project:** It was one of the major collaborative projects undertaken by many countries to sequence the whole human genetic material.

55. **Ideogram** is a schematic diagrammatic representation of all the 23 chromosomes showing all the bands and subbands.

56. **Inborn error of metabolism:** It is an inherent defect of metabolism due to abnormal enzyme.

57. **Incest:** It is the mating between two first degree relatives.

58. **Index case:** The individual in a family who is affected by a genetic disorder and serves as the first point of genetic study.

59. **Intron:** It is a region of DNA which forms a part of the precursor RNA but removed during transcription and does not form the part of mature mRNA.

60. **Inversion:** It is a type of chromosomal anomaly wherein a part of a chromosome or a DNA sequence is reversed.

61. **Isochromosome:** It is a type of chromosomal anomaly in which a particular chromosome is deleted such that the two arms of the isochromosome are mirror image of each other.

62. **Karyotype** is the written description of the normal or abnormal chromosomal complement of an individual in a standard arranged form as per the International System for Human Cytogenetic Nomenclature (ISCN) guidelines.

63. **Kilobase:** One kilobase is equal to 1000 bases.

64. **Knockout mutation:** It is the complete loss of function of a particular gene.

65. **Lagging strand:** During the replication process, it is the strand which is synthesized in 3′ to 5′ direction from short pieces synthesized in 5′ to 3′ direction and joined together using an enzyme called DNA ligase.

66. **Leading strand:** It is the synthesis of the DNA strand in 5′ to 3′ direction during DNA replication.

67. **Lethal mutation:** It is a mutation which leads to the death of an individual or organism.

68. **Linkage:** Two closely placed loci on the same chromosome transmitted together during meiosis for gamete formation.

69. **Linkage disequilibrium:** Occurrence of two or more alleles together at closely linked loci more often than is considered as a chance.

70. **Locus control region (LCR):** A region near the β-like globin genes responsible for timing and tissue specificity of their expression during development.

71. **Malformation:** Structural defect of an organ results from an abnormality during *in utero* development

72. **Marker chromosome:** A small, extra and distinct abnormal chromosome fragment.

73. **Meiosis:** It is the type of cell division during gamete formation leading half of the somatic number of chromosomes and gamete will be haploid.

74. **Messenger RNA (mRNA):** A single-stranded molecule complementary to one of the strands of double stranded-DNA formed during transcription and involves in the protein synthesis.

75. **Metacentric:** It is a term used to describe chromosomes centrally placed centromere resulting in two equal sized arms.

76. **Metaphase:** The stage of cell division in which the chromosomes come in a line on the equatorial plate.

77. **Microarray:** Comparative complementary genomic hybridization of target DNA and thousands of short sequences of DNA on a small grid.

78. **Microdeletion:** Loss of small part of chromosome detectable by FISH, microarray or MLPA.

79. **Missense mutation:** It is a point mutation that results in a change in an amino acid code sequence and leads to formation of new amino acid.

80. **Mitochondrial DNA:** Mitochondria possess its own DNA that leads to synthesis of various enzymes of respiratory chain complex.

81. **Mitochondrial inheritance:** Transmission of a mitochondrial disorder exclusively through mother.

82. **Mitosis:** Cell division for replication of somatic cells resulting in two daughter cells with same no of chromosome.

83. **Mixoploidy:** The presence of different cells with a different genotype in a person.

84. **Monosomy:** Loss of one of a chromosome of homologous pair of chromosomes so that there is one chromosome less than the diploid number of chromosomes.

85. **Mosaicism:** The presence of two or more cell lines in an individual or tissue either at the chromosomal or gene level.

86. **mRNA splicing:** It is the removal of intervening introns in the primary mRNA resulting in the formation of the mature mRNA from exons.

87. **Multifactorial:** Disease is caused by multiple genetic variants with the added effect of an environmental factors.

88. **Mutagen:** It is a natural or artificial agent (ionizing radiation, chemical or physical agent) causing changes in the genetic material of an individual.

89. **Mutant:** A gene which has got change in sequence or mutation.

90. **Mutation:** It is a heritable change in the DNA, either a single variation in the DNA sequence or in the number or structure of a chromosome.

91. **New mutation:** The occurrence of a variation in a gene for the first time.

92. **Next generation sequencing:** It is a high throughput parallel sequencing technology which allows the rapid analysis of genetic material.

93. **Non-disjunction:** It is the failure of a pair of homologous chromosomes to separate during mitosis or meiosis.

94. **Nonsense mutation:** It is mutation which leads to the formation of a stop codon thus prematurely terminating the protein synthesis.

95. **Non-synonymous mutation:** A mutation which is responsible for the change nucleotide sequence leading to change in the coded protein.

96. **Normal allele:** The gene or DNA sequence which does not contain a mutation.

97. **Nuchal translucency:** It is the assessment of the quantity of fluid collecting within the nape of the neck of the fetus by an ultrasound scan during the first trimester.

98. **Nucleotide:** Nucleotide is composed of a nitrogenous base, pentose sugar and a phosphate group which leads to formation of nucleic acid.

99. **Null allele:** It is a mutation which leads to the complete loss in function.

100. **Obligate carrier:** It is an individual having a higher possibility of carrying a particular mutation after seeing a pedigree.

101. **Penetrance:** The proportion of individuals with mutation for a dominant gene who shows either mild or severe symptoms.

102. **Pericentric inversion:** A chromosomal inversion involving the centromere.

103. **Pharmacogenetics:** It is the study of genetic constitution of a person in drug metabolism which can affect an individual's drug response.

104. **Point mutation:** It is a single base change in the DNA sequence which can be a substitution, insertion or deletion.

105. **Polygenic inheritance:** Disorders in which both environmental and genetic causative factors play role.

106. **Polymerase chain reaction:** It is the repeated cyclic reaction using the oligonucleotide primers and DNA polymerase to get amplicons of target DNA sequence.

107. **Polymorphism:** It is the existence of two or more different genetic variations in a population in such frequencies that the rarest of them could be pathogenic.

108. **Positional candidate gene:** It is a gene located in a chromosome region bearing a causative gene of the disease under research.

109. **Predictive testing:** The test which is done prior to the appearance of symptoms of the disease.

110. **Preimplantation genetic diagnosis:** It is the ability to detect the presence of a genetic disorder in an embryo during *in vitro* fertilization technique before implantation.

111. **Premutation:** Unstable mutation in a gene which can undergo expansion to cause a disease.

112. **Prenatal diagnosis:** Test during a pregnancy to diagnose whether the fetus is affected by a genetic condition.

113. **Proband:** It is the affected individual in the family who comes to take medical attention.

114. **Promoter:** It is the small initiator sequence for the binding of the RNA polymerase to initiate transcription.

115. **Proposita:** It is a female proband individual.

116. **Propositus:** It is a male proband individual.

117. **Proto-oncogene:** It is the gene that gets changed to an oncogene by mutations and cause cancer.

118. **Pseudoautosomal:** Genes do not undergo inactivation and behave like autosomal genes as they are located on the pseudoautosomal regions of sex chromosome Xp, Xq, Yp, Yq.

119. **Pseudodominance:** Autosomal recessive disorder appears to be having dominant transmission of a disorder when an individual homozygous for a recessive gene and asymptomatic carrier partner has affected offspring.

120. **Pseudogene:** It is a DNA sequence which is similar to a known gene but is inactive.

121. **Pseudomosaicism:** Mosaicism which is present in the cells during cell culturing in prenatal diagnosis due to artifacts but is not present in the fetus.

122. **Recessive:** Phenotype which is expressed in a person who is in homozygous state for a gene.

123. **Recombinant DNA molecule:** It is the combination of two different foreign DNA sequences.

124. **Recombination:** It is the pairing between two linked loci on homologous chromosomes.

125. **Replication:** It is the process of getting similar type of the double stranded DNA.

126. **Restriction fragment:** It is the DNA fragment which is formed by a restriction endonuclease.

127. **Restriction fragment length polymorphism (RFLP):** It is a polymorphism which occurs due to the presence or absence of a specific restriction fragment site.

128. **Reverse transcriptase:** It is the enzyme that is involved in the synthesis of a DNA from an RNA.

129. **Reverse transcriptase PCR (RT-PCR):** RT-PCR is a type of PCR synthesize a cDNA from mRNA by using a particular primer.

130. **Ribonucleic acid (RNA)** is a single stranded macromolecule made of nucleic acids adenine, thymine, cytosine and guanine on a ribose sugar backbone linked by phosphodiester bond.

131. **Sanger sequencing:** It is a DNA base sequencing technique involving inclusion of dideoxynucleotides which terminate the chain during *in vitro* replication process.

132. **Screening:** It is the detection of unrecognized disease in apparently healthy asymptomatic population by means of clinical examinations or tests.

133. **Semi-conservative:** It is the process of DNA replication in which only one strand of copy of DNA molecule is newly synthesized.

134. **Sense strand:** It is the strand of the DNA to which the mRNA is similar.

135. **Sequence:** It is a part of DNA nucleotides bases.

136. **Sequencing:** It is the process of ascertaining the order of bases in a given DNA part.

137. **Sickle cell disease:** Hemolytic anemia due to homozygous state for hemoglobin S.

138. **Sickle cell trait:** Heterozygous state of hemoglobin S not causing clinical phenotype.

139. **Silent mutation:** It is a point mutation in a genetic code which does not change the amino acid in the polypeptide chain.

140. **Sister chromatids:** Sister chromatids are 2 identical copies of a chromosome formed during cell division.

141. **Sister chromatids exchange (SCE):** Exchange of genetic material between two sister chromatids in mitosis.

142. **Skewed X-inactivation:** Non-random non-functioning of X-chromosome in a female.

143. **Somatic cells:** They are the non-germline cells in an individual's body.

144. **Somatic mosaicism:** It is the occurrence of two different cell lines with different genotype in a somatic tissue.

145. **Splicing:** It is the excision of introns and the joining of exons in RNA during the transcription.

146. **Submetacentric:** The type of chromosomes in which the centromere is slightly away from the center.

147. **Syndrome:** A syndrome is a well-characterized constellation of major and minor anomalies that occur together in a predictable fashion presumably due to a single underlying etiology.

148. **Tandemly repeated DNA sequences:** Tandem repeats of non-coding DNA sequences which can be either scattered or limited in their position in the genetic material.

149. **Target DNA:** It is the carrier DNA to get recombinant DNA by inserting the foreign DNA.

150. **Telomere:** It is the distal end of a chromosome arm.

151. **Template strand:** It is one strand of the double strand DNA that is complementary to mRNA.

152. **Teratogen:** Any agent taken during first trimester of pregnancy causing congenital malformations in the fetus.

153. **Thalassemia intermedia:** It is a less severe form of the β-thalassemia disease and requires lesser number of transfusions.

154. **Thalassemia major:** Hemolytic anemias caused due to the under production of one of the globin chains due to homozygous nature of mutation.

155. **Thalassemia minor:** β-thalassemia featured by asymptomatic, mild, microcytic and hypochromic anemia due to heterozygous state of an individual for the gene.

156. **Transfer RNA (tRNA):** It is the RNA which adds the amino acids codon to the polypeptide chain during the process of protein formation.

157. **Translocation:** It is the exchange of genetic material from one chromosome to another non-homologous chromosome.

158. **Triploid:** A cell which contains three times the haploid number of chromosomes (i.e. 3N).

159. **Trisomy:** It is the presence of an additional chromosome to the normal number of chromosomes (i.e. 2N + 1).

160. **True fetal mosaicism:** Chromosomal mosaicism which is truely present in the fetus.

161. **Tumor suppressor gene:** It is the gene which losses its function of protecting the cell from becoming malignant, due to a mutation, leads to the proliferation of tumor cells.

162. **Unbalanced translocation:** It is a translocation where there is seen a loss or gain of the genetic material resulting in abnormal phenotype.

163. **Uniparental disomy:** When a single parent transmits both the homologous chromosome to a person.

164. **Uniparental heterodisomy:** Uniparental disomy due to transmission of two different homologous chromosomes from a single parent.

165. **Uniparental isodisomy:** Uniparental disomy occurs due to transmission of two copies of a single chromosome of a homologous pair from single parent.

166. **Variable expressivity:** It is the difference in the severity of the clinical features either intrafamilial or interfamilial in an autosomal dominant disorder.

167. **Whole exome sequencing (WES):** It is a technique of sequencing of all the coding regions in the whole genome using next generation sequencing.

168. **Whole genome sequencing (WGS):** It is a technique of sequencing the individual's whole genomic DNA including non-coding DNA sequences also.

169. **X-linked dominant:** Genes present on the X-chromosome which express in heterozygous females and hemizygous male.

170. **X-linked recessive:** These are genes which are carried by asymptomatic females and manifest in hemizygous males.

Appendix

The increase in the information of human medical genetics should be reached to both the medical students and the physician. So there are some important websites and databases, tables and flowcharts available for them for easy reference of the genetic disorders. The websites and databases are meant for experienced persons in the subject. So these should be used carefully under the guidance of experts.

Websites and Clinical Databases

1. **General Genetic Databases Websites:**
   - Online Mendelian Inheritance in Man (OMIM)
     http://www.ncbi.nlm.nih.gov/omim/
   - Genetic Reviews
     http://www.ncbi.nlm.nih.gov/books/NBK1116/
   - PubMed
     http://www.ncbi.nlm.nih.gov/pubmed
   - Orphanet
     http://www.orpha.net/
   - London Medical Databases online
     http://www.fdna.com/london-medical-databases-online/
   - Gene Clinics and Gene Tests
     www.geneclinics.com
   - Pictures of Standard Syndromes and Undiagnosed Malformations (POSSUM)
     www.possum.net

2. **Human Genome Databases Websites:**
   - 1000 Genomes Project
     http://1000 genomes.org/

- Exome Aggregation Consortium (ExAC)
  http://exac.broadinstitute.org/
3. **Cytogenetic Databases Websites:**
   - Decipher Website
     http://decipher.sanger.ac.uk/
4. **Human Genetics Databases Societies:**
   - American Society of Human Genetics
     http://www.ashg.org/
   - American College of Medical Genetics
     www.acmg.net
   - British Society for Genetic Medicine
     http://www.bsgm.org.uk/
   - European Society of Australasia
     http://www.hgsa.org.au/

Other sites for getting information on individual genes, diagnosis of medical conditions, various genetic mutations, ethical issues:

- National Center for Biotechnology Information.
  www.ncbi.nlm.nih.gov
- Genetic Testing Registry. For individual genes, diagnosis of medical conditions.
  www.ncbi.nlm.nih.gov/gtr/
- Genetics Home References.
  www.ghr.nlm.nih.gov
- National Human Genome Research Institute, about human genetics and ethical issues.
  www.genome.gov
- Human Gene Mutation Database.
  www.hgmd.cf.ac.uk
- Database of Genomic Variants.
  http://dgv.tcag.ca/dgv/app/home
- Gene Letter. An online magazine of genetics
  www.geneletter.com

ISCN symbols and abbreviated terms used in description of chromosomes and chromosomal abnormalities are listed in Table 1.

For further details please refer, An International System for Human Cytogenomic Nomenclature (1). (*Courtesy:* Dr Usha R Dutta, CDFD, Hyderabad).

TABLE 1: ISCN symbols and abbreviated terms used in description of chromosomes and chromosomal abnormalities

Symbol	Description
arrow (-> or →)	from–to, in detailed system
brackets, square ([ ])	Surround number of cells or genome build
Cen	Centromere
Chr	Chromosome
Colon, single (:)	Break, in detailed system
comma (,)	Separates chromosome numbers, sex chromosomes, and chromosome abnormalities, separates locus designations
Decimal point (.)	Denotes sub-bands
Del	Deletion
Der	Derivative chromosome
Dic	Dicentric
Dup	Duplication
Fra	Fragile site
I	Isochromosome
Ins	Insertion
Inv	Inversion
Mar	Marker chromosome
Mos	Mosaic
P	Short arm
Pter	Terminal end of short arm
Q	Long arm of chromosome
R	Ring chromosome
Rob	Robertsonian translocation
slant line, single (/)	Separates clones, or contiguous probes or mosaicism
T	Translocation
minus sign (–)	Loss; decrease in length; locus absent from a specific chromosome
plus sign (+)	Additional normal or abnormal chromosomes; increase in length locus present on a specific chromosome
semicolon (;)	Separates altered chromosomes and break points in structural rearrangements involving more than one chromosome; separates probes on different derivative chromosomes
FISH	Fluorescence *in situ* hybridization

TABLE 2: All types of chromosomal abnormalities along with examples and karyotype

Numerical Abnormalities		
Abnormality	Description/Example	Karyotype
Autosomal (trisomy)	Trisomy occurs due to an extra chromosome which originates from meiotic non-disjunction or abnormal meiotic recombination, e.g. Trisomy 21, 18 and 13	○ 47,XY,+21 (Down Syndrome) ○ 47,XY,+18 (Edward syndrome) ○ 47,XY,+13 (Patau syndrome)
Sex chromosomal	Presence of an extra X chromosome, e.g. Klinefelter, triple X syndrome	○ 47,XXY (Klinefelter) ○ 47,XXX (Triple X)
Monosomy	Absence of one X chromosome which occurs due to anaphase lag, e.g. Turner syndrome	45,X (Turner)

Contd.

TABLE 2: All types of chromosomal abnormalities along with examples and karyotype *(Contd.)*

Numerical Abnormalities		
Abnormality	*Description/Example*	*Karyotype*
Triploidy	Presence of an additional haploid set of chromosomes which occurs due to a failure in meiotic division.	69,XYY/69,XXY/69,XXX
Tetraploidy	Tetraploidy occurs when two diploid cells fuse	92,XXYY/92XXXX/92,XXXY
Structural Abnormalities		
Interchromosomal rearrangements		
Reciprocal translocations	A two-way exchange of non-homologous material between long arm of chromosome X at region 1, band 2 and short arm of chromosome 20 at region1, band 3	46,X,t(X;20)(q12;p13)
Robertsonian translocations	Translocation occurs between two acrocentric chromosomes 14 and 15.	45,XY,rob(14;15)(q11.1;q11.1)
Intrachromosomal rearrangements		
Inversion	When two breaks occur on a single chromosome, the segment between them gets inverted and reunites to form an inversion.	○ 46,XX,inv(3)(p23q26) ○ Two breaks occur on chromosome 3 on the short arm of chromosome 3, region 2, band 3 and another at long arm of chromosome 3, region 2, band 6. The segment between them gets inverted and reunites to form an inversion.
Ring chromosome	Two terminal breaks occur on either ends of the chromosome and reunites to form a ring.	○ 46,XX,r (9)(p22q31) ○ Two terminal breaks occur one on short arm of chromosome 9, region 2, band 2 and another on long arm of chromosome 9, region 3, band 1 and these ends of the both breaks reunite to form a ring.
Deletion	Occurs due to loss of a chromosome segment.	○ 46,XX,del(3)(p14p24) ○ Occurs due to loss of chromosome 3 segment between 3p14 and 3p24 region.
Duplication	Occurs due to gain of an extra chromosome segment.	○ 46,XY,dup(9)(q25q22) ○ Occurs due to gain of an extra segment between 9q25 and 9q22 on chromosome 9.
Isochromosome	Losing one arm of the chromosome and duplication of the other arm forming a mirror image is called an isochromosome	○ 46,X,i(X)(q10) ○ Losing short arm of the one of the chromosomes X and duplication of the long arm forming a mirror image leading to isochromosome anomaly.

Courtesy: Dr Usha R Dutta, CDFD, Hyderabad

	Syndrome	Description
1.	**Apert syndrome**	Sporadic, craniostenosis, midface hypoplasia, syndactyly of 2,3,4 mitton hands, hearing loss, congenital heart disease.
2.	**Aicardi syndrome**	X-linked dominant inheritance, microcephaly, coloboma, developmental delay, agenesis of the corpus callosum, and infantile spasms.
3.	**Aagenaes syndrome**	Paucity of bile duct with cholestasis, lymphedema of legs.
4.	**Alstrom syndrome**	ALMS1 gene, obesity, hypogonadism, retinal degeneration, deafness, diabetes mellitus.
5.	**Aarskog syndrome**	FGD1 gene, short stature, dysmorphic face, Widow's sign, clinodactyly, shawl scrotum, behavior problems.
6.	**Bardet-Biedl syndrome**	Previously Laurence-Moon-Bardet-Biedl, autosomal recessive (AR), obesity, postaxial polydactyly, hypogonadism, low IQ, pigmentary retinopathy.
7.	**Beckwith-Wiedemann syndrome**	Autosomal dominant (AD), macrosomia and hemihypertrophy, macroglossia, hypoglycemia, omphalocele, pits and ear creases, Wilms tumor, hepatoblastoma, normal IQ
8.	**Bartter syndrome**	Autosomal recessive disorder, excessive Cl, K and Na ion wasting in thick ascending limb of loop of Henle. Hypochloremic, hypokalemia, metablolic alkalosis, hypercalciuria, normal BP.
9.	**Bloom syndrome**	Leukemia, lymphoma, and solid tumors.
10.	**CHARGE syndrome**	AD, coloboma, tetralogy, aortic arch, conotruncal defects, choanal atresia, growth retardation, genitourinary defects, ear/deafness
11.	**Crouzon syndrome**	AD, craniostenosis, brachycephaly (coronal suture), frontal bossing, ocular proptosis, squint, hearing loss, hypoplasia of maxilla, dental abnormalities, cleft lip/palate, congenital heart disease, patent ductus arteriosus and coarctation of aorta.
12.	**Carpenter syndrome**	Craniaosynostosis, obesity, polydactyly, syndactyly, midface hypoplasia, hearing loss, mental retardation, congenital heart disease.
13.	**Dandy-Walker syndrome**	Posterior fossa cyst & hydrocephalus, cerebellar vermis hypoplasia, enlarged fourth ventricle, obstruction hydrocephalus, macrocephaly
14.	**Fetal alcohol syndrome**	Facial dysmorphism, smooth philtrum, thin vermillion border, small palpebral fissures, microcephaly, global cognitive delay performance, low IQ 50–115 (normal 100), attention deficit hyperactive disorder, difficulties with language and number processing, memory and sequencing skills, hearing loss.
15.	**Holt-Oram syndrome**	AD,TBX5 gene, absent thumb or radius, 1st-degree heat block, atrial septal defect.
16.	**Klinefelter syndrome**	47XXY, delayed puberty with infantile testes (< 2.5 cm), tall, long arms and legs, gynecomastia, osteopenia osteoporosis, behavioral problems.
17.	**Kartagener syndrome**	Triad of bronchiectasis + sinusitis + situs inversus.
18.	**Marfan syndrome**	AD, FBN1gene, fibrillin, upward lens subluxation, dilatation of ascending aorta + aortic regurgitation, dissection of ascending aorta,

Contd.

	Syndrome	Description
		mitral valve prolapse, pectus carinatum, pectus excavatum, wrist & thumb sign, decreased U:L ratio, span-ht ratio > 1.05, scoliosis, arachnodactyly, high arched palate, pneumothorax, lumbosacral dural ectasia, family history positive.
19.	**Meckel-Gruber syndrome**	AR, occipital encephalomyelocele, microcephaly with sloping forehead, cerebral or cerebellar hypoplasia, cleft palate, talipes, renal dysplasia, cryptorchidism.
20.	**Miller-Dieker syndrome**	Microdeletion 17p, microcephaly with bitemporal narrowing, lissencephaly, heterotopias, mental deficiency. Furrowing of central forehead, mid-facial hypoplasia, low set ears, small nose, broad nasal bridge.
21.	**Oculoauriculo-vertebral spectrum Goldenhar syndrome, facioauriculo-vertebral syndrome**	Sporadic inheritance, Abn 1st and 2nd brachial arches, sporadic (2% recurrence), hemifacial macrosomia hemivertebrae, normal IQ, microtia, preauricular tags or pits, epibulbar dermoids, coloboma, mandibular hypoplasia.
22.	**Pierre Robin sequence**	Micrognathia, retrognathia, glossoptosis, cleft palate.
23.	**Pendred syndrome**	Goiter with sensory neural deafness.
24.	**Sotos syndrome**	Cerebral gigantism, AD, large for gestational age, macrocephaly, frontal prominence, hypotonia, seizures, developmental delay and behavioral difficulties. Enlarged ventricles in neuroimaging.
25.	**Stickler syndrome**	AD, flat face, scooped out nasal bridge, U-shaped cleft palate, robin sequence, myopia, risk of retinal detachment, hearing loss, hyperextensible and enlarged joints.
26.	**Smith-Lemli-Optiz syndrome**	AR, cholesterol synthesis defect. DHCR7 (7-dehydrocholesterol-7 reductase) gene. microcephaly, ptosis, low IQ, scaphocephaly, inner epicanthic folds, anteverted nostrils, low birth weight, marked feeding problems, abnormal genitalia.
27.	**Swyer syndrome**	XY karyotype, pure gonadal dysgenesis, normal female int. & ext. genitalia, primary amenorrhea, I.
28.	**Trisomy 13, Patau syndrome**	Cleft lip or palate, coloboma, polydactyly, scalp defects (e.g. cutis aplasia), congenital cardiac malformation, apneic spells, holoprosencephaly, polycystic kidney, usually die by 1y
29.	**Trisomy 18, Edwards syndrome**	Small for gestational age, microcephaly, short sternum, rocker bottom feet, horseshoe kidneys, congenital heart defects, flexion deformities of extremities, hypertonia. Usually die by 1 mo, Low IQ.
30.	**Turner syndrome**	XO, 15% are mosaic, short stature and gonadal dysgenesis, congenital lymphedema, edema over fingers and toes, shield chest, cubitus valgus, low posterior hairline, webbed neck, primary amenorrhea, streak ovaries, horseshoe kidney, bicuspid aortic valve, coarctation, valvular aortic stenosis, normal IQ, but difficulties with visuospatial orientation, hydrops fetalis, cystic hygromas, excessive loose skin around neck in infants.

Contd.

TABLE 3: Common genetic syndromes *(Contd.)*

	Syndrome	Description
31.	**Treacher Collins syndrome**	AD, symmetric downslanting eyes, abnormal deformed ears, lower eyelid colobomas, zygomatic hypoplasia.
32.	**VATER/VACTERL Association**	Vertebral, anal atresia, ventral septal defect, tracheoesophageal fistula, horseshoe or ectopic kidney, limb anomalies, polydactyly, forearm defects, absent thumbs.
33.	**Waardenburg syndrome**	AD, PAX-3 mutation, heterochromia, white forelock, sensorineural hearing loss 15–25%
34.	**Wiskott-Aldrich syndrome**	X-linked recessive, primary immunodeficiency, thrombocytopenia, small-sized platelets, recurrent infections, eczema, lymphoma.
35.	**Zellweger (cerebro-hepatorenal)**	Autosomal recessive, peroxisomal disorder, hypotonia, developmental delay, low IQ, abnormal head shape and dysmorphic face, stippled calcifications of the patella.

Courtesy: Dr Komal Uppal, Dr Suvarna Ghanashammagar

TABLE 4: Some of the relatively common and well-recognized syndromes associated with Intellectual disability are listed. (*Courtesy*: Dr Prajnya Ranganath, NIMS, Hyderabad, Dr Suvarna Ghanashammagar MGM Medical College, Maharashtra)

Name of the syndrome	Etiology	Associated salient features
Chromosomal anomalies (detectable by conventional cytogenetic techniques, i.e. karyotyping)		
Down syndrome	Free trisomy 21 (in around 95%); translocation involving chromosome 21 and another chromosome (in around 3–4%); mosaic trisomy 21 (in around 1%)	Typical facial dysmorphism (upslanting eyes, epicanthic folds, depressed nasal bridge, low-set ears, protuberant tongue), congenital cardiac anomalies, gastrointestinal and renal anomalies, and hypothyroidism
Cri du chat syndrome	Chromosome 5p deletion (the deletion may be gross or sub-microscopic ranging from 0.5 Mb to 40 Mb in size)	Facial dysmorphism (round face, hypertelorism, micrognathia, epicanthal folds and low-set ears), microcephaly, hypotonia, severe psychomotor retardation and intellectual disability, and a characteristic high-pitched cat-like cry (especially in the newborn period).
Submicroscopic chromosomal anomalies (detected by molecular cytogenetic techniques like FISH/MLPA/chromosomal microarray)		
1p36 deletion syndrome	Chromosome 1p36 microdeletion	Facial dysmorphism (deep set eyes, straight eyebrows, large anterior fontanel, pointed chin, mid-face hypoplasia), microcephaly, ear anomalies, orofacial clefting, hypotonia, congenital heart disease, renal anomalies, hearing loss and seizures.

Contd.

Name of the syndrome	Etiology	Associated salient features
Wolf-Hirschhorn syndrome	Chromosome 4p16 microdeletion	Pre- and post-natal growth restriction, microcephaly, distinctive facial features with a "Greek warrior helmet" appearance, preauricular tags & pits, cleft lip/palate, and congenital heart disease.
Williams-Beuren syndrome	Chromosome 7q11 microdeletion	Distinctive facial dysmorphism (previously called elfin facies—periorbital fullness, bulbous tip of nose, thick lips), cardiac anomalies especially supravalvular aortic stenosis, over-friendly behavior, hypercalcemia, renal anomalies, and nephrocalcinosis.
WAGR (Wilms tumor-aniridia-genitourinary anomalies-mental retardation) syndrome	Chromosome 11p13 microdeletion	Aniridia and other associated eye anomalies such as iris hypoplasia, congenital cataract, and glaucoma, Wilms tumor by the age of 4 years in up to 90% of affected children, genital abnormalities, seizures, and obesity.
Prader-Willi syndrome	Chromosome 15q11–q13 microdeletion (paternal copy deletion) in ~70–75%; uniparental disomy of the maternal copy or imprinting center defects in the remaining cases	Obesity, mild facial dysmorphism (almond-shaped and up-slanting eyes), hypogonadism with small penis and cryptorchidism and pubertal delay, short stature.
Angelman syndrome	Chromosome 15q11–q13 microdeletion (maternal copy deletion) in ~ 70%; uniparental disomy of the paternal copy, UBE3 A gene mutation or imprinting center defects in the remaining cases	Ataxic gait, tremors of limbs, inappropriate happy demeanour like frequent laughing and excitability, seizures, and microcephaly.
Smith-Magenis syndrome	Chromosome 17p11 microdeletion	Facial dysmorphism (mid-face retrusion, deep-set eyes, broad and square-shaped face, broad nose, relative prognathism and downturned upper lip), self-injurious behavior, and sleep disturbances.
DiGeorge syndrome	Chromosome 22q11 microdeletion	Congenital heart disease particularly conotruncal malformations, cleft palate, facial dysmorphism (bulbous nose, micrognathia),immune deficiency, hypocalcemia, thymic hypoplasia.
Single gene disorders (detectable by molecular genetic tests such as gene sequencing)		
Fragile X syndrome	CGG trinucleotide repeat expansion in FMR1 gene (X-linked)	Long facies, large ears, macro-orchidism, autism

Contd.

Name of the syndrome	*Etiology*	*Associated salient features*
Tuberous sclerosis	Mutation in TSC1 or TSC2 gene (autosomal dominant)	Hypopigmented macules on the skin, adenoma sebaceum, cortical tubers and other brain lesions, cardiac rhabdomyoma, autism, seizures, renal angiomyolipoma
RASopathies-Noonan syndrome and Noonan-like syndromes (such as cardiofaciocutaneous syndrome and Costello syndrome)	Mutation in *PTPN11*(in around 50%) and some other genes (autosomal dominant)	Short stature, facial dysmorphism (ptosis, downslanting eyes, hypertelorism, low-set ears), webbed neck, cardiac anomalies (especially hypertrophic cardiomyopathy and pulmonic stenosis)
Rett syndrome	Mutation in *MECP2* gene (X-linked)	Autism, stereotypic behavior, and neurological deficits
Rubinstein-Taybi syndrome	Mutation in *CREBBP* or *EP300* gene (autosomal dominant)	Prenatal and postnatal growth restriction, microcephaly, dysmorphic facies (high-arched eyebrows, overhanging columella, down-slanting palpebral fissures and a grimacing smile), broad thumbs and halluces, congenital heart disease, and eye abnormalities.
Cornelia de Lange syndrome	Mutation in *NIPBL, RAD21,* or *SMC3* gene (autosomal dominant) or in *HDAC8* or *SMC1A* gene (X- linked)	Typical facial dysmorphism (synophrys, long eyelashes, short nose with anteverted nares), microcephaly, growth retardation, hirsutism, upper-limb reduction defects and congenital heart defects.
Coffin-Siris syndrome	Mutation in *ARID1A*, *ARID1B*, and in some other genes (autosomal dominant)	Aplasia or hypoplasia of distal phalanx of the fifth digit (little finger), facial dysmorphism, hirsutism, hypertrichosis, cardiac defects, gastrointestinal and genitourinary defects, and intracranial anomalies.
Kabuki syndrome	Mutation in *KMT2D* gene (autosomal dominant) or in *KDM6A* gene (X-linked)	Typical facial dysmorphism (long palpebral fissures with eversion of the lateral third of the lower eyelid), large ears, arched and broad eyebrows), cleft lip/palate, persistent fetal fingertip pads, congenital cardiac defects, and anal atresia.
Seckel syndrome and microcephalic osteody-splastic primordial dwarfism (MOPD)	Mutations in *ATR, PCNT,* and in some other genes (autosomal recessive)	Primordial growth failure with prenatal and postnatal growth retardation, very severe short stature (usually more than 5 SDs below mean), severe microcephaly (usually more than 5 SDs below mean), bird-like facies.

Clinical photographs of children with some syndromes associated with typical facial features are shown in Figure 1.

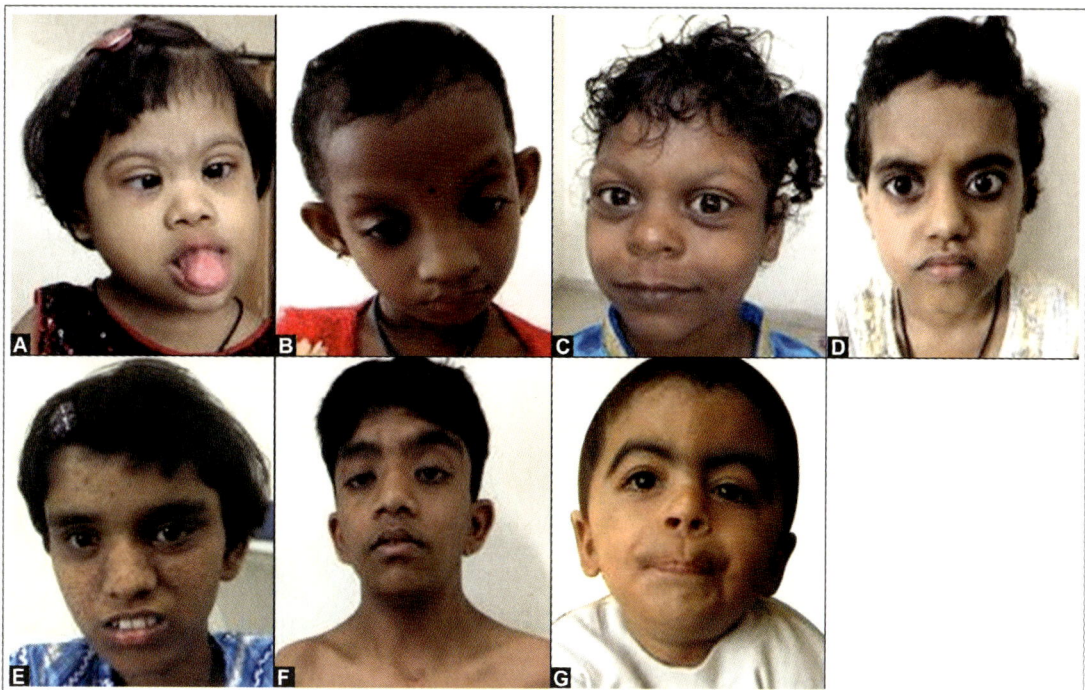

Figure 1: Clinical photographs of children with some syndromes associated with typical facial features. (*Courtesy:* Dr Prajnya Ranganath, NIMS, Hyderabad) **(A)** Child with Down syndrome with upslanting eyes, epicanthic folds, depressed nasal bridge, low-set ears, and protuberant tongue; **(B)** Child with Wolf-Hirschhorn syndrome with the typical 'Greek warrior helmet' appearance; **(C)** Child with Williams syndrome with periorbital fullness, bulbous tip of nose, and thicklips; **(D)** Child with Smith-Magenis syndrome with mid-face retrusion, deep-set eyes, broad and square-shaped face, broad nose, relative prognathism and downturned upperlip; **(E)** Child with tuberous sclerosis with adenoma sebaceum lesions seen on both cheeks; **(F)** Boy with Noonan syndrome with the typical facial dysmorphism (ptosis, downslanting eyes, hypertelorism, low-set ears), and webbed neck; **(G)** Child with Cornelia de Lange syndrome with synophrys, long eyelashes, short nose with anteverted nares and upturned tip of nose, and long philtrum.

TABLE 5: Revised Ghent criteria for the diagnosis of MFS (*Courtesy:* Dr Shruti Bajaj, Sir HN Reliance Foundation Hospital, Mumbai)	
In the absence of family history	
1. Ao (Z ⩾ 2) and EL = MFS	3. Ao (Z ⩾ 2) and systemic score 7 = MFS
2. Ao (Z ⩾ 2) and *FBN1* = MFS	4. EL and *FBN1* with known Ao = MFS
In the presence of family history	
1. EL and family history of MFS based on above definition = MFS	
2. Systemic score 7 and family history of MFS based on above definition = MFS	
3. Ao (Z ⩾ 2 for > 20 years age, and ⩾ 3 for <20 years of age) and family history of MFS based on above definition = MFS	
MFS—Marfan syndrome; Ao—Aortic diameter at the sinus of Valsalva as indicated by the Z score or aortic root dissection; EL—Ectopialentis; *FBN1*—fibrillin-1 mutation; *FBN1* with known Ao, fibrillin-1 mutation that has been identified in an individual with aortic aneurysm.	

CALCULATION OF THE SYSTEMIC SCORE

Maximum total points = 20, score ⩾ 7 indicates systemic involvement

Wrist and thumb sign = **3** (Wrist or thumb sign = **1**)

Pectus carinatum = **2** (Pectus excavatum or chest asymmetry = **1**)

Hindfoot deformity = **2** (Pes planus = **1**)

Pneumothorax = **2**

Dural ectasia = **2**

Protrusioacetabuli = **2**

Reduced US: LS and increased arm:height and no severe scoliosis = **1**

Scoliosis or thoracolumbar kyphosis = **1**

Reduced elbow extension = **1**

Facial features (3/5): Dolichocephaly, enophthalmos, downslanting palpebral fissures, malar hypoplasia, retroganthia = **1**

Skin striae = **1**

Myopia > 3 dioptres = **1**

Mitral valve prolapse (all types) = **1**

Approach to different metabolic abnormalities in metabolic disorders (Figures 2 to 5). (*Courtesy:* Dr Chaitanya A. Datar, KEM Hospital, Pune)

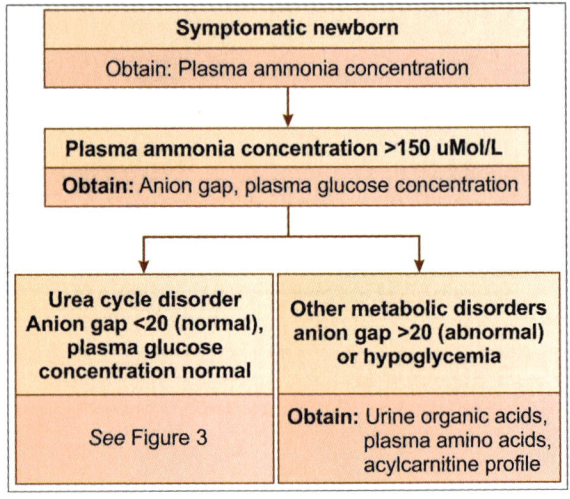

Figure 2: Approach to hyperammonia in inborn error of metabolism

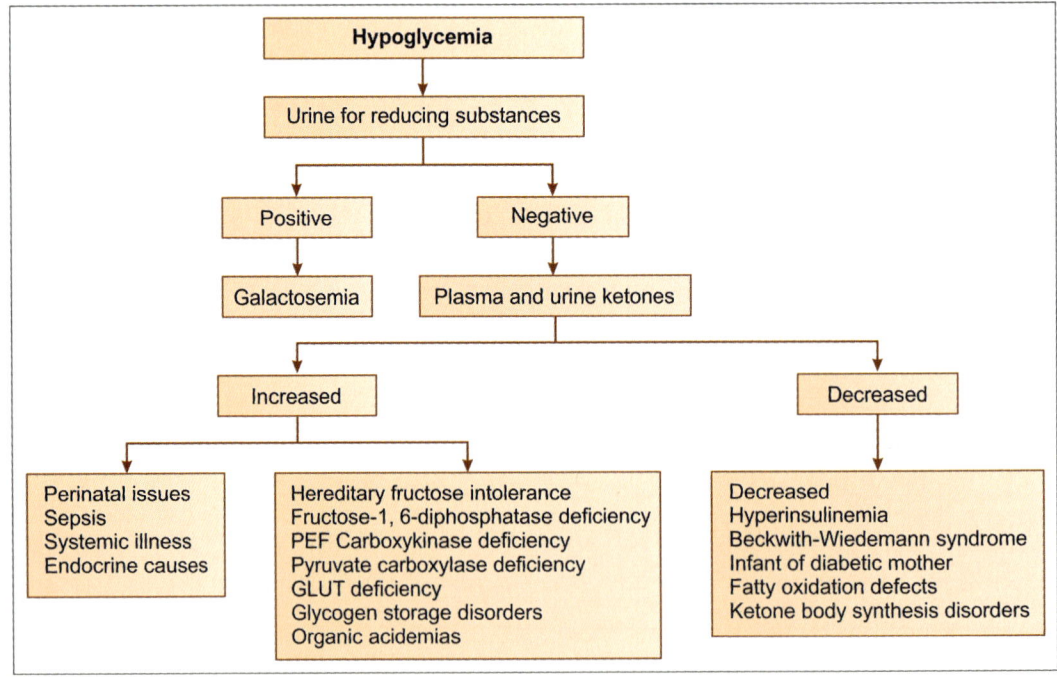

Figure 3: Approach to hypoglycemia in a newborn baby

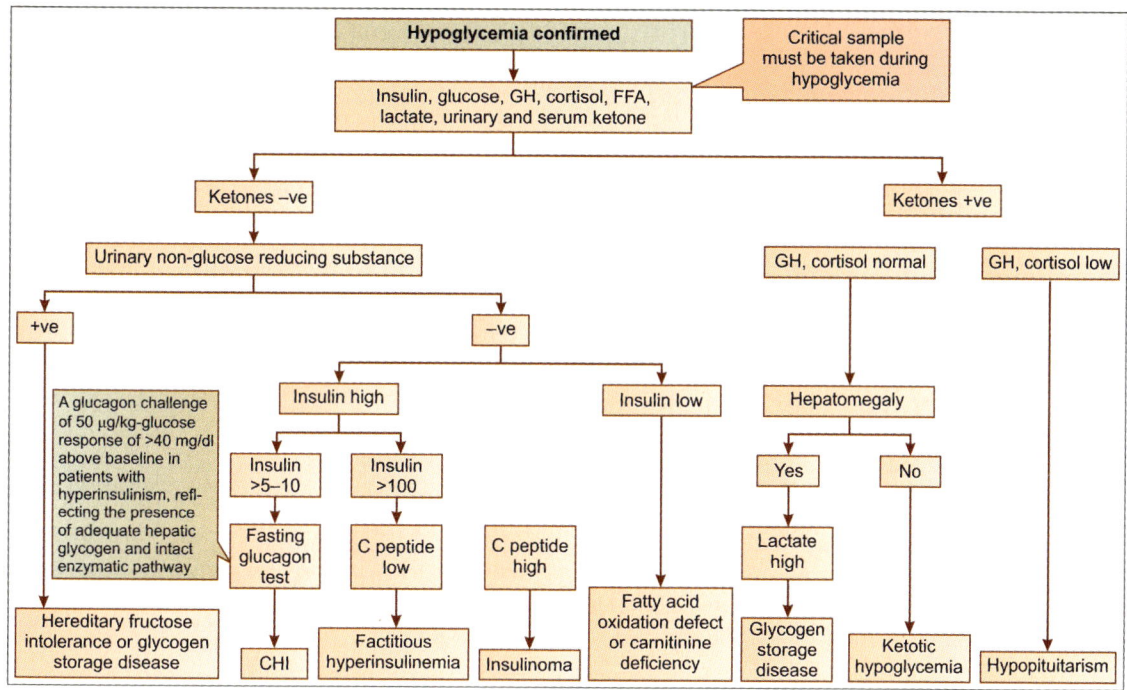

Figure 4 : Approach to hypoglycemia in a newborn baby
CHI—Congenital hyperinsulinemia; FFA—Free fatty acid; GH—Growth hormone

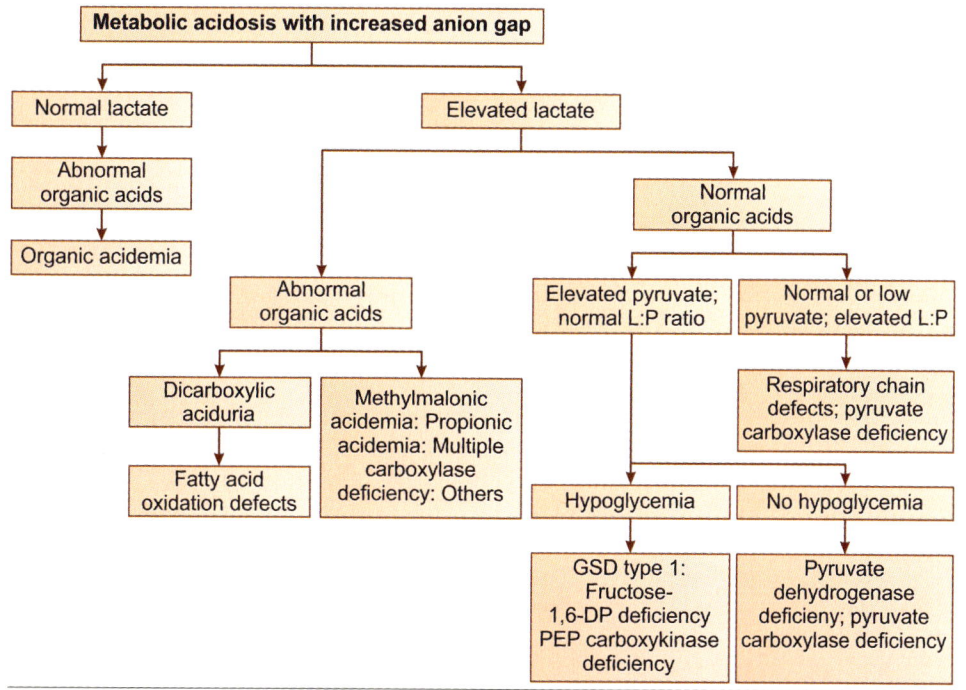

Figure 5: Approach to metabolic acidosis with increased anion gap in a newborn baby
L:P—Lactate–pyruvate ratio

TABLE 6: Biochemical laboratory findings of metabolic disorders (*Courtesy*: Dr Komal Uppal)

Sl. No.	Investigation	Amino acido-pathies	UCD	OAA	FAO	Mito-chondrial disorders	Hyper-insuli-nemia/hyper-ammonia syndrome	Transient hyper-ammonia of neonate
1.	WBC/RBC	N	N/↓	N/↓	N	N	N	N
2.	LFT	N	N	N	N/↓	N/↓	N	N
3.	Plasma glucose	N/↓	N	N/↓	↓	↓	↓	N
4.	Acidosis	+/-	+/-	+	+	+/-	–	–
5.	Serum lactate	N	N	N/++	N/++	N/++	N	N
6.	Serum NH3	N	+++	++/+++	++	++	++	++
7.	Ketosis	+	–	++	++	–	–	–

UCD—Urea cycle defect; OAA—Organic acidemia; FAO—Fatty oxidation defect, LFT—Liver function test; WBC—White blood cell; RBC: Red blood cell

Diagnosis of hyrdrops fetalis with lysosomal storage disorder (Figure 6). (*Courtsey:* Dr Siyaram Didel, AIIMS, Jodhpur)

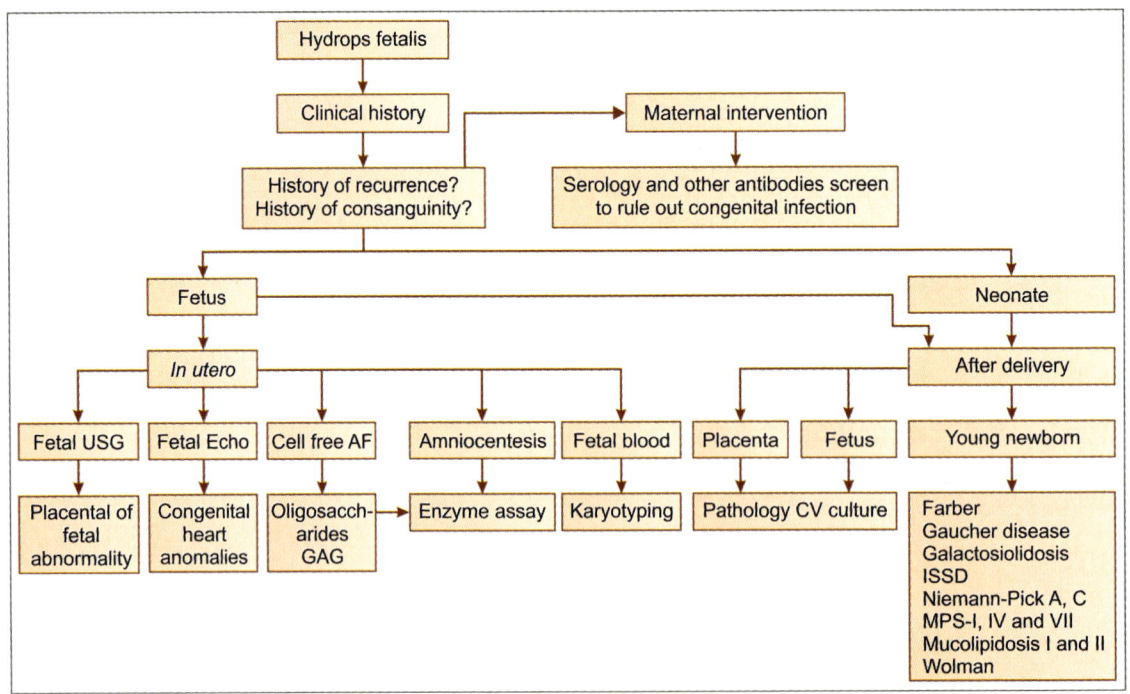

Figure 6: Diagnosis of hyrdrops fetalis with lysosomal storage disorder
USG—Ultrasound; AF—Amniotic fluid; GAG—Glycosaminoglycans;
ISSD—Infantile free sialic acid storage disorder; MPS—Mucopolysaccharides

TABLE 7: Management of isolated soft marker based on likelihood ratio (*Courtesy:* Dr Seema Thakur, Fortis Hospital, Delhi-NCR)

Soft marker	Aneuploidy risk	Positive likelihood ratio	Management
First trimester NT >3 mm or above the 99th centile for CRL	○ Aneuploidy risk increases with size of NT – 7% if <3 mm and 30%: 3.5–4.5 mm ○ Also associated with Noonan syndrome, multiple pterygium syndrome, skeletal dysplasias, congenital heart disease, and other anomalies.	-	1. Genetic counseling 2. Offer cfDNA or CVS 3. Second-trimester detailed anatomic survey and fetal cardiac ultrasonography.
First trimester cystic hygroma	If septate, approximately 50% are aneuploidy	-	1. Genetic counseling 2. Offer CVS 3. Second-trimester detailed anatomic survey and fetal cardiac ultrasonography 4. Fetal death: 90%. 5. In 10% of cases the hygromas resolve
Second trimester echogenic intra-cardiac focus	LR: 1.4–1.8 for Down syndrome seen in 15–35% of Down syndrome and 4–7% of euploid fetus	0.95	If aneuploidy screen: Low-risk, no further testing
Second trimester pyelactasis	LR: 1.5–1.6 for Down syndrome	1.08	1. If aneuploidy screen: Low-risk, no further testing 2. Repeat ultrasonography in third trimester for potential urinary tract obstruction
Second trimester echogenic bowel	LR: 5.5–6.7 for Down syndrome Associated with aneuploidy, intra-amniotic bleeding, cystic fibrosis (CF), CMV		1. Further counseling 2. Offer CMV, CF, and aneuploidy screening or diagnostic testing
Second trimester increased nuchal fold thickness >/=6 mm	LR 11–18.6 with 40–50% sensitivity and for Down syndrome	3.79	1. Detailed anatomic survey 2. Genetic counseling 3. Diagnostic testing
Second trimester ventriculomegaly–10–15 mm	LR 25 for Down syndrome	3.81	1. Genetic counseling 2. Second-trimester detailed anatomic ultrasound evaluation 3. Consider diagnostic testing for aneuploidy and CMV 4. Repeat ultrasound in third trimester

Contd.

Soft marker	Aneuploidy risk	Positive likelihood ratio	Management
Second trimester short femur length <2.5 centile for gestational age	LR 1.2–2.2 for Down syndrome. Can be associated with aneuploidy, IUGR, short limb dysplasia	0.61	1. Genetic counseling 2. Detailed anatomic survey to exclude skeletal dysplasia
Absent/hypoplastic nasal bone ◦ nasal bone ◦ length less than 10th centile ◦ less than 2.5 mm and biparietal diameter to nasal bone ratio 10 or11	Sensitivity 48.9–68.9%		1. Genetic counseling 2. Invasive testing
Aberrant right subclavian artery	Sensitivity 17.9–47.5%	3.94	1. Genetic counseling 2. NIPT/Invasive
cfDNA—Cell-free DNA; CVS—Chroinic villi sampling; NT—Nuchal translucency; CRL—Crown rump length; CMV—Cytomegalovirus; IUGR—Intrauterine growth retardation			

TABLE 8: Various fetal abnormalities and their management. (*Courtesy:* Dr Seema Thakur, Fortis Hospital, Delhi-NCR)

Anomaly	Management	Counseling regarding prognosis	Recurrence risk
Ventriculomegaly- Dilatation of atrium of lateral ventricle ◦ Mild (10–12 mm) ◦ Moderate (13–15 mm) ◦ Severe (>15 mm).	◦ Detailed level 2 USG ◦ Fetal Echocardiography ◦ Amniocentesis for FISH + CMA, PCR for TORCH	◦ Prognosis is poor if associated anomalies are detected. ◦ Prognosis for isolated ventriculomegaly is based on the size of the ventricular atrium ◦ **Isolated mild/moderate:** Survival 97–98% and neurodevelopmental delay in 10% of cases, this may not be higher than the background rate ◦ **Isolated severe:** Survival 60–80%, mental handicap 40–50%.	Isolated <1% **Trisomy:** 1% above age related risk **Infections:** No increased risk of recurrence **Genetic syndrome:** As per syndrome

Contd.

Anomaly	Management	Counseling regarding prognosis	Recurrence risk
NTD—Neural tube defects open spina bifida, meningomyelocele, anencephaly, encephalocele and iniencephaly.	○ Quadruple test/triple test to detect open NTD ○ Invasive testing not recommended in case of isolated NTD	1. Anencephaly, Iniencephaly: Lethal: Termination is advised 2. Open NTD: Termination if diagnosis before 20 weeks. If patient wants to continue or pregnancy >20 weeks—risks of physical handicap and bladder or bowel involvement should be informed. This condition can be corrected by surgery and hence referral to a higher center should be done. Outcome of surgery varies from normal to severe handicap.	1. Previous one isolated NTD: 5%. 2. Previous two isolated NTD: 10%. 3. Syndromes: As per syndrome 4. **Prevention:** Supplementation of the maternal diet with folate (5 mg/day) for 3 months before and 2 months after conception reduces the risk of recurrence by about 75%.
Cystic hygroma (CH) or hygromacolli is characterized by increased accumulation of fluid in the fetal neck. This may be septated or nonseptated	○ Detailed level 2 ultrasound ○ Fetal echocardiography ○ Chorionic villi sampling/amniocentesis for FISH + microarray ○ Follow-up scans every 4 weeks to detect resolution or appearance of hydrops	○ Fetal death: 90%. ○ In 10% of cases the fetal karyotype is normal, there are no other obvious defects and the hygromas resolve during pregnancy. In these cases the prognosis is good.	○ **Isolated or part of Turner syndrome:** No increased risk of recurrence. ○ **Syndromes:** As per syndromes
Congenital diaphragmatic hernia (CDH): CDH is due to defect in diaphragm and can be left sided or right sided. Left-sided diaphragmatic hernia is more common. Ultrasound diagnosis is based upon presence of cystic lesion in thorax, absent	○ Detailed level 2 ultrasound ○ Fetal echocardiography ○ CVS ○ Amniocentesis for FISH+ microarray ○ Assessment of severity is by measurement of contralateral lung area in a transverse section of the chest to head circumference ratio (LHR).	1. If associated anomalies or large diaphragmatic hernia or detected before 20 weeks, parents should be counselled and reproductive decision option should be left on parents 2. Isolated diaphragmatic hernia is correctable after surgery and	**Isolated:** No increased risk. **Trisomy:** 1%. **Syndromes:** As per syndromes.

Contd.

Anomaly	Management	Counseling regarding prognosis	Recurrence risk
stomach bubble, mediastinal shift. There may be associated poly-hydramnios.	o LHR <1- Poor prognosis, LHR: 1–1.4- o Moderate, LHR o >1.4 indicates good prognosis	hence delivery should be planned in tertiary care hospital	
Posterior urethral valves: The cardinal signs of posterior urethral valve is dilatation of urinary bladder and posterior urethra termed keyhole sign. The bladder wall is hypertrophied.	o Detailed level 2 ultra-sound to detect associated anomaly and also assess for kidneys echogenicity/cysts and oligoamnios. These indicate poor renal function o Fetal echocardiography o Chromosomal microarray to exclude aneuploidy/copy number variations.	o In severe cases presenting before 20 weeks, parents should be counselled and reproductive decision option should be left on parents o In mild cases or cases presenting late in preg-nancy, serial assessment for fetal renal function by ultrasound and fetal urine analysis for electrolytes and B_2 microglobulin	o Trisomy–1% o Isolated—No increased risk of recurrence
Skeletal dysplasia (SKD) should be considered in any fetus with short limbs on USG. To exclude lethal SKD is most important issue to guide the parents to take right reproductive decision. o Long bones <5th centile o Thoracic circum-ference less than 5th centile forgest. o Femur/FL <1 o BPD/HC: Normal or increased size for pregnancy o Defective minerali-zation, fractures	Detailed ultrasound to detect skeletal dysplasia by ultrasound features mentioned above	Lethal skeletal dysplasia: Parents should be counselled and reproductive decision option should be left on parents.	o Osteogenesis imperfecta: Generally sporadic, 5% recurrence risk due to gonadal mosaicism o Thanatophoric dysplasia—not increased significantly. o Short rib polydactyly 25% o Asphyxiating thoracic dystrophy 25%
Hydrops Fetalis is abnormal collection of fluid with at least two of the following:	Detailed level 2 USG o Fetal Echocardiography o Amniocentesis—FISH + chromosomal	o Depends on underlying cause and severity of the heart failure.	o Trisomy: 1% o Monogenic disorders: 25–50%

Contd.

Anomaly	Management	Counseling regarding prognosis	Recurrence risk
○ Generalized skin thickness of >5 mm, ○ Edema ○ Ascites ○ Pleural effusion ○ Pericardial effusion ○ Placental enlargement	microarray, poly-merase chain reaction for toxoplasma, cytomegalovirus	○ If the cause of NIH cannot be determined, the perinatal mortality is approximately 50% ○ Among live born infants, neonatal mortality with non-immune hydrops fetalis is reported to be as high as 60%. ○ Chylothorax—mortality may be as low as 6% Associated anomalies, almost two-thirds do not survive ○ Treatable causes of hydrops, such as fetal arrhythmia or infection with parvovirus B_{19} have a better prognosis	○ Syndromes: As per syndromes. ○ Infections: No increased risk of recurrence

FISH—Fluorescent *in situ* hybridization; CMA—Cytogenic microarray; PCR—Polymerase chain reaction; TORCH—Toxoplasmosis, rubella, cytomegalovirus, herpes; BPD/HC—Biparietal diameter, head circumference

TABLE 9: Recurrence risk for isolated malformations: (*Courtesy:* Dr Seema Thakur, Fortis Hospital, Delhi-NCR)

Malformation	Recurrence risk
Anencephaly/NTD	5% if one sib and 10% if 2 sibs affected
Cleft lip and palate	4–5%
Cardiac malformations	3–4%
Club foot	2–4%
Congenital diaphragmatic hernia	2%
Omphalocele	<1%
Posterior urethral valve	No increased risk of recurrence